Pediatric Ultrasonography

Edited by Gabriel Kalifa

With Contributions by
C. André, F.-E. Avni, F. Brunelle, L. Cadier,
J.-Y. Cohen, A. Couture, Ph. Devred, M. Dewald,
D. Eurin, J.-L. Ferran, L. Garel, G. Lalande,
D. Lallemand, B. Le Bihan, P. Le Dosseur, J. Leclere,
J.-Ph. Montagne, S. Neuenschwander, D. Pariente,
J. Poncin, M. Spehl-Robberecht

With 413 Figures in 752 Separate Illustrations and 17 Tables

Springer-Verlag
Berlin Heidelberg NewYork Tokyo

Editor:

Dr. Gabriel Kalifa
Service de Radiologie
Hôpital Saint-Vincent-de-Paul
74, av. Denfert Rochereau
F-75674 Paris Cédex 14

Title of the original French edition: *Echographie pédiatrique*, 2ème édition

ISBN-13: 978-3-642-82212-4 e-ISBN-13: 978-3-642-82210-0
DOI: 10.1007/978-3-642-82210-0

Library of Congress Cataloging-in-Publication Data.
Echographie pédiatrique. English. Pediatric ultrasonography.
Translation of: Echographie pédiatrique. Includes bibliographies and index.
1. Children—Diseases—Diagnosis. 2. Diagnosis, Ultrasonic. I. Kalifa, G. II. André. C. (Christine) III. Title. [DNLM; 1. Ultrasonic Diagnosis—in infancy & childhood. WS 141 E18]
RJ51.U45E2413 1985 618.92′007543 85-14830

Softcover reprint of the hardcover 1st edition 1986

Typesetting: H. Hagedorn, Berlin. Offsetprinting: Brüder Hartmann, Berlin

2121/3020-543210

Contributors

André, Christine
Chef de Clinique Assistant. Service de Radiologie.
Hôpital Saint-Vincent-de-Paul. 74, av. Denfert Rochereau.
75674 Paris Cédex 14, France

Avni, Freddy
Assistant de Radiologie. Service de Radiologie.
Institut E. Cavell. 32, rue E. Cavell. 1180 Bruxelles, Belgium

Brunelle, Francis
Chef de Clinique Assistant. Service de Radiopédiatrie.
Hôpital Bicêtre. 78, av. Général Leclerc. 94270 Le Kremlin, Bicêtre, France

Cadier, Laurent
Chef de Clinique Assistant. Service de Radiopédiatrie.
Hôpital des Enfants. 168, cours de L'Argonne. 33000 Bordeaux, France

Cohen, Jean-Yves
Chef de Clinique Assistant. Service de Radiologie.
Pavillon de la Mère et l'Enfant. C.H.U. de Nantes. Quai Moncousu.
44035 Nantes, France

Couture, Alain
Chef de Clinique Assistant. Service de Radiopédiatrie.
Hôpital Saint-Charles. Rue Auguste Broussonnet. 34000 Montpellier, France

Devred, Philippe
Chef de Clinique Assistant. Service de Radiologie Pédiatrique.
C.H.U. Timone. 13385 Marseille Cédex 4, France

Dewald, Michel
Chef de Clinique Assistant. Service de Radiopédiatrie.
Hôpital Charles Nicolle. 1, rue Germont. 76000 Rouen, France

Eurin, Danièle
Attachée du Service de Radiologie.
Hôpital Charles Nicolle. 1, rue Germont. 76000 Rouen, France

Ferran, Jean-Louis
Adjoint de Radiologie. Service de Radiopédiatrie.
Hôpital Saint-Charles. Rue Auguste Broussonnet. 34000 Montpellier, France

Garel, Laurent
Chef de Clinique Assitant. Service de Radiologie.
Hôpital des Enfants Malades. 149, rue de Sèvres. 75730 Paris Cédex 15, France

Lalande, Guy
Assistant des Hôpitaux, ex-Chef de Clinique Assistant. Service de Radiologie.
Hôpital Saint-Vincent-de-Paul. 74, av. Denfert Rochereau.
75674 Paris Cédex 14, France

Lallemand, Denis
Professeur de Radiologie. Service de Radiologie.
Hôpital des Enfants Malades. 149, rue de Sèvres. 75730 Paris Cédex 15, France

Le Bihan, Brigitte
Attachée du Service de Radiologie.
Hôpital Saint-Vincent-de-Paul. 74, av. Denfert Rochereau.
75674 Paris Cédex 14, France

Le Dosseur, Patrick
Radiologiste des Hôpitaux. Maître de Conférences Agrégé.
Service de Radiopédiatrie. Hôpital Charles Nicolle. 1, rue Germont.
76000 Rouen, France

Leclere, Jérôme
Assistant de Radiologie.
Institut Gustave Roussy. Rue Camille Desmoulins. 94800 Villejuif, France

Montagne, Jean-Philippe
Chef des Clinique Assistant. Service de Radiologie.
Hôpital Trousseau. 8-28, av. du Dr Arnold Netter. 75571 Paris Cédex 12, France

Neuenschwander, Sylvia
Chef de Clinique Assistant. Service de Radiologie.
Hôpital Trousseau. 8-28, av. du Dr Arnold Netter. 75571 Paris Cédex 12, France

Pariente, Danièle
Chef de Clinique Assistant. Service de Radiologie.
Hôpital des Enfants Malades. 149, rue de Sèvres. 75730 Paris Cédex 15, France

Poncin, Jocelyne
Chef de Clinique Assistant. Service de Radiologie.
Hôpital Jean Verdier. Avenue du 14 juillet. 93140 Bondy, France

Spehl-Robberecht, Marianne
Adjoint du Service de Radiologie.
Hôpital Universitaire Saint-Pierre. 322, rue Haute. 1000 Bruxelles, Belgium

Preface

The aim of this work was not an exhaustive review of all pediatric echographic problems but a presentation of our daily experience with ultrasonography in pediatric practice. Several teams of pediatric radiologists from France and Belgium have combined their experiences to produce a practical book. The different authors have been chosen for their specific experience and their special area of work. The different chapters express therefore personal opinions. Unresolved questions are posed and ultrasonographic examinations are used in the diagnosis of different diseases, while the discoveries and ideas of the individual authors are described. Some fields are not included, such as echocardiography.

Gabriel Kalifa

Contents

Chapter 1

Antenatal Diagnosis by Ultrasonography

E. F. Avni

1 Introduction

Ultrasound (US) examination has become the main method for an objective and precise evaluation of a pregnancy [11]. This examination, unharmful for the mother and the fetus [2], is easy to perform and allows not only rapid estimation of the gestational age, determination of the number of fetuses, and appreciation of the fetal welfare, but also detection of abnormalities of the fetoplacental unit.

With the help of highly developed US technology our knowledge of the physiological and anatomical development of the fetus has become more and more accurate and has been completed by the discovery of unsuspected aspects [4, 41]. These improvements allied to a growing experience lead to more accurate and precise diagnoses. Anomalies of various systems and organs have already been described, which has resulted in peri- and even prenatal treatment. It opens a new era in human therapeutics [5, 24, 31–33, 66].

The diagnosis of a malformation should be made with great caution after careful evaluation and control examination. There should be complete coordination between the radiologist, obstetrician, and pediatrician so that rapid and adequate steps can be taken [22]. This chapter first considers US examination of a normal pregnancy and the way to judge it. Normal fetal anatomy is then illustrated. The second part deals with pathological conditions, especially fetal malformations. Finally, the implications of the discoveries are discussed.

2 Ultrasonography of a Normal Pregnancy

2.1 Timing of Successive Examinations

Three examinations are useful and sufficient [11, 61]:

The first at 10–12 weeks of amenorrhea confirms most precisely the gestational age and the number of fetuses.

The second around 20–25 weeks: The fetal biometry is objectivated by the measurements of the biparietal diameter (BPD), thoracic transverse diameter (TTD), abdominal transverse diameter (ATD), and the femoral length. All these values are compared with standards. Fetal anatomy, movements, and heart beats are observed. Some anomalies of the neurological system and the urinary tract can already be excluded (e.g., anencephaly or renal agenesis). The estimation of amniotic fluid volume and visualization of the placenta complete the examination.

The third examination around 30–32 weeks confirms the good evolution of the pregnancy based on the same measurements. A detailed analysis of the fetal anatomy is made at this time and more precise structures can be delineated (e.g., renal pyramids or cardiac chambers). Again, estimation of amniotic fluid, placentar analysis, and determination of the presentation complete the examination.

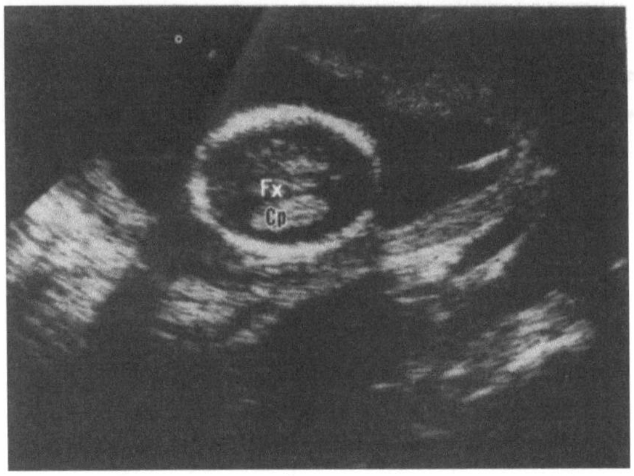

Fig. 1. Biparietal diameter at 15 weeks amenorrhea. *Cp*, Choroid plexus; *Fx*, cerebral falx.

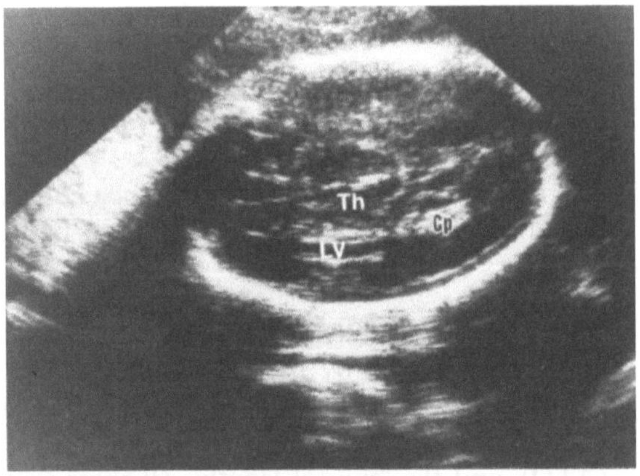

Fig. 2. Biparietal diameter at 31 weeks. *LV*, Lateral ventricle; *Cp*, choroid plexus; *Th*, thalamus.

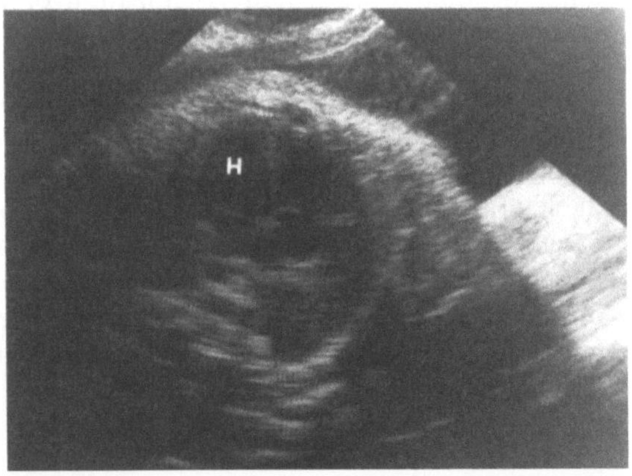

Fig. 3. Thoracic transverse diameter: view of four chambers of the heart *(H)*.

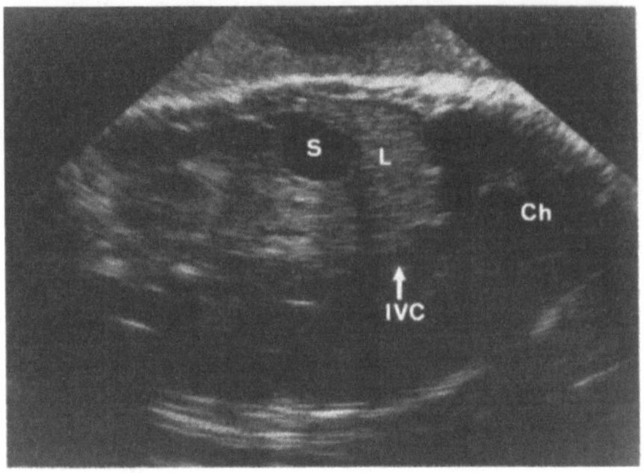

Fig. 4. Sagittal scan of the fetal trunk. *Ch*, Chest; *L*, liver; *S*, stomach; *IVC*, Inferior vena cava.

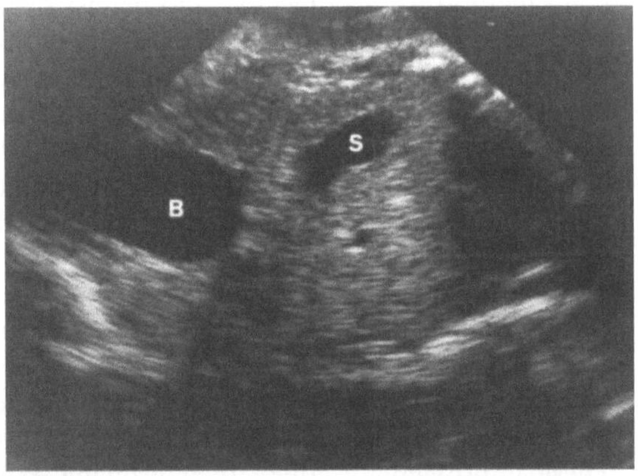

Fig. 5. Sagittal scan of the fetal trunk. *S*, Stomach; *B*, bladder.

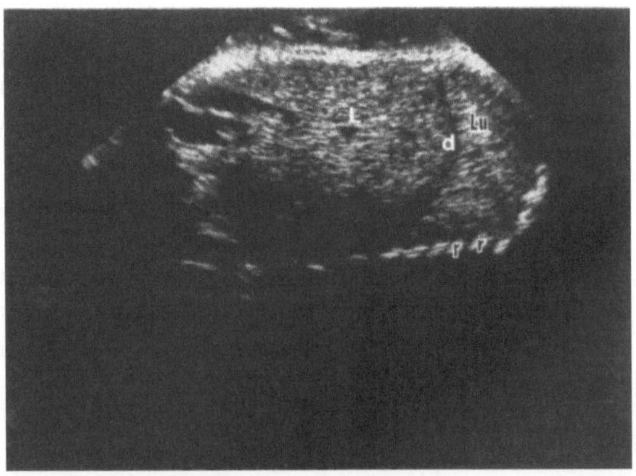

Fig. 6. Sagittal scan of the fetal trunk. *L*, Liver; *Lu*, lung; *d*, diaphragm; *r*, ribs

2.2 Normal Fetal Anatomy

2.2.1 Central Nervous System

Until the beginning of the second trimester, most of the central nervous system (CNS) is composed of the lateral ventricles and choroid plexuses (Fig. 1). Afterwards there is a relative decrease in the size of the ventricles as compared with the growing brain mantle [36]. The evolution and development of the cerebral structures can be followed and at the end of the second trimester more definitive structures can be identified (lateral ventricles, thalami, cerebellum) (Fig. 2) [19, 30, 38].

2.2.2 Chest

The heart, its chambers and rhythm, and the great vessels are mainly studied (Fig. 3) [52]. M mode recording can be obtained. The pulmonary parenchyma appears as a bright uniformly echogenic "mass." Respiratory movements are visualized in real time (Fig. 6) [37].

2.2.3 Abdomen

The analysis of the abdomen is easier thanks to "cystic" landmarks such as the bladder, stomach, gallbladder, and vessels (Figs. 4 and 5). The stomach and bladder can be identified as early as week 18 [34] and should be systematically sought (Figs. 4 and 5). With the use of high frequency real-time transducers the "solid" organs of the abdomen can be delineated: the liver, kidneys, adrenal, spleen, and (less easily) the pancreas are visualized [20, 39] (Figs. 6–8). At the end of the pregnancy the intestines become filled with more echogenic meconium, which makes delineation more difficult.

2.2.4 Skeletal System

The calvarium and face (Fig. 9), the spine (Fig. 10), and the ribs and extremities (Fig. 11) can be detailed as early as the beginning of the second trimester. Their development can be followed and measurements can be compared to standard charts for the long bones and the orbital diameters [8, 17, 37, 48, 49].

2.2.5 Gender

Fetal gender may sometimes be visualized as early as week 20 of amenorrhea [16].

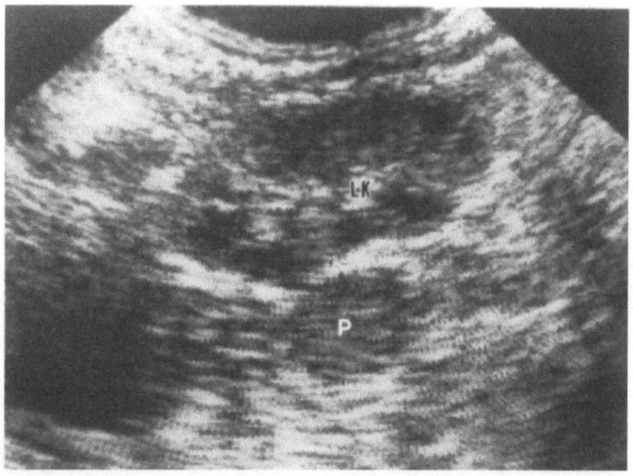

Fig. 7. Sagittal scan showing the left kidney *(LK)*. Note the corticomedullary differentiation. *P*, Tail of the pancreas.

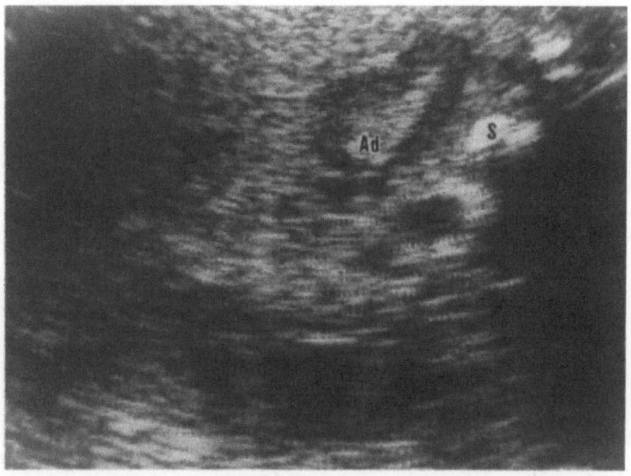

Fig. 8. Transverse scan of fetal abdomen showing the adrenal gland *(Ad)* and the spine *(S)*.

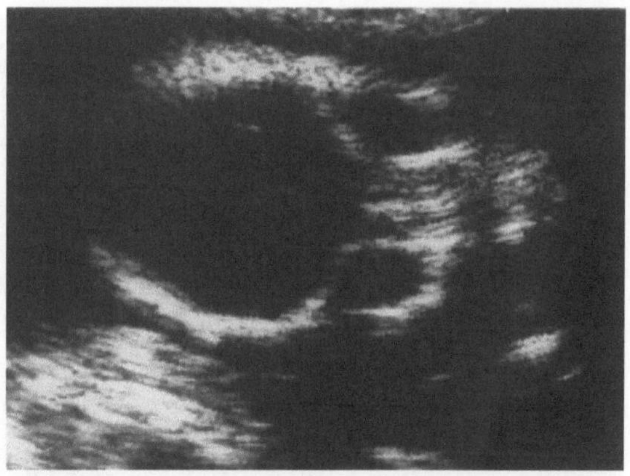

Fig. 9. Facial bones "en face" (19 weeks).

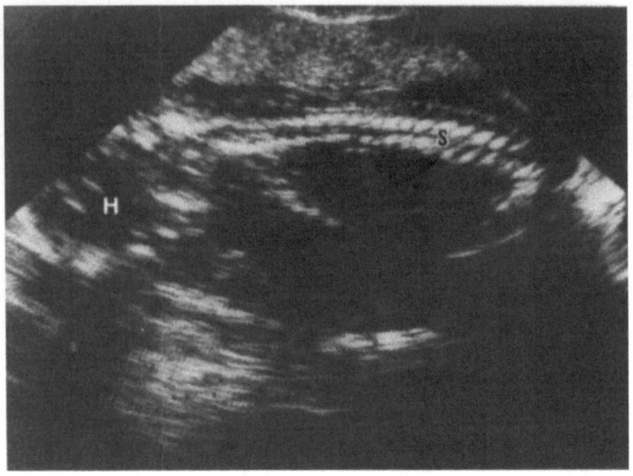

Fig. 10. Fetal longitudinal scan (19 weeks) showing the spine *(S)* and the head *(H)*.

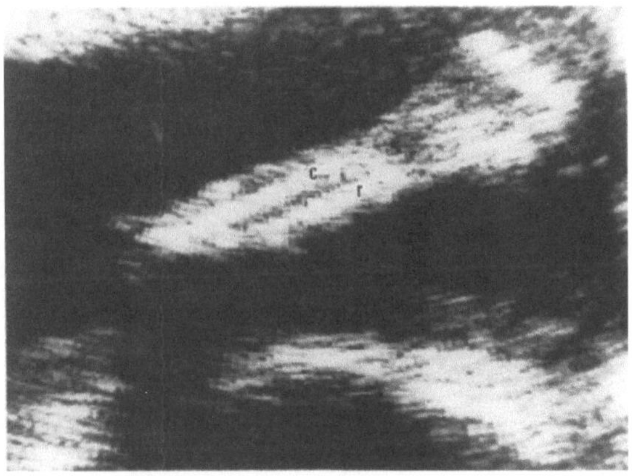

Fig. 11. Forearm and wrist, *r*, Radius; *c*, Cubitus.

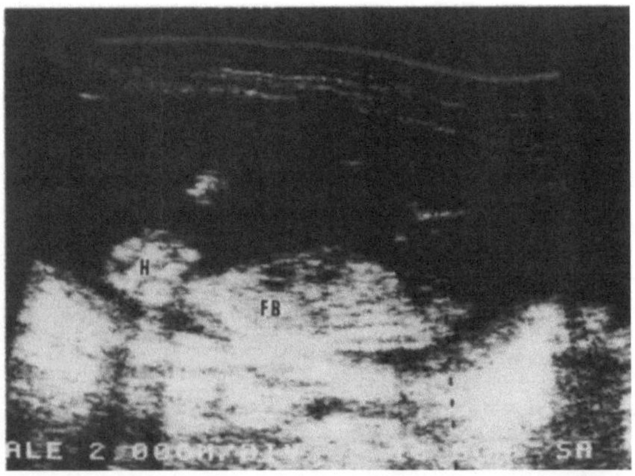

Fig. 12. Sagittal scan at 15 weeks showing anencephaly. *H*, Cerebral pole; *FB*, Fetal body.

2.3 Conclusions from Examinations

In the vast majority of cases, the examination confirms the normal evolution of a normal pregnancy. Yet, in some cases the conclusions are different: the first abnormal condition is that of retarded growth; the second abnormal condition (the two can be associated) corresponds to cases where an anatomical abnormality has been detected.

3 Abnormal Pregnancies

3.1 Intrauterine Growth Retardation

Growth is retarded when the measurements are significantly lower on the percentile charts than at a previous examination and/or when the measurements are under the 10th percentile for the estimated gestational age. The abdomen and thoracic diameters are lower long before any growth retardation of the BPD [13].

Detecting retarded growth is of great clinical significance since these fetuses are fragile and the end of their gestation is at high risk [71]. The rate of death in utero is high among these fetuses and their delivery must be carefully monitored. US is the main examination in such cases; it may also provide important additional information such as eventually associated fetal malformations, placentar anomalies, or oligoamnios.

3.2 Fetal Anatomical Malformations

Theoretically, a great number of malformations can be diagnosed in utero [34, 57–59] (Table 1). However, at least three elements greatly influence their detection:

1. The equipment: high frequency real-time transducers are more suitable for a detailed and easy anatomical study.
2. The experience, knowledge, and savoir faire of the examiner help to discriminate between normal and abnormal but also between normal and atypical images.
3. The nature of the abnormality: cystic masses are more evident than solid tumors or skeletal malformations.

US examination is per se a good method for detecting malformations. Its accuracy can be

Table 1. Antenatal diagnosis between July 1979 and May 1983 (17000 examinations).

CNS	
Hydrocephalus	4
Triploidy	1
Spina bifida	1
Isolated	1
With porencephaly	1
Anencephaly	4
Anencephaly with meningocele	1
Encephalocele	1
Cerebral hemorrhage	1
Chest and neck	
Cystic hygroma (Turners syndrome)	1
Bronchogenic cyst	1
Pleural effusion	2
Transitory	1
Hydrops fetalis	1
Heart rhythm anomalies	3
Transient bradycardia	2
<Nuchal encirclement	1
Cardiac complex malformation with aneurysm of pulmonary artery and hypoplastic left heart	1
Abdomen (urinary tract excluded)	
Ascites	4
Fetal death	1
Maternal diabetes	1
Urinary tract obstruction	1
Turners syndrome	1
Omphalocele	2
Ovarian cyst	1
Urinary tract	
Renal agenesis bilateral	1
Renal hypoplasia	1
Multicystic dysplastic kidney	2
Unilateral hydronephrosis	3
Ureteropelvic junction	4
Ureterovesical junction	3
Ectopic ureterocele	1
Bilateral hydronephrosis	7
Triploidy	1
Transitory hydronephrosis	2
Posterior urethral valves	2
So-called megacystic megaureters	2
Megabladder (transitory)	3
Solitary renal cyst	1
Musculoskeletal system	
Spina bifida (with hydrocephalus)	1
Axillary cystic hygroma	1

greatly improved by anamnestic and environmental factors. Patients affected by these factors can be gathered in a "high risk" pregnancy group (Table 2). These patients are monitored not only by US but also by an amniocentesis [59]. This will produce objective biochemical elements (α-fetoprotein) and chromosomal studies (Table 3) [25]. It may confirm clinical suspicion of an anomaly and further orient the examination. Finally, abnormal variations in the volume of the

Table 2. High-risk pregnancies (modified from [57]).

Maternal age > 35 years
Former history of chromosomal aberrations
Among the children
Personal
Familial
More than three miscarriages
Personal or familial history of hereditary disease
Former history of malformations (e.g., spina bifida)

Table 3. Causes of an increase in α-fetoprotein (modified from [57, 68]).

Hydrocephalus and CNS malformations
Omphalocele
Duodenal atresia
Cystic hygroma
Turner's syndrome
Hypospadias
Pilonidal sinus
Fetal death
Multiple pregnancies
Rhesus incompatibility
Contamination by fetal blood
Trisomy 13, 18, 21
Hydrops fetalis

Table 4. Malformation associated with polyhydramnios (modified from [1]).

Idiopathic	80%
CNS anomalies	3%
Hydrops fetalis	1.4%
Intestinal obstruction	1%
Diaphragmatic hernia	0.6%
Cardiac pathology	1%
Ectopic testis	1%
Various	12%

Table 5. Malformations associated with oligoamnios (modified from [57]).

Idiopathic
Bilateral obstructive uropathies
IUGR
Loss of amniotic fluid
Pregnancies beyond term

amniotic fluid are associated with specific types of malformation (Tables 4 and 5) [1, 34, 57].

3.2.1 Central Nervous System (CNS)

CNS malformations concern about 20% of all malformations seen at birth (Table 6). They may be associated with an increase in the α-fetoprotein and amniotic fluid. The vast majority are diagnosed during the third trimester. Up to now, few (anencephaly, encephalocele, congenital hydrocephalus) can be diagnosed during the second trimester. The first objective element of an eventual pathology is an abnormal biparietal.

Table 6. Congenital anomalies found at birth[a].

	For 1 000 births
Anencephaly	0.45
CNS + spina bifida	0.5
Hydrocephalus	0.34
Cardiovascular anomalies	0.38
Facial anomalies	0.88
Digestive system anomalies	0.18
Urogenital system anomalies	0.59
Osteoarticular system anomalies	1.88
Multiple anomalies and syndromes	1.16
Undefined	0.19

[a] Belgian Health and Family Ministery, Inspection of public hygiene (Demographic and biomedical information, 1981)

3.2.1.1 Malformations Associated with Small Biparietal

Anencephaly. This frequent malformation (0.44‰) is due to nondevelopment of the encephalum and appears early in the development. Its diagnosis is easy; the consequence may be an early abortion. The main US characteristics are a nonmeasurable BPD after 14 weeks of amenorrhea and absence of lateral ventricles [19] (Fig. 12).

Acrania. It is a rare condition where the vault does not develop and where no measurable biparietal can be obtained [47].

Microcephaly. The biparietal is less than the 10th percentile for the gestational age with normal ATD and TTD. Hydrocephaly is a possible associated malformation and craniostenosis should be suspected when there is an abnormal calvarium configuration [42].

Encephalocele, Meningocele, and Myelomeningocele. These malformations result either from intracranial hyperpression or from a persistent opening of the neural tube. A careful examination is necessary to detect small masses. An encephalocele appears as a solid, lamellated mass floating in the amniotic fluid next to the head (Fig. 13) [19, 50, 60]. (Myelo)meningoceles are more liquid masses and can be located anywhere along the neural tube.

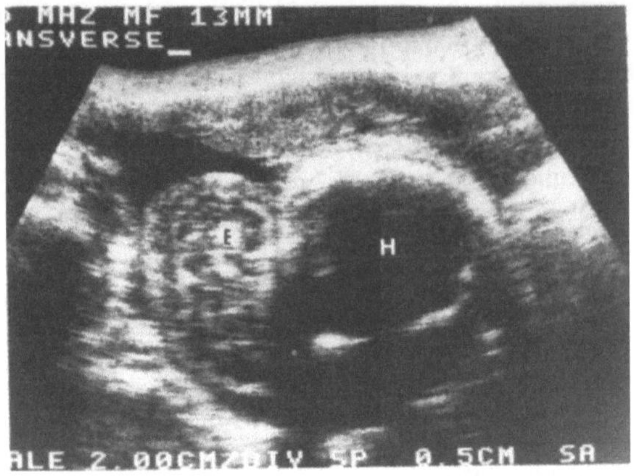

Fig. 13. Encephalocele *(E)* at 30 weeks. Biparietal diameter under 10th percentile. *H,* Head.

It is mandatory to look for associated hydrocephalus or spine malformations. A spina bifida is characterized by widening of the spinal canal on longitudinal scans and by crescent-like opening of the spine on the transverse scan (Fig. 14). Small masses especially at the lumbosacral junction can be difficult to visualize [19].

3.2.1.2 Malformation Associated with Normal or Increased BPD

Hydrocephalus and Ventricular Malformations. The diagnosis of hydrocephalus is based on the value of the fraction between the lateral ventricle and the corresponding hemisphere (LVW/HW) value. This value varies greatly: from 70% at 14 weeks to 30% near term [36, 57]. Early diagnosis of hydrocephalus is therefore difficult and should be made with caution. BPD can be within normal limits until very late in the pregnancy. However, it is possible that with improvement of our knowledge and technology the diagnosis will be made earlier and will be more accurate [34].

Localized dilatations or malformations of the ventricles can also be observed and in utero diagnosis of the Dandy-Walker deformity can be made [19]. The discovery of an intracranial malformation should be followed by careful examination of the spine for an associated anomaly (Fig. 14) [8].

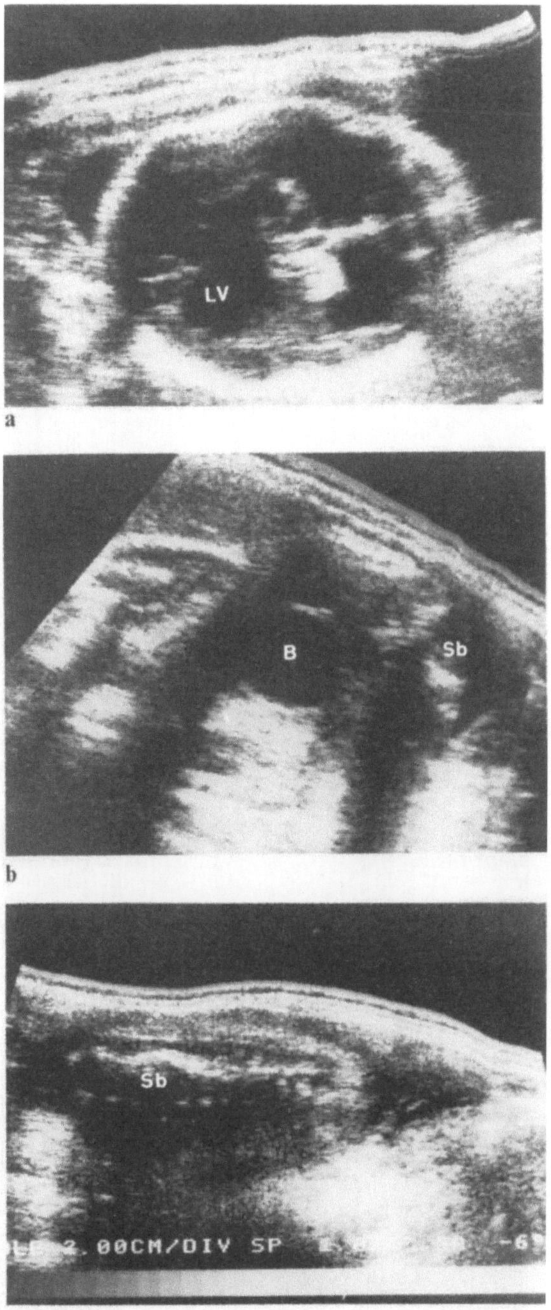

a

b

c

Fig. 14a–c. Hydrocephalus with spina bifida (without meningocele). **a** Biparietal diameter with marked dilatation of lateral ventricles *(Lv)*. **b** Spina bifida *(Sb)* shown by transverse scan. *B*, Bladder. **c** Spina bifida *(Sb)* shown by sagittal scan.

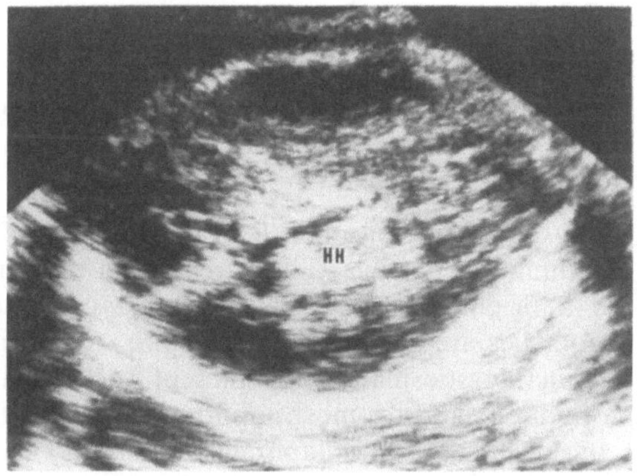

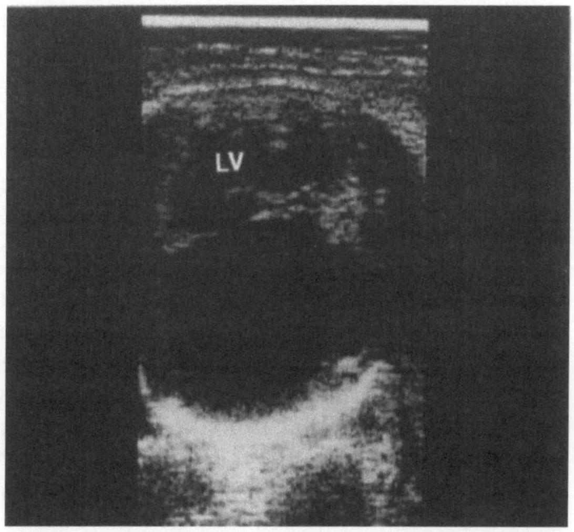

Fig. 16. Porencephaly at 35 weeks. Asymmetrical dilatation of lateral ventricles *(LV)*. No cerebral mantle with the most dilated ventricle.

Hydranencephaly, Porencephaly, and Cerebral Hemorrhage. These conditions are infrequent but their diagnosis is possible and becoming and more precise [45]. They probably all result from vascular impairment at one stage of the neurological development. Intracerebral hemorrhage is characterized the substitution of the normal hypoechoic cerebral tissue by hyperechoic areas (Fig. 15) [51]. Porencephaly could be the consequence of intracerebral hemorrhage and probably results from a vascular thrombosis. US examination shows asymmetrical dilatation of the ventricles with irregular borders (Fig. 16).

Vascular Malformations and Tumors. Aneurysm of Galien's vein is characterized by a cystic mass related to a tubular vascular structure. Intracranial teratoma and posterior fossa cyst have been diagnosed [35, 43].

3.2.2 Chest and Neck

Neck Masses. These include teratomas and cystic hygromas whose visualization is easy, but sometimes the differential diagnosis with CNS malformations is difficult (Fig. 17) [53, 60, 62].

Lungs. The lack of air in fetal lungs makes US examination possible. The parenchyma appears as a bright, uniform, echogenic mass. Cystic anomalies are again easy to visualize. An intrathoracic cystic mass can represent varied malformations and the most important diagnosis to consider is that of a diaphragmatic hernia. This pathology constitutes a surgical emergency at birth. It is characterized by intrathoracic cystic masses and absence of visualization of the thoracoabdominal limit [57]. The other diagnoses to consider are cystadenomatoid malformation, neuroenteric cyst, cystic hygroma, and bronchogenic cyst (Fig. 18) [14, 34, 64].

Pleural effusions can also appear as cystic areas. They are uni- or bilateral and we have observed a transitory pleural effusion. They can be associated with hydrops fetalis or heart failure (Fig. 19) [7, 12].

Heart. Real-time and M mode examinations are mandatory to characterize abnormalities. Gross malformations can be identified [40] but their detection requires cautious study. A precise diagnosis is usually difficult to make (Fig. 20). Transitory rhythm irregularities can be measured by M mode recordings (e.g., fetal primary bradycardia).

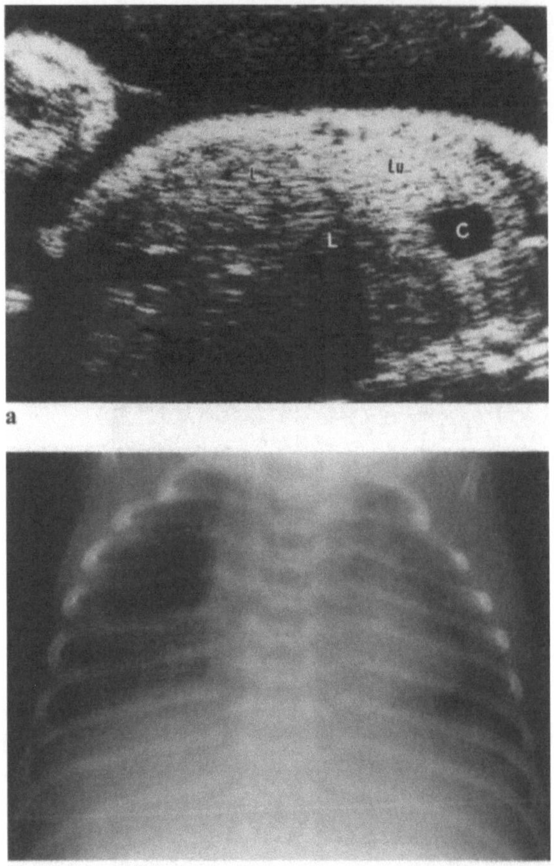

Fig. 18a and b. Bronchogenic cyst (30 weeks). **a** Right parasagittal scan. *L,* Liver; *Lu,* lung; *C,* 13 mm cyst. **b** Preoperative chest roentgenogram.

3.2.3 Abdomen

In cases of abdominal masses, it is mandatory to search for the normal anatomical landmarks so

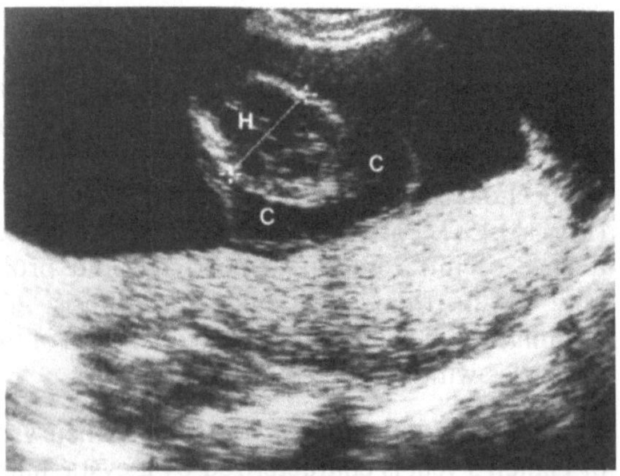

Fig. 17. Transverse scan at 15 weeks showing cystic hygroma of the neck (Turners's syndrome). *C,* Cyst; *H,* Head.

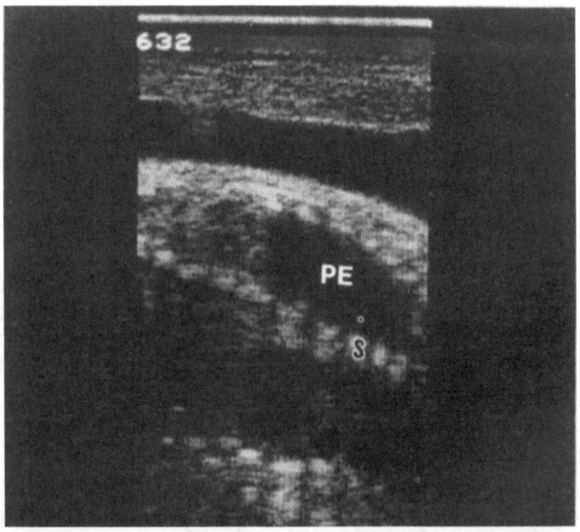

Fig. 19. Hydrops fetalis (30 weeks) with bilateral pleural effusion *(PE). S,* Spine.

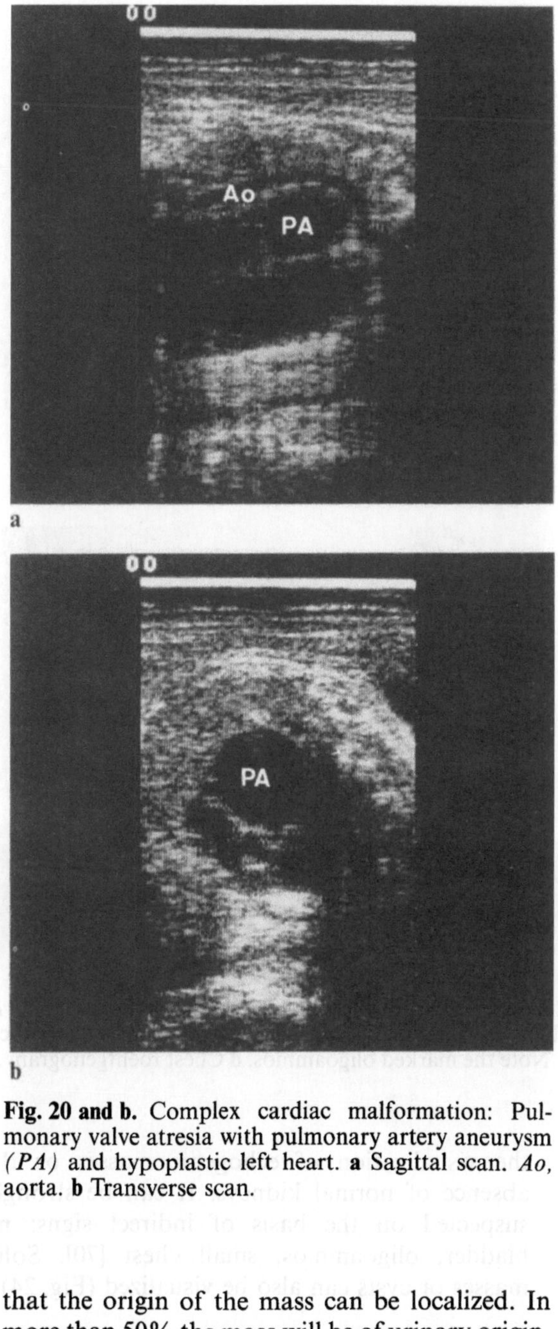

Fig. 20 and b. Complex cardiac malformation: Pulmonary valve atresia with pulmonary artery aneurysm *(PA)* and hypoplastic left heart. **a** Sagittal scan. *Ao*, aorta. **b** Transverse scan.

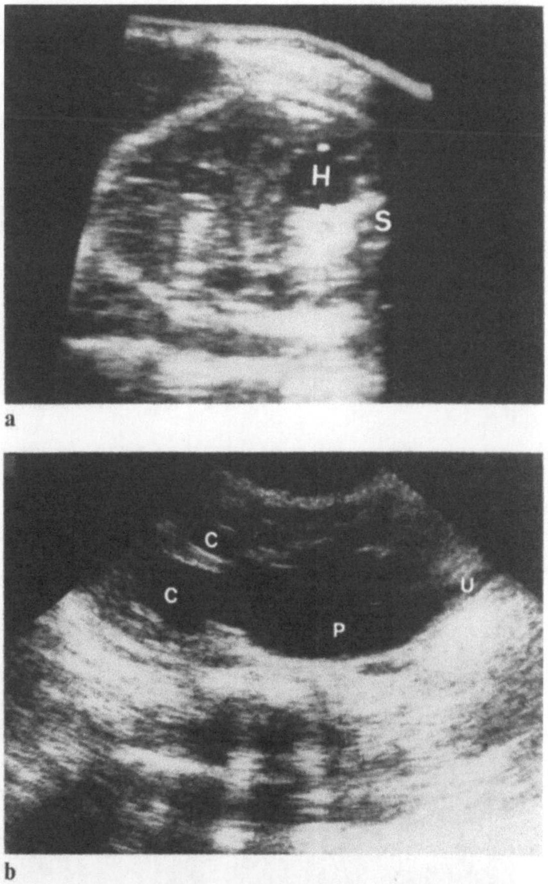

Fig. 21 a and b. Obstruction of the ureteropelvic junction. **a** Transverse scan at 35 weeks. *H*, Hydronephrosis; *s*, Spine. **b** Sagittal scan of left kidney at birth. *P*, Left kidney pelvis; *C*, calyces; *U*, ureter.

that the origin of the mass can be localized. In more than 50% the mass will be of urinary origin, less usually it will be intestinal, biliary, or varia.

3.2.3.1 Urinary Masses [6, 9, 28, 69]

Renal anomalies can be diagnosed during the second trimester (as early as the 20th week) especially obstructive uropathies. The anomalies can be separated into two categories: uni- or bilateral masses.

Unilateral Masses. A unilateral cystic mass corresponds most often either to a multicysic dysplastic kidney or to a ureteropelvic junction obstruction (Fig. 21). Both pathologies are characterized by unique or multiple cystic areas along the lumbar spine. Hydronephrosis can be transitory and control examinations will show the eventual persistence of a dilatation. Variable recurrent and disappearing hydronephrosis should suggest reflux. Other dilatations usually result from ureterovesical junction obstruction but a dilated ureter is sometimes difficult to identify.

Bilateral Masses. In cases of bilateral cystic masses, the bladder and the gender of the fetus

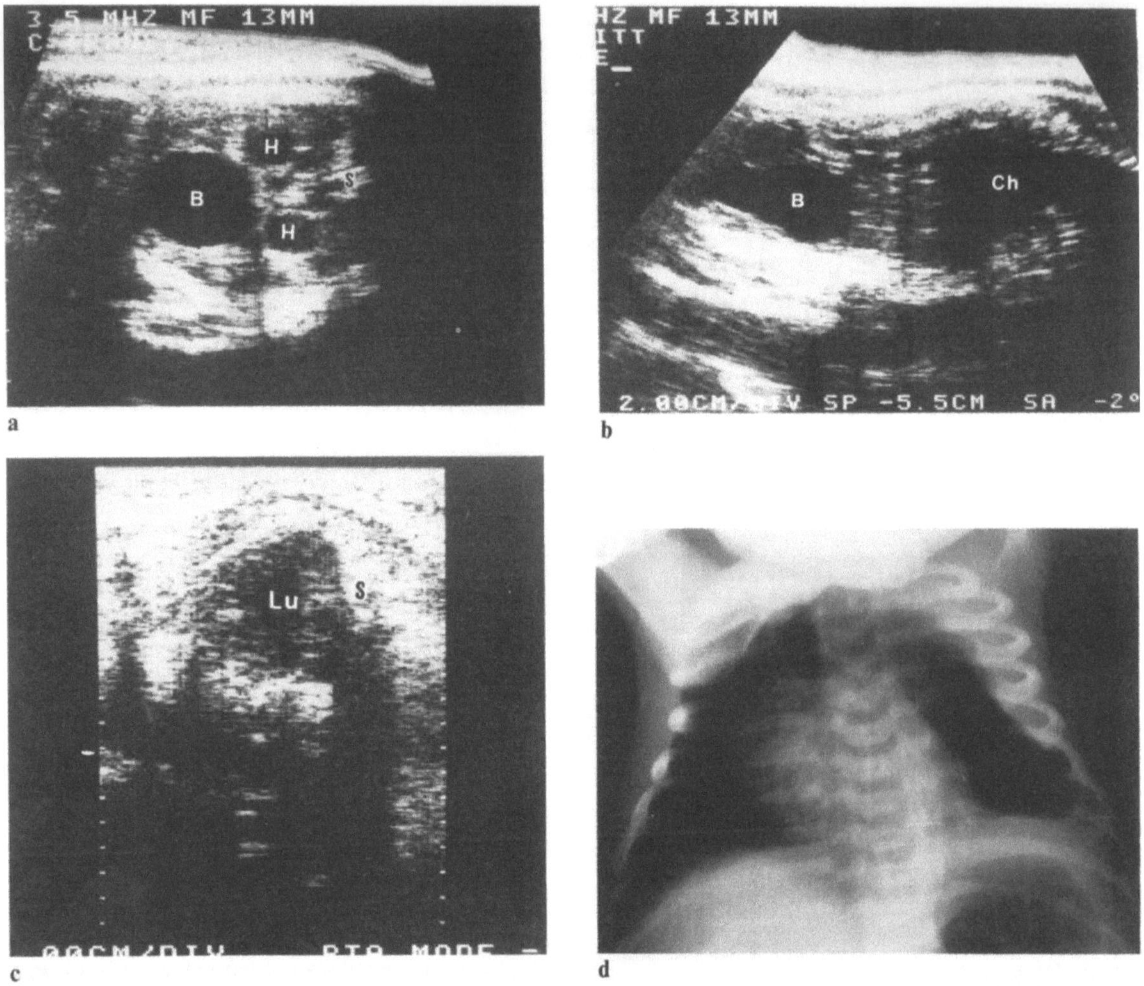

Fig. 22a–c. Posterior urethral valves (32 weeks). **a** Transverse scan showing bilateral hydronephrosis *(H)*. *B*, Bladder; *S*, spine. **b** Sagittal scan. *Ch*, Chest; *B*, bladder. Note the size and the form of the bladder. **c** Transthoracic diameter *(DTT)* under 10th perantile. *S*, Spine; *Lu*, lung. Note the marked oligoamnios. **d** Chest roentgenogram at birth. Massive bilateral pneumothorax.

should be studied. Bilateral hydronephrosis and persistent megabladder in a male fetus orients the diagnosis towards posterior urethral valves (PUV) (Fig. 22). In those cases, the chest diameter and the amniotic fluid should be measured or estimated and followed as indicators of lung hypoplasia and urine production. Not all cases of megabladder result from PUV: an enlarged bladder and hydronephrosis can result from massive reflux. When the masses are too big, their origin is more difficult to precise.

3.2.3.2 Other Urinary Tract Anomalies

These essentially concern polycystic kidney disease [27] and renal agenesis (Fig. 23) [15], which are usually part of Potter's syndrome. This diagnosis is more difficult to make since it is based on the visualization of echogenic masses or the absence of normal kidneys. It can be strongly suspected on the basis of indirect signs: no bladder, oligoamnios, small chest [70]. Solid masses or cysts can also be visualized (Fig. 24).

3.2.3.3 Digestive Masses

The majority of these masses result from intestinal obstruction. The stomach is the main landmark to look for. These obstructions are usually associated with polyhydramnios.

In the case of nonvisualization of the stomach, esophageal atresia can be suspected, while a double cystic image in the abdomen will orient the diagnosis toward duodenal atresia (Fig. 25). Numerous dilated tubules will orient the diagnosis toward a more distal obstruction [3, 46, 63].

The diagnosis of intestinal obstruction cannot be made on a single examination. Fluid-filled intestinal loops can be a physiological phenomenon, especially in late pregnancy [44]. Repeat demonstration of dilated loops in successive examinations in conjunction with polyhydramnios will confirm the diagnosis. A duplication cyst also has to be considered in the differential diagnosis.

3.2.3.4 Other Abdominal Masses

A cystic mass is more difficult to identify when a urinary or digestive origin is excluded. It can be from biliary origin or an ovarian cyst (Fig. 26) [10, 23]. Pseudomasses with calcification can result from meconium peritonitis [54].

3.2.3.5 Abdominal Wall Anomalies

Polyhydramnios is a persistent accompanying anomaly, which can be diagnosed early (20–25 weeks). An omphalocele is characterized by a solid mass continuous with the abdomen (Fig. 27). The mass is well defined and is concomitant with a small abdominal diameter. In the case of laparoschisis, the preabdominal wall will be less well defined [25, 26].

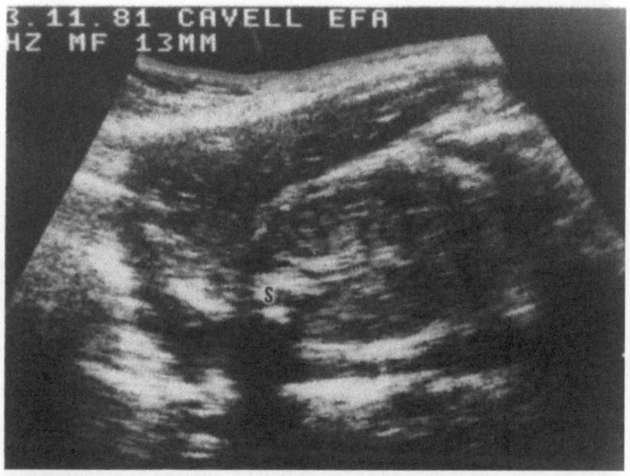

Fig. 23. Transverse abdominal scan showing bilateral renal agenesis (Potter's syndrome) at 30 weeks with marked oligoamnios. *S*, Spine.

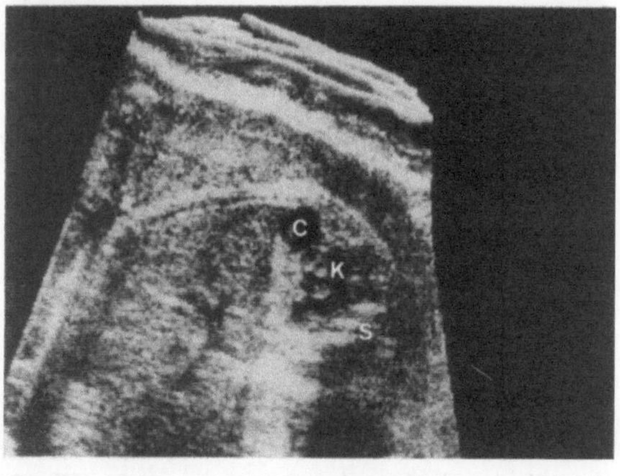

Fig. 24. Transverse scan showing solitary renal cyst. *K*, Right kidney; *C*, cyst; *S*, spine.

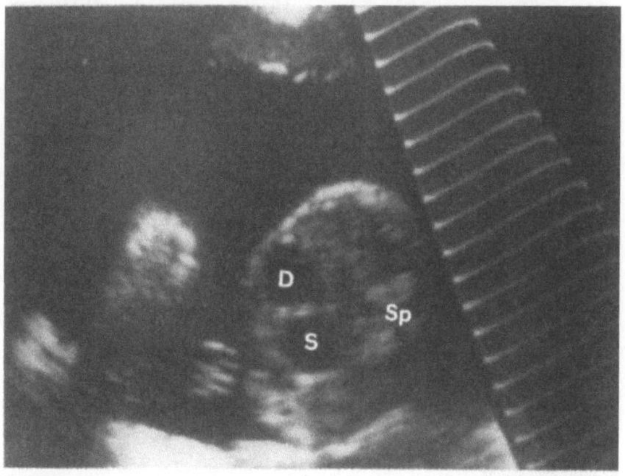

a

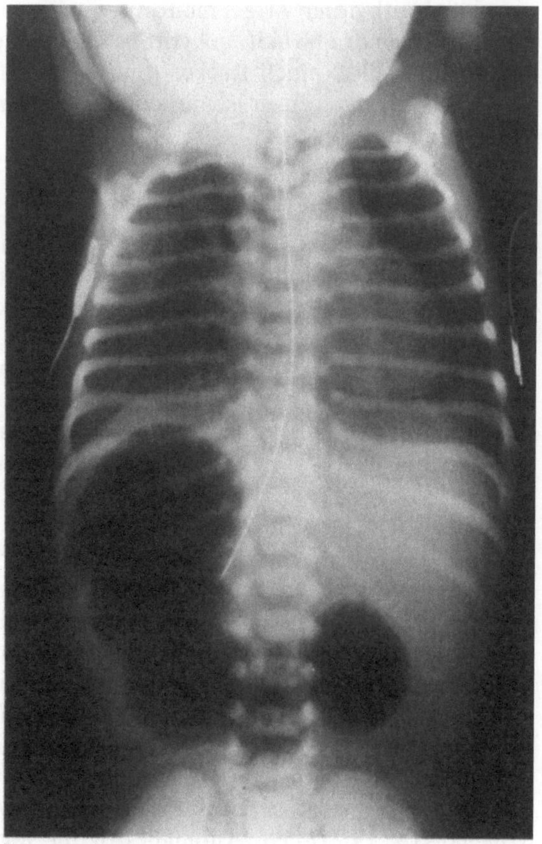

b

Fig. 25 a and b. Duodenal atresia.
a Transverse scan showing polyhydramnios at 30 weeks. *S*, Stomach; *D*, duodenum; *Sp*, spine.
b Plain film of liver at birth. (Courtesy of L. Cadier, Bordeaux).

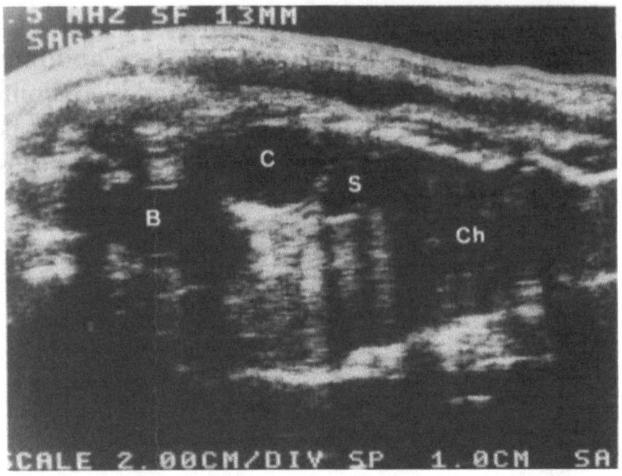

Fig. 26. Sagittal scan at 36 showing ovarian cyst *(C)*. *Ch*, Chest; *S*, stomach; *B*, bladder.

Anomalies of the abdominal wall can be seen associated with urinary tract malformations as in prune-belly syndrome [65]. In hydrops fetalis, the abdominal wall is much thicker (more than 20 mm). This can be seen in isoimmunization or in maternal diabetes [21].

3.2.3.6 Ascites and Hydrocele

In most cases ascites is characterized by a perihepatic collection of fluid (Fig. 28). It results from urinary tract or intestinal obstruction; in utero infection or isoimmunization are less usual [29]. It is imperative to make sure that it is not the normal hypoechogenic rim that can be seen under the abdominal wall [56]. Hydrocele is usually transitory [67].

3.2.4 Musculoskeletal System

Skeletal malformations are the most frequent congenital anomalies seen at birth (30%). Their visualization depends on the part involved and the size of the anomaly. Measurement of the femur is now part of our routine examination and dwarfism should be easy to detect, although it is still difficult due to varied fetal presentation.

Fractures or absence of limbs can also be detected [18, 19, 57–59]. Anomalies of the face (hypo telorism, clefts) can be measured and malformations of the spine are relatively easy to detect. The search for spina bifida is important especially when there is previous familial history (5% recurrence) [19].

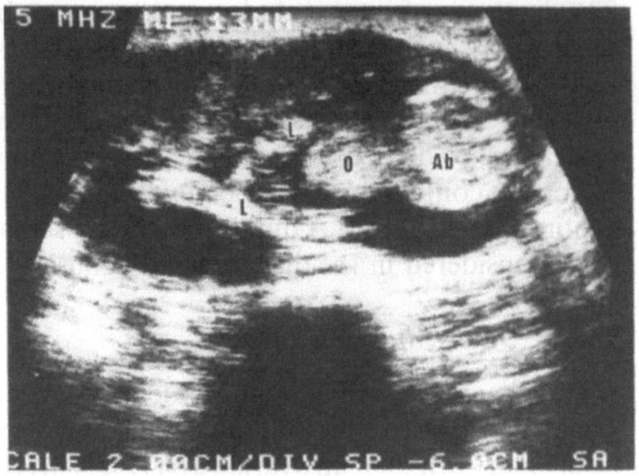

a

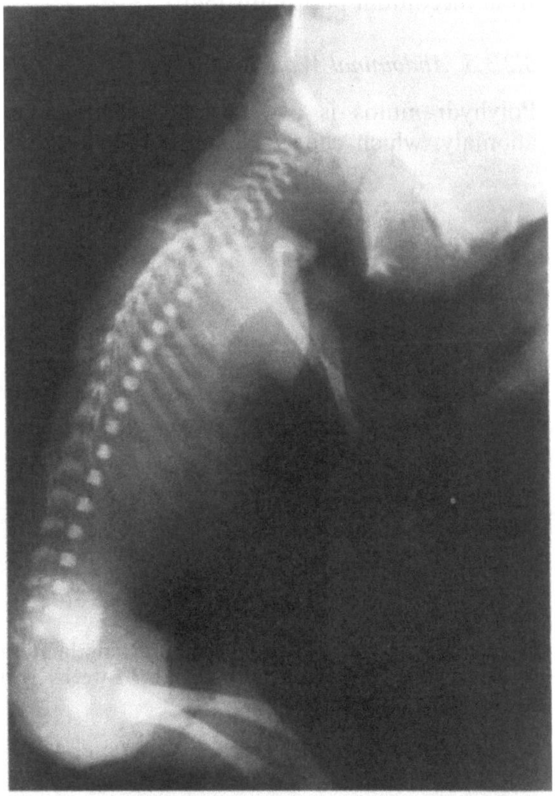

b

Fig. 27 a and b. Omphalocele at 25 weeks. **a** Transverse scan. *Ab*, Abdomen; *O*, omphalocele; *L*, legs. **b** Fetogram.

3.2.5 Soft Tissue Masses

Soft tissue masses are easy to visualize and are usually cystic hygromas or teratomas (Fig. 29) [53].

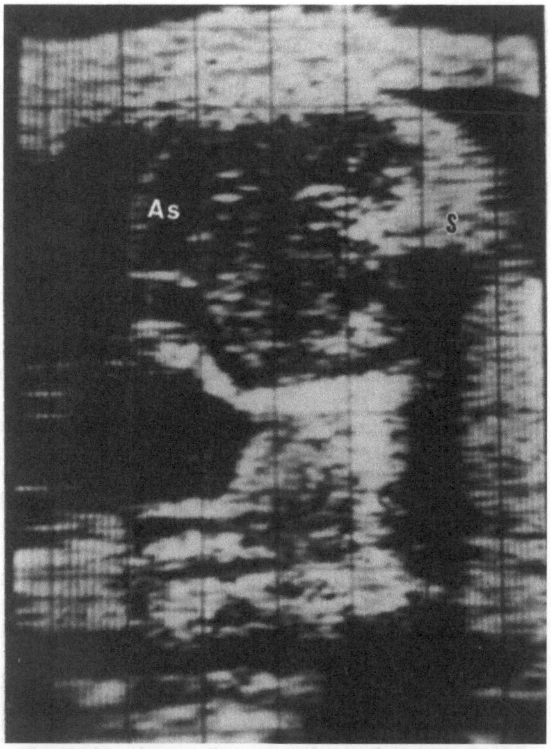

Fig. 28. Transverse scan showing fetal ascites (case of maternal diabetes) at 36 weeks. *As*, Ascites; *S*, spine.

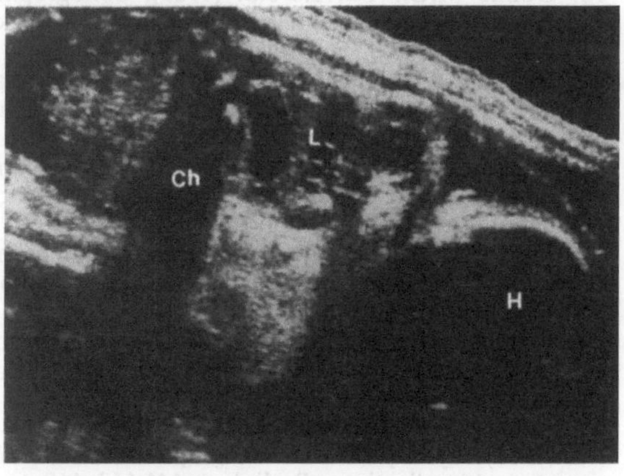

Fig. 29. Sagittal scan showing right axillary lymphangioma *(L)*. *Ch*, Chest; *H*, head.

4 What to do in Case of Fetal Malformation

Any suspicion of fetal malformation has to be confirmed by a careful control examination. Ultrasonography is an easy, safe, and rapid examination and can therefore be repeated. The lesion should be evaluated as precisely as possible and its eventual evolution should be observed. It is also important to look for indirect signs. US examination should be completed by analysis of the amniotic fluid through amniocentesis (with measurement of α-fetoprotein, bilirubin, and chromosomal studies). This will help to obtain the most accurate diagnosis [68].

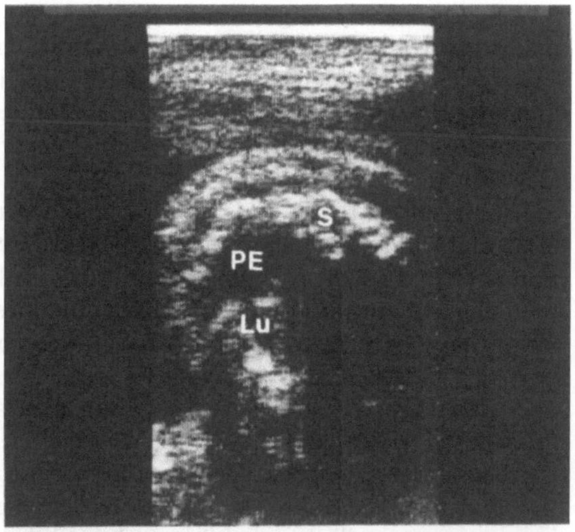

a

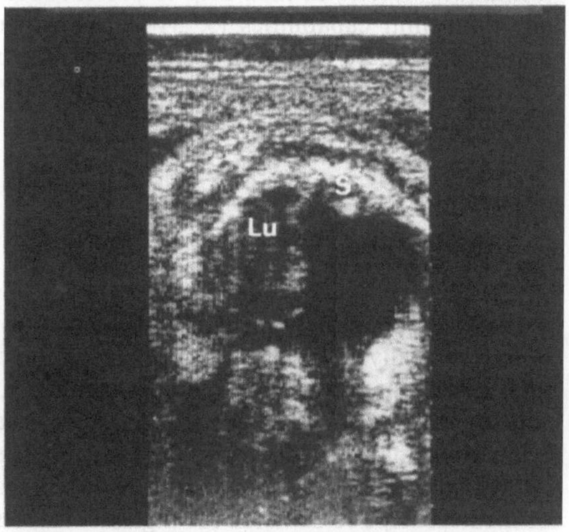

b

Fig. 30 a and b. In utero puncture of a pleural effusion *(PE)*. Same case as in Fig. 19. Transverse scans. **a** Prepuncture, bilateral effusion. **b** After drainage of the left effusion. *S*, Spine; *Lu*, lung. (Courtesy of F. Rodesch).

5 Implications of the Diagnosis

Up to now the role of US was to survey the pregnancy and to detect eventual fetal anomalies, both physiological and anatomical.

Sometimes, early diagnosis of a lifethreatening malformation leads to an early abortion [34]. In cases where intrauterine growth retardation is diagnosed, careful monitoring of the pregnancy has to be carried out until the end of the delivery [24, 69].

The role of US is also to detect those malformations that will require emergency surgical correction at birth. In some pathological cases US leads to in utero treatment, usually under US guidance. There have been attempts to correct totally or partially hydrocephalus, obstructive uropathies, and diaphragmatic hernias and to drain pleural effusions (Fig. 30). Not all treatments have been successful, but this opens a new area in therapeutics and it is reasonable to think that further improvements will be rapidly made to these techniques which will then help to preserve fetal developmental capabilities [5, 31–33]. Furthermore, better understanding of fetal development will lead to better indications for in utero treatment.

6 Conclusions

Prenatal US examination is still in full evolution both technically and scientifically. Observation of fetal evolution, physiological and morphological, will increase our knowledge and experience. Numerous malformations can already be precisely diagnosed. The examination helps surgical or medical steps to be taken for high-risk babies. Findings of a fetal anomaly should be made with extreme caution. Every diagnosis should be based on certainty or great prohability to avoid undesirable consequences.

References

1. Acton M.B., Weir P.E., Beucher N.A. (1981). The US aspects of polyhydramnios. Aust. Radiol. 25:62–67
2. Adamovics A., Edmonds P.D. (1981). US irradiation of mouse tissues in vivo and human amniotic cells in vitro. Ultrasound Med. Biol. 7:83–86
3. Bean W.J., Calonje M.A., Aprill C.N. (1978). Anal atresia: a prenatal US diagnosis. J. Clin. Ultrasound 6:111–112
4. Birnholz J.C., Stephens J.C., Faria M. (1978). Fetal movement patterns: a possible means of defining neurologic developmental milestones in utero. Am. J. Roentgen 130:537–540
5. Birnholz J.C., Frigoletto F.D. (1981). Antenatal treatment of hydrocephalus. New Eng. J. Med. 304:1021
6. Blanc C.E., Koff S.A., Bowerman R.A., Barr M. (1983). Non-obstructive fetal hydronephrosis: sonographic recognition and therapeutic implications. Radiology 147:95–99
7. Bovicelli L., Rizzo Nicola et al. (1981). US real time diagnosis of fetal hydrothorax and lung hypoplasia. J. Clinic. Ultrasound 9:253–259
8. Campbell S., Pryse Davies J., Coltart T., Seller M.J., Singer J.D. (1975). Us in the diagnosis of spina bifida. Lancet 1:1965
9. Chin R.H., Filly R.A. (1983). US diagnosis of fetal genito-urinary tract anomalies. Urolog. Radiol. 4:115–123
10. Crade M., Gilloly L., Taylor K.W. (1980). In utero demonstration of an ovarian cystic mass by US. J. Clin. Ultrasound 9:251–253
11. Creteur V., Schmitz C., Brombart J.C. (1981). Controle échographique de la grossesse normale. J. Belge Radiol. 64:343–349
12. Defort T. (1979). Antenatal diagnosis of congenital chylothorax. J. Clin. Ultrasound 6:47
13. Deter R.L. (1982). Intrauterine growth retardation: a review. J. Clin. Ultrasound 10:9–16
14. Donn S.M., Martin J.N., White S.J. (1982). Antenatal US findings in cystic adenomatoid malformation. Pediatr. Radiol. 10:180–182
15. Dubbins P.A., Kurtz A.B. et al. (1981). Renal agenesis: spectrum of in utero findings. J. Clin. Ultrasound 9:189
16. Dunne M.G., Currals J.S. (1983). Sonographic determination of fetal gender before 25 weeks gestation. Am. J. Roentgen. 140:741–743
17. Filly R.A., Gilbus M.S. (1982). US of the normal and pathologic fetal skeleton. Radiol. Clin. N. Am. 20:311–323
18. Filly R.A., Golbus M.S., Carey J.C. (1981). Short limb dwarfism: US diagnosis by measurement of femoral length. Radiology 138:653
19. Fiske C.E., Filly R.A. (1982). US evaluation of the normal and abnormal fetal neural axis. Radiol. Clin. N. Am. 20:285–296
20. Flaningan D., Buttny J. (1977). US imaging of normal intrauterine fetal anatomy. J. Clin. Ultrasound 5:134
21. Fleischer A.C., Killiam A.P., Boehm F.H. et al. (1981). Hydrops fetalis: sonographic evaluation & clinical implications. Radiology 141:163–168
22. Fletcher J.C. (1981). The fetus as a patient: ethical issues. JAMA 246:772–773
23. Frank J.L., Hill M.C., et al. (1981). Antenatal observation of a choledocal cyst by US. Am. J. Roentgen. 137:166
24. Garrett W.J., Kossof G. (1976). Selection of patients by US echography for fetal and immediate neonatal surgery. Aust. Paediatr. J. 12:313
25. Goldberg M.F., Oakley G.P. (1979). Interpreting elevated amniotic fluid and FP levels in clinical practice. Am. J. Obstet. Gynecol. 133:126
26. Guilian B.B., Alvear D.T. (1978). Prenatal US diagnosis of fetal gastroschisis. Radiology 129:473
27. Habif D.V., Berdon W.E., Ming Neng Y. (1982). Infantile polycystic kidney disease: in utero diagnosis. Radiology 142:475–477

28. Hadlock F.P., Deter R.L., Carpenter R. et al. (1981). Sonography of fetal urinary tract anomalies. Am. J. Roentgen. 137:261–267
29. Hadlock F.P., Deter R.L., Garcia Pratt (1980). Fetal ascites non-associated with Rh incompatibility. Am. J. Roentgen. 134:1225
30. Hadlock F., Deter R.L., Park S. (1981). Real time sonography: ventricular and vascular anatomy of the fetal brain in utero. Am. J. Roentgen. 136:133–137
31. Harrisson M.R., Bussack M.A., Churg A.M. (1980). Correction of congenital diaphragmatic hernia in utero. Surgery 88:260–268
32. Harrisson M.R., Golbus M.S., Filly R.A. et al. (1982). Fetal surgery for congenital hydronephrosis. New Engl. J. Med. 306:591
33. Harrisson M.R., Golbus M.S., Filly R.A., Naka Yama D.K., Callen P.W., De Lorimier A., Hricak H. (1982). Management of the fetus with congenital hydronephrosis. J. Pediatr. Surgery 17:728–742
34. Hobbins J.C., Graunin P.A., Berkowitz R.L., Silverman R., Mahoney M.J. (1979). US in the diagnosis of congenital anomalies. Am. J. Obstet. Gynecol. 134:331
35. Hoff N., Mackay I.M. (1980). Prenatal US diagnosis of intracranial teratoma. J. Clin. Ultrasound 8:247
36. Jeanty P., Dramaix M., Wilmet D., Delbecke, Rodesch F., Struyven J. (1981). US evaluation of fetal ventricular growth. Neuroradiology 21:127–131
37. Jeanty P., Kirkpatrick C., Dramaix-Wilmet M., Struyven J. (1981). US evaluation of fetal limb growth. Radiology 140:165
38. Johnson M.L., Dunne M.G., Mack L.A., Rashbaum C.L. (1980). Evaluation of fetal intracranial anatomy by static and real time US. J. Clin. Ultrasound 8:311–318
39. Johnson M.L., Hattan R.A., Rees G.K. (1982). The normal fetus. Sem. Roentgen. XVII-3:182–189
40. Kleinman C.S., Domerstein R.L. et al. (1982). Fetal Echocardiography for evaluation of in utero congestive heart failure. New Engl. J. Med. 306:568
41. Kurjak A., Latin V., Breyer B. (1978). Clinical application of fetal breathing movements. In: Proceedings of the fifth conference on fetal breathing, Nijmegen
42. Kurz A.B., Wapner R.J., Rubin C.S. et al. (1980). US criteria for in utero diagnosis of microcephaly. J. Clin. Ultrasound 8:11–16
43. Lee T.G., Newton B.W. (1979). Posterior fossa cyst prenatal diagnosis by US. J. Clin. Ultrasound 4:20
44. Lee T., Warren B. (1977). Antenatal Us demonstration of fetal bowel. Radiology 124:471
45. Lee T.G., Warren B. (1977). Antenatal diagnosis of hydranencephaly by US. J. Clin. Ultrasound 5:271
46. Lees R.F., Alford B.A. et al. (1978). Sonographic appearance of duodenal atresia in utero. Am. J. Roentgen 131:701
47. Mannes E.J., Crelin E.S., Hobbins J.S., Visconi G.N., Alcebo L. (1982). Sonographic demonstration of fetal acrania. Am. J. Roentgen. 139:181–182
48. Mayden K.L., Tortora M., Berkowitz R.L., Bracken M., Hobbins J.C. (1982). Orbital diameters: a new parameter for prenatal diagnosis and dating. Am. J. Obstet. Gynecol. 144:289–297
49. Miskin M., Baim R., Allen L., Benzie R. (1979). US assessment of fetal spine before 20 weeks of gestation. Radiology 132:131
50. Miskin M., Rudd N., Dische M., Benzie R., Pirani B. (1978). Prenatal diagnosis of occipital encephalocele. Am. J. Obstet. Gynecol. 130:585
51. Myung-Sup Kim, Morteza K.E. (1982). Sonographic diagnosis of cerebroventricular hemorrhage in utero. Radiology 142:479–480
52. Nisand I., De Geeter B. (1980). Echocardiographie foetale. Ultrasons 1:243–248
53. Philips H.E., Mc Gahan J.P. (1981). Intrauterine fetal cystic hygroma: sonographic detection. Am. J. Roentgen 136:799
54. Ram P.C., Bowie J.D. (1983). Prenatal US diagnosis of meconium peritonitis. Prenat. Diagn. 3:65–68
55. Roberts C. (1978). Intrauterine diagnosis of omphalocele. Radiology 127:262
56. Rosenthal S.J., Filly R.A., Callen P.W., Sommer F.G. (1979). Fetal pseudo ascites. Radiology 131:195
57. Rumack C.M., Johnson M.L., Zunkel D. (1981). Antenatal diagnosis. Clin. Ultrasound 8:210–230
58. Sabbagha R.E. (1980). US evaluation of fetal congenital anomalies. Clin. Obstet. Gynecol. 7:103–119
59. Sabbagha R.E., Shkolnik A. (1980). Us diagnosis of fetal abnormalities. Sem. Perinat. 4:213–227
60. Sabbagha R.E., Tamura R.K., Dal Compo S., Sherman E., Salvino C., Shkonik A., Gerbie A. (1980). Fetal cranial and craniocervical masses: US characteristics and differential diagnosis. Gynecology 138:511–517
61. Sabbagha R.E., Tamura R.K., Del Campo S. (1982). Fetal dating by US. Sem. Roentgen XVII-3:190–197
62. Schoenfeld A., Edelstein R., Joel Cohen S.J. (1978). Prenatal US diagnosis of fetal teratoma of the neck. Br. J. Radiol. 51:742
63. Szymour Zenlyn (1981). Prenatal diagnosis of oesophageal atresia. J. Clin. Ultrasound 9:453–454
64. Shanto H., Wilson R., Collea J. (1976). Fetal cystic hygroma – preparation US findings. Radiology 121:449
65. Shih W.J., Greenbaum L.D., Baro C. (1982). In utero sonogram in Prune Belly syndrome. Urology 20:102–105
66. Touloukian R., Hobbins J.C. (1980). Maternal US in the antenatal diagnosis of surgically correctable fetal abnormalities. J. Pediatr. Surg. 15:373–377
67. Vanesian R., Grossman M., et al. (1978). Antepartum US diagnosis of congenital hydrocele. Radiology 126:765–766
68. Van Regemorter N., Defleur V., Delbeke D., Vamos E., Rodesch F. (1983). Alphafoetoprotein (AFP), concanavalin A nonreactive AFP and specific acetylcholinesterase in amniotic fluid from pathological pregnancies. Eur. J. Gynecol. Obstet. (in press)
69. Walzer A., Koenigsberg M. (1980). Prenatal evaluation of partial obstruction of the urinary tract. Radiology 135:93

70. Wolf E.L., Berdon W.E. (1977). Diagnosis of oligoamnios related pulmonary hypoplasia (Potter syndrome). Radiology 125:769

71. Yerushalmy Y. (1970). Relation of birth weight, gestational age and rate of intrauterine growth to perinatal mortality. Clin. Obstet. Gynecol. 13:107

Chapter 2

Ultrasonography of the Head in Infancy

A. Couture and L. Cadier

1 Introduction

The first clinical applications of echoencephalography were made 20 years ago. For a long time, mode A ultrasonography was the only method for detection of the midline and measurement of ventricular size. Leksell [1] was the first to show that one could define midline cerebral structures by ultrasound. Significant progress was made using the "bistable" method and this permitted Sjogren [2] and Lombroso [3] to appreciate easily the morphology of the cerebral ventricles: it was in this way that early hydrocephalus was diagnosed and confirmed by pneumoencephalography. With the apparition of the grayscale, Kossof and Garret [4] accurately described the echoanatomy of the normal brain of an infant. They accurately isolated the ventricular system, taking precise measurements. However, they also defined certain parenchymal structures such as the thalamus, caudate nucleus, internal capsule, corpus callosum and the brain stem. More recently, the realization of horizontal transosseous sections by Morgan [5] and Johnson [6] permitted interesting comparisons with CT scan. The merits of this transosseous method compared with CT scan were widely discussed with the conclusion that, with regard to appreciation of ventricular size, the sensitivity of the methods was identical. However, the transosseous approach demands a meticulous technique. To identify both ventricles correctly, perpendicular projection of the ultrasound beam with respect to the ventricular wall is required [7]. The modification of direction due to the configuration of the cranial vault, often results in images that are difficult to interpret: these physical factors explain the fact that the posterior and frontal regions are poorly accessible or not at all accessible via US examination.

In addition, the cranial vault and in particular its thickness absorbs a large part of the ultrasonographic energy, which makes appreciation of small intracranial structures difficult. Cerebral parenchymal structures are much better defined by CT scan (Fig. 1). These facts, as well as the remarkable anatomical information gained by CT scan, explain the role of echoencephalography as a supplementary or screening method. These difficulties were recently eliminated by use of the anterior and posterior fontanelles as acoustic windows, which allows

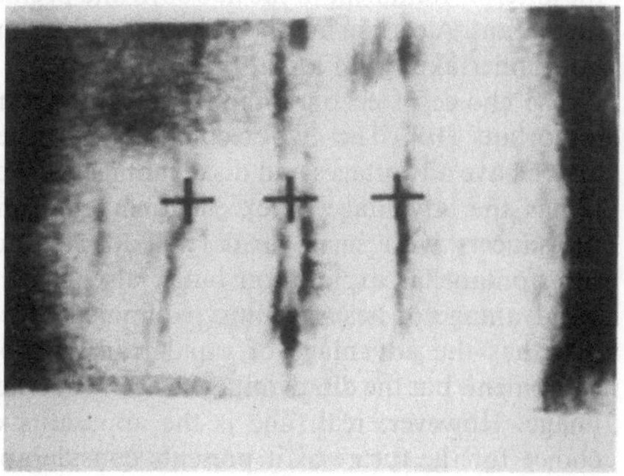

Fig. 1. Transosseous section, perpendicular to the orbitomeatal line. The middle portion of the dilated lateral ventricles is easy to measure but the frontal and occipital horns are not visible. Detailed examination of the cerebral parenchyma is not possible.

elimination of the bony barrier. Along with Ben Ora in the United States [8] we were among the first groups to use the transfontanellar acoustic window [9]. In fact, this technique has considerable advantages because it assures not only identification of the entire ventricular system, but also a panoramic vision of the entire cerebral parenchyma and the posterior fossa.

2 Instruments

2.1 Examination Technique and Practical Considerations

The great majority of examinations are carried out using a gray-scale mode B apparatus. This is a static apparatus with sectorial sweep and a jointed limb, well – adapted for pediatric use. The image is transcribed on an oscilloscope and the final pictures are taken with a polaroid camera. Simultaneously, the curve of A-mode echoes is visualized on the screen. High frequency transducers (5 mHz) are usually used. The use of a 7 mHz transducer is necessary for studying more superficial zones as well as in small premature infants. The choice of transducer depends on a compromise between correct penetration of cerebral tissue by US waves and satisfactory visualization of the image. Finally, it is imperative to use transducers with small heads (6 mm) due to the small size of the anterior fontanelle in the newborn and premature infant. A certain number of examinations are also undertaken with a real-time apparatus.

The choice of echographic equipment is very important [10]. The two techniques described above have advantages and disadvantages: Mode B has the advantage of excellent imaging and transducers with small heads well-adapted for transfontanellar exploration but it also has the disadvantage of heavy, clumsy equipment; Real time has the advantage of rapid transportable equipment, but the disadvantage of a less detailed image. However, real time is the apparatus of choice for the future as it presents considerable advantages in being practical for use in a neonatal intensive care unit.

The technique of echographic examination is always identical and presents no difficulties [9].

1. The newborn never receives premedication; if necessary, a bottle will calm the child.
2. Maintenance of correct temperature is assured by an overhead infrared lamp pointed toward the child.
3. If the baby's clinical condition permits, the child is placed in a vertical "baby-relax" position, the head well centered and immobilized by foam cushions (Fig. 2).
4. The examination is rarely carried out in the incubator; but when necessary, the transducer can be introduced into the incubator.
5. In cases of severe neonatal distress, the portable real-time apparatus allows the examination to be carried out in the neonatal intensive care unit.
6. The transducer is applied to the anterior fontanelle with a gel interface that allows penetration of the US waves. The curve of gain compensation is calculated so that the amplitude of echoes is similar in areas proximal and distal to the transducer.
7. Coronal and sagittal sections are undertaken using rotatory movements of the transducer which allows a panoramic sweep. Certain sections should be systematic: six coronal sections to explore the ventricular system and cerebral tissue anteroposteriorly, and three sagittal sections, one median in the axis of the third and fourth ventricles and the other two slightly oblique and lateroposterior in the axis of the lateral ventricles.

If the static mode B apparatus is used, the examination takes approximately 10–15 min.

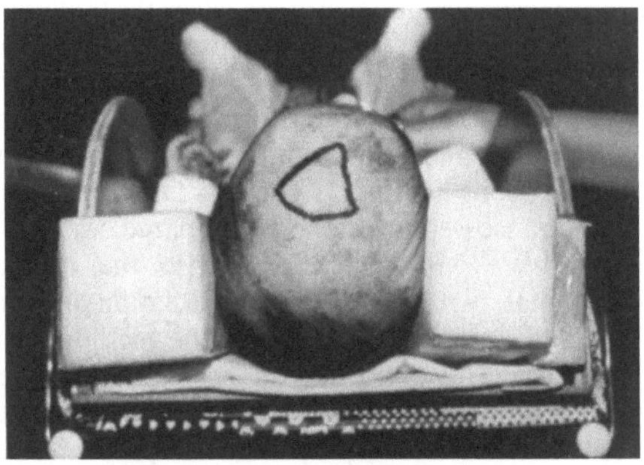

Fig. 2. Procedure for transfontanellar section.

3 Normal Echoencephalographic Anatomy (Fig. 3)

The lateral ventricles serve as essential anatomical landmarks. They have the shape of small echo-free triangles with an internally oriented base and rectilinear walls. A median longitudinal section will frequently show median cystic structure (cavum septi pellucidi and cavum vergae) in the premature infant, as well as the third ventricle, followed by the fourth ventricle. The cerebral cisterns are not visible except for the large cistern at the base of the skull which is sometimes seen as an echo-free triangular image: one can always

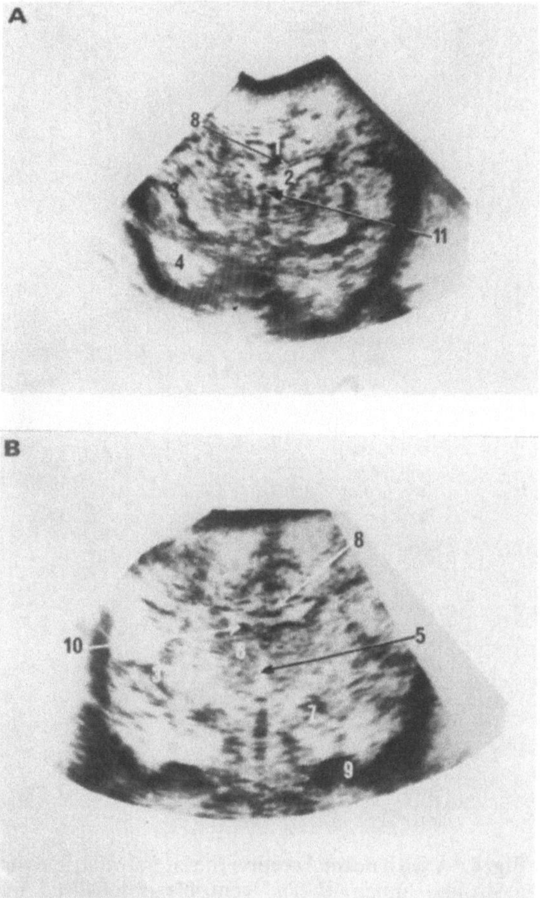

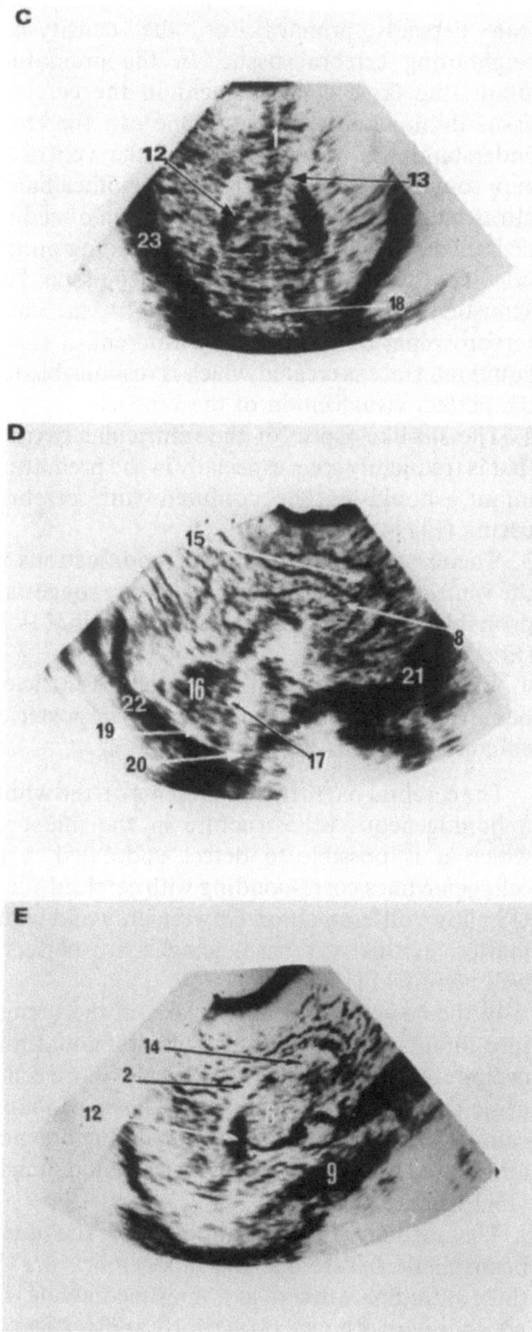

Fig. 3 A–E. Normal appearance on echoencephalogram. **A** Frontal section just anterior to the foramen of Monro; **B** Frontal section at the level of the third ventricle; **C** A more posterior frontal section; **D** Medial sagittal section; **E** Paramedial sagittal section along the axis of the lateral ventricle.
1, Interhemispheric sulcus; *2*, Lateral ventricle; *3*, Sylvian fissure; *4*, Temporal lobe; *5*, Third ventricle; *6*, Thalamus; *7*, Hippocampal circumvolution; *8*, Corpus callosum; *9*, Roof of the petrous temporal; *10*, Choroid plexus; *11*, Septum lucidum; *12*, Glomus of the choroid plexus; *13*, Intersection of the lateral ventricle; *14*, Caudate nucleus; *15*, Pericallous circumvolutions; *16*, Vermis; *17*, Fourth ventricle; *18*, Posterior fossa; *19*, Cisterna magna; *20*, Occipital foramen; *21*, Anterior fossa; *22*, Occipital bone; *23*, Temporal bone.

identify this cistern when it is dilated [11]. The choroid plexus can be seen within the lateral ventricular cavities as two linear, regular, symmetrical and very echogenic structures.

Four elements must be emphasized:

1. For demonstration of the lateral ventricles, the sensitivity of US examination is superior to that of CT scan especially in the premature infant. In fact, these two techniques depend on totally different physical characteristics: the visualization of a ventricular cavity by CT scan depends primarily on the density of neighboring cerebral tissue. In the premature infant, the large water content in the cerebral tissue diminishes its density. One can therefore understand that visualization of the ventricles may sometimes be mediocre. On the other hand, ultrasonography depends on the notion of acoustic impedance which is variable depending on the velocity of US waves within a specified tissue. The acoustic impedance of cerebral tissue and cerebrospinal fluid being very different, a solid-liquid interface is created which is responsible for the perfect visualization of the ventricle.
2. The slit-like aspect of the ventricular cavities that is frequently seen, especially in the premature infant, should not be confused with cerebral edema (Fig. 4).
3. The existence of physiologic modifications in the ventricular volume from day to day suggests a probable cyclical secretion of cerebrospinal fluid (Fig. 5).
4. Finally, the fact that the lateral ventricles, being liquid structures, do not result in posterior enhancement is as yet unexplained.

The cerebral parenchyma presents on the whole a homogeneous echostructure in the midst of which it is possible to detect undulated, very echogenic lines corresponding with cerebral sulci. US allows differentiation between gray and white matter: in this way basal ganglia are perfectly well identified [12].

In the newborn and particularly in the premature infant, the central parts of the frontal and occipital lobes appear physiologically more echogenic than the peripheral parts. This is probably caused by a neuronal maturational phenomenon and should not be confused with a recent parenchymal hematoma (Fig. 6).

The median line is composed of the interhemispheric fissure and the falx cerebri; on US these structures are seen as a thick medial line [13] which is very echogenic anteriorly and vertical. It separates the frontal lobes, the occipital lobes posteriorly and overrides the corpus callosum in the middle. Only coronal or frontal oblique sections can show these structures because on sagittal sections the US beams are parallel to them. The sulci of the internal hemispheric circumvolutions branch out from this central line [14].

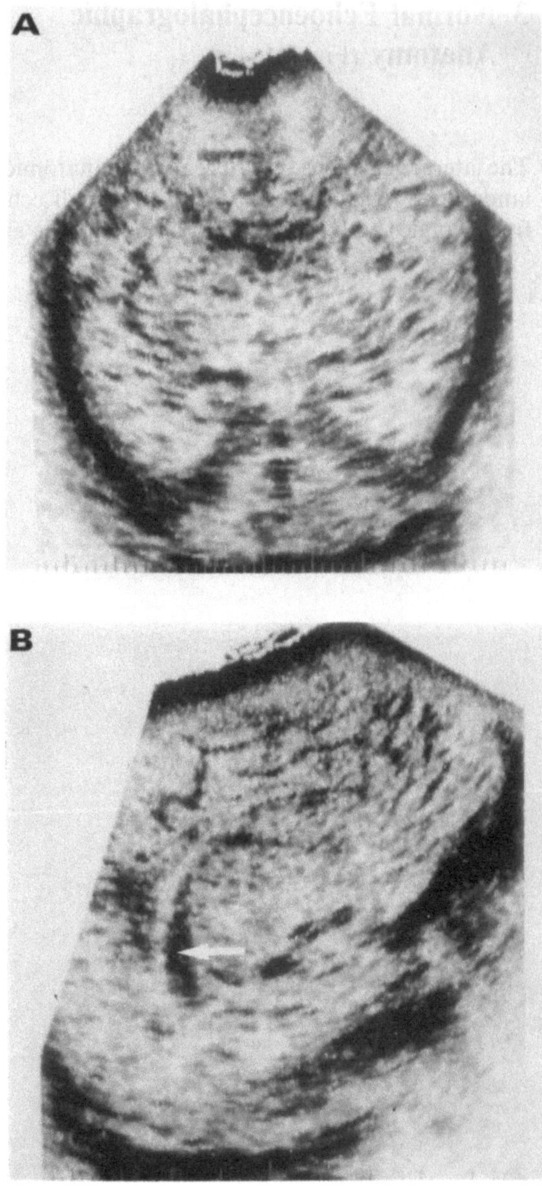

Fig. 4. **A** On a normal section the lateral ventricles have a slit-like lumen. **B** The ventricle is localized by a longitudinal paramedial section using the hyperechogenic choroid plexus as a point of reference (*arrow*).

The principal elements in the posterior fossa are easily identified due to their distinct echostruc-

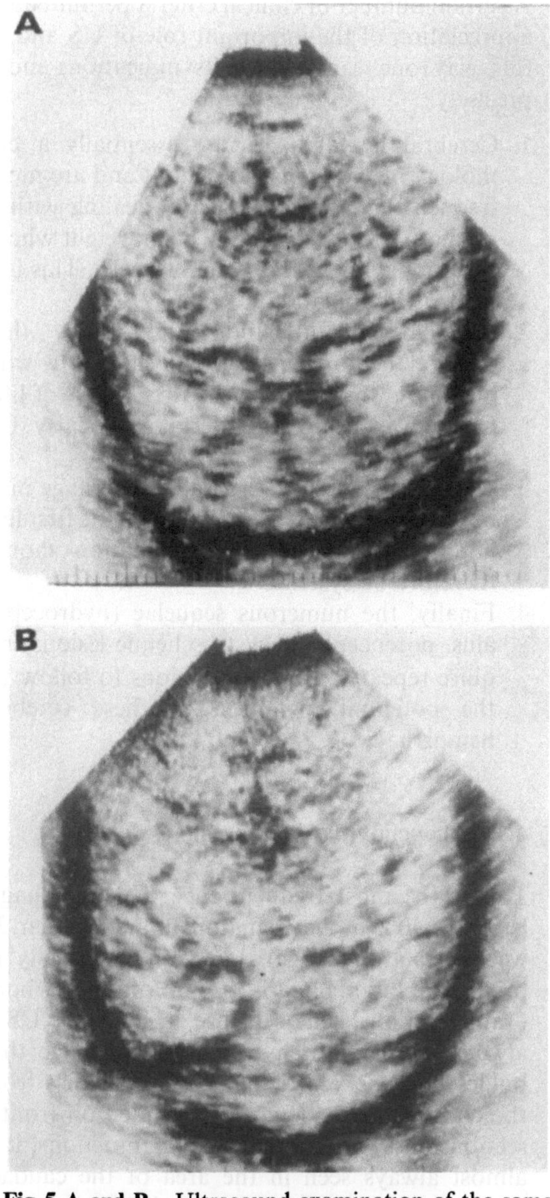

Fig. 5 A and B. Ultrasound examination of the same child with a 48-h interval between sections.
A The ventricles are slit-like; **B** The ventricles are easily distinguished.

tural differences: the intense echogenicity of the cerebellum is limited on its anterior aspect by a large, vertical, nearly echo-free band which represents the brain stem. The anterior view of the fourth ventricle is very difficult to distinguish from the posterior view of the brain stem. On the other hand, the small echo-free triangle with its apex pointing posteriorly, which represents the fourth ventricular cavity, can be easily distinguished amid the marked echogenicity of the cerebellar vermis (Fig. 3 D).

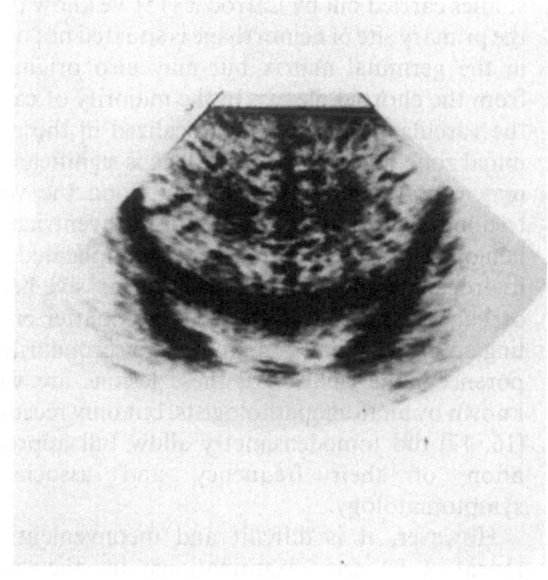

Fig. 6. The central zone of the frontal lobes is often much more echogenic than the peripheral zones in the healthy newborn.

Bone landmarks are very echogenic, permitting orientation as to the level of the section: anterior fossa with the orbital roofs, the greater and lesser wings of the sphenoid and sphenoid bone, the sella turcica, petrous pyramids and temporal bones in the middle fossa, and finally the parietal bone, lambdoid sutures, and occipital bone in the posterior fossa.

Precise measurement of the ventricular cavities may be made, using either a transosseous frontal section, suprameatal and perpendicular with respect to the orbitomeatal baseline or using a transfontanellar coronal section. The measurement is that of the transverse diameter of the middle part of the lateral ventricles. Normal values for a term newborn are between 8 and 13 mm, and for a premature infant at 32 weeks of gestation between 5 and 12 mm. For the third ventricle, the transverse diameter is always less than 5 mm at whatever gestational age. The anteroposterior diameter of the fourth ventricle is difficult to measure.

4 Cerebral Hemorrhages

Intracerebral hemorrhage is one of the principal causes of mortality and morbidity in the newborn especially in the premature infant. Since the studies carried out by Larroche [15] we know that the primary site of hemorrhage is situated not only in the germinal matrix but may also originate from the choroid plexus. In the majority of cases the vascular lesion remains localized in the germinal zone, but if the hemorrhage is significant it may rupture the ependyma and flood the ventricular cavities, thus causing an intraventricular hemorrhage which is frequently complicated by hydrocephalus. Finally, in cases of massive hemorrhage, it may penetrate the white matter creating an intracerebral hematoma and secondarily a porencephalic cavity. All these lesions are well known by anatomopathologists, but only recently [16, 17] did tomodensimetry allow full appreciation of their frequency and associated symptomatology.

However, it is diffcult and inconvenient to repeat CT scan examinations in the premature infant [18] who is often in poor general condition, which explains the pediatrician's reluctance to perform these examinations. In comparison, the development and improvement of US technique via the fontanelle has motivated numerous groups to use this method as a screening for cerebral lesions in newborns, in particular in the diagnosis of hemorrhagic lesions.

In the last few years, the progress in CT scan and US imaging has totally reversed the diagnostic approach toward hemorrhagic lesions and has permitted:

1. The incidence of cerebral hemorrhage in the premature infant to be established;
2. The different types of lesions to be understood;
3. The complications to be recognized without diagnostic delay;
4. Medical treatment to be started aimed at delaying or avoiding the definitive step of placing a ventriculoperitoneal shunt.

A certain number of clinical criteria permit better appreciation of the important role of US and in this way one can deduce its indications more precisely.

1. Cerebral hemorrhages are essentially a pathology of the premature infant and are more frequent and severe if one is dealing with a premature infant with low birth weight whose gestational age is less than 32 weeks. This is a high-risk population.
2. All experimental studies [19] show that cerebral hemorrhage occurs very early with maximum frequency in the first 2 days of life. One must therefore undertake an early US examination.
3. On the other hand, cerebral hemorrhage may be totally asymptomatic [20, 21] in the first few hours of life. The US examination should therefore be systematic.
4. Finally, the numerous sequelae (hydrocephalus, porencephalic cyst, ischemic lesions) require repeated US examinations to follow up the potential evolution of these cerebral hemorrhages.

4.1 Subependymal Hemorrhage

This is the most frequent type of hemorrhagic lesion (> 50% in the premature infant less than 32 weeks gestational age). It occurs essentially in premature infants and is rare in a term newborn (Table 1). Localized or diffuse, its image on US is always the same: a hyperechogenic image that bulges into the ventricular cavity, distinct from the choroid plexus (Fig. 7). Rounded on frontal sections and linear on longitudinal sections, it is almost always seen in the area of the caudate nucleus at the level of the germinal matrix and

Table 1. Incidence of hemorrhage in 384 high-risk premature infants.

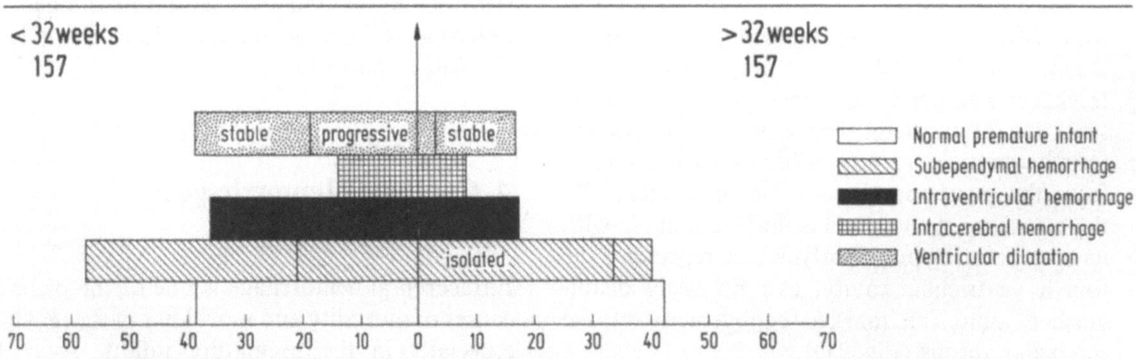

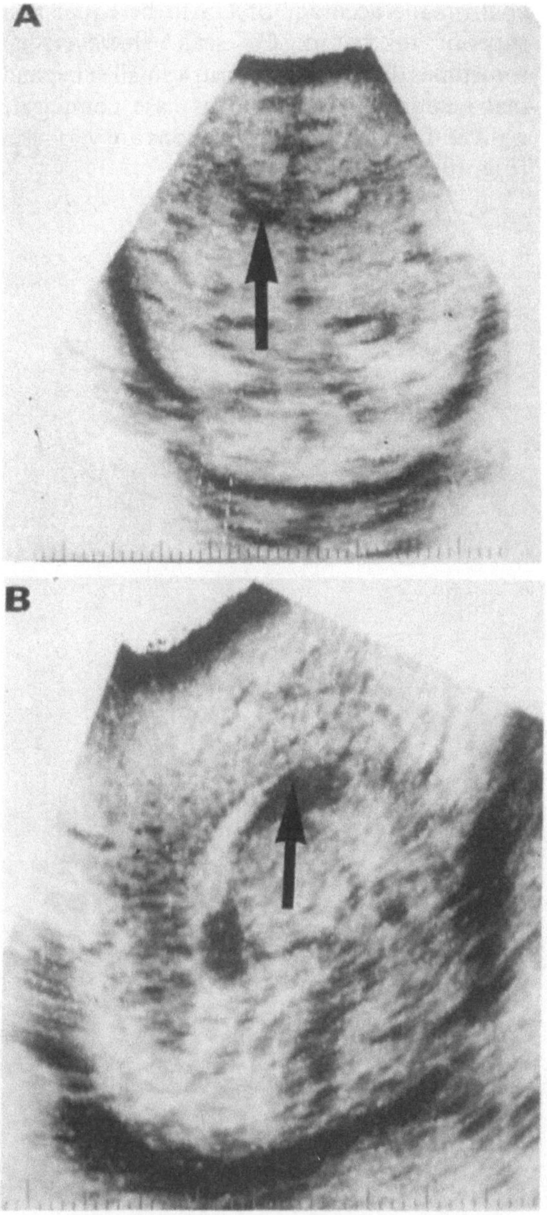

Fig. 7. A Coronal section and **(B)** right longitudinal paramedial section in a premature 6 days old infant with neurological distress. Unilateral right subependymal hemorrhage (*arrow*). The ventricular lumen is diminished and the hyperechogenic aspect is due to a recent hemorrhage.

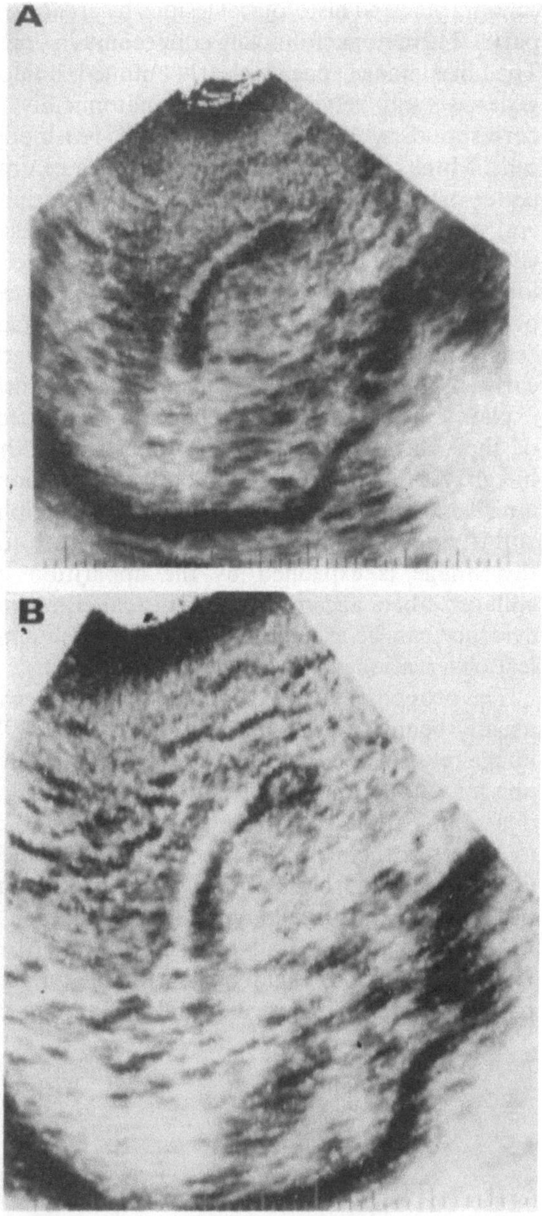

Fig. 8 A and B. Evolution on ultrasound of a subependymal hemorrhage in a premature 8 days old infant. **A** A hyperechogenic image bulging into the ventricular cavity at 8 days of age; **B** A typical target-like image at 30 days of age.

close to the foramen of Monro. The subependymal hemorrhage is sometimes unilateral, small and isolated, but may often be large, bilateral, and associated with an intraventricular hemorrhage especially in the premature infant less than 32 weeks gestational age.

On US examination its evolution is quite characteristic: the central necrosed area becomes progressively less echogenic surrounded by a hyperechogenic shell. The ultrasonic image disappears definitively in 1 or 2 months (Fig. 8). More rarely the evolution is towards the creation of a small porencephalic cavity which accurately delineates the site of original hemorrhage. The explanation of these evolutive images is clearly explained by Enzmann [22]. He achieved a correlation of echographic and histological lesions by creating a parietal hematoma following craniotomy in dogs. The initial image appears clearly outlined, homogeneous, and very echogenic. Anatomically it corresponds with aggregates of intact red blood cells. Three or four days later one notes a central region surrounded by a hyperechogenic peripheral wall. These modifications on US correlate with the loss of red blood cell integrity. These cells loose their biconcave form, lyze, and the liberated plasma progressively infiltrates between intact cells. These anatomical modifications take place early in the center of the hemorrhage which explains the progressively hypoechogenic aspect of the central region. On the other hand, the integrity of peripheral red blood cells is more durable, thus explaining the existence of a peripheral hyperechogenic wall. The persistence of this image is explained by the apparition of collagen fibers and reticulum. This experimental evidence can be exactly superimposed with clinical observations made in the human (Fig. 9).

The prognosis of subependymal hemorrhage is usually benign. In the majority of cases, the US image returns to normal. However, in some cases one may note a moderate but stable ventricular dilatation. In this case one may be dealing with a minimal intraventricular hemorrhage which passed unnoticed, but this image justifies systematic follow-up of subependymal hemorrhages.

Diagnosis of subependymal hemorrhage from US examination is usually easy. In this type of pathology, recent American publications [23, 24] confirm the accuracy of US to be equal if not superior to that of CT scan. However, it is sometimes difficult to confirm a small subependymal hemorrhage and in this case comparative right and left longitudinal sections are very useful (Fig. 10).

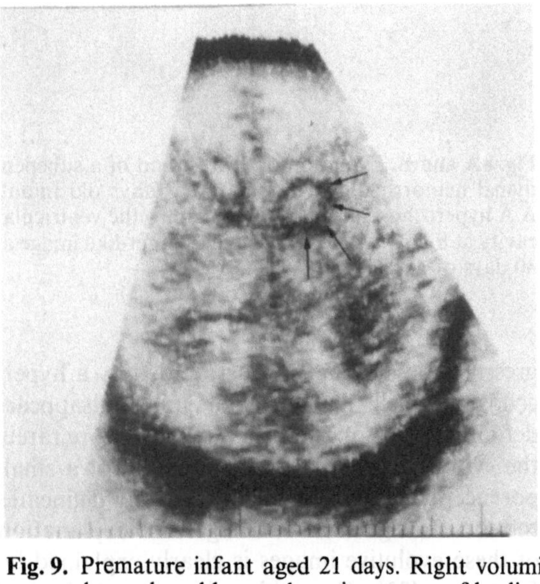

Fig. 9. Premature infant aged 21 days. Right voluminous subependymal hemorrhage in process of healing.

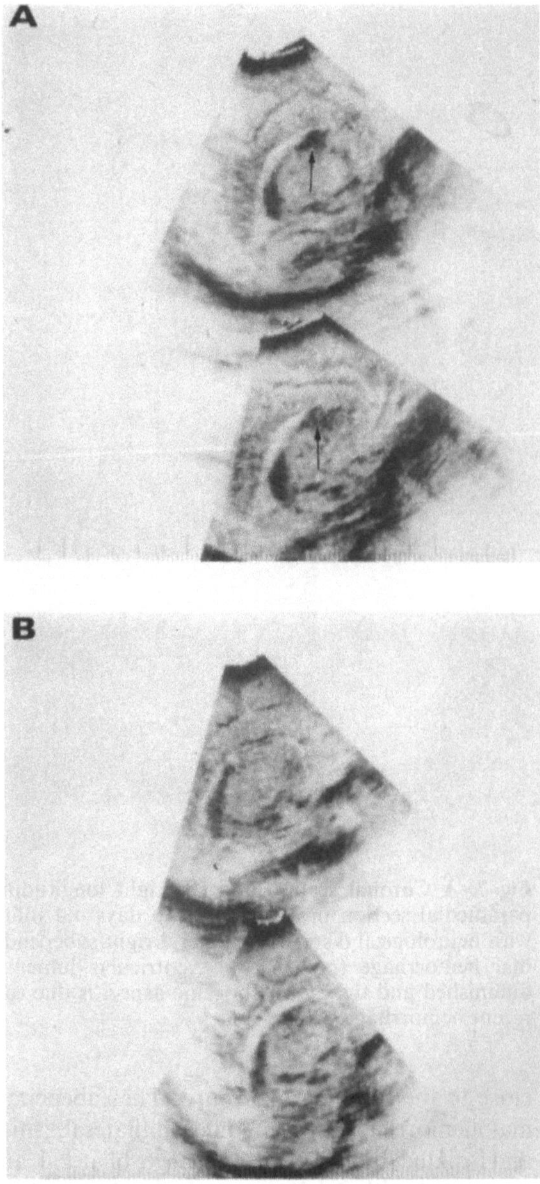

Fig. 10 A and B. Use of longitudinal comparative sections. **A** Paramedial section of the left ventricle shows moderate subependymal hemorrhage. **B** In the paramedial section of the right ventricle, the germinal zone is normal (arrow).

4.2 Intraventricular Hemorrhage [25, 26]

This is a serious lesion and its early diagnosis is fundamental to prevent the evolution toward cerebral atrophy or hydrocephalus. The intraventricular hemorrhage is seen on US as dense irregular echoes within the echo-free lumen of the lateral ventricles. The diagnostic difficulties are variable:

1. If the newborn is examined early and if the hemorrhage is moderate, the diagnosis is difficult: during an initial examination it is in factdifficult to ascertain the presence of fine echoes in nondilated ventricles whose lumen may be virtual for physiological reasons especially in the premature infant (Fig. 11). This means that the following indirect signs become very important: poor visibility of the ventricular cavities, the presence of echoes within normal cavities (cavum vergae and cavum of the septum lucidum), presence of subependymal hemorrhage, disappearance of choroid plexus oscillations [27] which can only be confirmed by real-time ultrasonography. In the majority of cases, follow-up shows the appearance of biventricular dilatation which is stable and evokes a secondary cerebral atrophy.
2. If the child is examined a little later and if the hemorrhage is massive, ventricular dilatation is nearly always present and the diagnosis is obvious (Figs. 12 and 13). In fact, the formation of a durable clot is rapid and can be seen as an irregular, voluminous, echogenic mass resting on the floor of the dilated ventricles. This clot then dissolves slowly (1–2 months), the echoes incline (Fig. 14) and cover the ventricular walls in the form of linear hyperechogenic images. Posthemorrhagic hydrocephalus occurs as a rule.

The follow-up of intraventricular hemorrhages is indispensable and allows one to judge:

1. The type of hydrocephalus by study of the volume of the third and fourth ventricles as well as that of the large basal cistern in order to differentiate between a noncommunicating and a communicating hydrocephalus. This allows a surgical or medical procedure to be carried out under the best conditions possible depending on the level of blockage (Fig. 15), i.e., repeated lumbar punctures in the case of communicating hydrocephalus or insertion of a ventricular reservoir in the case of noncommunicating hydrocephalus.
2. The prognosis for cerebral tissue integrity following ventricular shunt. In general the subtentorial cavities (third and fourth ventricles) rapidly return to normal but a durable dilatation of the lateral ventricles persists (Fig 16).
3. The exact estimation of cerebral atrophy sometimes being the only manifestation on US of a previous intraventricular hemorrhage that passed unnoticed. The measurement of the lateral ventricles acts as a precise criterion with respect to evolution but is often falsely reassuring as measurements are undertaken at levels (middle area of the ventricular body) where possibilities of expansion are most limited. This also applies to the third

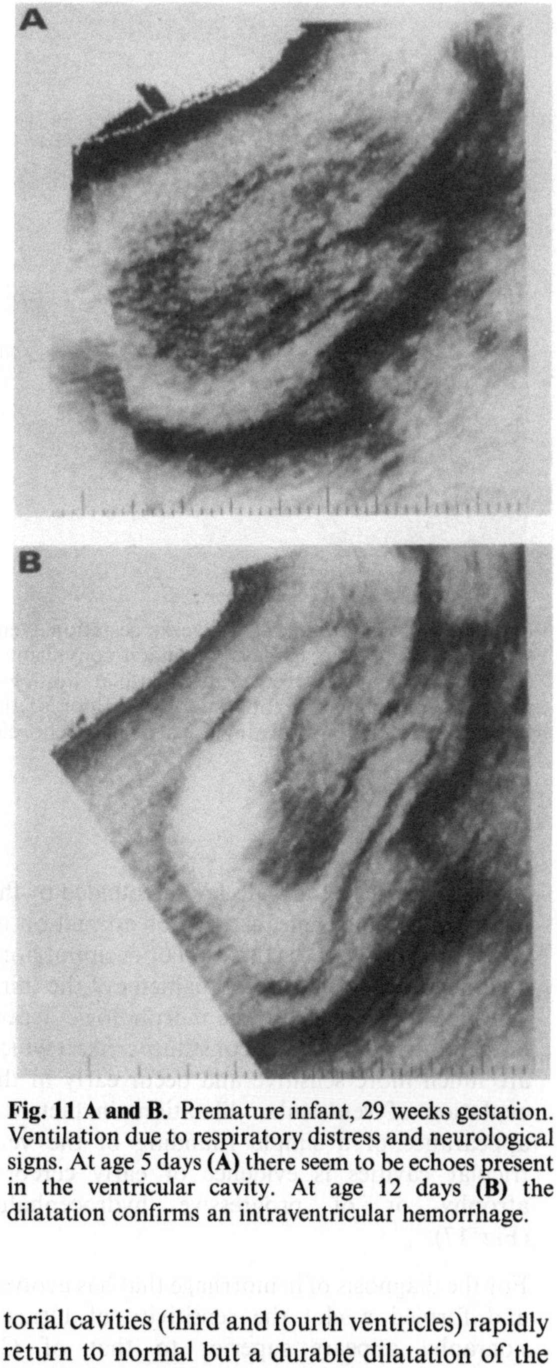

Fig. 11 A and B. Premature infant, 29 weeks gestation. Ventilation due to respiratory distress and neurological signs. At age 5 days **(A)** there seem to be echoes present in the ventricular cavity. At age 12 days **(B)** the dilatation confirms an intraventricular hemorrhage.

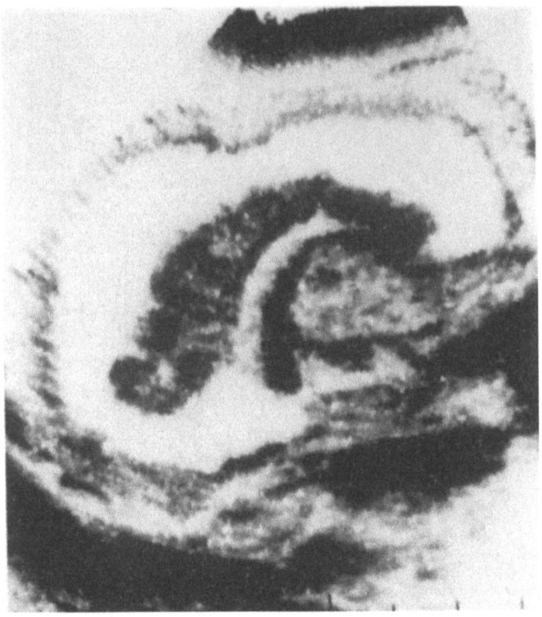

Fig. 12. A premature infant, 32 weeks gestation. Ventilated from age 1 to 12 days. Neonatal convulsions, severe hypotonia, and severe ventricular dilatation were present. A voluminous clot rests on the floor of the frontal horn and is easily distinguished from the choroid plexus.

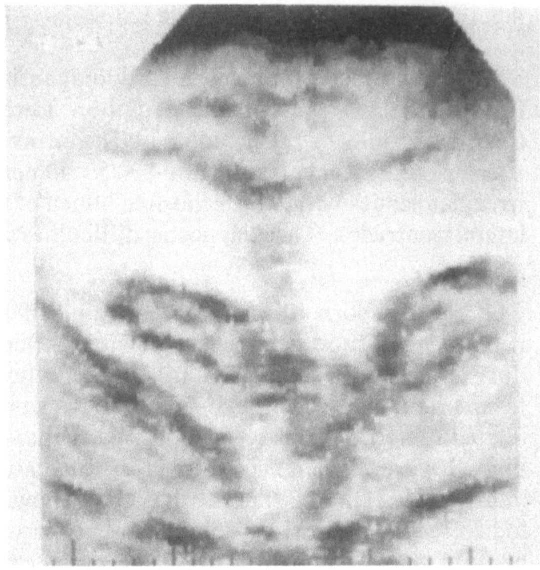

Fig. 13. The intraventricular hemorrhage may be massive, resulting in a ventricular "cast". Blood clots may occur within the ventricular bodies, the third ventricle, or the foramen of Monro.

ventricle whose lateral walls are surrounded by the basal ganglia. This means that for estimation of cerebral atrophy, the estimation of occipital horn volume, the anteroposterior diameter of the third ventricle, and especially the morphologic aspect of the ventricular cavities constitute criteria which are much more sensitive and occur early in the evolution of ventricular dilatation: in fact, the appearance of a simple rounding of the ventricular cavities is evidence of early cerebral atrophy or of progressive hydrocephalus (Fig. 17).

For the diagnosis of hemorrhage that has evolved and formed a clot the sensitivity of ultrasonography appears superior to that of CT scan. In fact, these two forms of imaging depend on totally different physical properties: the density of a clot as seen on CT scan depends above all on the concentration of hemoglobin, whereas ultrasonography depends on the notion of variable acoustic impedance depending on the velocity of US waves within the tissue being examined. The organization of a clot by reticuloendothelial cells and the progressive increase in liquid content of a hemorrhage diminishes the concentration of hemoglobin, thus explaining the fact that isodense clots are invisible on CT scan [24, 28]. On the other hand, it is known that blood causes a higher acoustic impedance

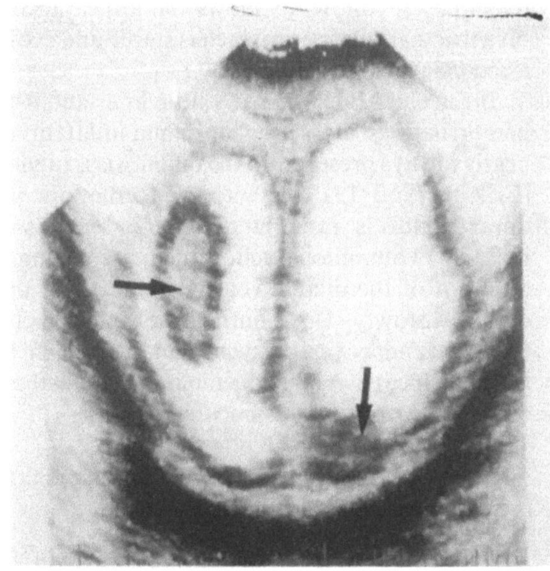

Fig. 14. Typical evolution of a hemorrhage with clot. Hydrocephalus appears early. The clot breaks up and dissolves progressively (arrow). In this way, it slopes and sinks, lining the walls of the occipital horns before disappearing (arrow).

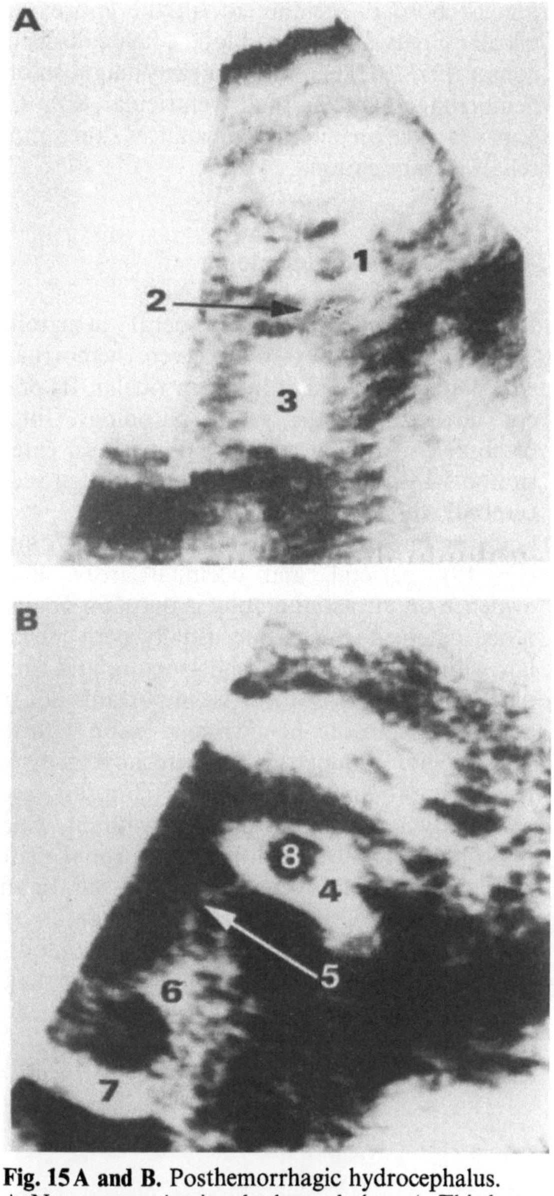

Fig. 15 A and B. Posthemorrhagic hydrocephalus. **A** Noncommunicating hydrocephalus. *1*, Third ventricle; *2*, Aqueduct of Sylvius; *3*, Fourth ventricle. **B** Communicating hydrocephalus. *4*, Third ventricle; *5*, Aqueduct of Sylvius; *6*, Fourth ventricle; *7*, Cisterna magna; *8*, Pars intermedia.

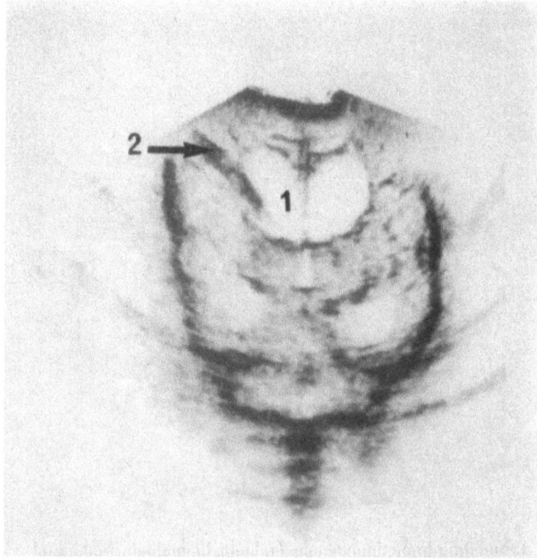

Fig. 16. Premature infant aged 30 days. A ventriculoperitoneal shunt performed at 15 days of age for tetraventricular hydrocephalus. The third and fourth ventricles are of normal size. The lateral ventricles remain significantly dilated *(1)*. Right-sided shunt *(2)*.

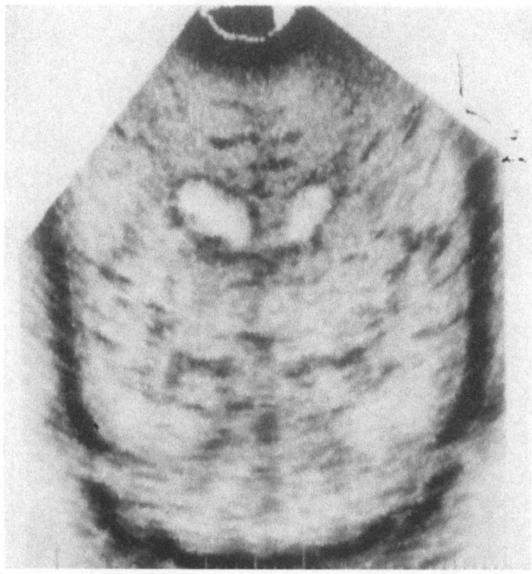

Fig. 17. Bilateral cerebral atrophy more marked on the right. The ventricular bodies present a typically rounded appearance.

than cerebral tissue or cerebrospinal fluid, which explains the creation of interfaces responsible for echogenic zones (Fig. 18).

The same physical properties seem to apply to the presence of fresh blood in the ventricles. However, identification of echoes within normal-sized ventricles remains very difficult to confirm even with highly selective apparatus. It is indispensable to carry out strict coronal sections and comparable sagittal sections: initial bilateral extensive bleeding is rare and the visualization of a localized or asymmetric hyperechogenicity is of prime importance. One must also repeat the examinations at short intervals to detect the appearance of initial clots which facilitates the

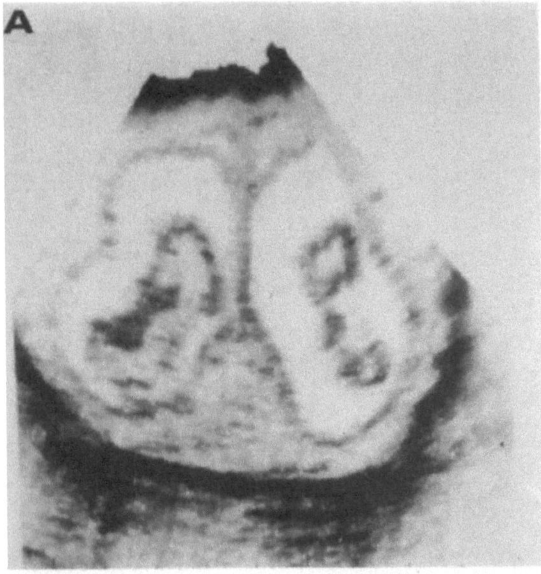

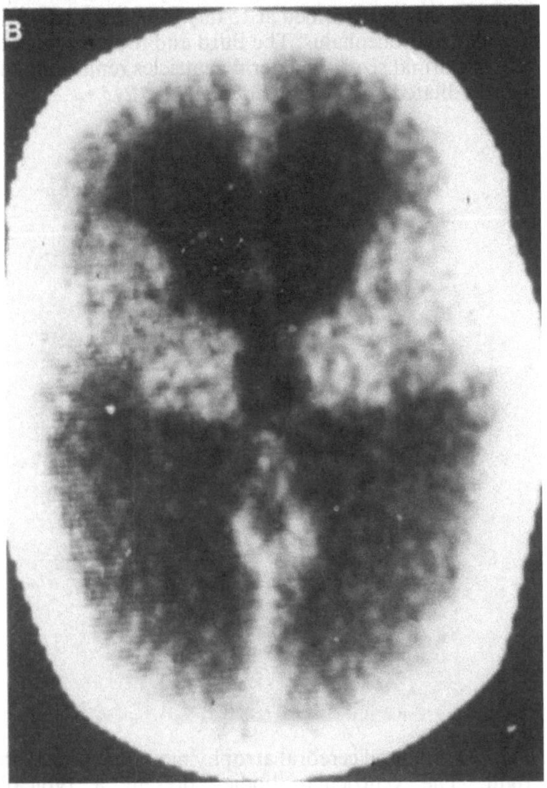

Fig. 18 A and B. A premature infant aged 10 days. Clotted hemorrhage on US **(A).** On CT scan 48 h later **(B),** the clots are invisible (courtesy of P. Castan).

diagnosis. Finally, it is certain that the differential diagnosis between intraventricular hemorrhage and a normal choroid plexus is difficult. One should be alerted by a large choroid plexus with regular borders seeming to fill the entire ventricular cavity as, in fact, blood often collects on contact [27, 30]. Therefore, for early diagnosis of a hemorrhage with normal ventricular size CT scan is in certain circumstances the most reliable examination.

4.3 Intracerebral Hematoma

Rarely isolated, an intracerebral hematoma occurs in the context of a severe hemorrhage either subependymal or intraventricular. Its presence always indicates severe pathology. Intracerebral hematoma corresponds with an extension of a subependymal hemorrhage into the cerebral white matter.

Its preferential localization is in the frontal (Fig. 19), parietal, and occipital areas. Early evidence on ultrasonography is that of a voluminous hyperechogenic zone usually periventricular, with heterogeneous echostructure and irregular borders [31–34]. It is important not to confuse this serious hemorrhagic lesion with the physiologic, symmetrical hyperechogenicity of the occipital and frontal lobes (Fig. 20), seen essentially in the healthy premature infant, which is probably related to different neuronal maturation with respect to neighboring tissue. In any case, repeated US examinations can define the diagnosis by showing echostructural modifications when one is dealing with a hemorrhagic

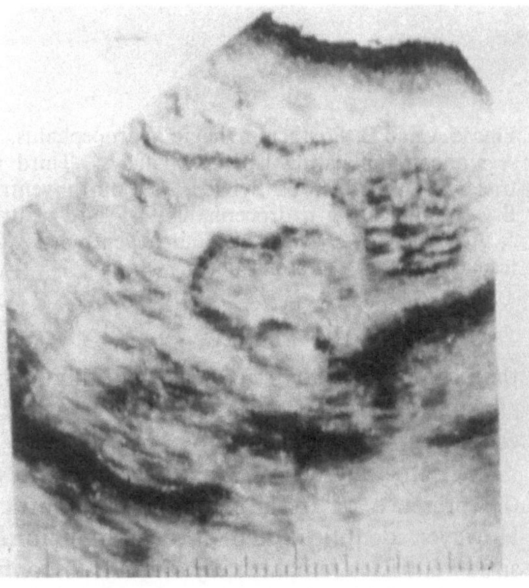

Fig. 19. Right frontal hematoma in the process of cavitation. Moderate dilatation of the lateral ventricle.

lesion. The sensitivity of CT scan in the detection of intracerebral hematomas is less precise. Flodmark [35] noted 6 false negative results in a group of 21 anatomically confirmed hematomas.

US follow-up is indispensable because destructive cavitating images develop rapidly between 7

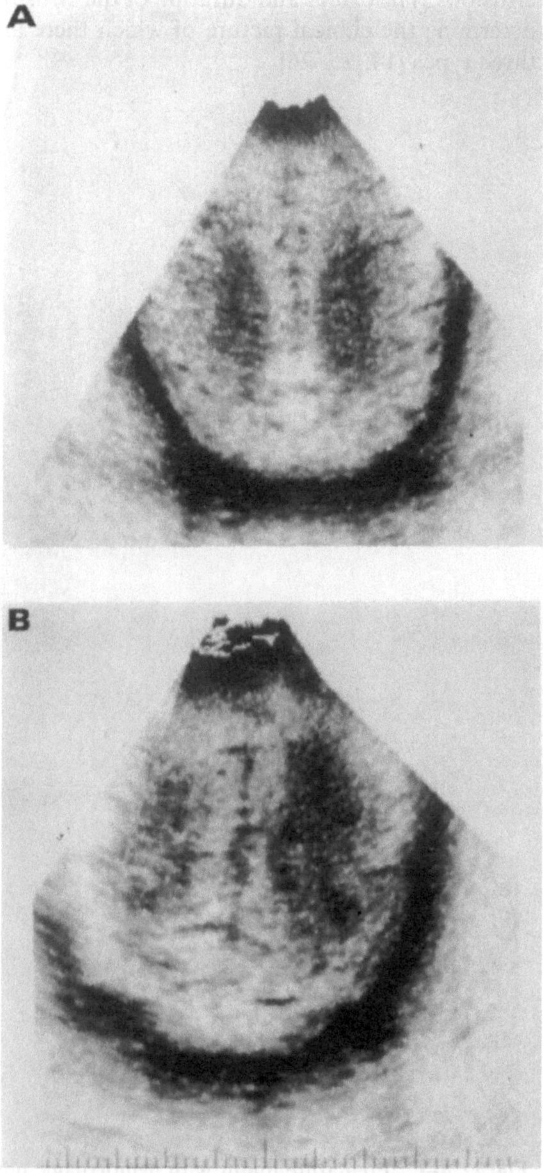

Fig. 20 A and B. Two premature infants with neurological signs.
A Physiological hyperechogenic occipital image at 9 days of age. This difficult diagnosis was made at age 15 days due to the static nature of these images.
B Left occipital hematoma. The diagnosis is made due to the asymmetrical echostructure of the occipital regions.

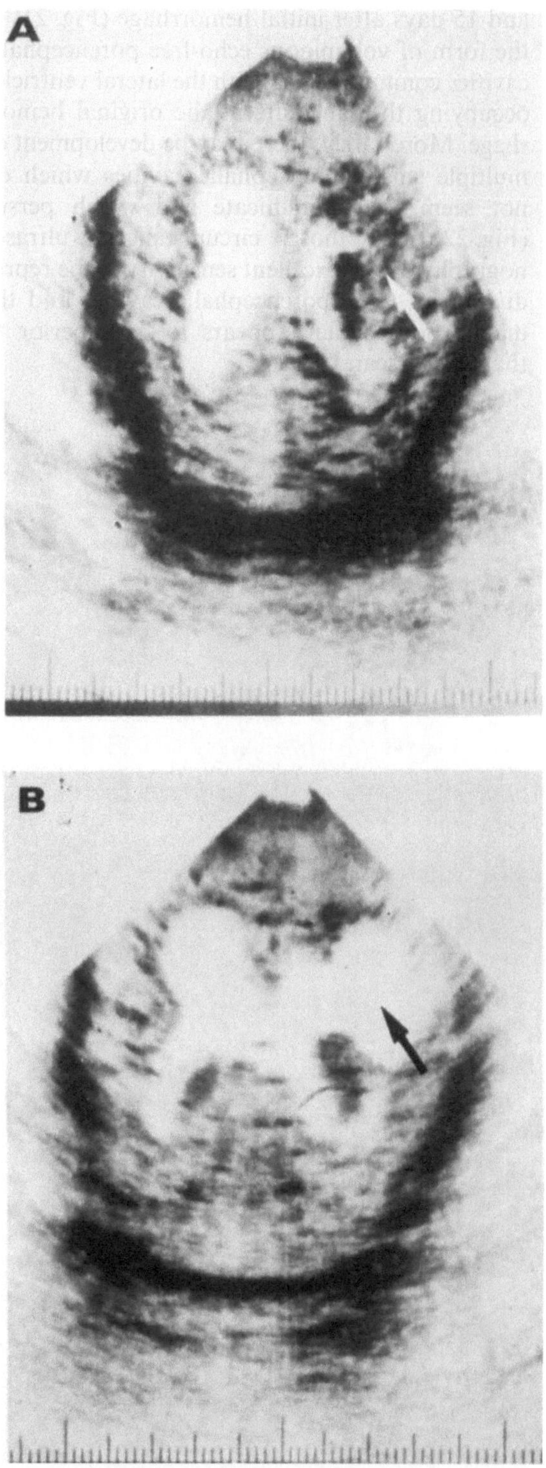

Fig. 21 A and B. Premature infant (36 weeks gestation) with neurological distress. Voluminous left heterogenous parieto-occipital collection of fluid **(A)**. Seven days later the porencephalic cavity communicates with the ventricle **(B)**.

and 15 days after initial hemorrhage (Fig. 21) in the form of voluminous echo-free porencephalic cavities communicating with the lateral ventricles occupying the same site as the original hemorrhage. More rarely, there may be development of multiple small porencephalic cavities which do not seem to communicate and which persist (Fig. 22). In those circumstances, ultrasonography has an excellent sensitivity in the reproduction of these porencephalic cavities and the diagnostic accuracy appears to be superior to that of CT scan [27, 36].

4.4 Subdural Hematoma

Subdural hematoma occupies a place among the etiologies of severe neonatal neurological distress in the newborn and in the infant which is not negligible [37, 38]. Diagnosis and treatment should be as early as possible as these lesions may become irreversible. Obstetrical or postnatal trauma dominate as etiological causes of subdural effusions. The extent and duration of the effusion determine the clinical picture of which there are three types [14, 25, 26]:

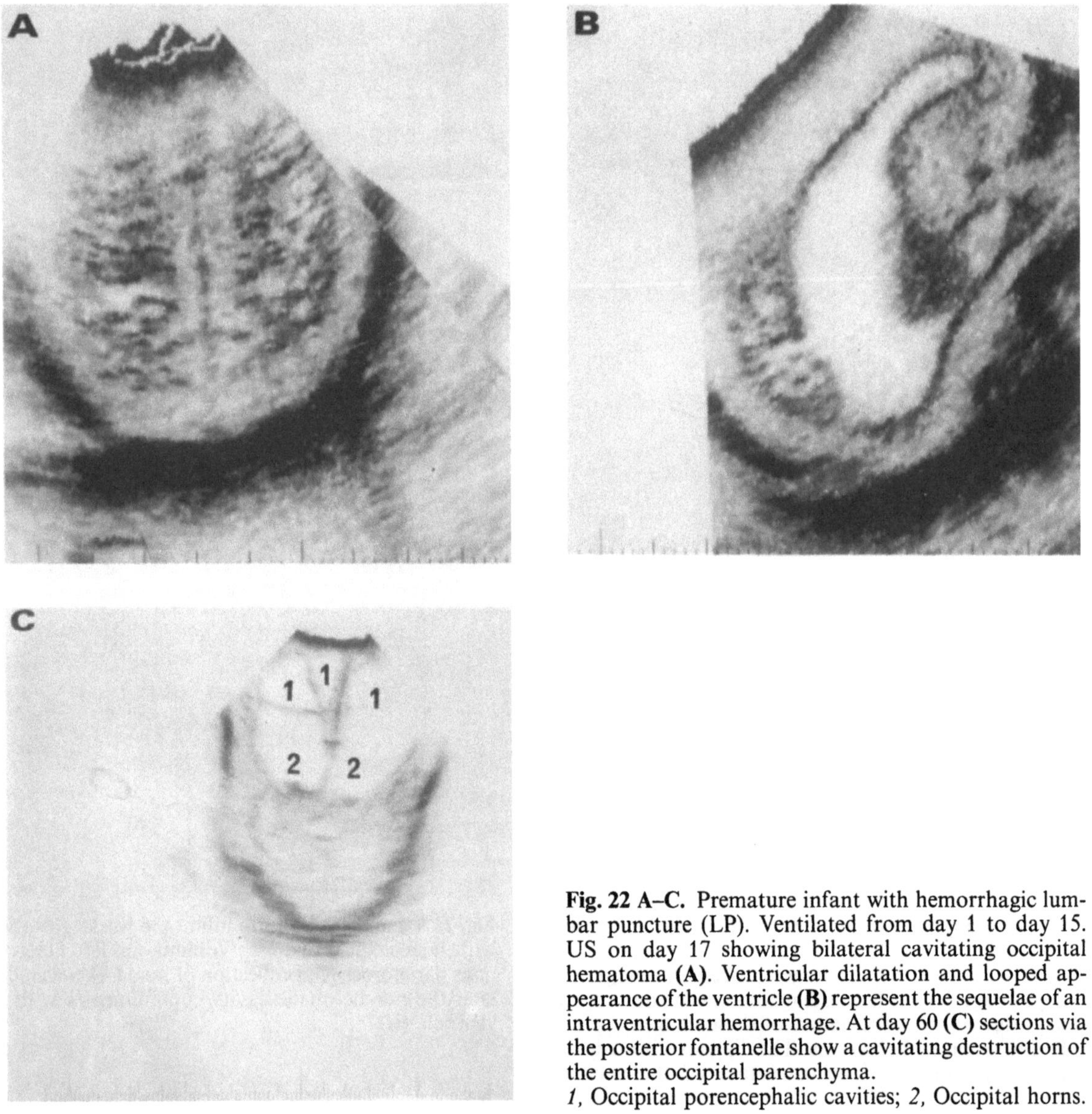

Fig. 22 A–C. Premature infant with hemorrhagic lumbar puncture (LP). Ventilated from day 1 to day 15. US on day 17 showing bilateral cavitating occipital hematoma **(A)**. Ventricular dilatation and looped appearance of the ventricle **(B)** represent the sequelae of an intraventricular hemorrhage. At day 60 **(C)** sections via the posterior fontanelle show a cavitating destruction of the entire occipital parenchyma.
1, Occipital porencephalic cavities; *2*, Occipital horns.

1. *Massive acute effusion.* This is rare and diagnosis is difficult. On US the echostructure of the effusion may be misleading as it is similar to that of the surrounding cerebral parenchyma. Indirect signs are therefore very valuable in aiding diagnosis: a space-occupying lesion in the pathological hemisphere resulting in deviation of the interhemispheric fissure toward the normal hemisphere and disappearance of the homolateral ventricular cavity. The contralateral ventricular cavity whose dynamics are disturbed is dilated (Fig. 23).

2. *Chronic voluminous effusion.* At a late stage with development of a hygroma, the diagnosis is obvious when confronted with a voluminous echo-free image which separates cerebral tissue from bone (Fig. 24).

3. *Moderate effusion.* Detection by ultrasonography depends on its localization and requires use of a high-frequency transducer (7 mHz) which is indispensable for exploration of superficial structures. The diagnosis is easy if the effusion is interhemispheric and bilateral, which is the most common presentation. This results in a double image with separation of the interhemispheric fissure in a V shape (Fig. 25): this sign on US is specific and very sensitive even in a small effusion. It must, however, be distinguished from the double image with edges parallel to the midline, which represents a cortical atrophy.

However, the diagnosis is much more difficult or even impossible when the collection of fluid is situated along the convexity. The range of inclination of the transducer does not permit visualization of this area.

One must also specify that ultrasonography and CT scan do not permit precision with respect to either the nature of the effusion (blood, hygroma, or empyema) or the exact localization (subarachnoid or subdural) [39].

In any case, echoencephalography seems to provide reliable elements for detection of voluminous as well as small effusions. US also allows follow-up of the evolution and progressive disappearance of the subdural collections of fluid. However, CT scan remains the examination of choice to define precisely the extent of a superficial collection of fluid.

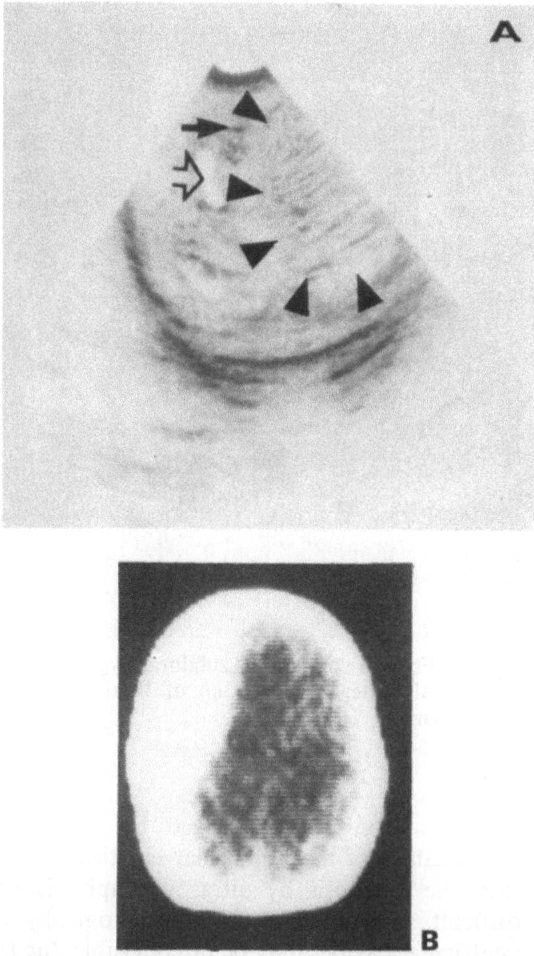

Fig. 23 A and B. Term newborn with focal neurological signs on the right. Right subdural hematoma. Voluminous mass effect with displacement of the interhemispheric sulcus, dilatation of the controlateral ventricle and disappearance of the homolateral ventricle **(A)**. At day 2, confirmation on CAT (Courtesy of P.Castan) **(B)**. Death at day 3, and diagnosis confirmed by autopsy.

4.5 Indications and Limitations

The transfontanellar technique has a certain number of limitations.

1. It represents an examination in the context of an exploration localized in time. Closure of the anterior fontanelle does not usually permit a good quality examination of the ventricles and especially of the cerebral parenchyma after 1 year of age.

2. The absence of image specificity is the second drawback [40]. Although it is clear that very hyperechogenic zones are without doubt due to hemorrhagic lesions, as yet there is no well-defined echographic representation for certain lesions such as edema or ischemia. In fact, when one is dealing with cerebral edema, parenchymal echostructure is not modified and the diag-

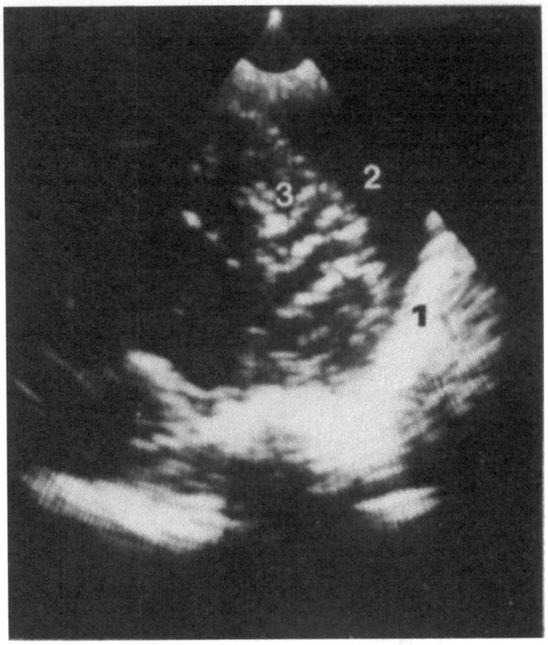

Fig. 24. Frontal voluminous subdural hygroma. *1*, Frontal bone; *2*, Collection of fluid; *3*, Frontal parenchyma.

nosis may only be envisaged by absence of visualization of the ventricular cavities. To confirm the diagnosis by ultrasonography is very difficult as we know that physiologically the ventricular cavities may be rarely visible due to a probable cycle in secretion of cerebrospinal fluid. Ischemiclesions have no early pattern on US except if voluminous and extended infarction occurs (Figs. 26 and 27).

In fact, the initial examination is most often falsely reassuring and, in children who have suffered from-severe neurological distress, signs of periventricular leukomalacia can be seen in the form of porencephalic cavities at the level of the outer aspect of the ventricular body [41–43] (Fig. 28). In any case, early diagnosis of cerebral ischemia and periventricular leukomalacia is difficult because on CT scan these lesions are manifested by isodense images which, as we know, may be physiological in the premature infant [35].

3. As already mentioned, to confirm the diagnosis of intraventricular hemorrhage in normal-sized ventricles at an early stage is also difficult despite encouraging studies by Bejar [27]. In addition, subarachnoid hemorrhage often passes unnoticed and the approach to the posterior fossa is difficult.

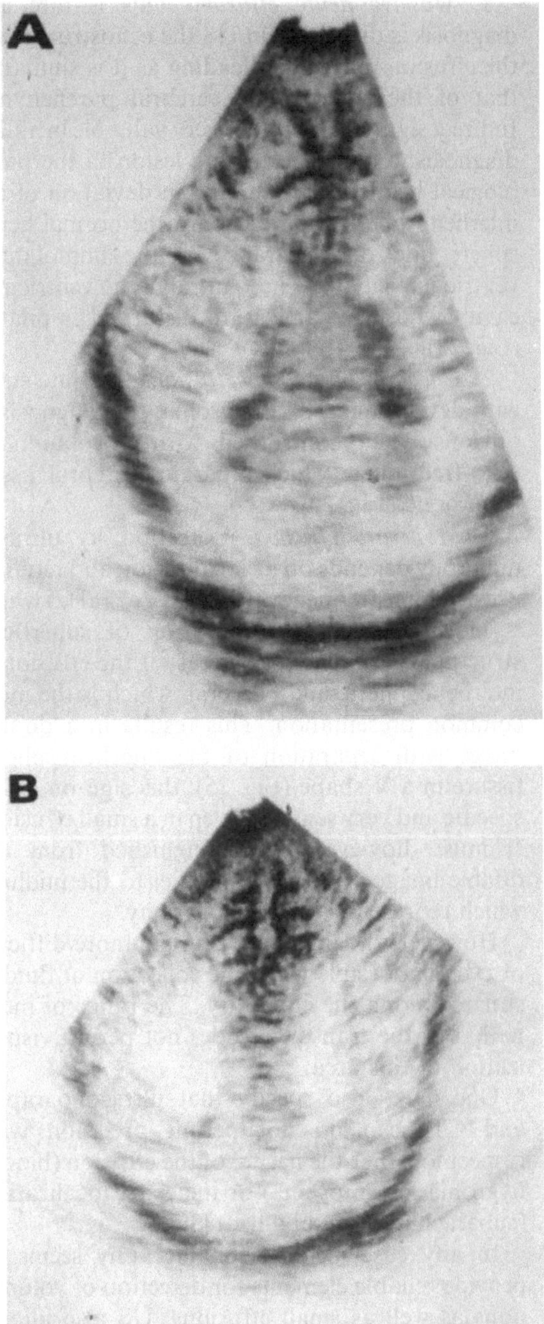

Fig. 25. A Premature infant with purulent meningitis. Subdural effusion with V-like separation of the interhemispheric sulcus. **B** Doubled parallel appearance of the sulcus indicates cerebral atrophy.

However, despite these limitations, the future for cerebral ultrasonography in diagnosis of hemorrhage is easily forseeable. Today US examination, which is absolutely inocuous, renders con-

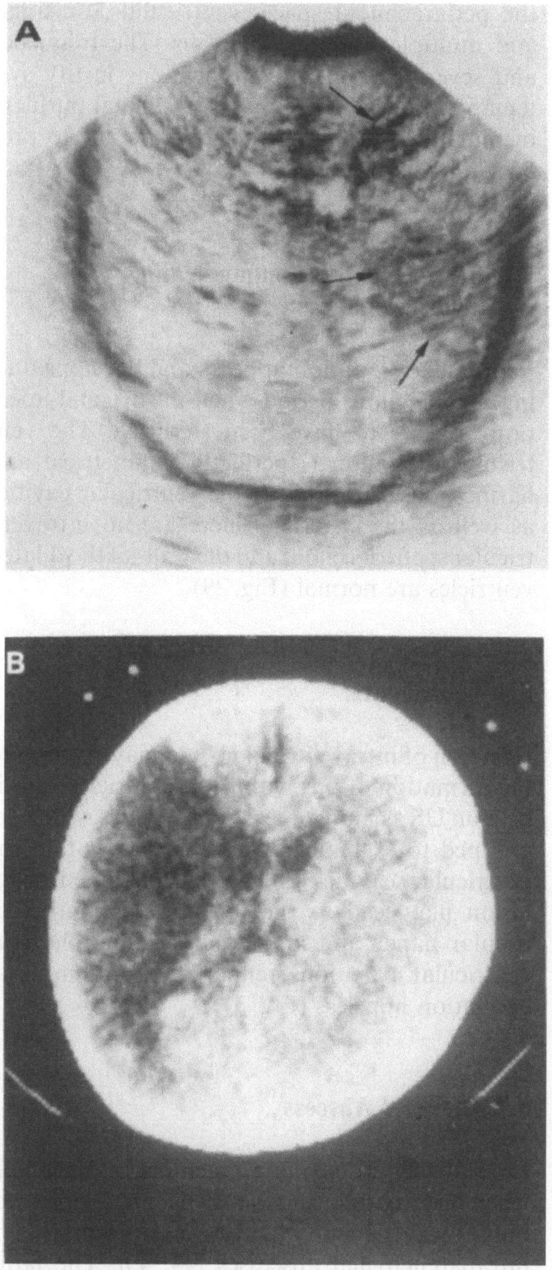

Fig. 26 A and B. Infant aged 3 months with localized neurological signs. **A** US examination shows a vast zone of heterogeneous echostructure (*arrow*); **B** CT scan visualizes an area of decreased density. The final diagnosis ist that of extensive carotid thrombosis.

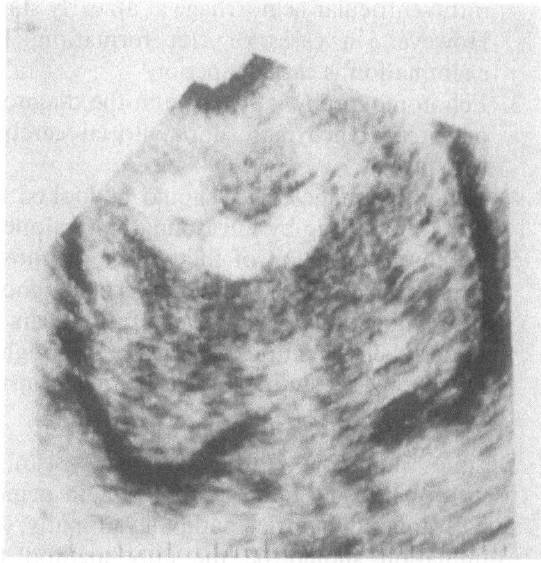

Fig. 27. Stillborn. Severe neurological signs. Heterogeneous aspect of the entire cerebral parenchyma due to areas of ischemia and diffuse hemorrhage.

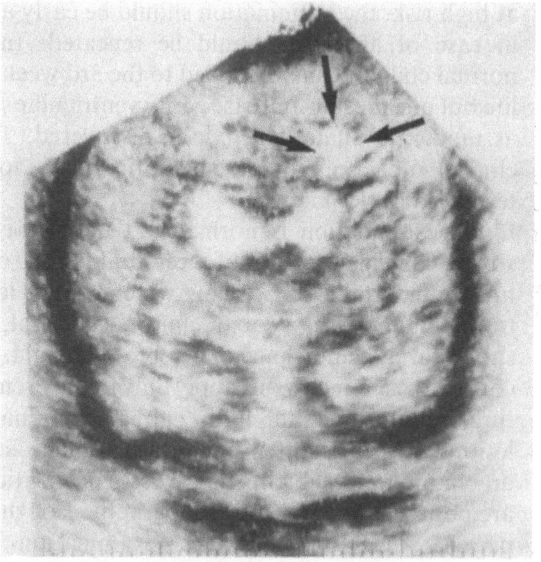

Fig. 28. Severe neonatal hypoxic ischemia. Apgar score of 2. Meconium in the amniotic fluid. US at day 5 normal. At day 30, moderate ventricular dilatation and evidence of porencephalic cavities at the external edge of the left ventricle.

siderable service with ease of utilization which CT scan cannot equal. There are numerous important conclusions with regard to the sensitivity of echoencephalography versus CT scan in the diagnosis of different hemorrhagic lesions:

1. Subependymal hemorrhage is well identified by ultrasonography. CT scan presents no advantages over US in this domain.
2. Compared with mode B ultrasound, CT scan is more beneficial in the diagnosis of

intraventricular hemorrhage at an early stage. However, in cases of clot formation, US examination is easily superior.

3. Echotomography is sensitive in the diagnosis of intraparenchymal supratentorial cerebral hematoma.
4. A porencephalic cavity should be looked for and followed up by ultrasonography alone.
5. Subdural collection of fluid poses diagnostic problems with both techniques. The diagnosis of a moderate or massive effusion can be undertaken by ultrasonography, although a more precise study should be made using CT scan.

Despite numerous difficulties, CT scan is useful for the detection of subarachnoid hemorrhages and subtentorial pathology. Finally, US examination should be the only method for detection and follow-up of ventricular dilatation.

In conclusion, systematic examination of premature infants using ultrasonography as the method of choice should be undertaken. In a child at high risk, the examination should be early and in case of anomaly should be repeated. In a normal child, it can be delayed to the 3rd week of life but one must in any case verify ventricular size as moderate dilatation may be discovered. The clinical impact of moderate dilatation in the long terms is not yet known.

If the examination is normal and if there is a strong clinical suspicion of a cerebral lesion, one must undertake CT scan which may lead to the diagnosis of a subarachnoid, subdural, or subtentorial hemorrhage or cerebral ischemia. Of course, these conclusions apply only to the premature infant. In a full term baby, hemorrhagic lesions are more often subdural, primary subarachnoid, and subtentorial. These localizations are poorly studied by ultrasonography. For these patients, CT scan is the examination of choice. Future progress in US technique and development of portable real-time apparatus will ensure new modifications in the strategy of neonatal diagnosis.

5 Cerebral Infectious Pathology

Neonatal infectious pathology often leads to meningeal infection, which may lead to serious complications: hydrocephalus due to occlusion of the periarachnoid space, ventriculitis, or single and multiple cerebral abscesses. The frequence and severity of these complications justify systematic follow-up by US of all neonatal purulent meningitides and in particular those due to proteus [44, 45].

5.1 Postmeningitis Communicating Hydrocephalus

Ventricular dilatation appears and develops during the infectious period when the original infection appears to have been sterilized. The ventricular dilatation is perfectly symmetrical and harmonious, affecting all the ventricular cavities as well as the cisterna. There are no intraventricular septa or echoes and the walls of the dilated ventricles are normal (Fig. 29).

5.2 Ventriculitis

Infection of intraventricular fluid may give rise to the formation of pus within the ventricles: this is seen on US as more or less dense echoes which are grouped to a greater or lesser extent within the ventricular cavities (Fig. 30). Subsequent evolution may lead to the formation of intraventricular bands and may result in multiple, true ventricular partitions rendering all attempts at derivation hopeless (Fig. 31).

5.3 Cerebral Abscess

Enterobacterial neonatal meningitis, especially when due to proteus or klebsiella, predisposes not only to ventriculitis but also to the formation of intraparenchymal abscesses [44, 45]. The latter may be discovered as an isolated event presenting as a focal space-occupying lesion which on US is seen as a shift of interhemispheric structures.

The two factors responsible for the masslike effect are the abscess itself and the edema which generally surrounds it. Cerebral edema is not visible on US, whereas CT scan delineates well the perilesional hypodensity which indicates the presence of edema (Fig. 32). However, the image of the abscess itself can be perfectly analyzed by US: the more or less thick shell is clearly more echogenic than the center, which represents the pouch of pus and is practically echo-free.

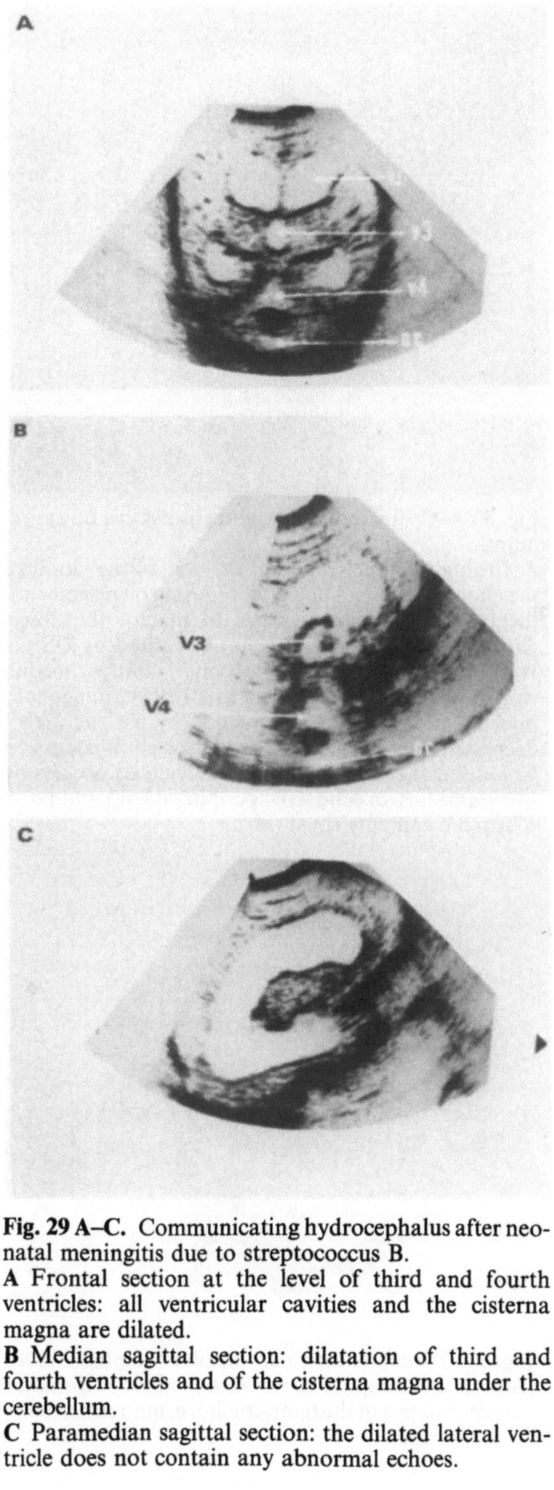

Fig. 29 A–C. Communicating hydrocephalus after neonatal meningitis due to streptococcus B.
A Frontal section at the level of third and fourth ventricles: all ventricular cavities and the cisterna magna are dilated.
B Median sagittal section: dilatation of third and fourth ventricles and of the cisterna magna under the cerebellum.
C Paramedian sagittal section: the dilated lateral ventricle does not contain any abnormal echoes.

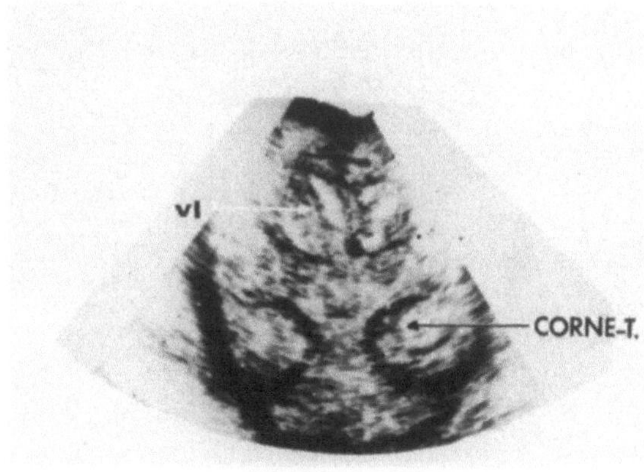

Fig. 30. Ventriculitis seen on a frontal section. Presence of echogenic agglomerates representing pus in the dilated ventricular cavities. *vl,* Frontal horn; *CORNE-T,* temporal horn.

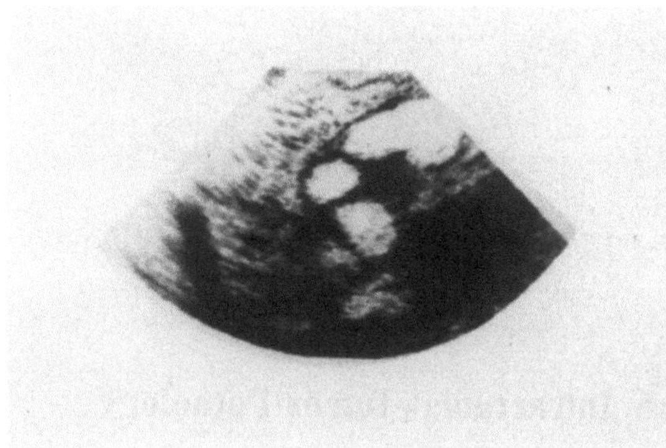

Fig. 31. Ventriculitis (sequelae) on a paramedian sagittal section. The lateral ventricle is multiloculated.

These images, as the lesion evolves, have been well described by Enzmann using experiments on dogs [47].

In the newborn, and particularly if the infection is due to proteus, there may be multiple abscesses sometimes associated with an intraventricular suppuration in the case of pyocephalus (Fig. 33).

Systematic US follow-up of these neonatal infections should permit, in the future, early detection of these infectious foci. CT scan has already enabled great progress to be made in the diagnosis of cerebral abscess when there is clinical suspicion. Now systematic US examinations permit early intervention even before the appearance of clinical signs which often signal the presence of lesions that are already severe.

It is now possible to institute a simple and precise surveillance of antibiotic therapy and, if necessary, to guide needle puncture with drainage and in situ antibiotic administration.

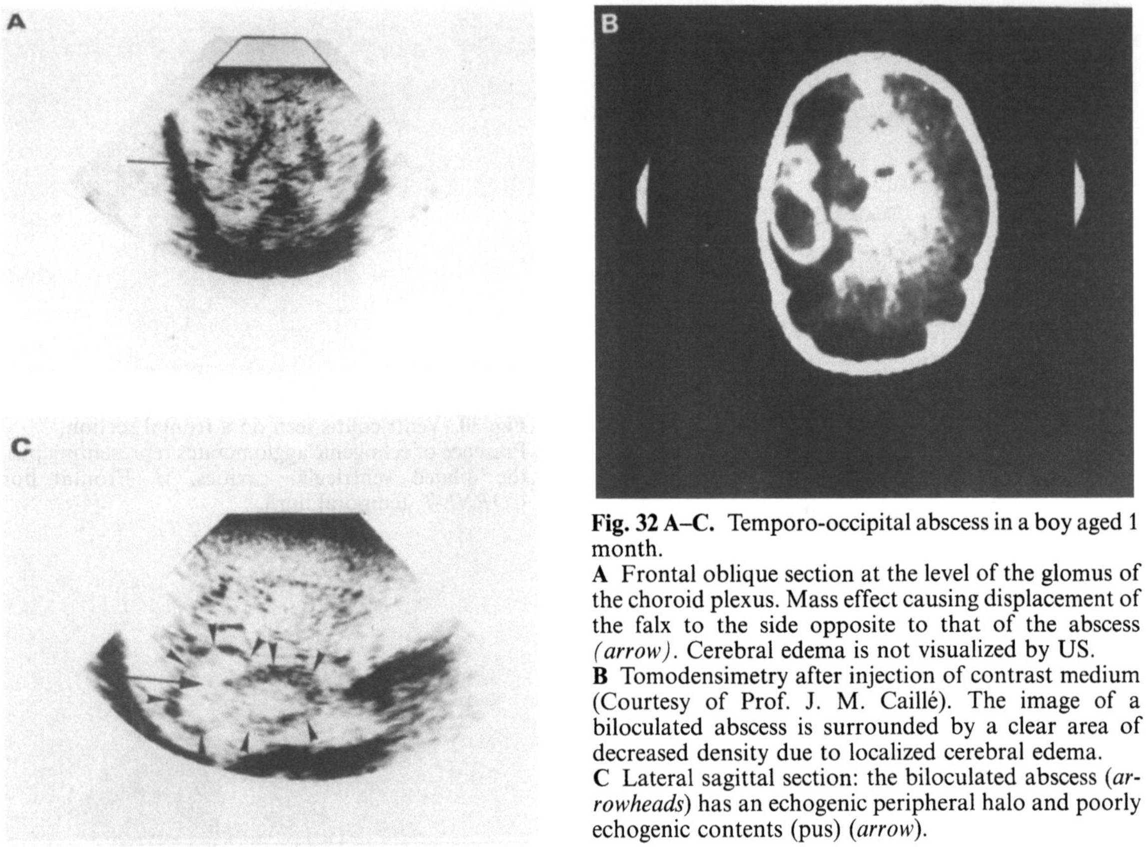

Fig. 32 A–C. Temporo-occipital abscess in a boy aged 1 month.
A Frontal oblique section at the level of the glomus of the choroid plexus. Mass effect causing displacement of the falx to the side opposite to that of the abscess *(arrow)*. Cerebral edema is not visualized by US.
B Tomodensimetry after injection of contrast medium (Courtesy of Prof. J. M. Caillé). The image of a biloculated abscess is surrounded by a clear area of decreased density due to localized cerebral edema.
C Lateral sagittal section: the biloculated abscess (*arrowheads*) has an echogenic peripheral halo and poorly echogenic contents (pus) (*arrow*).

6 Intracranial Tumor Pathology

Cerebral tumor are very rare during the period of life when the anterior fontanelle is open [48]. They represent less than 0.5% in our series of 1200 transfontanellar echographic examinations. The reliability of the examination depends on the size of the anterior fontanelle and we consider a size less than 1 cm^2 insufficient for an accurate study of the tumor. In clinical practice this criterion therefore applies to infants less than 18 months of age.

The information gained by ultrasonography is concerned with the structure, boundary, and dimensions of the tumor, the topography of the tumor, and a study of its effects on neighboring structures and the accompanying phenomena.

6.1 Structure, Boundary, and Dimensions

Solid tumors, such as astrocytoma or glioblastoma, are seen as layers of very dense echoes which are always much more brilliant and intense than those of the surrounding normal brain (Fig. 34). For this reason the contours can be easily seen and the measurement of tumoral dimensions is precise.

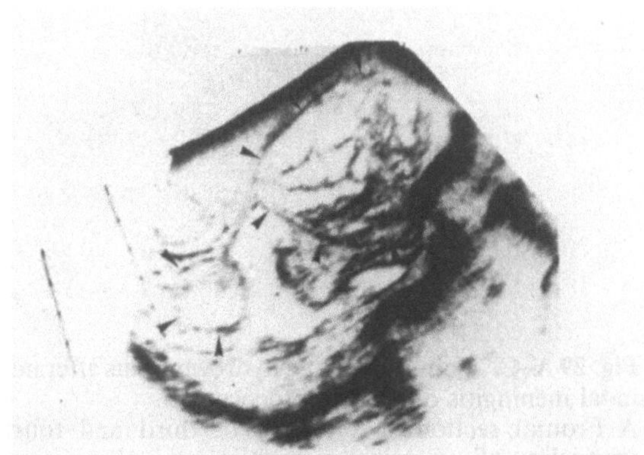

Fig. 33. Pyocephalus: paramedian sagittal section frontal and occipital (*arrowheads*) abscess formation. Presence of pus in the temporal horn, amputation of the frontal horn.

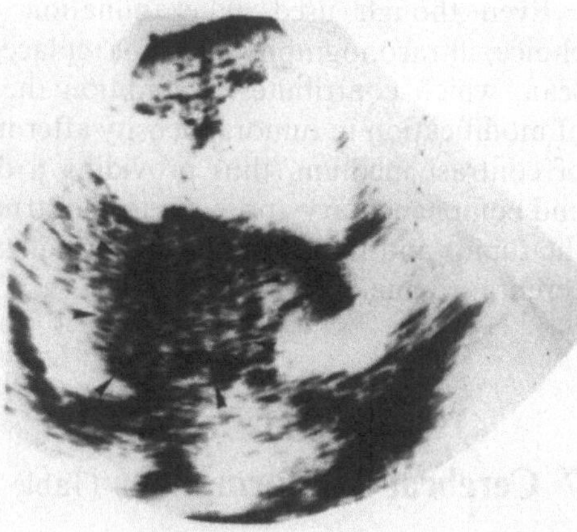

Fig. 34. Astrocytoma of the third ventricle in a girl aged 14 months.
Frontal section: the rounded tumor is composed of echoes that are more intense and compact than those of the surrounding parenchyma (*arrowheads*). Asymmetric dilatation of the lateral ventricles above the tumor.

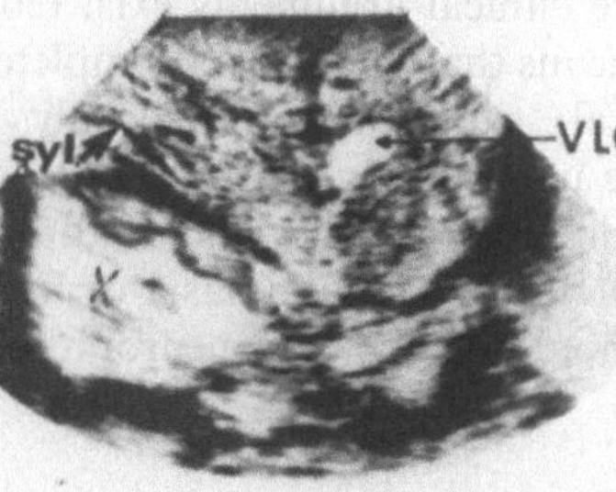

Fig. 35. Necrosed astrocytoma in a girl aged 17 days. Frontal section: voluminous encapsulated right temporal tumor. A large portion of this tumor is necrosed *(X)*. The fissure of Sylvius *(syl)* is deviated, the falx is displaced contralaterally, and the ipsilateral ventricle is not visible. *VLG;* Left lateral ventricle.

Zones of necrosis within the tumor result in echo-free layers (Fig. 35). The posterior reenforcement of these echoes is not more marked than that behind other liquid structures of the brain (ventricles).

The problem of hemorrhage within the tumor is more difficult as fresh blood is seen as a very echogenic layer not very different from the tumor itself, therefore rendering differentiation difficult (Fig. 36) [11]. However, the associated hemorrhage seems to have less well defined boundaries than the tumor itself.

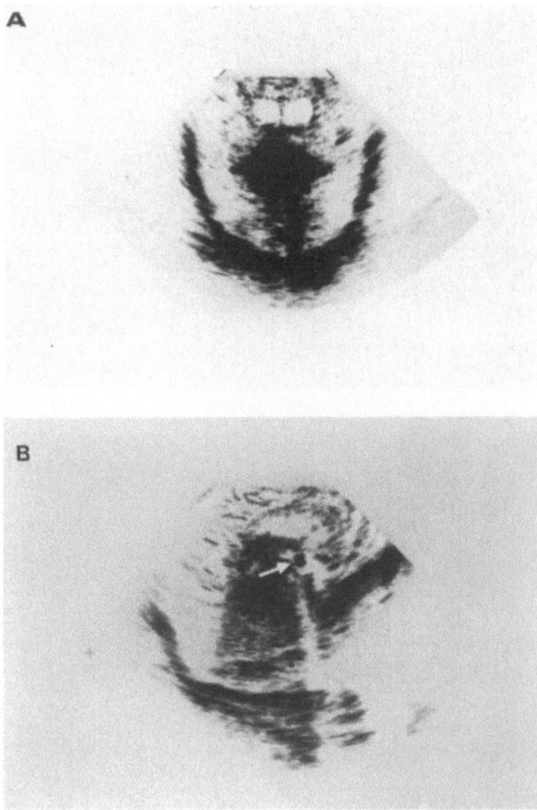

Fig. 36 A and B. Glioma infiltrating the brain stem with hemorrhage within the tumor in a 5-month-old girl. **A** Frontal section: a voluminous medial echogenic mass extends from the floor of the lateral ventricles to the posterior fossa. It is not possible to distinguish tumor tissue from blood. **B** Median sagittal section: the posterior region of the third ventricle is elevated and displaced anteriorly by the tumor arising from the posterior fossa and invading the anterior fossa.

6.2 Topography

When the tumor is small and the normal brain architecture is not too disrupted, it is usually easy to determine the point of origin of the tumor (Fig. 37). This may be much more difficult if the tumor is voluminous. Therefore, it is sometimes in possible to determine a localization that is more precise than simply regional (Fig. 34).

6.3 Impact of the Tumor and Accompanying Phenomena

The masslike effect is shown on US examination as reliably as on CT scan [11]. It is therefore easy to highlight (a) displacement of the

A

B

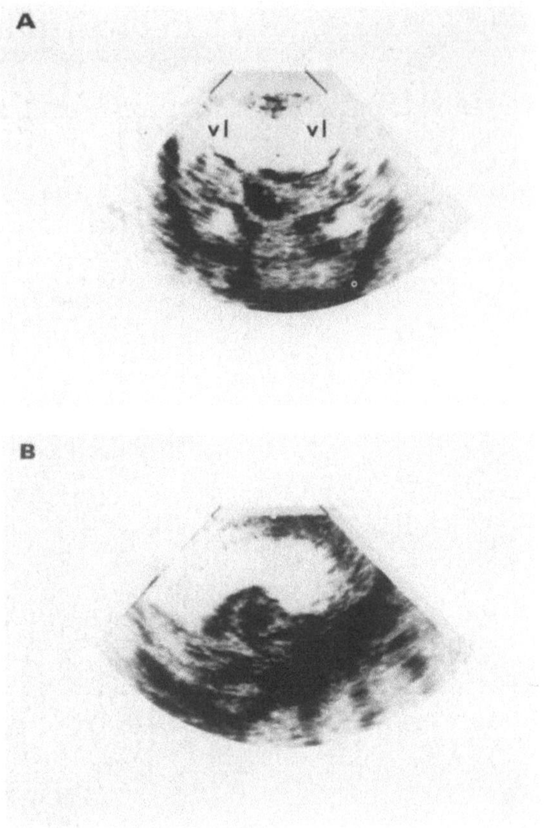

Fig. 37 A and B. Thalamic astrocytoma in a 7-month-old boy.
A Frontal section: a small right thalamic echogenic mass is seen causing lateral ventricular dilatation.
B Right paramedian sagittal section: tumor is entirely surrounded by thalamic tissue, limited posteriorly by the choroid plexus and superiorly by the floor of the lateral ventricle.

falx cerebri associated with the occlusion of a lateral ventricle in the case of a tumor located within a cerebral hemisphere (Fig. 35) and (b) a symmetrical supratentorial dilatation in the case of a posterior fossa tumor. On the other hand, it is much more difficult to confirm the presence of associated peritumoral edema which has little representation on US but which can be clearly seen on CT scan.

To conclude this section on cerebral tumors, transfontanellar echography may contribute very precise information. The ease with which the examination is carried out makes it the examination of choice in an infant with a patent fontanelle. Two reasons justify this attitude: an eventual decompression procedure would in this way be well guided and later follow-up rendered easier whatever the treatment undertaken.

Even though used as examination of first choice, ultrasonography does not replace the CT scan, which contributes in addition the notion of modification in tumoral density after injection of contrast medium, thus providing a different and complementary approach to the structure of the tumor and finally permitting visualization of cerebral edema.

7 Cerebral Malformations (Table 2)

7.1 Midline Facial Malformations

These malformations are very variable, some are obvious such as ethmocephalus, cebocephalus or midline slit with hypotelorism [49], others are more subtle. Even if the majority (especially severe morphological anomalies) evoke an underlying cerebral malformation, no specific and definitive clinical arguments exist [50]. In practice this means that one should complete a neuroradiological exploration (especially echography) before undertaking plastic surgery in these newborn infants. On the whole, all midline lesions (hypotelorism, nasal aplasia or hypoplasia, cleft lip) should be explored neuroradiologically.

7.2 Midline Cerebral Malformations

Us examination seems to be and should be sufficient to explore all midline cerebral malformations: cyclops, holoprosencephaly, agenesis of the septum pellucidum, total or partial agenesis of the corpus callosum.

Table 2. Cerebral malformations: 63 cases.

Myelomeningocele	22
Aqueduct of Sylvius – stenosis	10
Agenesis of the corpus callosum (3 partial)	9
Dandy-Walker deformity	6
Congenital toxoplasmosis	4
Aneurysm of the vein of Galen	3
Arachnoid cyst	3
Agenesis of the septum pellucidum	3
Lipoma of the corpus callosum	1
Congenital porencephaly	1
Tuberous sclerosis	1

A lobar or semilobar form of holoprosencephaly, which is a severe malformation usually incompatible with life, can be easily diagnosed from US examination [49]. In the lobar form there is a single ventricular cavity associated with a fusion of the gray nuclei and the thalami (Fig. 38). In its semilabor form one can see an attempt at ventricular division at the occipital horns. The diagnosis is very important as familial cases exist and genetic counseling may be required [51].

Early echographic exploration is necessary as cerebral modifications, especially progressive hydrocephalus which laminates the cerebral parenchyma, may render the diagnosis more difficult (Fig. 39).

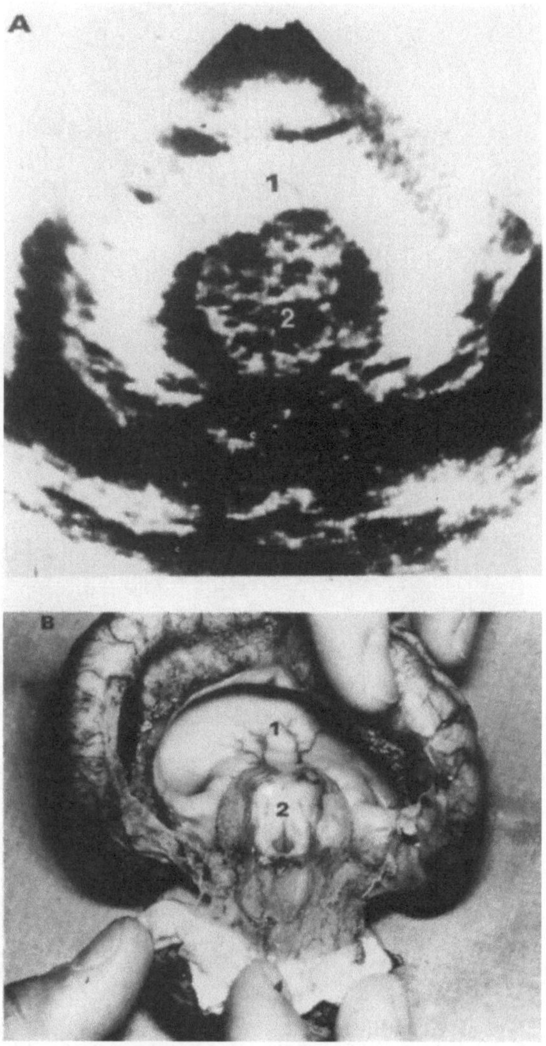

Fig. 38 A and B. Holoprosencephaly. Presence of a single dilated ventricular cavity *(1)*. Fusion of the basal nuclei *(2)* and absence of the interhemispheric sulcus *(3)*. Death at 2 days of age. Confirmation at autopsy.

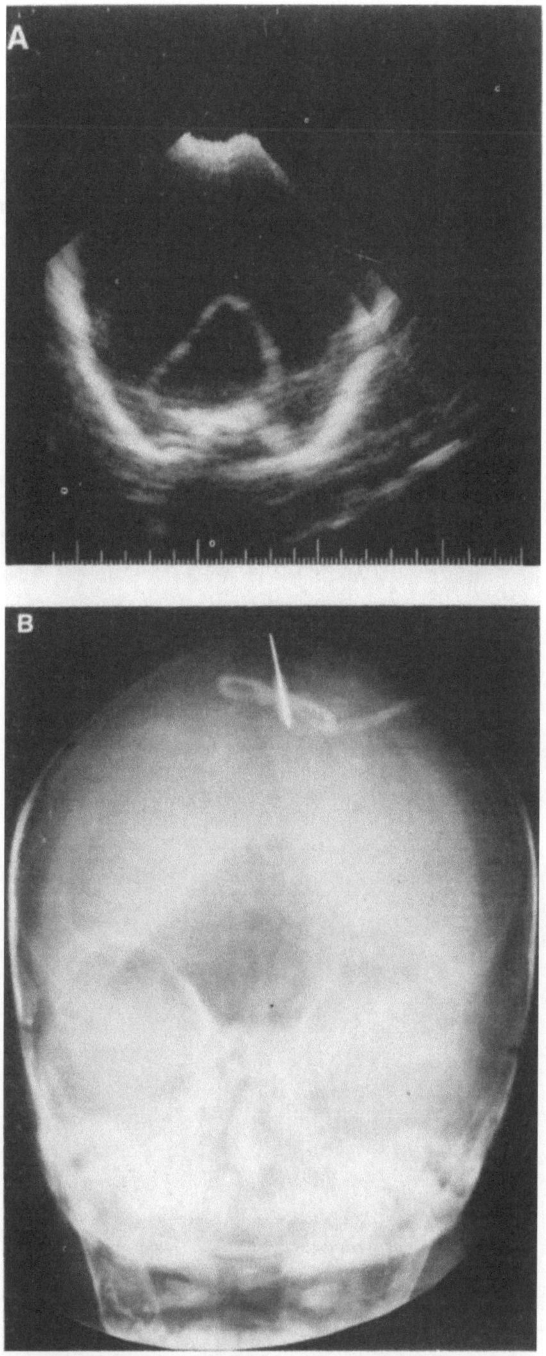

Fig. 39 A and B. Infant aged 14 months with macrocephaly, severe psychomotor delay, and problems with thermoregulation.
A US examination shows a totally liquid brain without evidence of cerebral parenchyma and the diagnosis of hydranencephaly is made.
B Air encephalography carried out at 5 months of age shows a single ventricular cavity. The final diagnosis is that of holoprosencephaly.

For the present ultrasonography may be considered the only exploration that should be carried out in the case of partial or total agenesis of the corpus callosum. In fact US delineates the classic neuroradiological signs which are as follows:

1. An abnormal gap between the frontal horns and lateral ventricles whose internal walls are inverted and concave superiorly and medially;

2. Besides the dilatation of the occipital horns and lateral ventricles one notes the ascending expansion of the third ventricle interposed between the lateral ventricles and reaching the interhemispheric fissure (Fig. 40).

These signs are responsible for the image of the "bull's head" [52, 53]. These images have also been widely confirmed on CT scan and encephalography [54, 55].

US also contributes two supplementary elements [52]. The first is the nonvisibility of the corpus callosum itself, which in the normal infant

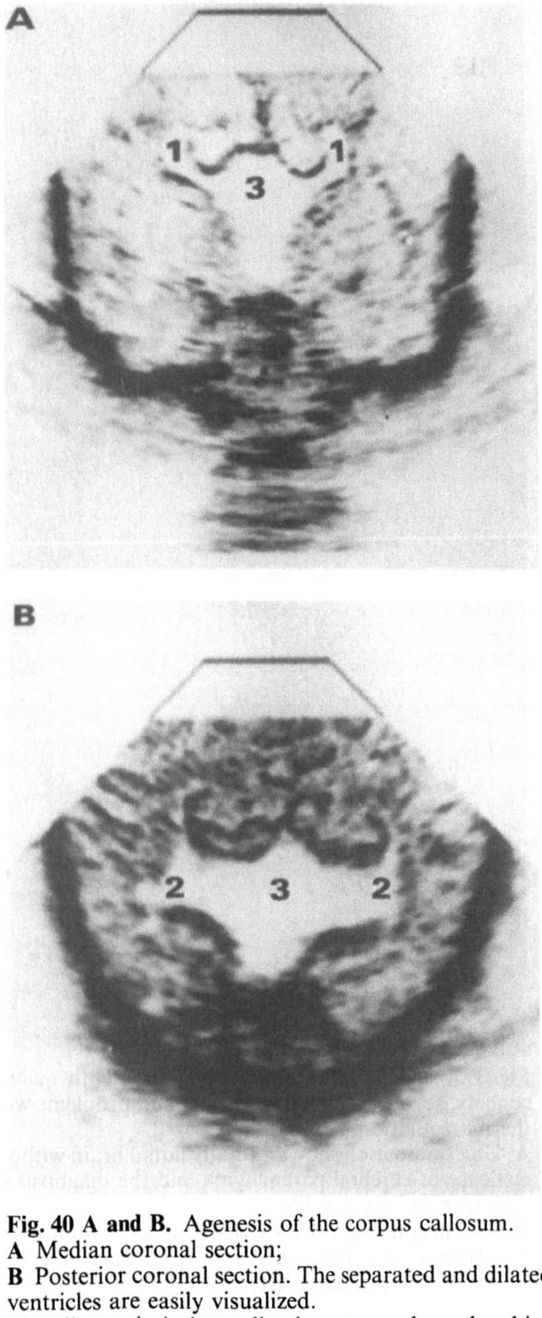

Fig. 40 A and B. Agenesis of the corpus callosum.
A Median coronal section;
B Posterior coronal section. The separated and dilated ventricles are easily visualized.
The diagnosis is immediately suspected as the third ventricle is high and dilated. *1*, Lateral ventricles; *2*, Occipital horns; *3*, Third ventricle.

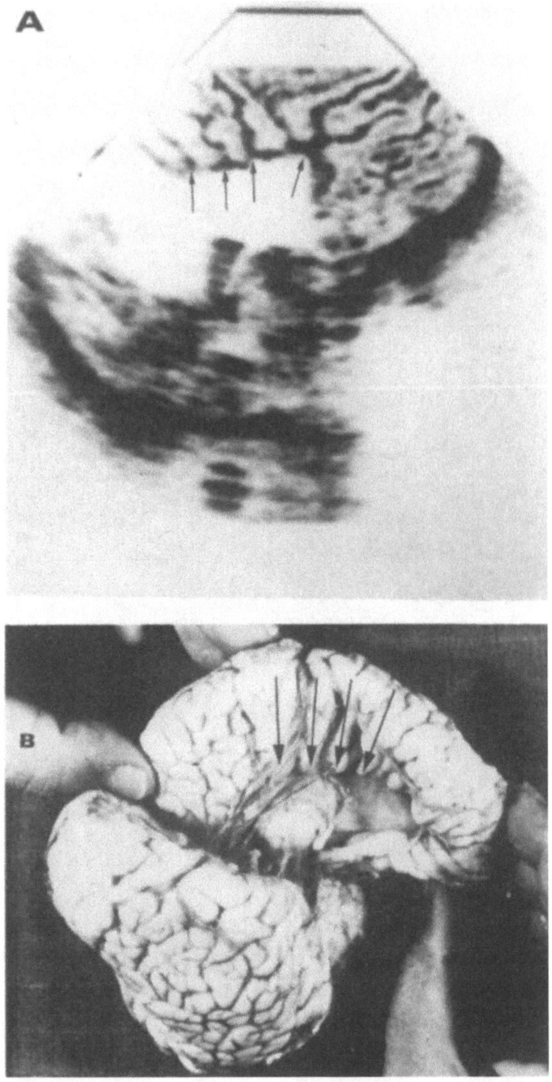

Fig. 41 A and B. Total agenesis of the corpus callosum: longitudinal median section passing through the axis of the third ventricle **(A)**.
The sulci are large and echogenic and converge towards the roof of the third ventricle (*arrows*). The anatomical appearance is also typical **(B)**.

is always identifiable. The second is the radial distribution of the sulci on the internal aspect of the hemispheres around the third ventricle on median sagittal section (Fig. 41).

While studying anatomical sections, Loiser and Alvord [56] noted this radial distribution and underlined the fact that this distribution is only seen when the corpus callosum is absent. This sign therefore appears to be pathognomonic of the malformation and very useful in the diagnosis of partial agenesis (Fig. 42) which usually poses well-known diagnostic difficulties particularly with tomodensimetry. Abnormalities of the septum pellucidum are also remarkably well diagnosed by ultrasonography.

The medial cava (cavum of septum lucidum and cavum vergae) are physiological images and are represented by an echo-free anterior or posterior median imade, closely surrounded by the lateral ventricles (Fig. 43). They can be seen in the majority of premature infants and then disappear progressively. The formation of cysts at this level [57], which may result in hydrocephalus due to obstruction of the foramen of Monro, is rare as their walls are very thin.

Agenesis of the septum pellucidum is a well-defined entity [58, 59]. On US one sees a single frontal cavity (Fig. 44). The differential diagnosis from holoprosencephaly is based on the presence and normality of the third ventricle, the existence of an interhemispheric fissure, and the absence of fusion of the basal nuclei. This primitive agenesis is rare whereas a secondary "agenesis" is much more common: the essential cause is hydrocephalus which results in excess pressure within the ventricular cavities and a progressive destruction of the septum due to multiple areas of necrosis (Fig. 45).

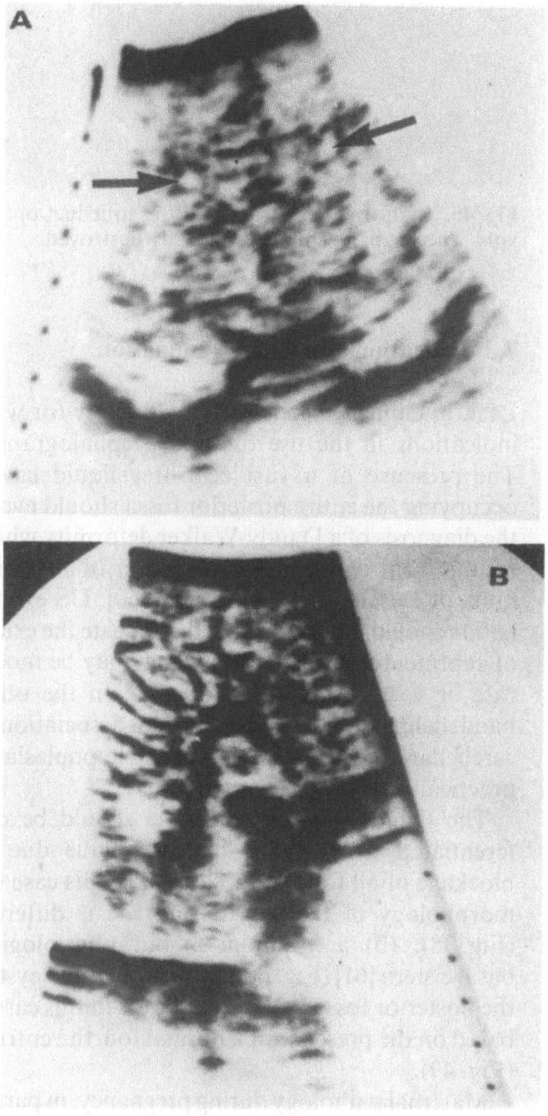

Fig. 42 A and B. Infant aged 1 month.
A Coronal section shows a separation of the ventricular bodies (*arrows*).
B Median longitudinal section shows pathognomonic radial distribution of the cerebral sulci indicating the presence of a partial posterior agenesis of the corpus callosum.

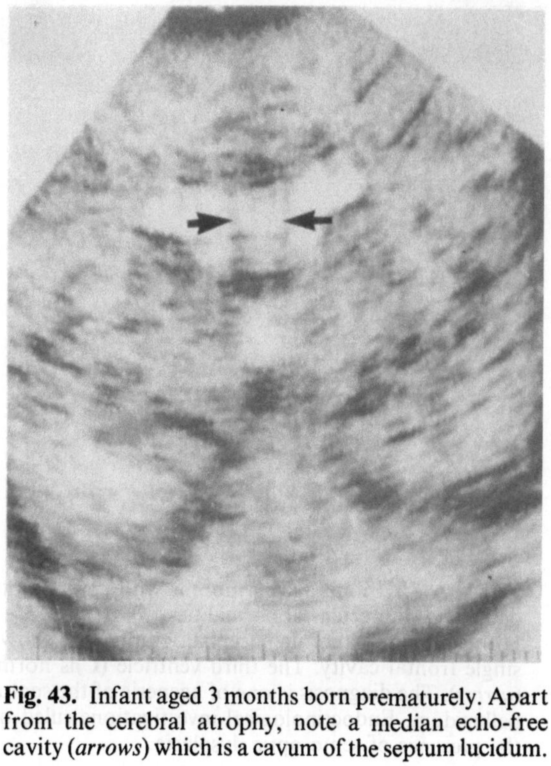

Fig. 43. Infant aged 3 months born prematurely. Apart from the cerebral atrophy, note a median echo-free cavity (*arrows*) which is a cavum of the septum lucidum.

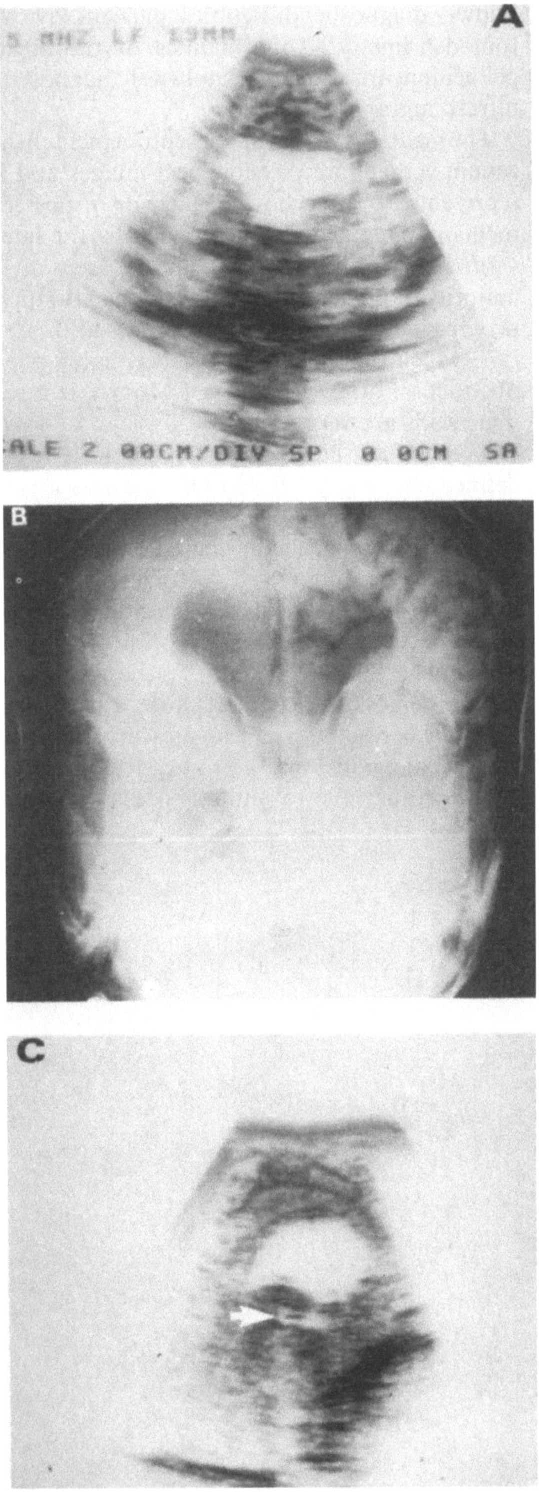

Fig. 44 A–C. Infant aged 7 months with psychomotor delay and no occular abnormalities.
Ultrasound **(A)** and air encephalography **(B)** show a single frontal cavity. The third ventricle **(C)**is normal (*arrow*). The diagnosis is one of agenesis of the septum pellucidum. Endocrinological investigations ruled out the presence of septo-optic dysplasia.

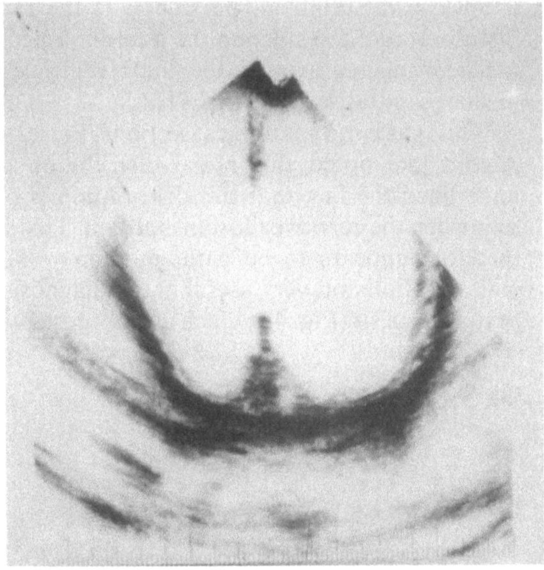

Fig. 45. Malformative stenosis of the aqueduct of Sylvius. The median septum is partially destroyed.

7.3 Indications for US Examination

Lack of clinical specificity should allow for wide indications in the use of echoencephalography. The presence of a vast echo-free liquid cavity occupying the entire posterior fossa should evoke the diagnosis of a Dandy-Walker deformity which results from congenital obstruction of the foramina of Luschka and Magendie [60]. US examination should, on the one hand, delineate the extent of supratentorial distension which may be moderate or very severe (Fig. 46) and, on the other hand, delineate the almost constant association of cerebellar vermis pathology either hypoplasia or practically total agenesis (Fig. 47).

The Dandy-Walker syndrome should be differentiated from: (a) a hydrocephalus due to blockage of all four ventricles but in this case the morphology of the fourth ventricle is different (Fig. 38); (b) a voluminous but physiological basal cistern [61] (Fig. 48); (c) an arachnoid cyst of the posterior fossa [62] the diagnosis in this case is based on the presence of a normal fourth ventricle (Fig. 49).

Maternal pathology during pregnancy, in particular viral infections (including cystomegalovirus, herpes virus), may be responsible for severe cerebral malformations such as congenital porencephaly which on US is characterized by multiple liquid cavities replacing the cerebral parenchyma (Fig. 50).

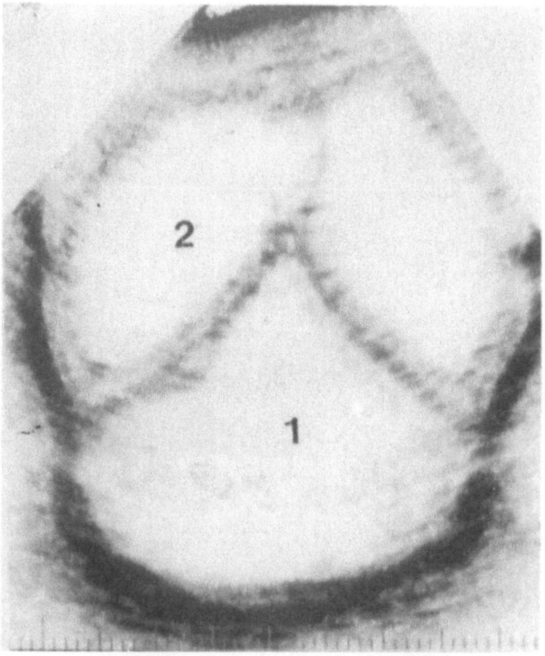

Fig. 46. Dandy-Walker deformity. Cerebral atrophy due to sever hydrocephalus. *1*, Cystic cavity of the fourth ventricle; *2*, Occipital horns.

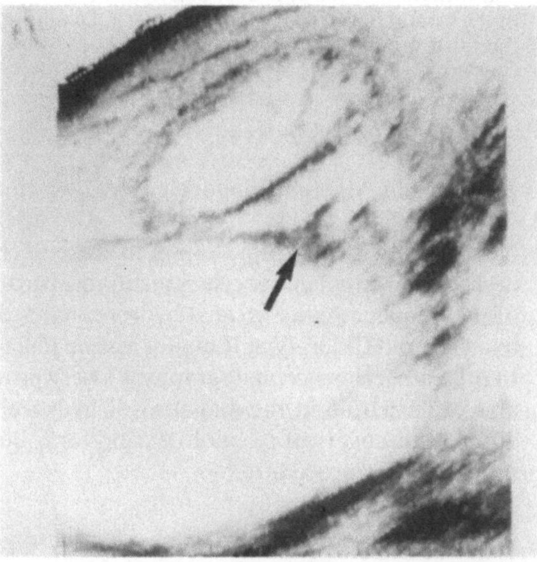

Fig. 47. On a longitudinal median section, cerebellar atrophy is easily visualized. The extreme dilatation of the fourth ventricle has practically destroyed the entire cerebellar parenchyma (*arrow*).

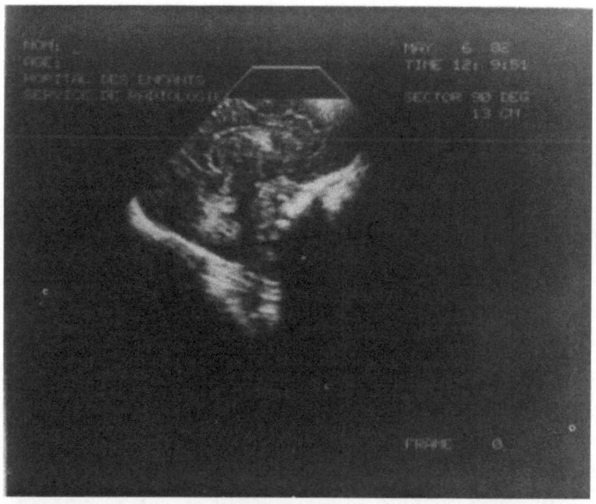

Fig. 48. Premature infant aged 15 days. The cystic cavity arising in the posterior fossa below the cerebellum is the cisterna magna.

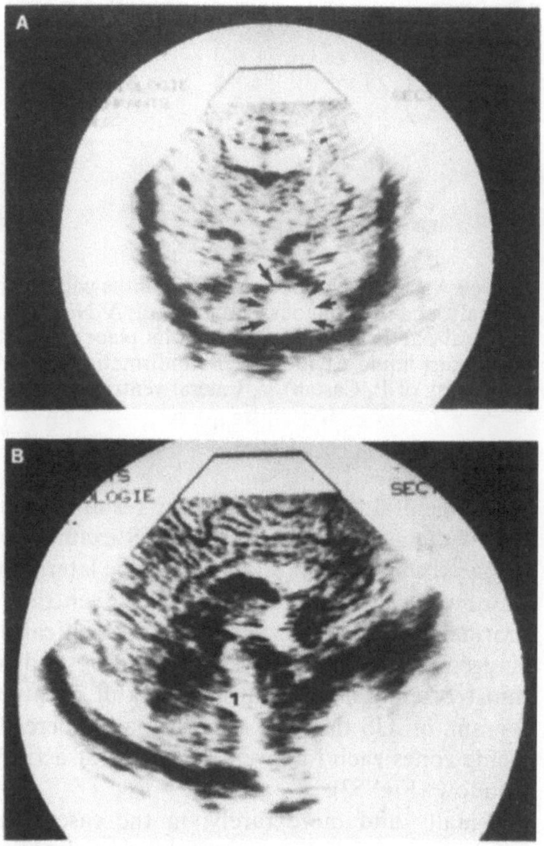

Fig. 49 A and B. Infant aged 3 months. Arachnoid cyst of the posterior fossa (*arrows*). The diagnosis is made by the presence of a lateral echo-free image **(A)** and a normal fourth ventricle *(1)* seen on a median longitudinal section **(B)**.

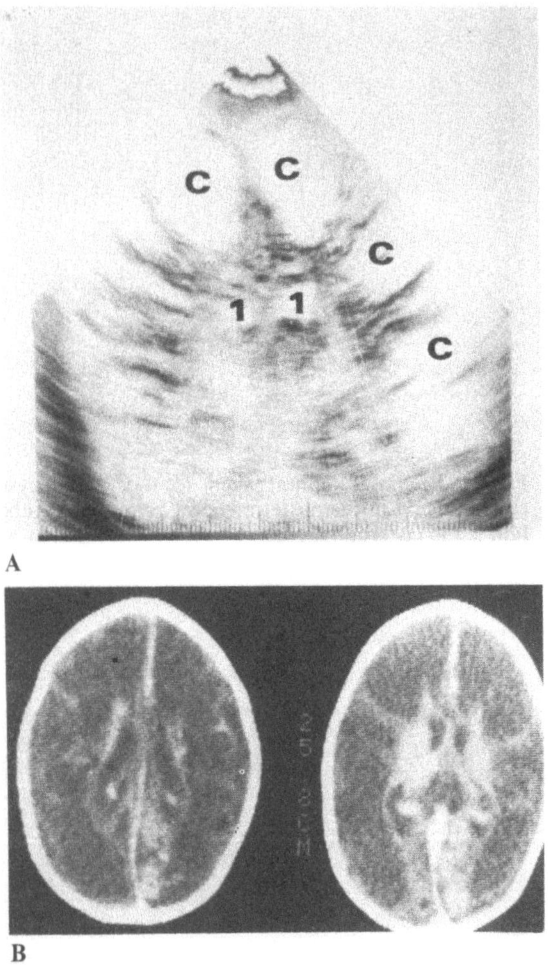

Fig. 50 A and B. Newborn aged 2 months with microcephaly and Continuous convulsions. **A** No normal cerebral parenchyma is visible. In its place one notes numerous liquid cavities (*c*), **B** confirmation by CAT (Courtesy of P. Castan). *1*, Lateral ventricles.

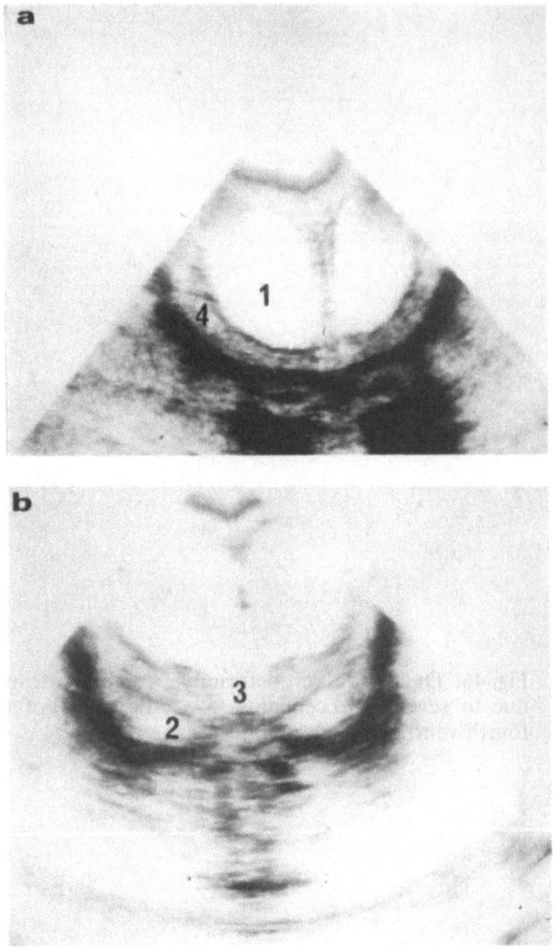

Fig. 51 a and b. Newborn aged 1 day. Stenosis due to malformation of the aqueduct of Sylvius. *1*, Dilatation of the frontal horns; *2*, Temporal horns; *3*, Dilatation of the third ventricle; *4*, Cerebral atrophy.

Congenital toxoplasmosis may result in stenosis of the aqueduct of Sylvius: US examination shows the significant dilatation of the lateral and third ventricles whereas the fourth ventricle is normal (Fig. 51). Periventricular calcifications suggest an infection by toxoplasmosis and are most often visible on a simple skull roentgenogram: on US they are seen as small hyperechogenic zones each followed by a cone of acoustic shadow (Fig. 52).

Finally and more rarely, in the case where clinical examination suggests tuberous sclerosis in an infant, ultrasonography may delineate rounded nodular hyperechogenic images which are periventricular in location and represent the classic phacomata (Fig. 53).

7.4 US and Myelomeningocele

Neuroradiological exploration in the case of children with myelomeningocele is justifiable because of the frequence of associated hydrocephalus due to an Arnold Chiari type II malformation [63, 64]. In this case, echoencephalography is a very profitable examination in the diagnosis of hydrocephalus, the discovery of its etiology, and for follow-up of a shunt procedure.

7.4.1 **Ventricular Dilatation** (Table 3)

Ventricular dilatation is very frequent. It is present even at birth before surgical closure of the lumbosacral lesion: dilatation is discovered in 14

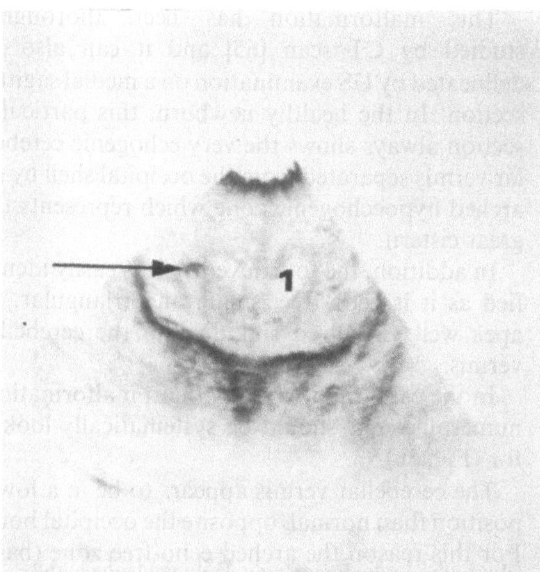

Fig. 52. Newborn aged 3 days with clinical hydrocephalus. Coronal section at the level of the dilated frontal horns *(1)*. Presence of calcification (*arrow*). Diagnosis of congenital toxoplasmosis.

Table 3. Initial cerebral ultrasound (21 cases).

Results	Normal	Biventricular dilatation	Triventricular dilatation
Neonatal	1	7	5
Early onset	0	3	2
Late onset	0	1	5

of 15 newborns suffering from lumbosacral meningoceles.

In addition, in the majority of cases, there are no clinical signs of hydrocephalus and head circumference is normal. This ventricular dilatation can affect the lateral ventricles as well as the third ventricle (Fig. 54). The third ventricle has a particular morphological appearance. On the one hand, one can visualize interthalamic commissure hypertrophy, which is seen as a voluminous echogenic rounded image in the center of the echo-free ventricular triangle (Fig. 55). On the other hand, the possibility of ventricular cavity expansion in its transverse diameter is poor and the increase in volume first appears in the longitudinal axis and occurs mainly in the anterior recess where dilatation may be very marked [67].

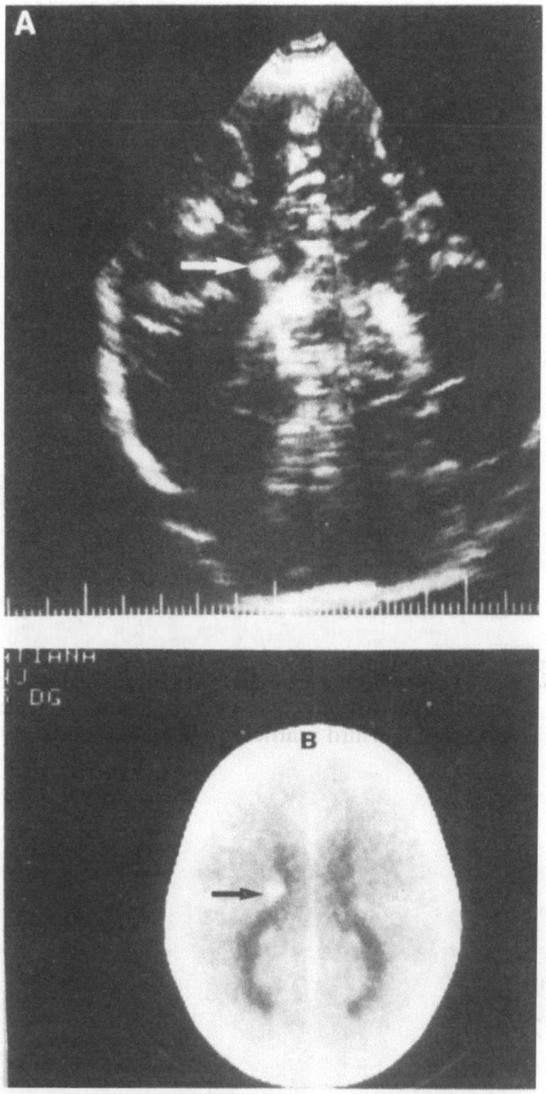

Fig. 53 A and B. Infant aged 14 months with psychomotor delay and convulsions. Depigmented spots led to suspicion of tuberous sclerosis.
On aposterior coronal section **(A)** one notes the presence of a rounded periventricular image which corresponds with a phakoma. Confirmation on CT scan **(B)** (Courtesy P. Castan).

7.4.2 Diagnosis of Arnold-Chiari Malformation

The Arnold-Chiari malformation associated with this pathology of spinal dysraphism is a type II malformation and is composed of herniation of the cerebellar vermis, herniation of the bulb and of the fourth ventricle, and deformation of its junction with the cervical portion of the spinal cord.

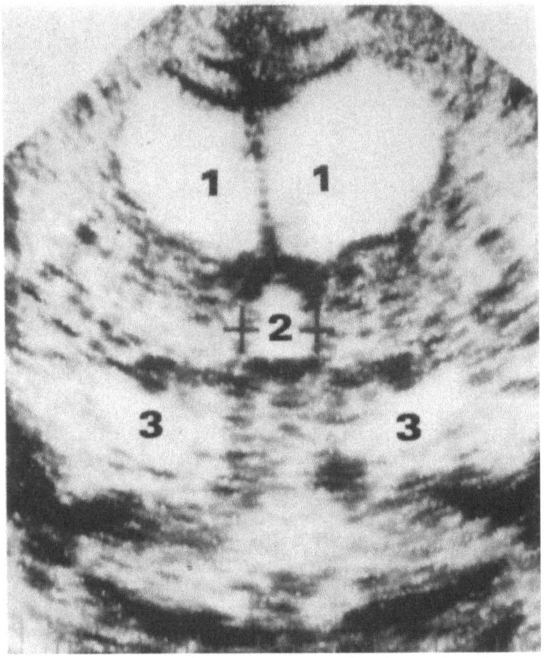

Fig. 54. Newborn aged 1 day with myelomeningocele. One notes a triventricular hydrocephalus. *1*, Lateral ventricles; *2*, Third ventricle; *3*, Temporal horns.

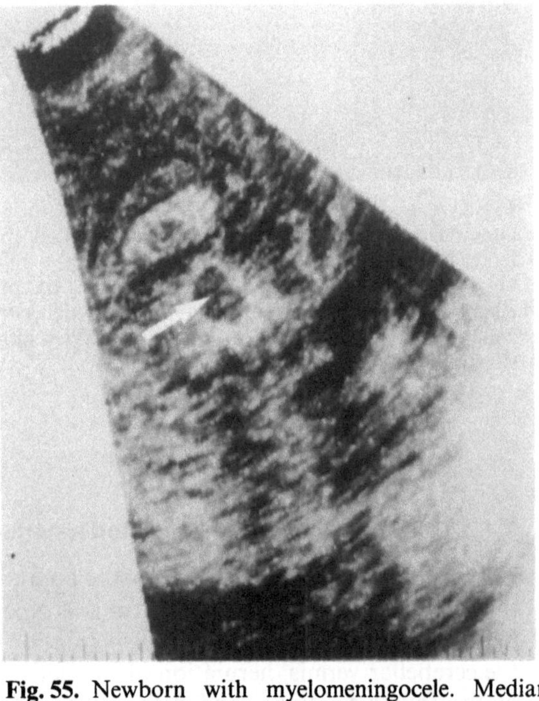

Fig. 55. Newborn with myelomeningocele. Median longitudinal section: a voluminous hyperechogenic rounded image within the third ventricle corresponds with hypertrophy of the pars intermedia (*arrow*).

This malformation has been thoroughly studied by CT scan [65] and it can also be delineated by US examination on a medial sagittal section. In the healthy newborn, this particular section always shows the very echogenic cerebellar vermis separated from the occipital shell by an arched hypoechogenic zone which represents the great cistern.

In addition, the fourth ventricle is easily identified as it is echo-free, small, and triangular, its apex well visualized sinking into the cerebellar vermis:

In the case of an Arnold-Chiari malformation, numerous signs should be systematically looked for (Fig. 56).

The cerebellar vermis appears to be in a lower position than normal, opposite the occipital bone. For this reason the arched echo-free zone (basal cistern) is never visualized. Finally, the fourth ventricle is displaced downward.

7.4.3 Follow-up of Shunt Function

As soon as a ventricular dilatation is discovered US examination permits follow-up of its evolution and decision with respect to a surgical shunt procedure. In the majority of cases, a ventriculoperitoneal shunt is used. Within the first week after surgery, the ventricular dilatation diminishes. The third ventricle also attains a normal size

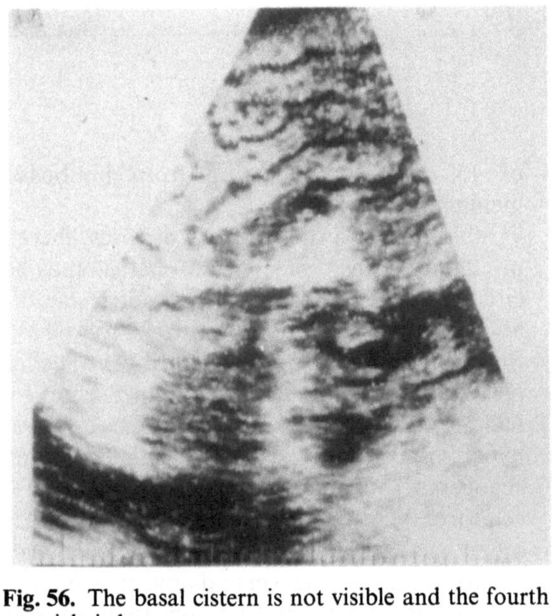

Fig. 56. The basal cistern is not visible and the fourth ventricle is low.

fairly rapidly and the lateral ventricles more gradually. At 8 days one notes an increase in size of the interhemispheric sulcus with parallel borders. This aspect is typical and constant in patients with a myelomeningocele. It is a sign of an increase in the subarachnoid space and for some authors this indicates the presence of cerebral atrophy (Fig. 57).

For ventriculoperitoneal shunts, complications occur in 50%–80% of cases according to various authors [66]. The most frequent complication is due to blockage in the shunt system. The clinical presentation is variable and may often be absent. For this reason it is necessary to carry out systematic checks by echography (Fig. 58).

Infection is the second most frequent complication of shunted myelomeningoceles. If infection is present from the onset, therapy should be altered to insertion of an external shunt with ventricular irrigation using specific antibiotics.

Semiologically, three types of image may be observed: (a) the presence of fine punctiform echoes due to small purulent collections of fluid; (b) the presence of fine linear floating echoes which represent filaments of nonlocalized pus (Fig. 59); (c) veritable ventricular loculations seen as echogenic septae (Fig. 60).

Subdural hematomas are now rare due to the use of ventriculoperitoneal shunts.

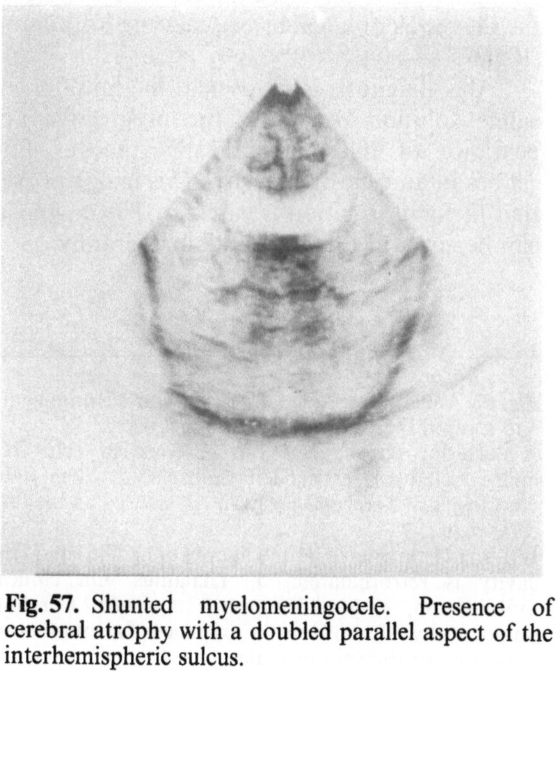

Fig. 57. Shunted myelomeningocele. Presence of cerebral atrophy with a doubled parallel aspect of the interhemispheric sulcus.

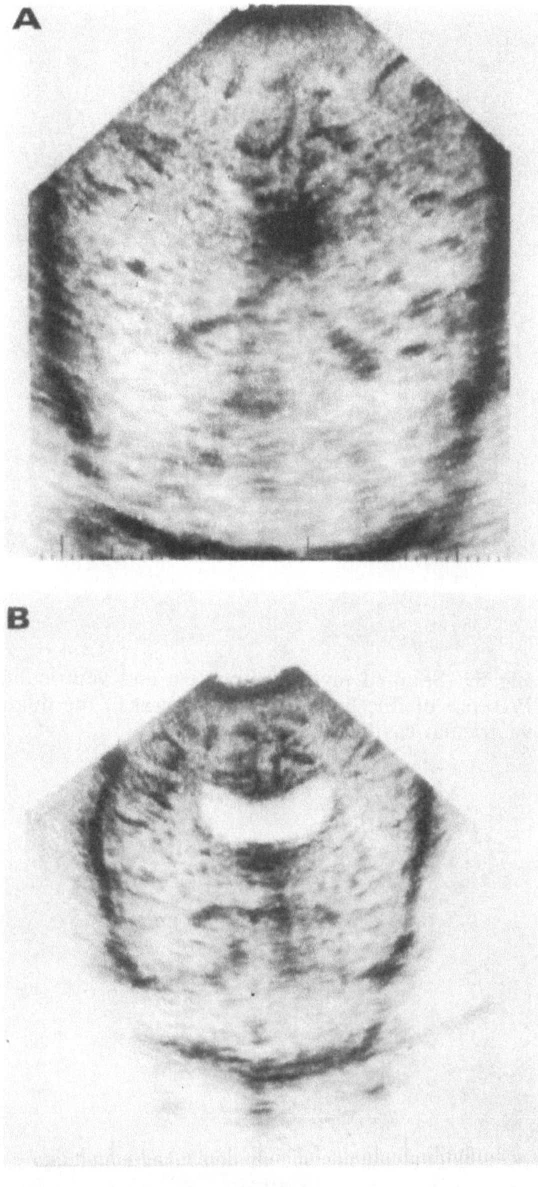

Fig. 58 A and B. Shunted myelomeningocele in infant aged 2 month.
Absence of ventricular dilatation **(A)**. Systematic follow-up at 4 months of age showed no clinical signs of hydrocephalus. Discovery of a blocked shunt at surgery **(B)**.

Finally, US examination is very useful in the diagnosis of an intraabdominal collection of cerebrospinal fluid [67] (Fig. 61).

In conclusion, ultrasonography is necessary in the initial investigation of a myelomeningocele and is sufficient alone to detect ventricular dilatation within the first days of life.

US examination may be used in follow-up of ventriculoperitoneal shunt function and may also

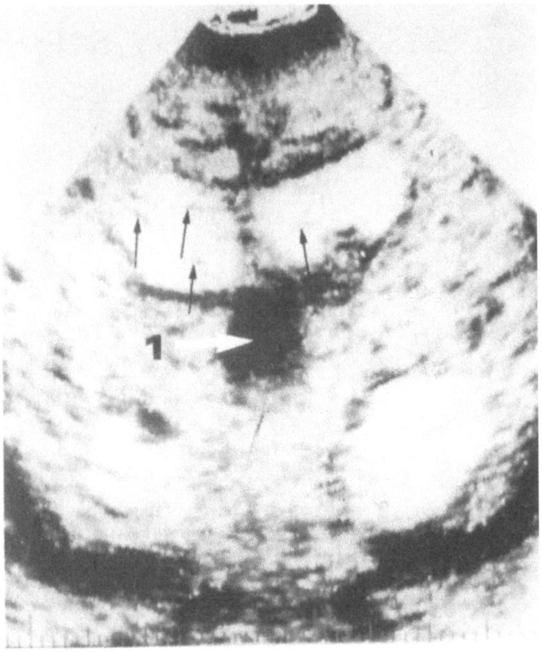

Fig. 59. Shunted myelomeningocele and ventriculitis. Presence of fine linear echoes (*arrows*) in the dilated ventricular cavities. *1*, Shunt tube.

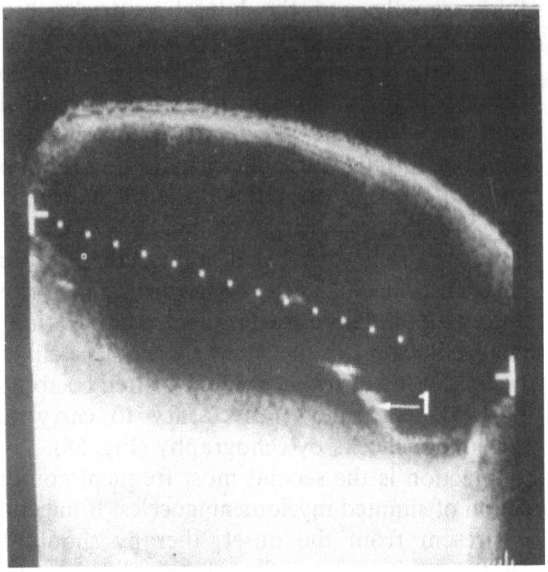

Fig. 61. Longitudinal section of the abdomen. An enormous liquid cavity is noted which corresponds with a collection of cerebrospinal fluid. *1*, Shunt tube.

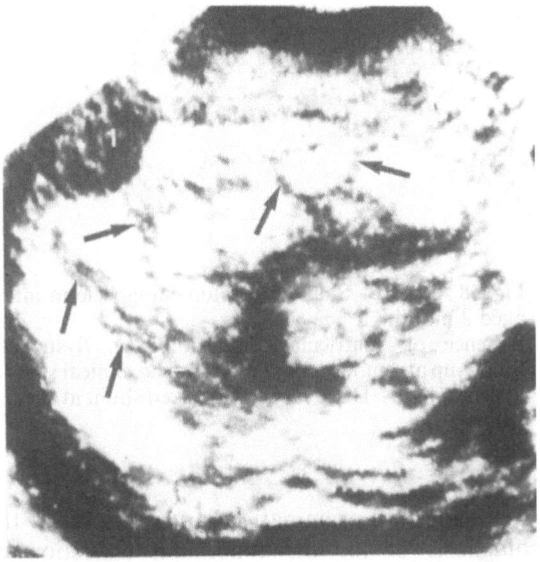

Fig. 60. Shunted myelomeningocele and pyocephalus. Serious evolution with multiple ventricular loculations (*arrows*) and a cerebral abscess *(1)*.

be useful in the diagnosis of complications before the appearance of clinical signs. It permits diagnosis of a cerebral malformation as well as delineating its vascular nature.

The presence of an echo-free retrothalamic voluminous median image, compressing the ventricular cavities and associated with an intracranial murmur on auscultation, should indicate the diagnosis of a cerebrovascular malformation (Fig. 62).

If this diagnosis is suspected, the injection of saline solution results in the progressive appearance of microbubbles appearing as fine echoes in an echo-free cavity. This image proves that the malformation is vascular. The diagnosis can be confirmed by cerebral angiography.

Fig. 62 A–C. Infant aged 17 days with cardiomegaly ▶ and a rapid increase in head circumference.
A Posterior coronal section. A rounded echo-free image *(4)* displaces the left ventricle *(2)*. The right ventricle is in a normal position *(3)* as well as the falx cerebri *(1)*.
B Longitudinal left paramedian section. The echo-free cavity is retrothalamic. *5*, Thalamus. On clinical examination, a cranial murmur is noted. Cerebral angiography **(C)** confirms the existence of a voluminous aneurysm of the vein of Galen.

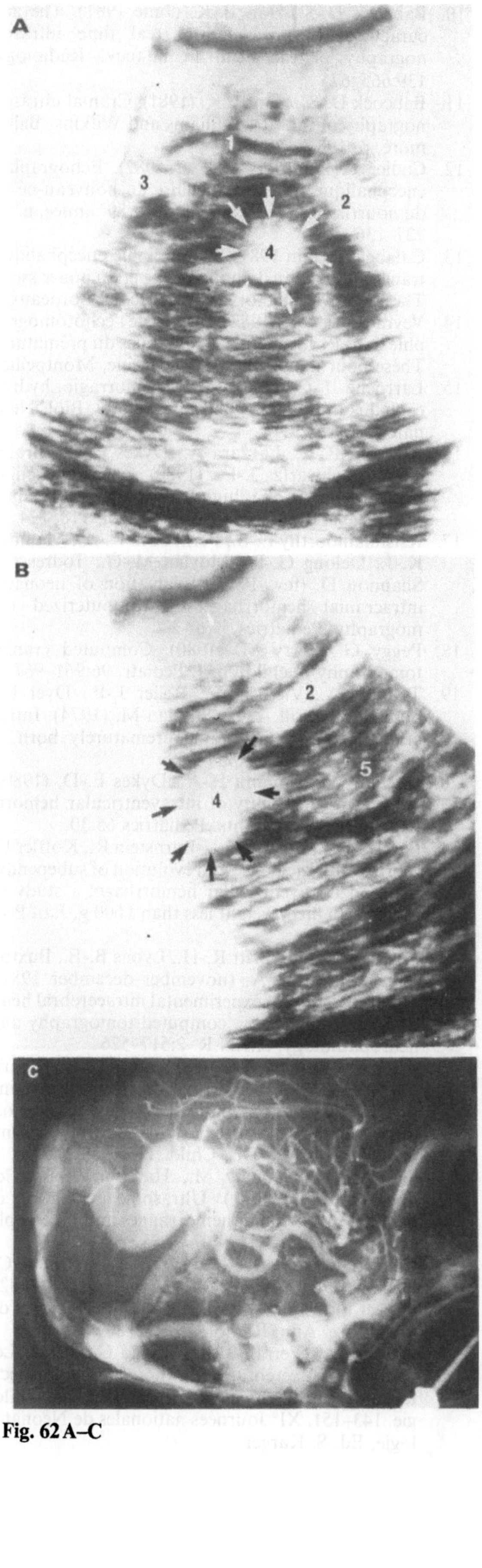

Fig. 62 A–C

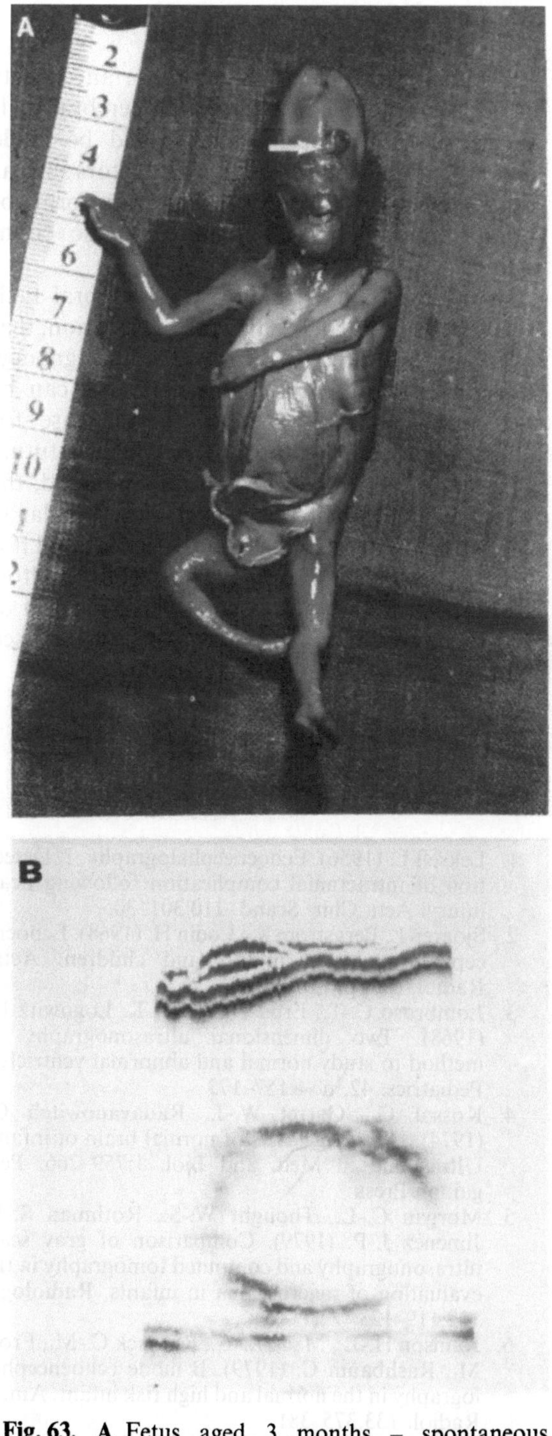

Fig. 63. A Fetus aged 3 months – spontaneous abortion. Cyclops (*arrow*). **B** Cranial ultrasound carried out in a basin of water shows the cerebral malformation characterized absence of cerebral parenchyma.

7.5 Conclusion

In conclusion, a number of important points should be noted. The diagnosis of cerebral malformations is important and should be made early, as prognostic and diagnostic factors such as the diagnosis of Trisomy 13 or certain forms of holoprosencephaly may require genetic counseling.

We know that the majority of cerebral malformations occur at the 6th week of gestation, that is to say within the first 3 months of pregnancy. Certain echographic in utero diagnosis can be made at an early stage: this is the case for anencephaly and hydrocephalus. For the future two factors are important: on the one hand, the possibility of in utero treatment, in particular in the case of hydrocephalus, on the other hand it is not impossible to imagine that certain malformations such as holoprosensephaly (Fig. 63) or the Dandy-Walker syndrome can be diagnosed within the first 3 months of pregnancy.

References

1. Leksell L. (1956). Echoencephalography. I. Detection of intracranial complication following head injury. Acta Chir. Scand. 110:301–305.
2. Sjogren I., Bergstrom K., Lodin H. (1968). Echoencephalography in infants and children. Acta. Radiol. (Suppl.) 278:4–83
3. Lombroso C.-T., Erba G., Yogo T., Logowitz N. (1968). Two dimensional ultrasonography: a method to study normal and abnormal ventricles. Pediatrics. 42, n° 1:157–173
4. Kossof G., Garret W.-J., Radavanowitch G. (1974). Ultrasonic atlas of normal brain of infant. Ultrasound in Med. and Biol. 1:759–766, Pergamon Press
5. Morgan C.-L., Thought W.-S., Rothman S.-J., Jimenez J.-P. (1979). Comparison of gray scale ultrasonography and computed tomography in the evaluation of macrocrania in infants. Radiology. 132:119–123
6. Johnson H.-L., Mack L.-A., Rumack C.-M., Frost M., Rashbaum C. (1979). B mode echoencephalography in the normal and high risk infant. Am. J. Radiol. 133:375–381
7. White D.-N. (1970). The six laws of echoencephalography. Neurology 20:435–444
8. Ben Ora A., Eddy L., Hatch G., Solida B. (1980). The anterior fontanelle as an acoustic window to the neonatal ventricular system. J. Clin. Ultrasound 8:65–67
9. Couture A., Ferran J.-L., Blum M., Montoya F., Germain M., Montoya P., Senac J.-P., Bonnet H. (1980). La coupe transfontanellaire en échoencéphalographie. Ann. de Radiol. 23, n° 8:649–654
10. Babcock D.-S., Han B.-K. (June 1981). The accuracy of high resolution, real time ultrasonography of the head in infancy. Radiology 139:665–675
11. Babcock D.-S., Han B.-K. (1981). Cranial ultrasonography of infants. Williams and Wilkins. Baltimore, p. 196
12. Cadier L., Diard F. (février 1982). Echographie encéphalique transfontanellaire du nouveau-né et du nourrisson. Médecine infantile. 89ᵉ année, n° 2, 227–136
13. Calabet A. (juin 1981). Echographie encéphalique transfontanellaire du nouveau-né et du nourrisson. Thèse pour le Doctorat en Médecine. Bordeaux
14. Veyrac C. (janvier 1982). Apport de l'échotomographie dans les hémorragies cérébrales du prématuré. Thèse pour le Doctorat en Médecine, Montpellier
15. Larroche J.-C. (1972). Post-hemorragic hydrocephalus in infancy: anatomical study. Biol. Neonate. 20:287–299
16. Ahmann P.-A., Lazzara A., Dykes F.-D., Brann A.-W., Schwartz J.-F. (1980). Intraventricular hemorrhage in the high risk preterms infants: incidence and outcome. Ann. Neurol. 118–124
17. Krishnamoorthy F.-S., Fernandez R.-A., Mamose K.-J., Delong G.-R., Moylan M.-G., Todres D., Shannon D. (fev. 1977). Evaluation of neonatal intracranial hemorrhage by computerized tomography. Pediatrics 59:n° 2
18. Peggy G., Ferry M. (1980). Computed cranial tomography in children. J. Pediatr. 96:961–967
19. Tsiantos A., Victorin L., Relier J.-P., Dyer N., Sundell H., Brill A.-B., Stahlan M. (1974). Intracranial hemorrhage in the prematurely born in infant. J. Pediatr. 85:854–859
20. Lazzara A., Ahmann P.-A., Dykes F.-D. (1980). Clinical predictability of intraventricular hemorrhage in preterm infants. Pediatrics 65:30
21. Papile L.-A., Burnstein J., Burnstein R., Koffler H. (april 1978). Incidence and evolution of subependymal and intraventricular hemorrhage: a study of infant with birth weight less than 1 500 g. J. of Ped. 92:529–534
22. Enzmann D.-R., Britt R.-H., Lyons B.-E., Buxton J.-L., Wilson D.-A. (november–december 1981). Natural history of experimental intracerebral hemorrhage: sonography, computed tomography and neuropathology. A.J.N.R. 2:517–526
23. Allan C.-W., Roveto A.-C., Sanyer L.-R., Courtney S.-E. (1980). Sector scan ultrasound imaging through the anterior fontanella. Its use in diagnosing neonatal periventricular, intraventricular hemorrhage. Amer. J. Dis.-Child. 134:1028–1031
24. Sauerbrei E., Digney M., Harrison P.-B., Cooperberg P.-L. (1981). Ultrasonic evaluation of neonatal intracranial hemorrhages and its complications. Radiology 139:677–685
25. Couture A., Ferran J.-L., Veyrac C., Guermoud C., Senac J.-P., Rodiere M., Montoya F. (1982). Aspect ultrasonore des hémorragies cérébrales du prématuré. Ann. Radiol. 25:1:72–80
26. Couture A., Ferran J.-L., Veyrac C. (1981). Les hémorragies cérébrales du nouveau-né: aspects techniques et diagnostic. In: Progrès en Néonatalogie. 143–151. XIᵉ Journées nationales de Néonatologie, Ed. S. Karger

27. Bejar R., Curbelo V., Coen W., Leopold G., James H. (1980). Diagnosis and follow-up of intraventricular and intracerebral hemorrhages by ultrasound studies of infant's brain through the fontanelle and sutures. Pediatrics 66:661–673
28. Messina A., Chernick N. (1976). Computed tomography: the "resolving" intracerebral hemorrhage. Radiology. 118:609–613
29. Wladihiroff J., Graft I., Talbert D. (1975). In vitro measurements of sound velocity in human fetal brain tissue. Ultrasound Med. Biol. 1:377
30. Fiske C.-E., Filly R.-A., Callen P.-W. (1981). The normal choroid plexus: ultrasonic appearance of the neonatal head. Radiology. 141:467–471
31. Cooke R.-W.-I. (1981). Factors associated with periventricular hemorrhage in very low birth weight infants. Arch. Dis. Child. 56:425–431
32. Edwards M.-K., Brown D.-L., Muller J., Grossman C.-B., Chua G.-T. (1981). Cribside neurosonography: real time sonography for intracranial investigation of the neonate. A. J. R. 136:271–276
33. Grant E.-G., Bortz F.-T., Schellinger D., McCullough D.-C. Sivasubramanian K.-N., Smith Y. (1981). Real time ultrasonography of neonatal intraventricular hemorrhage and comparison with computed tomography. Radiology 139:687–691
34. Levene M.-I., Wigglesworth J.-S., Dubowitz V. (1981). Cerebral structure and intraventricular hemorrhage in the neonate: a real time ultrasound study. Arch. Dis. Child. 56:416–424
35. Flodmark O., Becker L., Harwoodnash D., Fitzhardinge P., Fitz C., Chuang S. (1980). Correlation between C.T. and autopsy in premature and full term neonates that have suffered perinatal asphyxia. Radiology 137:93–103
36. Messina A.-V., Chernick N.-L. (1976). Computed tomography: the "resolving" intracerebral hemorrhage. Radiology. 118:609–613
37. Aicardi J., Goutieres F. (1971). Les épanchements sous-duraux du nourrisson. Arch. Franç. Ped. 28:233–47
38. Pinsard N., Choux M., Combes J.-C., Rebuffel P., Boyer M., Bernard R. (mai 1974). Hematomes sousduraux du nourrisson. Immex n° 5
39. Stroobandt G., Evrard P., Thauvoy C., Laterre C. (1981). Les épanchements péricérébraux du nourrisson à localisation sous-durale ou sous-arachnoïdienne. Neurochirurgie 27:49–57
40. Couture A., Ferran J.-L., Veyrac C., Senac J.-P., Germain H., Montoya F., Bonnet H. (1981). Apport de l'échoencéphalographie transfontanellaire chez le nouveau-né. Arch. Franç. Pédiatr. 38:481–487
41. Towbin A. (june 1970). Central nervous system damage in the human foetus and newborn infant. Amer. J. Dis. Child., Vol. 119, 529–542
42. Amstrong D., Norman G.-M. (1974). Periventricular leucomalacia in neonates complications and sequelae. Arch. of Disease in Childhood. 49:367–375
43. Volpe J. (August 1976). Perinatal hypoxie-ischemic brain injury. Pediatrics clinics of North America, vol. 23, n° 3
44. Pouplard F., Bouderlique C., Berthelot J., Limal J.-M., Larget-Piet L. (1980). Double abcès cérébral de la période néonatale. Pédiatrie 35, n° 7:619–623
45. Sann L., Lapras C., Duquesnel J.-C., Bourgeois J., Cottancin G., Bethenod H. (1980). L'abcès cérébral du nouveau-né. Pédiatrie 35, n° 7:625–630
46. Whelan M.-A., Hilal S.-K. (1980). Computed tomography as a guide in the diagnosis and follow-up of brain abcesses. Radiology 135, 3:663–671
47. Enzmann D.-R., Britt R.-H., Lyons B., Carroll B., Wilson D.-A., Buxton J. (1982). High resolution ultrasound evaluation of experimental brain abcess evolution: comparison with computed tomography and neuropathology. Radiology 142, 1:95–102
48. Harwood-Nash D.-C., Fitz C.-R. (1976). Neuroradiology in infants and children. Mosby, St-Louis
49. Manelfe C., Sevely A. (1982). Etude neuroradiologique des holoprosencéphalies. J. Neuroradiology 9:15–45
50. Robain O., Gorce F. (1972). Arhinencéphalie. Etude clinique anatomique et étiologique. Arch. Franç. Ped. 29:861–879
51. Deveze J., Jezequel Ch. (1971). Les cyclopes. Etude clinique et anatomique d'une cyclopie familiale. Arch. Franç. Ped. 28:321–337
52. Cadier L., Souyris S., Diard F. (1982). Agénésie complète du corps calleux: aspects échographiques a' propos de deux observations. Journal de Radiologie. (à Paraître)
53. Souyris S. (1981). Aspect échographique de l'agénésie du corps calleux. Thèse, Bordeaux
54. Coursault R., Delouvrier J.-J., Desbleds M.-T., Marsault C., Nahum H. (1981). Agénésie du corps calleux vue en tomodensitométrie. J. Radiol. 62:103–106
55. Probst F.-B. (1973). Congenital defect of the corpus callosum morphology and encephalographic appearances. Acta Radiologica, suppl. n° 331, Stockholm
56. Loeser J.-D., Alvord E.-C. (1968). Agenesis of the corpus callosum. Brain. 91:553–570
57. Cowley A.-R., Moody D.-M., Alexander E., Ball M.-R., Laster D.-W. (1979). Distinctive CT appearance of cyst of the cavum septi pellucidi. A. J. R. 133:548–550
58. Manelfe C., Rochiccioli P. (1979). CT of septo optic dysplasia. A. J. R. 133:1157–1160
59. Probst F.-P. (1979). The prosencephalies. Springer Verlag Edit., Berlin, Heidelberg, New York
60. Harwood-Nash D.-C., Fitz C.-R. (1976). Congenital malformations of the brain. In: Neuroradiology in infants and children. The Mosby company Edit., Saint-Louis, Vol. 3, p. 979–1053
61. Just N.-W.M., Goldenberg M. (may 1979). Computed tomography of the enlarged cisterna magna. Radiology 131:385–391
62. Archer C.-R., Darwish H., Smith K. (june 1978). Enlarged cisterna magnae and posterior fossa cysts simulating Dandy Walker syndrome on computed tomography. Radiology 127:681–686
63. Emery J.-L., Mac Kenzie N. (1973). Medullo cervical dislocation deformity (Chiari II deformity) related to neurospinal dysraphism. Brain 96:155–162
64. Peach B. (juin 1965). Arnold Chiari malformation. Anatomic features of 20 cases. Arch. Neurol. 12:613–621
65. Naidich T.-P., Pudlowski R.-M., Naidich J.-B. (march 1980). Computed tomographic signs of the

Chiari II malformation. III: ventricles and cisterns. Radiology. 134:657–663
66. Stark G-D., Drummond M.-B., Poneprasert S., Robarts F.-H. (1974). Primary ventriculo-peritoneal shunt in treatment of hydrocephalus associated with myelomeningocele. Arch. of dis. in childh. 49:112–117
67. Fried A.-M., Adams W.-E., Ellis G.-T., Hatfield D.-R., Walsh J.-W. (1980). Ventriculo-peritoneal shunt function: evaluation by sonography. A. J. R. 134:967–970
68. Couture A., Ferran J.-L., Senac J.-P., Castan-Tabouriech E., Bonnet H. (1981). Image ultrasonore d'un anévrysme de la veine de Galien. Arch. Franç. de Péd. 35:55–57

Chapter 3

Cervical Echography

J. Poncin, G. Lalande, and J.L. Ferran

1 Technique and Normal Anatomy

1.1 Technique

The echographic exploration of the cervical area is carried out on a child in the supine position with the neck slightly hyperextended using a pillow placed under the shoulders. Immobilization is sometimes difficult to obtain with the infant, especially since the feeding bottle cannot be used to calm the child because of the thyroid movements when swallowing. Sections that are transversal and longitudinal will be more closely spaced the younger the child. The US equipment is a 7 MHz transducer usually equipped with a manual scanning.

The use of a water pouch is difficult and does not seem to be any more efficient than a direct skin scan; however, it can be useful when the neck is very convex, which is quite rare in children, or when a highly protuberant nodule might cause the transducer to jerk abruptly. Nor does the use of real time appear to have any advantage over manual scanning: this method, however, allows recognition of the carotid beat so as to perceive better the change in diameter of the internal jugular vein during respiration and perhaps to locate more easily the left side of the esophagus.

Finally, it is worth noting the significance of making the gain vary, particularly when diagnosis a cyst.

1.2 Normal Echographic Anatomy (Figs. 1 and 2)

The thyroid gland is the main anatomic element; its two lobes, easily recognizable with homo-

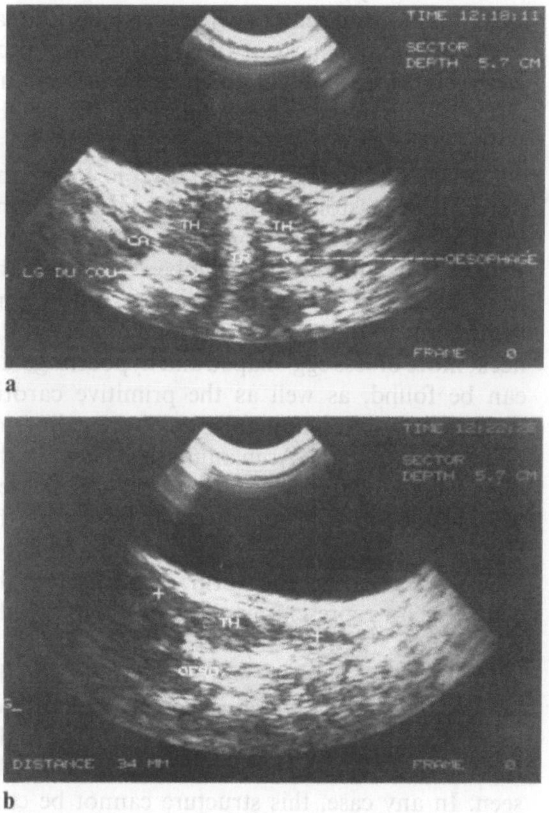

Fig. 1 a and b. Normal anatomy in an 8-year-old child. **a** Transverse section (only left and median regions are marked). **b** Longitudinal section (all longitudinal sections, except in Fig. 20, are presented with the same orientation, lower part to the left, upper part to the right). *TH*, Thyroid lobe; *IS*, Isthmus; *TR*, Trachea; *CA*, Carotid (primitive).

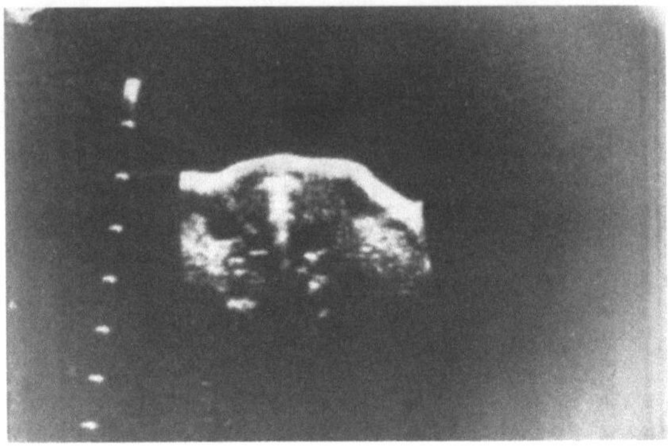

Fig. 2. Normal anatomy in a newborn. Transverse section.

geneous echogenicity, are usually symmetrical although occasionally there is a slight predominancy on the right side.

The very narrow isthmus is rarely visible in the foreground of the dense transverse tracheal echogram. Even in newborns, the thyroid is always visible in closely packed transverse sections, but at times it is more difficult to perceive in longitudinal sections. The thickness of the thyroid lobes progressively increases from about 8 mm at birth up to 15–20 mm in the young adult, with the weight of the thyroid increasing from 1.5 to 15 g.

Outside and in front of the thyroid lobes, the sternocleidomastoideus is always visible in the form of an ovoid, very elongated, hypoechogenic structure. Behind the thyroid lobe and outside the tracheal cone shadow, in a transverse section from the interior to the exterior, the long muscle of the neck, more or less egg-shaped and hypoechogenic, can be found, as well as the primitive carotid joined to the internal jugular vein, the caliber of which varies greatly. As in adults, it is between the long muscle of the neck in the rear and the left thyroid lobe in front that the left border of the hypoechogenic esophagus can be seen, which is easily perceived in the form of a rosette, the central echo representing the true cavity of the esophagus.

In the child, neither the parathyroids nor the nerves and vessels which make up the inferior thyroid artery and the recurrent nerve between the thyroid and the long muscle of the neck can be seen. In any case, this structure cannot be confused with a parathyroid adenoma if a parathyroid is considered pathological only when it exceeds 5 mm.

On a longitudinal section, slanting inwards, the thyroid lobe can be seen, roughly ovoid, slender at the ends, and then the image of the hypoechogenic long muscle of the neck, regularly elongated anterior to the spine, and molded to its lordosis. On a longitudinal section the vessels are clearly visible slightly inclined outwards.

2 Thyroid Pathology

Cervical echography, which is simple, provides the clinician with new information especially concerning morphology. In particular, it completes functional information given by the isotope study which has the disadvantage of not being able to be repeated often. This examination is required when confronted with an increase in thyroid volume, especially a goiter. However, it may in fact involve a nodule which in most cases is the thyroid gland but which may sometimes be a cervical mass whose thyroid nature is not clinically evident. Finally, echography can provide much information in certain circumstances where the local clinical examination does not show any anomaly.

2.1 Goiter

Among our patients, goiter is the most frequently required examination. It may be associated with clinical and biological signs of dysfunction of the thyroid. It can be discovered at any age and even in the neonatal period where it is sometimes *hard* to detect because of the cervical morphology in the newborn. In practice, whatever the cause the echographic aspect of a recent benign goiter in the infant is fairly clear: there is a more or less symmetrical and considerable increase in thyroid volume which is also homogeneous and not very dense (Fig. 3). After a period of evolution, the sclerotic, cystic, and hemorrhagic modifications alter the architecture of the gland. Heterogeneous multinodular aspects associating solid, mixed, and liquid nodules are signs of aging of the goiter, which is observed especially in older children (Fig. 4). In order of decreasing frequency we will study the different etiologies of goiter.

2.1.1 Pubertal Goiter

This type of goiter, is 6–9 times more frequent among girls and is moderate, regular, usually symmetrical, and homogeneous. While it is gener-

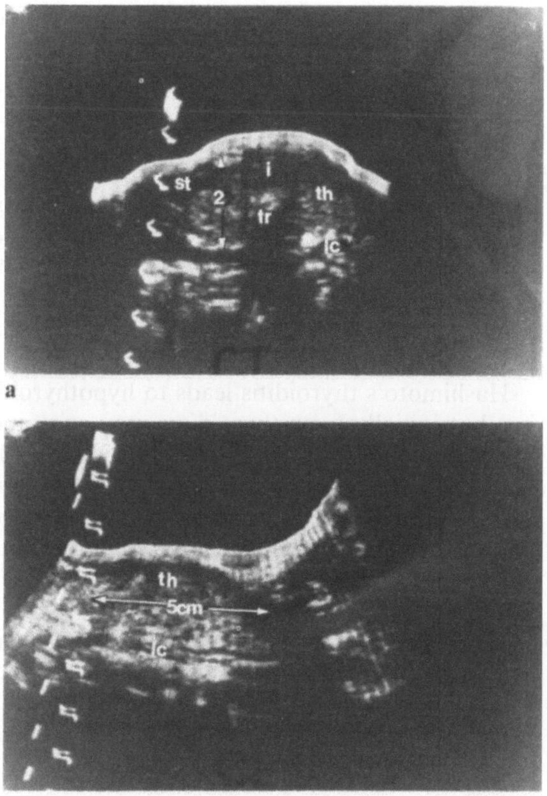

Fig. 3 a and b. Congenital goiter in a boy of 4 months, hypothyroid. Mother was treated with synthetic antithyroids.
a Transverse section of a homogeneous goiter affecting the isthmus.
b Longitudinal section of left lobe.

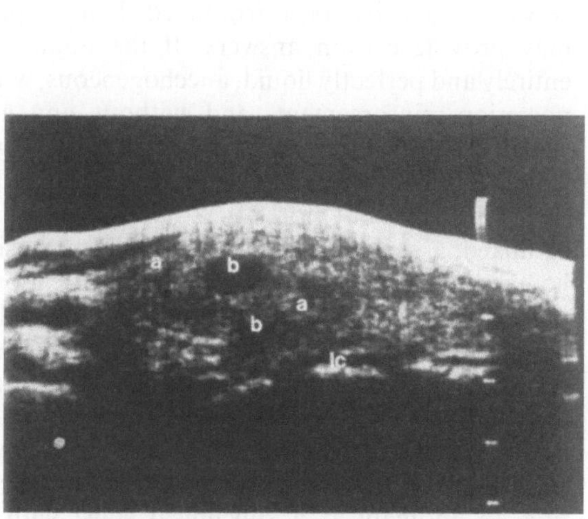

Fig. 4. Longitudinal section of a multinodular goiter in a 16-year-old girl. It is an old endemic goiter whose structure is modified, with compact nodules in the form of a resotte surrounded by a light halo *(a)* and semiliquid nodules without posterior reinforcement *(b)*.

ally isolated, it may be associated with minor signs of hyperthyroid. Its active evolutions is about 2 years. The sclerotic and cystic modifications which lead to non-regressive after-effects are most frequently found in the largest goiters.

2.1.2 Endemic Goiter

Usually euthyroid, most frequent in girls, it appears prior to puberty, at around 4–5 years of age and is rarely seen from birth. Iodine deficiency is the primary cause but nutritional problems and genetic predisposition may often be associated. The goiter initially has a homogeneous echostructure but may undergo an abrupt outburst at puberty and become nodular, cystic, or hemorrhagic.

2.1.3 Family-Linked Goiter, Hereditary Due to Hormonogenesis Disorders

The clinical and echographic appearance may highly resemble an endemic goiter. In severe forms, with hypothyroidism, it generally appears earlier, before the age of 2 years. Goiter, which is observed in Pendred's syndrome and is associated with deaf and dumbness, is initially homogeneous and might then take on a multinodular appearance.

2.1.4 Goiter in the Newborn

It is usually of moderate volume but may occasionally be revealed by a neonatal respiratory distress linked to mechanical compression of the trachea. Here, echography is of utmost importance because it permits distinction between goiter and another cervical mass, e.g., lymphangioma.

It may involve Graves' disease in a newborn whose mother suffered from Graves' disease, a hereditary goiter caused by hormonogenesis disorders, especially a goiter secondary to ingestion by the mother of "goitergeneous" substances during pregnancy (iodine, synthetic antithyroids).

2.1.5 Sporadic Goiter

These goiters for which no cause has been found and which occur outside endemic regions have an identical echographic appearance.

2.2 Thyroiditis (Figs. 5 and 6)

A diffuse increase in volume of the thyroid gland is the first visible symptom of thyroiditis.

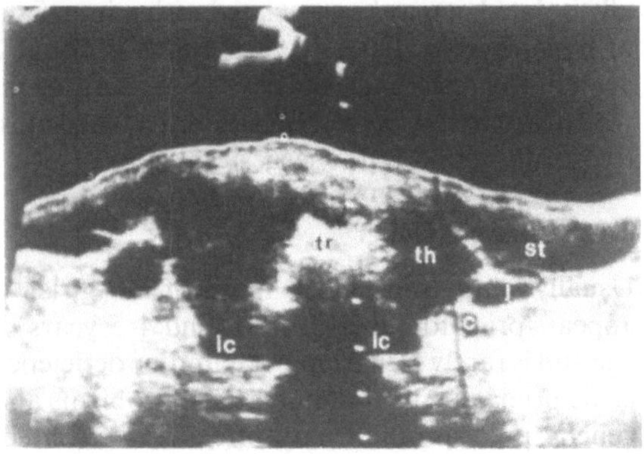

a

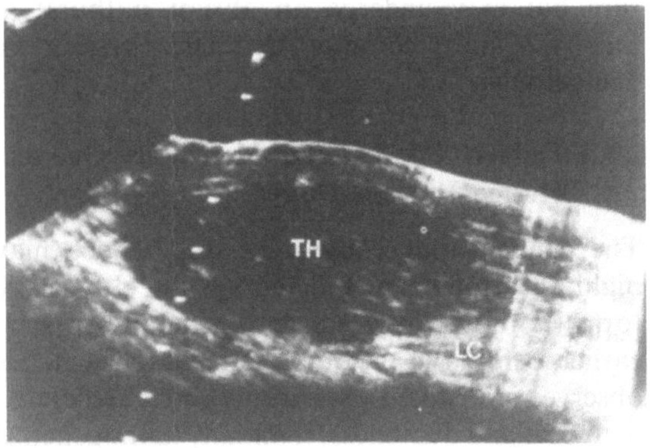

b

Fig. 5 a and b. Hashimoto's thyroiditis in a young adult. **a** Transversal section. **b** Left longitudinal section. Hypoechogenic structure of the thyroid resembling the muscles.

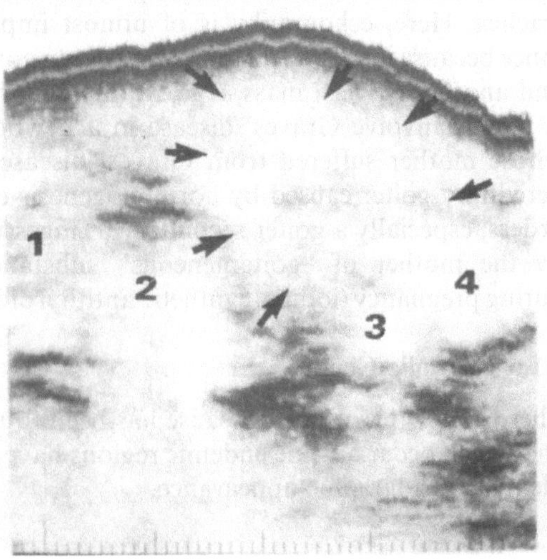

Fig. 6. Thyroiditis: localized form, in a 3.5-year-old child. Transverse section showing left cervical swelling, inflammatory; large hypoechogenic left lobe (*arrows*). *1*, Right thyroid lobe; *2*, Trachea; *3*, Left carotid; *4*, Left jugular vein.

In children, it is usually chronic juvenile lymphocytic thyroiditis or Hashimoto's thyroiditis as a response to an autoimmune mechanism chiefly observed in young girls of all ages, but particularly between 2 and 15 years, with a peak of frequency at 10 years. The echographic appearance is highly characteristic: the goiter is generally small, homogeneous, sometimes sensitive, even painful and above all hypoechogenic, and of the same echogenicity as the sternocleidomastoid muscle. It may evolve toward a modification of the thyroid structure and become more heterogeneous.

Hashimoto's thyroiditis leads to hypothyroidism but initially hyperthyroidism may exist and echography helps a great deal in the diagnosis. It may also sometimes be difficult to distinguish it from a tumoral process such as lymphoma especially since some ganglions may be found in both cases, but the lymphoid thyroid is generally much more lumpy.

De Quervain's subacute thyroiditis, which is rare in children, has the same appearance: moderate hypoechogenic goiter, either diffuse or localized, usually leading to restitutio ad integrum.

2.3 Thyroid Nodule

Thyroid nodule is rare in pediatric pathology. The question raised is its benignity or malignancy: 20%–40% of unique nodules in children are malignant, i.e., four times more frequent than in adults. This percentage is higher if the child's cervical region has been irradiated. Echography may provide certain answers. If the nodule is entirely and perfectly liquid, anechogeneous, with posterior reinforcement, and without any associated solid element whatsoever, even at high gain the diagnosis is that of a cyst with a benignity of 99% (Fig. 7), but more often the nodule is solid or mixed, associating a solid and liquid necrosis, hemorrhage or cysts (Figs. 8–10). Calcifications are visible in benign and malignant nodules. The hypoechogenic halo surrounding a solid nodule was originally considered to be benign until it was shown that certain neoplasms also had this halo.

Echography offers within this context two possibilities owing to its high sensitivity of detecting an anomaly at a subclinical stage with a diameter of 3–4 mm. The discovery of other nodules next to the palpated nodule raises the question of multinodular goiter in which malignancy is less frequently encountered. On the contrary, the discovery of regional lymphoid struc-

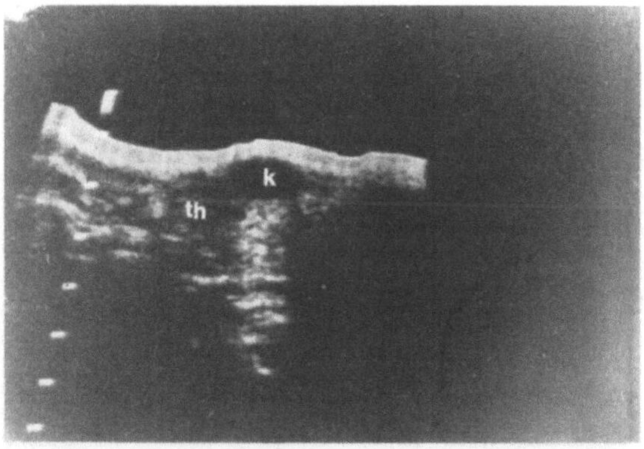

a

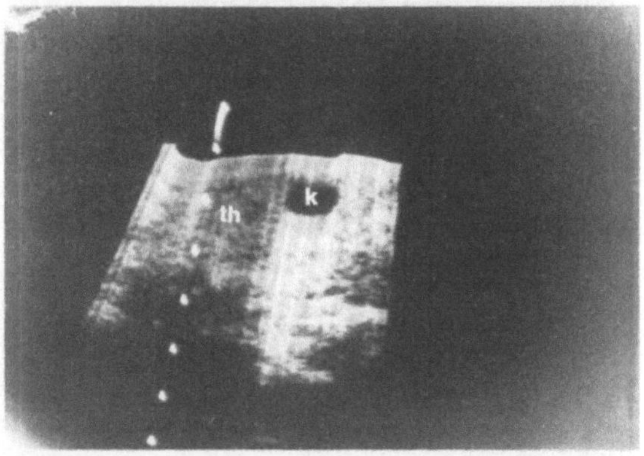

b

Fig. 7 a and b. Cyst *(K)*. Longitudinal section at increasing gain (b > a)
a Small liquid nodule and **(b)** same at high gain.

tures makes the nodules highly suspect of being malignant. Echography is the most efficient examination in the search for small thyroid nodules while assessing the cervical adenopathies which appear to be isolated.

Echography's major limit is its lack of specificity in differential diagnosis of benignity and malignancy. The cytologic puncture, which is essentially guided by echography and used when nodules appear solid or mixed and cold at the scintigraphy test, may improve the diagnosis and allow a better selection of surgical indications.

Fig. 8 a–d. Mixed nodule: differential diagnosis of cyst. ▶
a Transverse section at usual gain; **b** Transverse section at high gain; **c** Left longitudinal section at usual gain; **d** Left longitudinal section at high gain. This young patient underwent a right hemithyroidectomy 6 months earlier. A cold isolated nodule appears on the remaining lobe. On sections with usual gain (**a** and **c**), the lesion resembles a cyst: an echogenic nodule *(K)* with small posterior reenhancement *(arrow)*. When increasing the gain (**b** and **d**), a solid, evident component appears *(S)*. It is a papillary cancer.

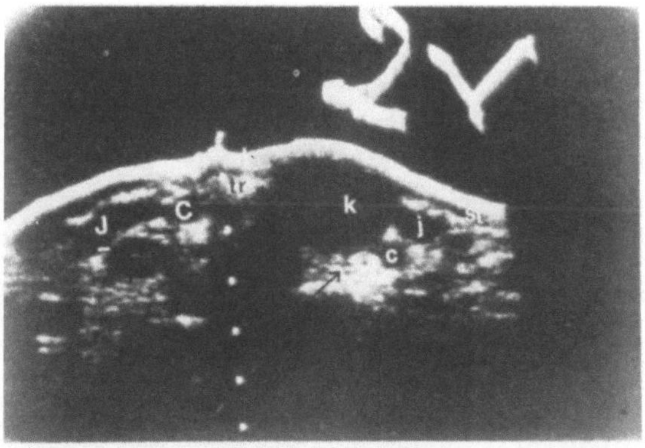

a

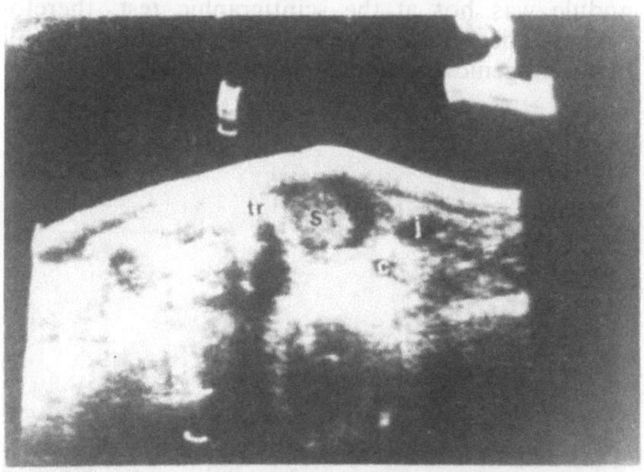

b

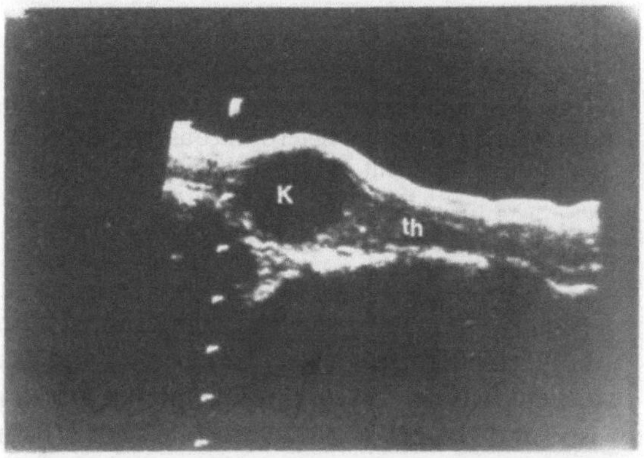

c

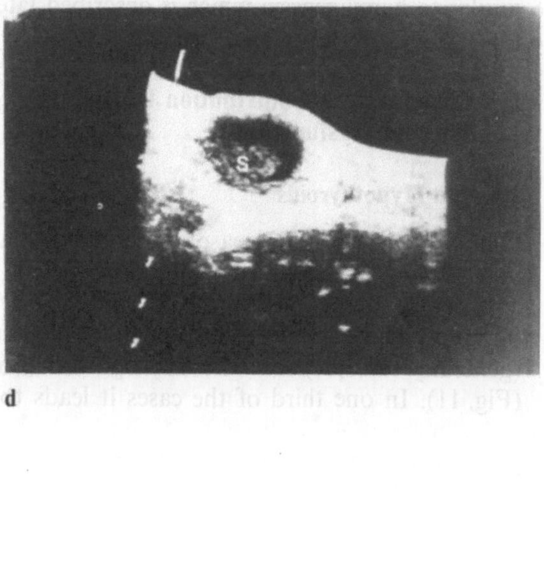

d

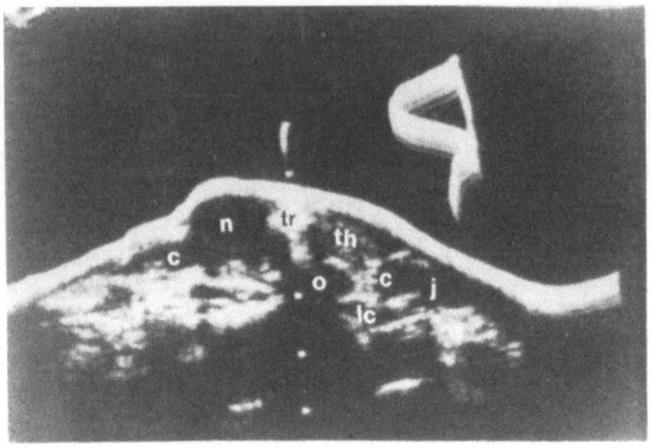

Fig. 9. Solid thyroid nodule in a 7-years-old girl The nodule was hot at the scintigraphic test, therefore benign (adenoma). Transverse section shows a solid hypoechogenic and homogeneous nodule.

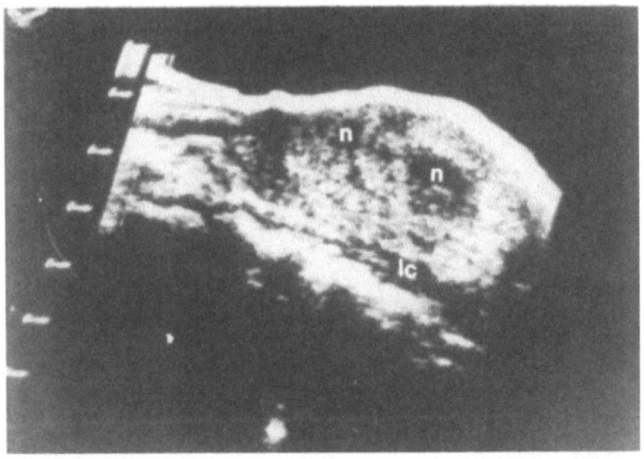

Fig. 10. Mixed nodule in a 6-year-old girl. Longitudinal section showing mixed heterogeneous nodule with a semiliquid component of hemorrhagic necrosis *(n)*.

Finally, after the operation, echography, being totally harmless, may easily be repeated and is an excellent way of surveying the remaining thyroid tissue and the cervical region. Following a hemithyroidectomy, the cervical morphology is similar to hemiagenesia which is described later.

2.4 Echography's Contribution During Thyroid Dysfunctions

2.4.1 In Hypothyroids

Echography may in this case contribute to diagnose etiology. In two thirds of the cases it leads to agenesis or dysgenesis of the thyroid: the echography discovers little or no thyroid tissue (generally ectopic) on the thyroglossal tract (Fig. 11). In one third of the cases it leads to a

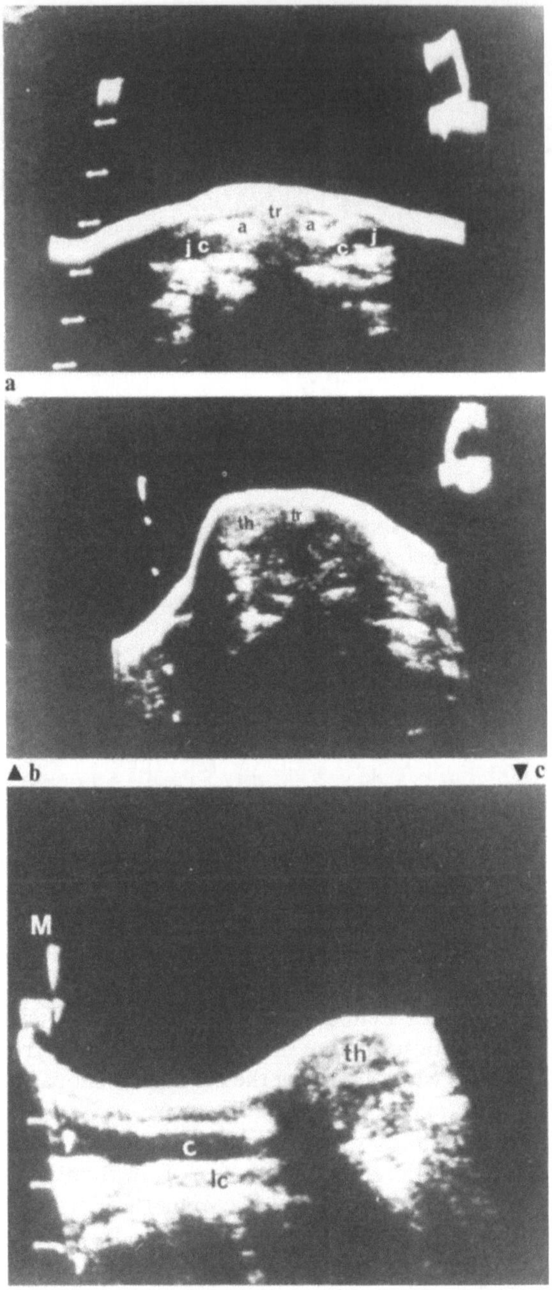

Fig. 11 a–c. Ectopic thyroid in a 5-year-old girl. An upper lateral and median cervical mass on the right side. **a** Transverse section through the usual center of the thyroid lodges (1 cm above the sternal manubrium). Absence of thyroid tissue in normal location: the site of the thyroid lodges is occupied by small gatherings of echoeas *(a)* which are not very precise. The carotids *(c)* are more internal than normal.
b Transverse section 4 cm above sternal manubrium. Palpated mass *(th)* corresponds to a homogeneous tubular structure.
c Longitudinal section through the right mass. Palpated mass *(th)* is located 5 cm from the sternal manubrium *(M)*. The carotid *(c)* is more internal than normal, anterior to the long neck muscle (lc).

hormonogenesis disorder: echography shows the thyroid gland as normally located or voluminous.

2.4.2 In Hyperthyroids

As described above, it may involve a hyperthyroid which has been transmitted by a basedowian mother: Basedow's or Graves' disease in a newborn or young infant is transitory, from 3 to 5 weeks; sometimes it lasts longer and may evolve over 2 years. The thyroid may be of normal volume or be the center of a generally moderate goiter.

Hyperthyroidism in an adolescent is often linked to Graves' disease, which might be locally associated with a goiter with two possible kinds of echostructure: either it is hypoechogenic, which raises the problem of differential diagnosis with thyroiditis at an early stage, or it is a goiter of normal or increased but homogeneous echogenicity. Less frequently an isolated, toxic adenoma is involved or an adenoma located within a goiter (sometimes plurinodular).

Echography provides a solution to the scintigraphic problem of a nodule which takes up the entire isotope in such a way that other nodules are not perceived. However, in echography, thyroid parenchyma is found exterior to the fixing region. Or is it a thyroid hemiagenesia? This congenital anomaly which affects little less than 1% of the population is easy to recognize: one thyroid lodge (mostly the left one) is small, without tissular echo and the important homolateral vessels are closer to the median line (Fig. 12).

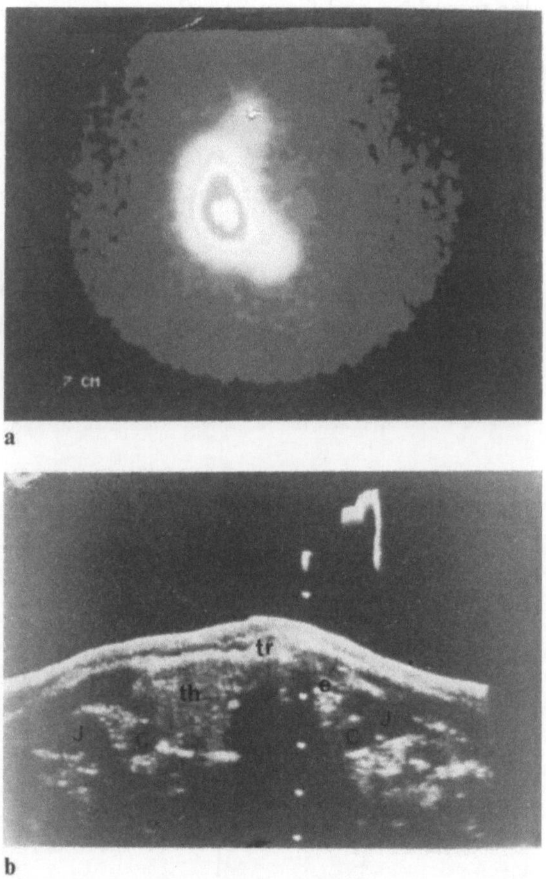

Fig. 12 a and b. Thyroid hemiagenesia.
a Scintigraphy with limited fixation of right lobe. Either a nodule or a hemi-agenesia takes up the entire isotope.
b Transverse section: right thyroid lobe is normal. Left thyroid lodge is very small and is occupied by some vague echoes *(e)*. The left carotid and jugular are closer to the median line anterior to the long neck muscle.

3 Parathyroid Pathology

Hyperparathyroidism in children is rare: it may be a primary or secondary hyperparathyroidism in chronic hypocalcemia or hypomagnesemia. Anatomically, hyperparathyroidism may be a response to an adenoma or hyperplasia which can be surgically treated.

Echography is an easy and efficient examination to locate certain elements before surgery. It permits recognition of one or several parathyroids which are increased in volume, the largest of which are more than 5 mm. A pathological parathyroid is perceived in the form of an oblong mass on the vertical axis; it is less echogenic than the thyroid tissue and generally separated from it by a dense fascia. It might lead to a cyst. This mass is located posterior to one thyroid lobe which is anterior to the long muscle of the neck and inside the primitive carotid (Fig 13). Here, the problem is to diagnose the physiological structures: the left side of the esophagus, the long muscle of the neck, and the inferior thyroid artery.

The limit of detection is the pathological parathyroid smaller than 5 mm and its unusual retroesophageal and mediastinal locations.

4 Other Cervical Masses

Echography may be of importance in diagnosing nonthyroid palpable cervical masses. This diagnosis is often made when confronted with the

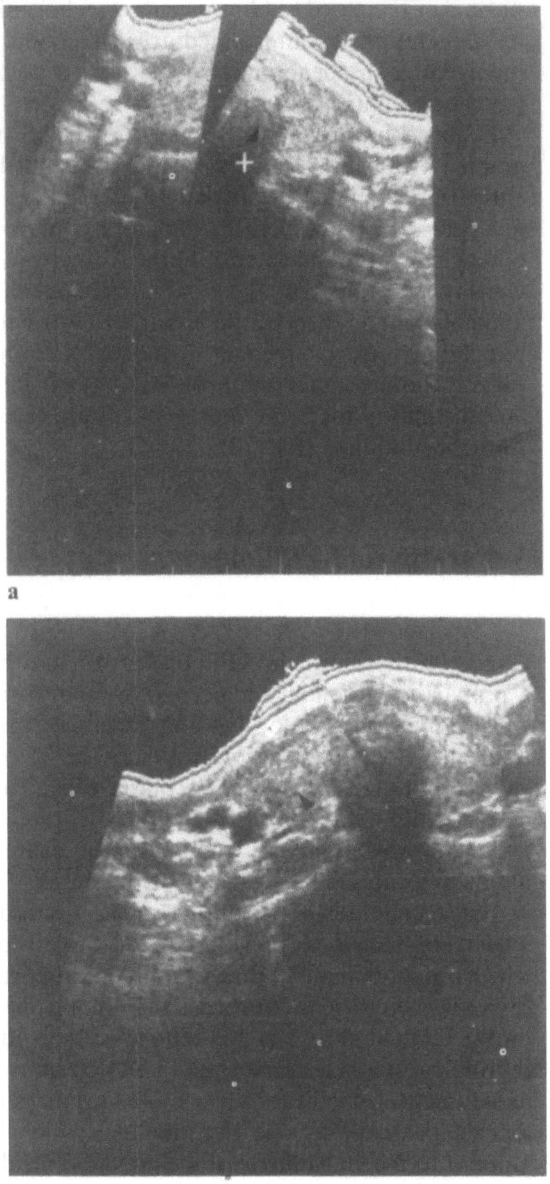

a

b

Fig. 13 a and b. Renal deficiency and tertiary hyperparathyroidism in a 15-year-old. Transverse sections. Appearance of a right parathyroid adenoma on the remaining parathyroid, the other three having been removed. The hypoechogenic nodule on the inside of the vascular bundle in front of the long neck muscle.

clinical aspect of the lesion: date of appearance, median or lateral topography, anterior or posterior to the sternocleidomastoid muscle, fistula or no fistula, positive transillumination. The contribution of echography is to distinguish these masses from the thyroid to which they may adhere and to approach the etiological diagnosis by analyzing the echostructure.

A lesion which is discovered at birth evokes, of course, a congenital anomaly which, however, may be revealed later, sometimes in the form of an inflammatory mass. Among these anomalies, two thirds are cysts of the thyroglossal tract and about one third are branchial cysts. Cystic lymphangiomas are exceptional.

4.1 Cysts of the Thyroglossal Tract

Diagnosis of the cyst is obvious when palpating a small mass which moves when swallowing, when it is median located along the thyroglossal tract at the same level as the hyoid bone, and when a fistulous trace is found on the skin.

Echography confirms the liquid nature of the mass and gives an objective view of the thyroid which is found in its normal location (Fig. 14). The echostructure may be more heterogeneous due to sudden and frequent inflammations, usu-

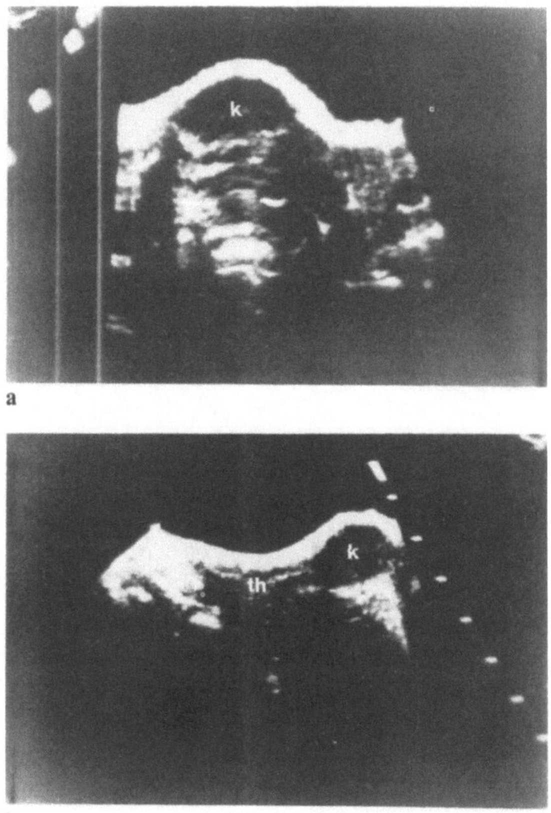

a

b

Fig. 14 a and b. Thyroglossal cyst in an infant of 5 months with a median inflammatory mass of the neck. **a** Transverse section above the thyroid. Liquid mass (*K*) with posterior reinforcement; it contains some echoes due to the acute infection.
b Oblique longitudinal section. The cyst is located above the normal thyroid (*th*).

ally occurring around 4–5 years of age. Generally, it is of moderate volume, 1–2 cm in diameter, sometimes more.

If there is no fistulous trace, the differential diagnosis is that of a dermoid cyst (Fig. 15), which is movable with the skin and of variable echostructure mostly solid and heterogeneous, or a lipoma which is rare and usually has an echogenic strata parallel to the cutaneous plane (Fig. 16). In all these cases the thyroid is normally located which permits distinction from ectopic thyroids where ablation is particularly disastrous.

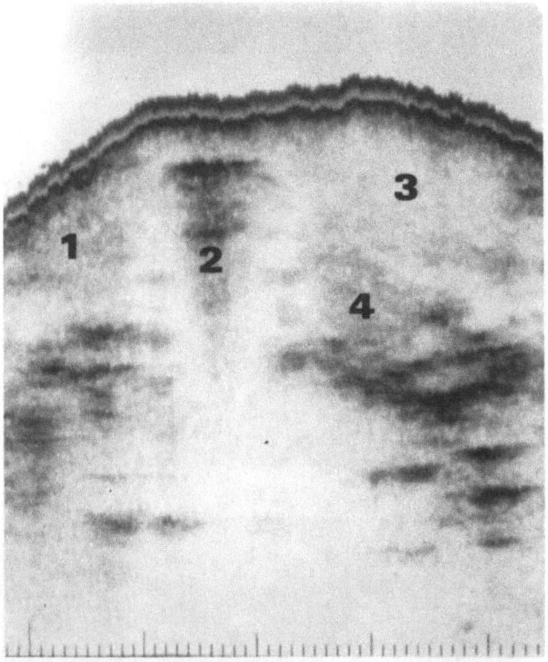

Fig. 15. Epidermoid cyst in a 6-year-old child. Appearance of a lateral cervical mass on the left side increasing rapidly in volume, clinically closely linked to the thyroid. Transverse section: an echogenic, homogeneous mass clearly defined in front of the left thyroid lobe from which it is separated.
1, Right thyroid lobe; *2*, Trachea; *3*, Tumor; *4*, Thyroid lobe.

4.2 Branchial Cysts

This abnormality of the second branchial arch is usually revealed much later. The echographic aspect is the same as the cyst of the thyroglossal tract, but the branchial cyst is more lateral, in front of the middle third of the sternocleidomastoid muscle. The existence of a cutaneous opening helps diagnosis and permits opacification which provides a better preoperative assessment of the extension. If discovered during an infection of the upper airways, it must not be confused with a lymph node: a solid hypoechogenic mass, mostly polycyclical and located around the vessels.

4.3 Cystic Lymphangiomas (Figs. 17 and 18)

The diagnosis is already suspected when confronted with the clinical aspects. The mass may be voluminous and in 90% of the cases is located posterior to the sternocleidomastoid muscle, in the supraclavicular dimple. It may overlap the median line and continue to the jaw angle or the shoulder. The cystic aspect of this mass, which is firm, sometimes soft and transilluminating, may be confirmed by echography. The lesion is generally made up of several cysts of different size separated by septa (more or less thin) and sometimes associating lymphoid structures (Fig. 17). A solid component may also be present (Fig. 18).

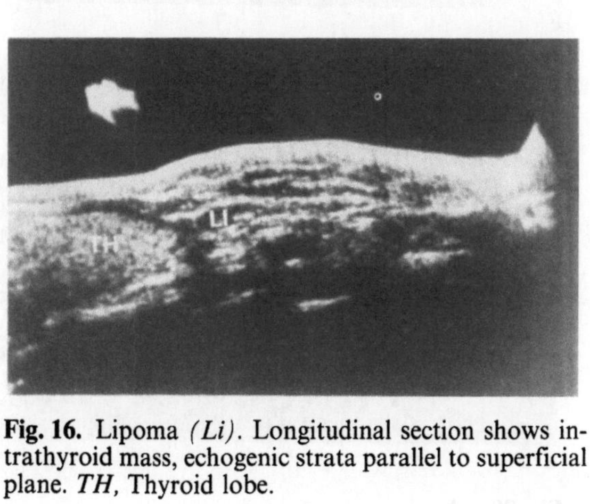

Fig. 16. Lipoma *(Li)*. Longitudinal section shows intrathyroid mass, echogenic strata parallel to superficial plane. *TH*, Thyroid lobe.

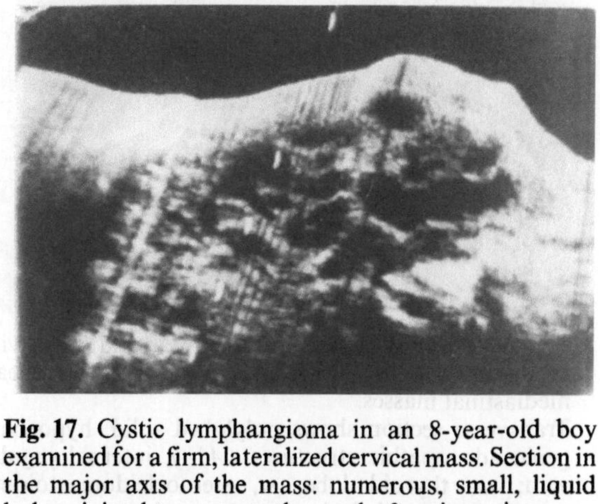

Fig. 17. Cystic lymphangioma in an 8-year-old boy examined for a firm, lateralized cervical mass. Section in the major axis of the mass: numerous, small, liquid lodges joined to one another and of various sizes.

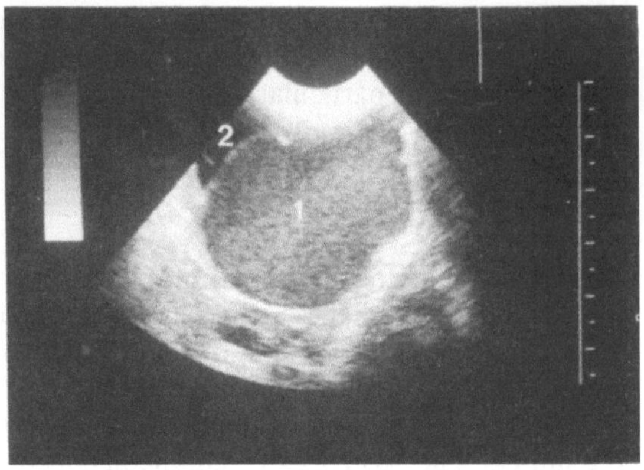

Fig. 18. Cavernous hemolymphangioma. Newborn, respiratory distress with laryngopharangeal compression caused by a voluminous submaxillary bluish tumor on the left side. Mixed mass with a solid mass *(1)* and liquid cavities *(2)*.

4.4 Malignant Cervical Tumors Exterior to the Thyroid

It is considered that one cervical mass out of seven in children is malignant – mostly lymphoid, particularly in the case of Hodgkin's disease or non-Hodgkin's lymphomas. It may involve an isolated or multiple mass which is usually located in the posterior cervical triangle of the sternocleidomastoid muscle. The echographic structure of these masses is usually the polycyclical and hypoechogenic lymph node surrounding the internal jugular vein (Fig. 19).

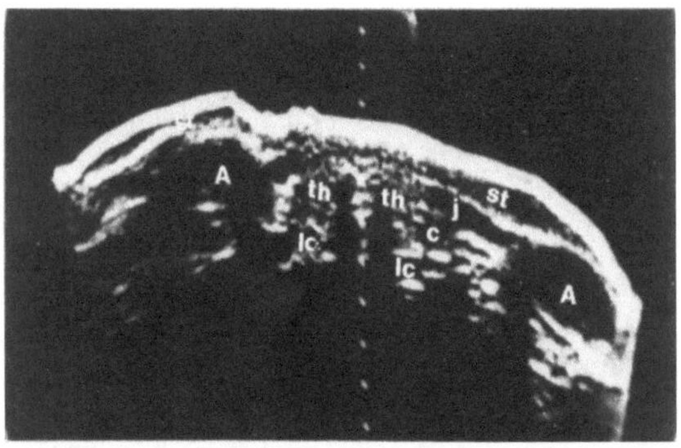

Fig. 19. Cervical masses in a 13-year-old boy with Hodgkin's disease. Radiography of thorax reveals mediastinal masses.
Transverse section shows polylobed solid, hypoechogenic adenopathic structures *(A)*. *j*, internal jugular vein; *th*, thyroid lobe; *st*, sternocleidomastoideus muscle; *c*, carotid; *lc*, long neck muscle.

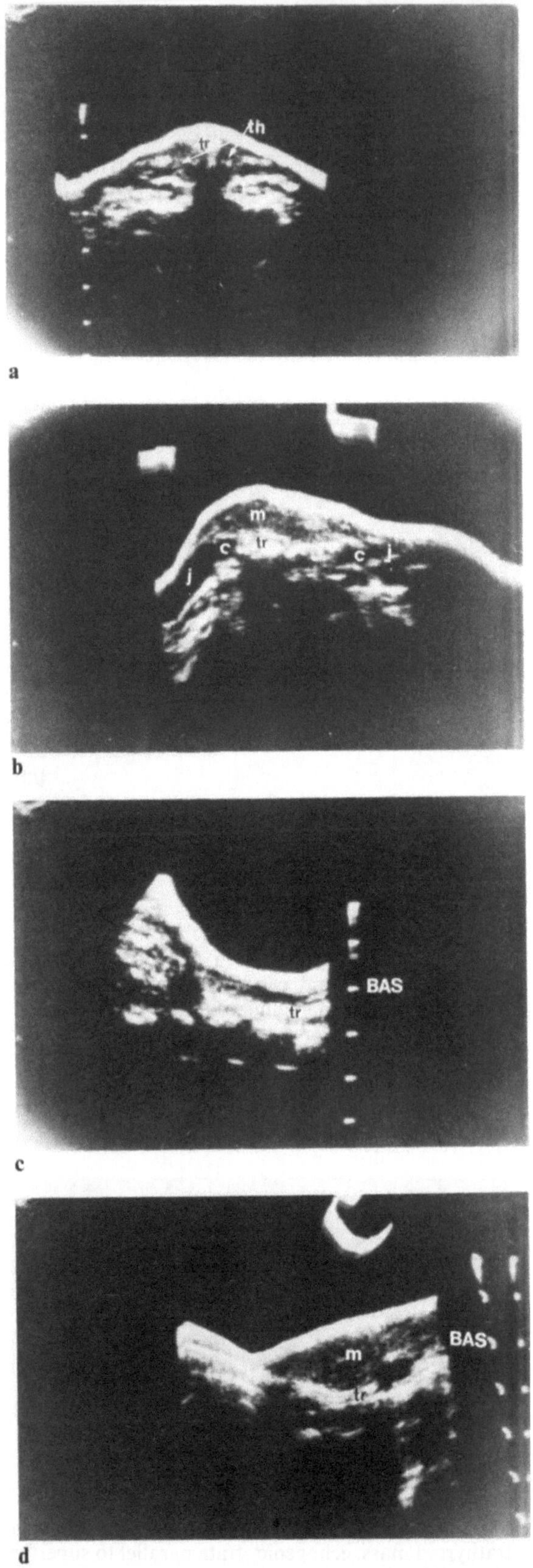

Fig. 20 a–d

4.5 Other Masses

It rarely involves a cervical thymus which moves when breathing; the echographic aspect is a homogeneous solid mass which increases when crying or breathing in (Fig. 20). A sternocleidomastoid mass in a newborn or young infant is most often linked to hematoma in the form of a fusiform liquid or semiliquid collection separating the cervical aponeurosis layers (Fig. 21).

Cervical echography, which is easy to carry out and without risk, provides a precise study of morphology and should play an increasing role in diagnosing cervical pathology in children.

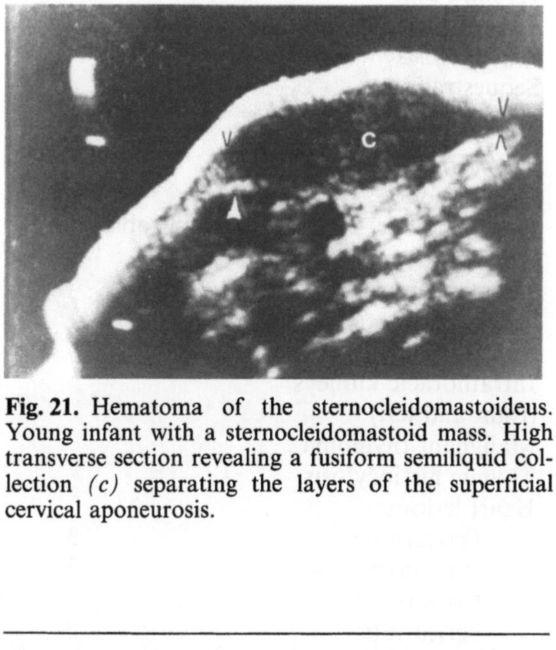

Fig. 21. Hematoma of the sternocleidomastoideus. Young infant with a sternocleidomastoid mass. High transverse section revealing a fusiform semiliquid collection *(c)* separating the layers of the superficial cervical aponeurosis.

◀ **Fig. 20 a–d.** Cervical thymus in a 15-month-old girl. Low median cervical mass appears when crying.
a and b Transverse sections 1 cm above the sternal manubrium: **a** when not crying and **(b)** when crying.
c and d Median longitudinal sections when crying.
In **a** the thyroid is normal and in **c** the median pretracheal *(T)* region is normal.
In **b** and **d** when crying a median, echogenic, homogeneous mass from the mediastinum *(M)* is visible (also not the habitual jugular turgescence).

References

Thyroid

1. Blum M., Passalaqua A.-M., Sackler J.-P., Pudlowski R. (1977). Thyroid echography of subacute thyroiditis. Radiology 125:795–798
2. Bruneton J.-N., Fenart D., Ettore F., Roux F., Abbes M., Demard F., Lapalus F. (1981). Apport de l'échographie en pathologie thyroidienne. JEMU 2:80–83
3. Clark O.-H., Okerlund M.-D., Cavalieri R.-R., Greenspan F.-S. (1979). Diagnosis and treatment of thyroid, parathyroid and thyroglossal duct cysts. J. Clin. Endocr. Metab. 48:983–988
4. Job J.-C., Pierson M. (1978). Endocrinologie pédiatrique et croissance. Flammarion Médecine Science. Paris
5. Sackler J.-P., Passalaqua A.-M., Blum M., Amorocho L. (1977). A spectrum of diseases of the thyroid gland as imaged by Gray Scale Water Bath Sonography. Radiology 125:467–472
6. Scheible M., Leopold G.-R., Woo V.-L., Gosink B.-B. (1979). High-resolution real time ultrasonography of thyroid nodules. Radiology 133:413–417
7. Van Herle A.-J., Rich P.-J., Britt-Marie Ljung, Ashcraft M.-W., Solomon D.-H., Emmet B., Keeler Ph. (1982). The thyroid nodule. Annals of Internal Medicine 96:221–232
8. Zollikofer Ch. L., Frank Th., Wewerka J. (1978). Ultrasonic evaluation of "Silent Regions" in the thyroid scintiscan. Nucl. Med. 17:16–23

Parathyroid

9. Moreau J.-F., Dubost C., Buy J.-N., Ferry J. (1981). Dépistage ultrasonographique pré-opératoire des adénomes parathyroidiens. Nouv. Presse Méd. 23:1923–1927
10. Willi U., Wieland P., Rickham P.-P., Otto R. (1982). Diagnostic ultrasonographique d'un adénome parathyroidien et d'un calcul rénal chez une fille de 15 ans. Ann. Radiol. 25:146–150

Cervical Masses

11. Bertin P., Pellerin D. (1982). Chirurgie de la tête et de cou. "In Pédiatrie" (Mozziconacci P. et Saudubray J.-M.). Flammarion Médecine Science. Paris
12. Pounds L.-A. (1981). Neck masses of congenital origin. Pediatrics clinics of North America. 28 (4):841–844
13. Zitelli B.-J. (1981). Neck masses in children. Adenopathy and malignant cells. Pediatrics clinics of North America. 28 (4):813–841

Chapter 4

Chest

L. Garel, D. Pariente, and D. Lallemand

Ultrasonography has some limitations for chest examinations because aerated lungs and bony thorax interfere with sound transmission. On this topic the literature is poor; by reference to our cases we would like to stress the indications and the limitations of chest sonography.

1 Material

The cases studied are indicated in the following list:

Chest wall lesions		
Breast abscess		2
Breast calcified fibroma		1
Breast lipoma		2
Breast hypertrophy		1
Chest wall lipoma		4
Chest wall lymphangioma		3
Chest wall hamartoma		2
Chest wall hematoma		1
Costal Ewing's tumor		3
Diaphragmatic lesions		
Diaphragm hypoplasia		10
Phrenic paralysis		1
(subphrenic abscess)		11
Pleural lesions		
Fluid collection (6 loculated collections)		13
Thickened pleura		2
Pleural malignant tumor (rhabdomyosarcoma, embryonic tumor)		2
Parenchymal lesions		
Hydatid cyst		14
Pulmonary consolidation		3
Aspergillosis		1
Sequestration		1
Hamartoma		1
Mediastinal lesions		
Lymph nodes (3 lymphomas, 2 metastatic nephroblastomas)		7
Normal thymus		6
Thymic hemorrhage (postcardiac surgery)		1
Superior vena cava ectasia		1
Intrathoracic kidneys (right and left)		2
Malignant thymoma		1
Thymic histiocytosis		1
Heart lesions		8
– Pericarditis	3	
– Rhabdomyoma	3	
– Constrictive pericarditis	2	
Lymphangioma (1 diagnosis in utero)		4
Pericardial cyst		2
Bronchogenic cyst		3
Neurenteric cyst		1
Neurogenic tumors		7
– Neuroblastomas	2	
– Ganglioneuromas	3	
– Meningocele	1	
– Neurofibroma	1	

2 Technique

We have mainly had experience with static B scanning. A 5-MHz short-focus transducer with a small contact surface is necessary. Patients are scanned by subcostal approach with cephalad angulation, by intercostal approach, and by supraclavicular and suprasternal approach with caudad angulation. Marked inspiration is often helpful in older children. Pressure on the ribs caused by the transducer is often very unpleasant, and it is advisable for the operator to delineate the intercostal space with his free hand to keep the cooperation of the child.

Various scanning positions are often useful: supine, prone, lateral decubitus, sitting, and upright. Double exposure may provide some information on the diaphragm mobility. Real-time scanning does simplify the understanding of the motion of the diaphragm, the heart, and the great vessels. Sector scanning in intercostal spaces is possible with no problems.

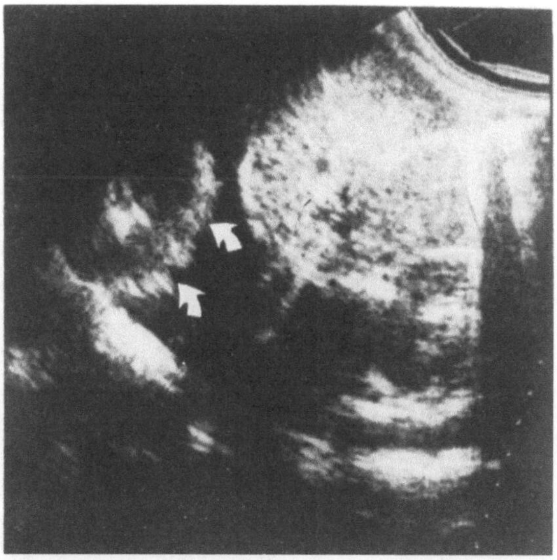

Fig. 1. Complete opacification of the left hemithorax in a 10-year-old boy (supine left subcostal longitudinal scan). Pleural effusion and solid tumor (*arrows*) are well separated (rhabdomyosarcoma).

3 Indications

Ultrasonography is the best procedure to evaluate the diaphragm and the juxta diaphragmatic regions. It is undoubtedly more flexible than computed tomography.

The indications of chest sonography are:
1. Work-up of an opaque hemithorax;
2. Diagnosis, localization of pleural and subphrenic effusions and guidance for aspiration or drainage;
3. Analysis of the echogenicity of lesions of the chest wall, the parenchyma and the mediastinum;
4. Evaluation of the diaphragm and the juxta diaphragmatic regions;
5. Diagnosis of pericardial lesions and intracardiac tumors.

3.1 Opacification of a Hemithorax (Figs. 1 and 2)

US examination is useful in discriminating solid tumor or parenchymal consolidation from pleural effusion.

3.2 Pleural Effusions (Figs. 3 and 4)

First, the diaphragm has to be recognized to differentiate pleural and subphrenic collections of fluid. A large pleural effusion can invert the diaphragm, so that in the supine position the fluid collection appears "in contact" with the kidneys. When the fluid collection is loculated, ultrasonography helps to localize it and guides the pleural tap or the thoracocentesis (six cases).

3.3 Analysis of Lesions of the Chest Wall, Parenchyma and Mediastinum

Ultrasonography, just as CT, can assess the extension of a chest wall lesion (Fig. 5). Analysis of the echogenicity of pulmonary and mediastinal masses is possible when there is no air between the mass and the transducer. The posterior echo accentuation, used as a criterion for cystic masses in the abdomen, is not valid in the chest, since the aerated lungs create reverberation artifacts. Hydatid cysts (14 cases, Fig. 6) are very well imaged by ultrasonography. Pulmonary consolidation cannot accurately be differentiated from thickened pleura or from pleural fluids such as chyle, blood, or pus (Fig. 7).

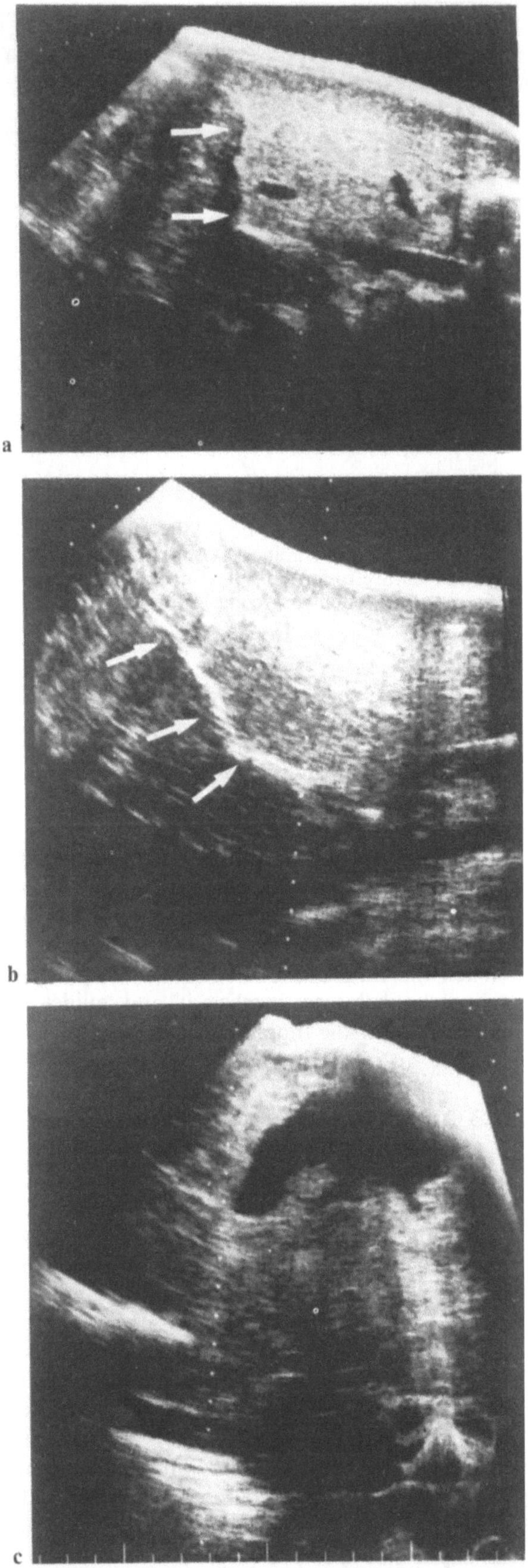

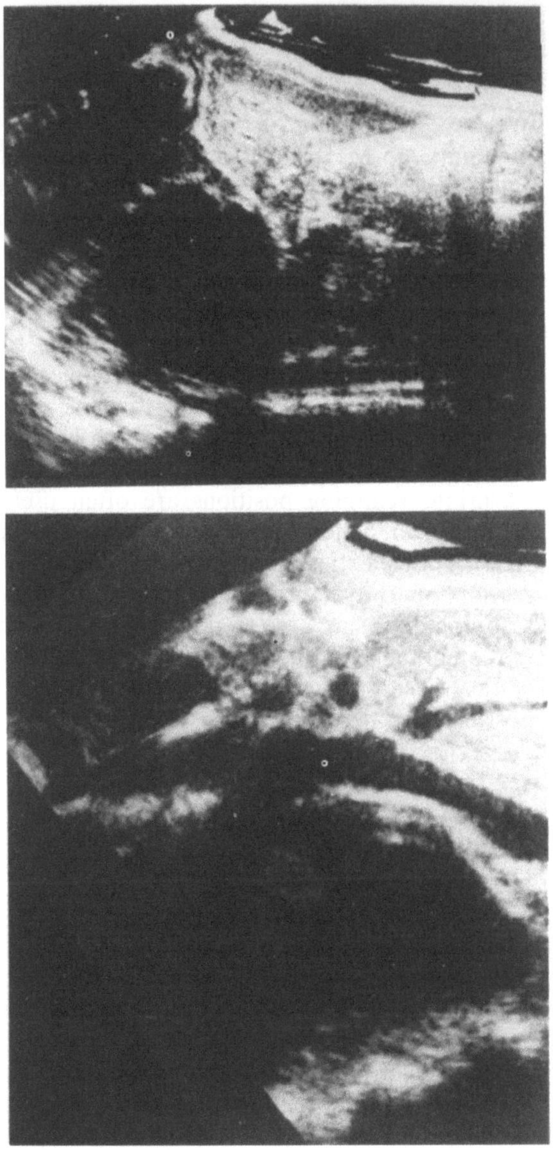

Fig. 3 a–d. Recurrent bilateral chylothorax in a 14-year-old girl.
a Left longitudinal scan: the diaphragm is inverted by the fluid collection. **b** Right longitudinal scan through the inferior vena cava: the diaphragm is also inverted.
c Longitudinal scan through the right kidney: the pleural fluid is "in contact" with the superior pole of the kidney.
d Transverse epigastric scan: there is evidence of bilateral pleural effusion (*arrows*).

Fig. 2 a–c. Complete opacification of the right hemithorax in an 11-year-old boy.
a Right subcostal longitudinal scan through the inferior vena cava (*arrow*). **b** Right subcostal longitudinal scan through the right kidney (*arrow*). **c** Intercostal transverse scan. Inversion of the hemidiaphragm by a supradiaphragmatic mass associated with a minimal pleural effusion (malignant thymoma) (*arrow*).

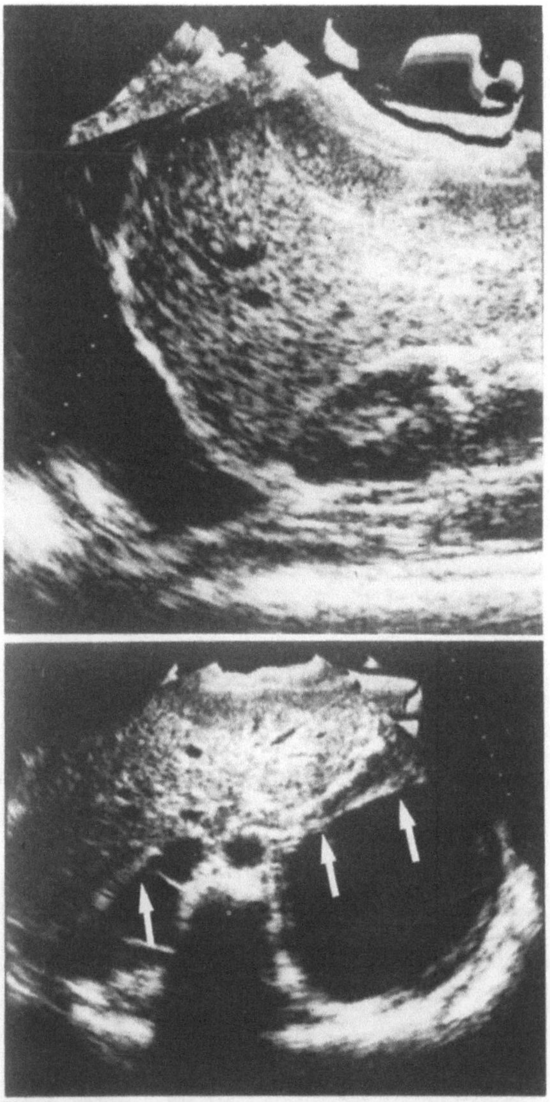

c

d

Fig. 3c and d

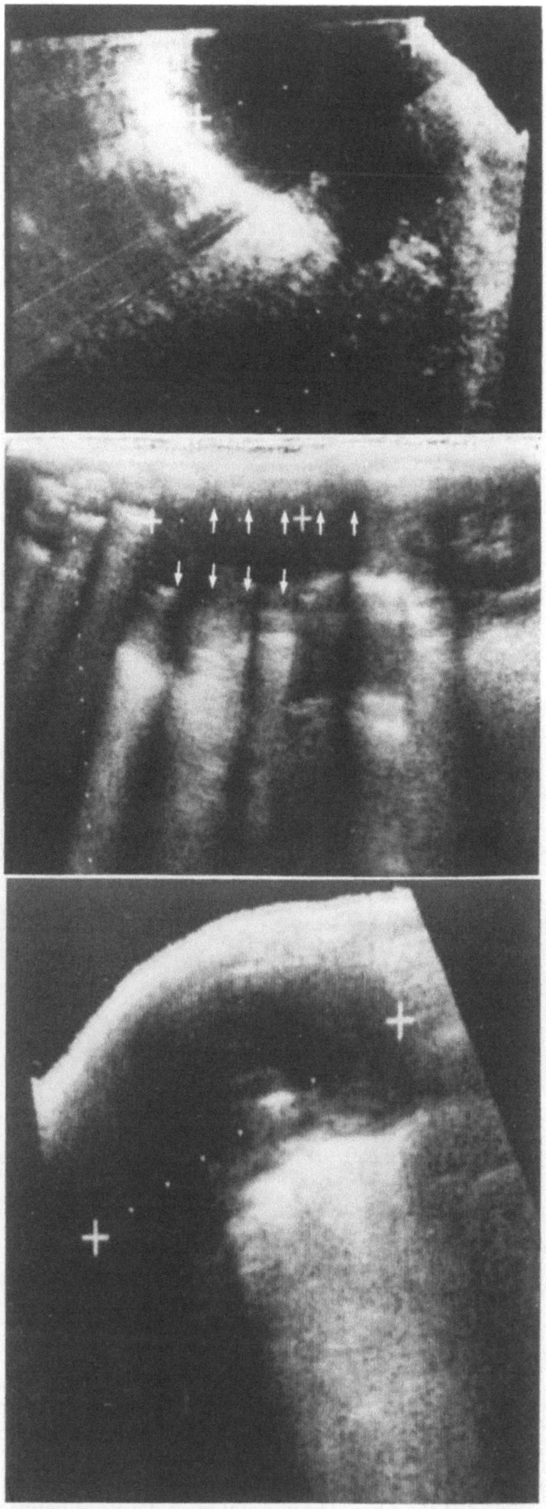

b

c

d

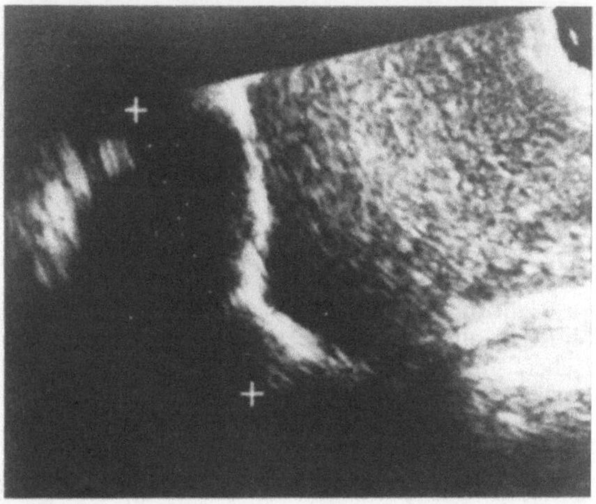

a

Fig. 4 a–d. Loculated pleural effusion following purulent effusion.
a and b Five-year-old child. Two right pockets of fluid remain: one is located just above the diaphragm (**a** right subcostal longitudinal scan) and the other in the 8th right intercostal space (**b** intercostal transverse scan). **c and d** 7-year-old child. **c** Prone longitudinal scan: the remaining pocket is in the left suprarenal region. **d** Prone transverse scan in the intercostal space showing the size of the loculated collection (8 cm).

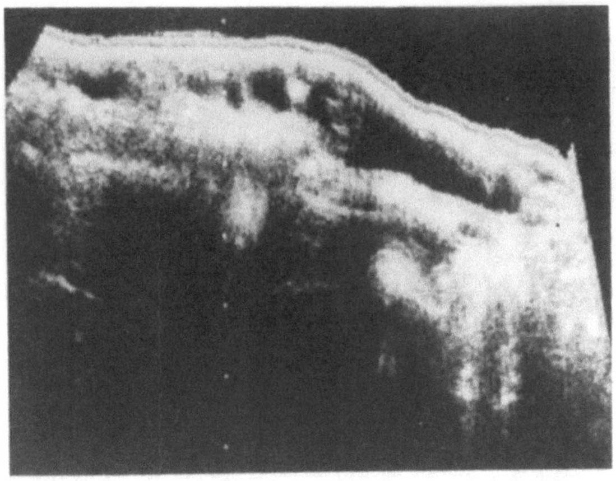

a

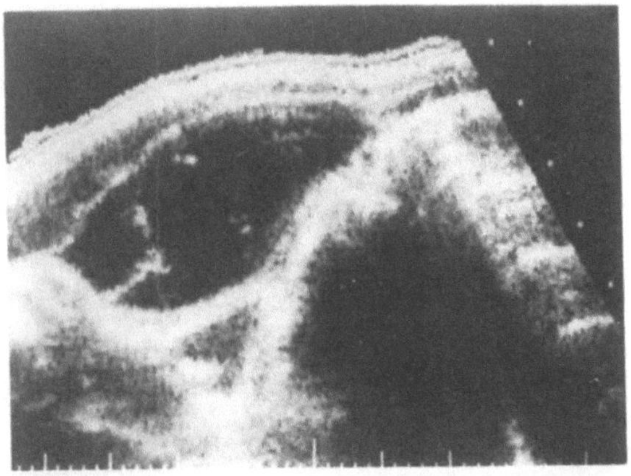

b

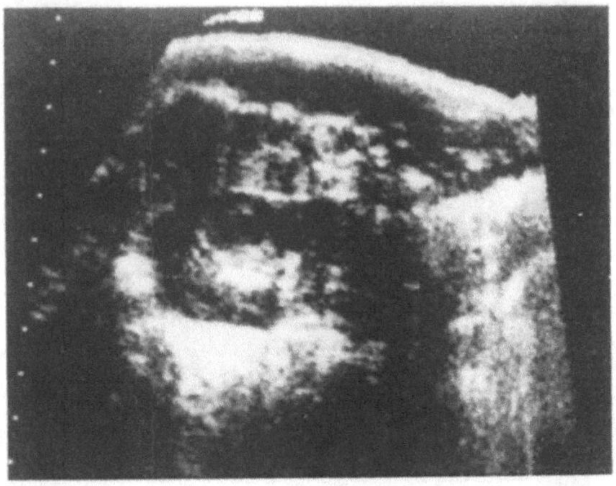

c

Fig. 5 a–c. Chest wall masses.
a and b Three-year-old girl. Lymphangioma of the right chest wall. Longitudinal **(a)** and transverse **(b)** scans show that the mass does not extend over the ribs.
c Three-year-old boy. Costal metastases of an Ewing's tumor of the tibia. The parietal mass develops between the rib and the left kidney (left longitudinal axillary scan).

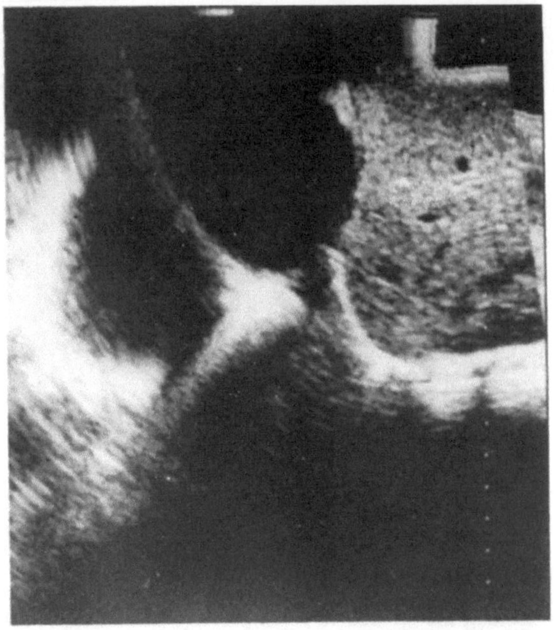

a

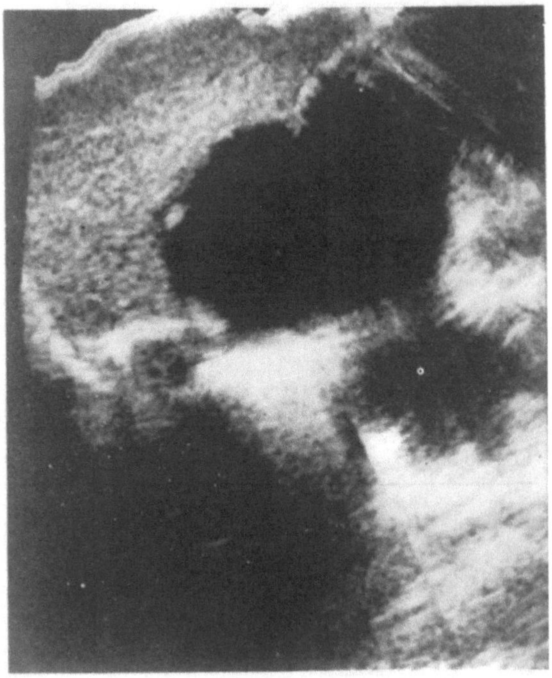

b

Fig. 6 a and b. Four-year-old girl born in North Africa. Opacity of the right lung base.
a Right subcostal longitudinal scan.
b Right subcostal transverse scan.
There are two supradiaphragmatic contiguous cystic masses which are hydatid cysts.

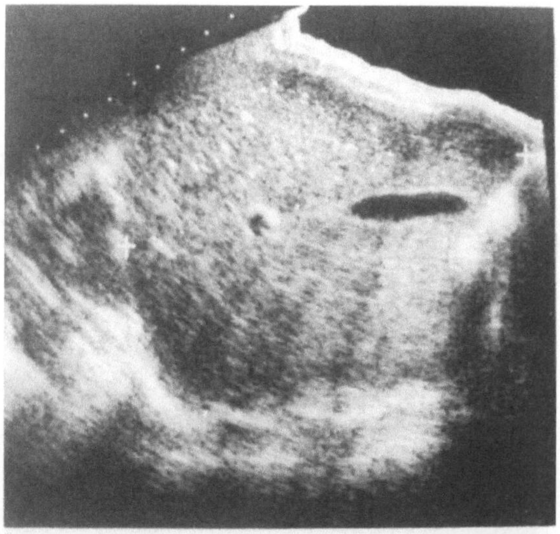

a

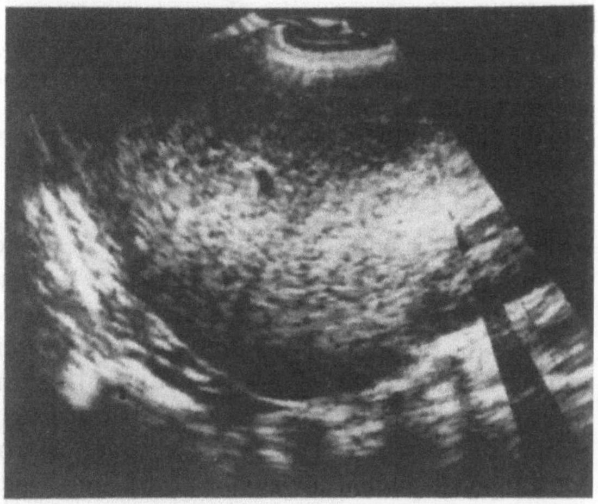

b

Fig. 7 a and b. Pulmonary consolidation.
a Nine-year-old child with immunodeficiency. Right subcostal longitudinal scan through the gallbladder. There is a supradiaphragmatic poorly echogenic mass: consolidation of the right lower lobe.
b Fourteen-year-old boy with hypogammaglobulinemia. Longitudinal scan through the right kidney. The supradiaphragmatic image represents thickening of the pleura plus pulmonary consolidation.

Fig. 8 a–e. Cystic lymphangioma. ▶
a Transverse intercostal scan in a 12-year-old boy: lymphangioma with thick septa in the anterior mediastinum.
b Left longitudinal subcostal scan in the same patient: there is also a pericardial effusion.
c–e 7-year-old boy with a lymphangioma in the posterior mediastinum.
c and d Prone longitudinal scan through the left kidney, the mass measures 14 cm.
e Transverse epigastric scan.
(**d** and **e** see p. 70)

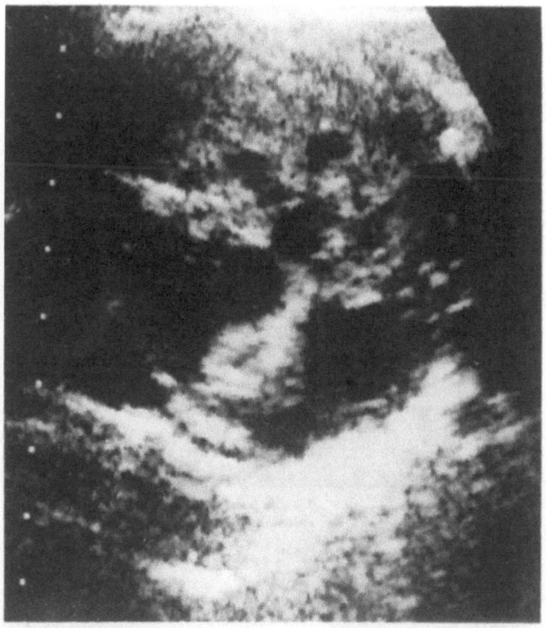

a

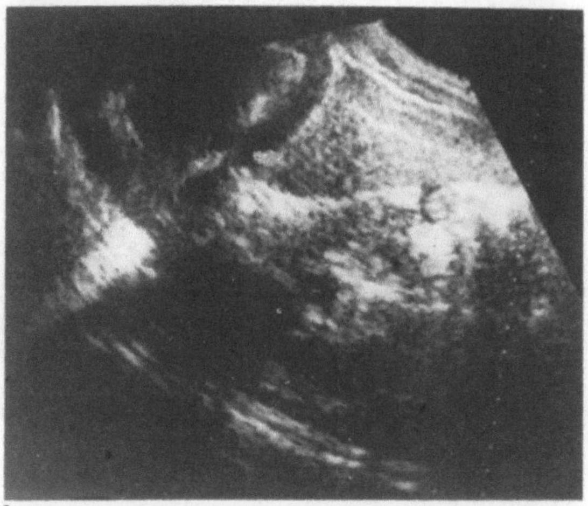

b

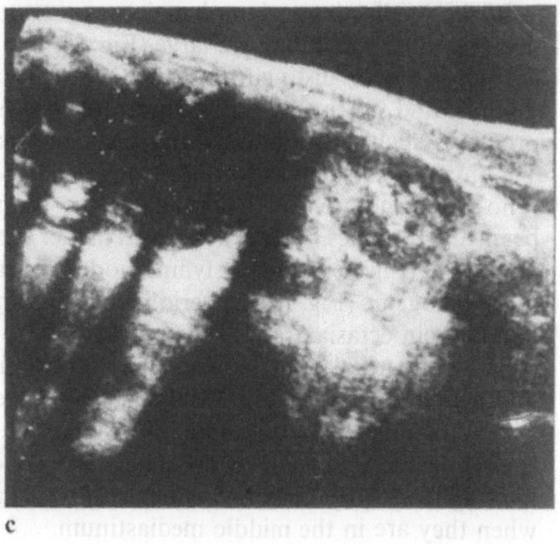

c

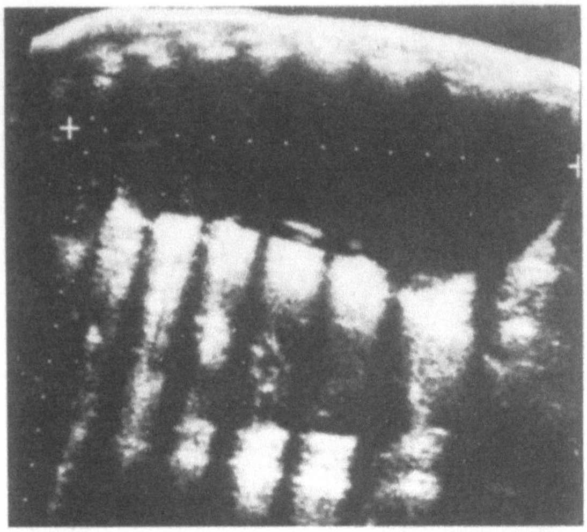

d

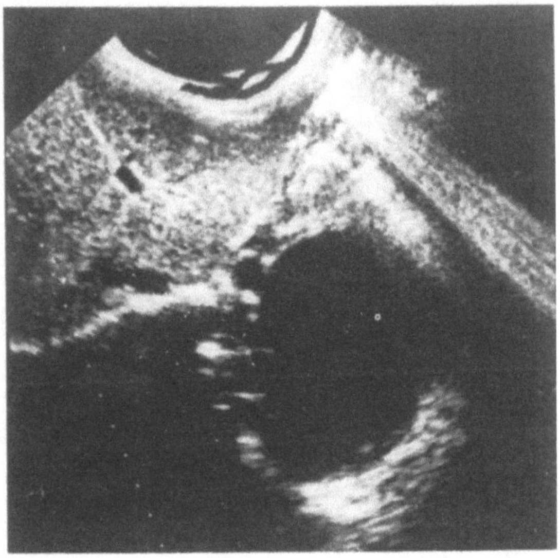

e

Fig. 8d and e

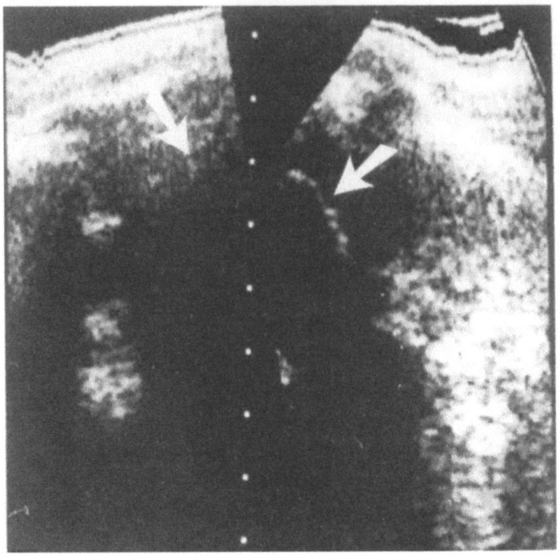

Fig. 9. Normal thymus in an 8-year-old child. Anterior transverse scan through the sternum (*dotted line*). On the left side: echo-free appearance of the gland due to low echo amplitude setting.
On the right side: the echo amplitude has been increased and the thymus appears finely echogenic (*arrow*).

In the mediastinum, lymphangiomas are well demonstrated when they are large (Fig. 8). But it is impossible to distinguish between a normal thymus and a thymic infiltration (in disease processes such as lymphoma and histiocytosis). The thymus is usually a homogeneous, relatively echo-free structure, but it attenuates the sound beam and becomes finely echogenic at higher echo amplitude (Fig. 9). Anterior lymph nodes appear more echogenic (Fig. 10). Superior vena cava and jugular vein ectasia are well diagnosed by US.

The pericardial cysts (Fig. 11), bronchogenic, and neurenteric cysts (Fig. 13) that we have seen were completely echo-free. However, a bronchogenic cyst can be an echogenic, solid-looking mass [10]. They are difficult to visualize when they are in the middle mediastinum.

Posterior mediastinum tumors correspond essentially to neurogenic tumors (Fig. 12). It is important when they are juxta diaphragmatic to localize the diaphragm to differentiate them from supra renal masses (Fig. 19 in Chap. 10). An intrathoracic kidney can be surprisingly recognized by US (Fig. 14). The diagnosis of meningocele should always be considered when confronted with a cystic mass in the posterior mediastinum (Fig. 15).

3.4 Diaphragm and Juxta Diaphragmatic Regions

To assess the diaphragm, ultrasonography is really more contributory than other imaging procedures, even CT, as the entire diaphragm can be displayed. A right subcostal approach shows the diaphragm through the liver on longitudinal, transverse, and oblique scans. Right diaphragmatic eventration is common (Fig. 16). Usually no treatment is needed as it can resolve spontaneously with growth. One must emphasize the importance of the evaluation of the posterior inframediastinal space and the celiac extension of mediastinal tumors (neuroblastomas, sarcomas) (Fig. 17).

Analysis of the position and mobility of the diaphragm is often useful, especially after surgery

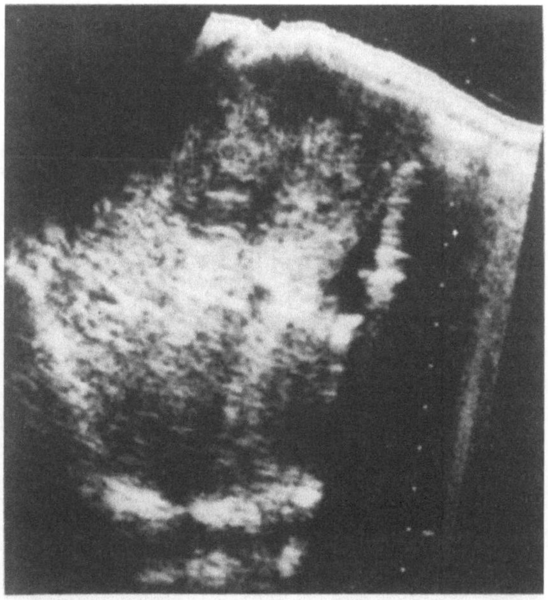

a

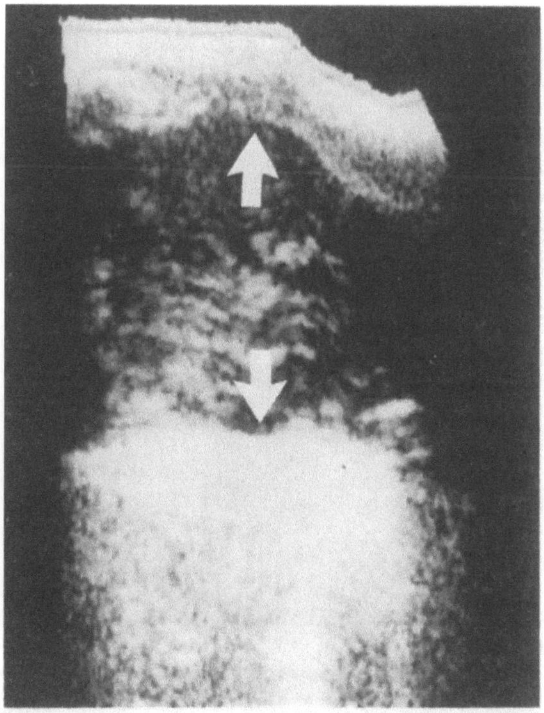

b

Fig. 10 a and b. Liver and mediastinum metastases of a Wilms tumor in a 5-year-old girl. **a** Longitudinal scan through the liver. **b** Left intercostal transverse scan.

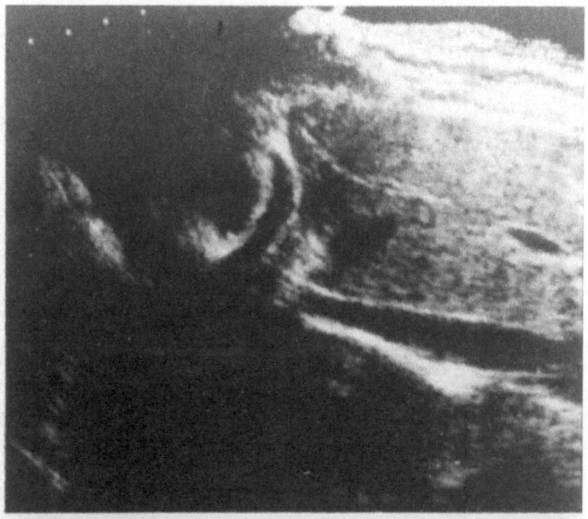

a

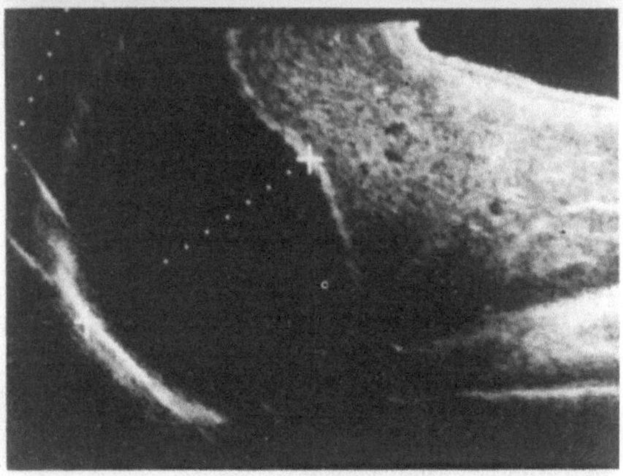

b

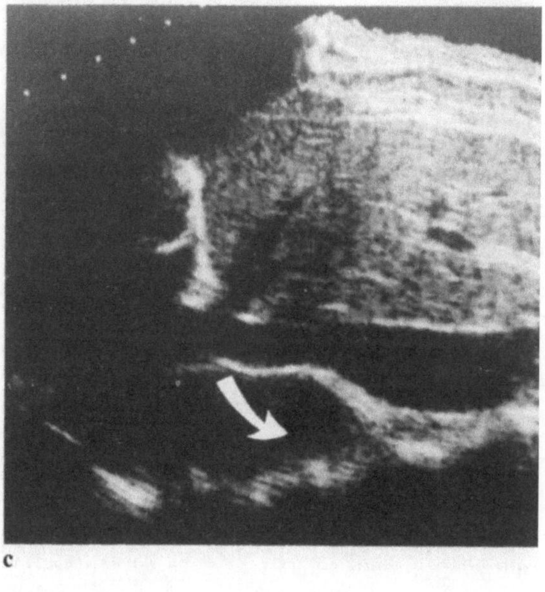

c

Fig. 11 a–c. Pericardial cyst in the right thoracic base discovered at the age of 13. Work-up before puncture at the age of 26.
a and b Longitudinal scan through the inferior vena cava. The cyst develops behind the right atrium.
c Longitudinal scan through the right kidney. Inversion of the diaphragm by the subpulmonic cyst.

◀ **Fig. 12 a–c.** Neurogenic tumors of the superior mediastinum.
a Right supra clavicular transverse scan in a 4-year-old boy showing a 3-cm poorly echogenic mass: ganglioneuroma.
b and c Longitudinal and transverse scans on the left side of the sternum showing a 3 cm echogenic mass above the aorta: neuroblastoma in a 7-month-old baby.

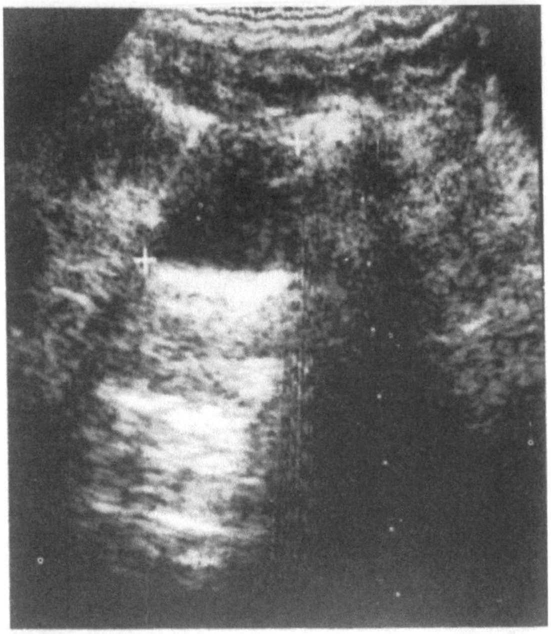

a

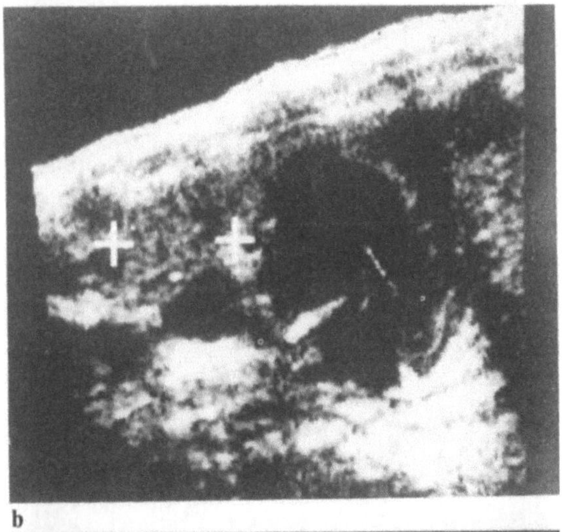

b

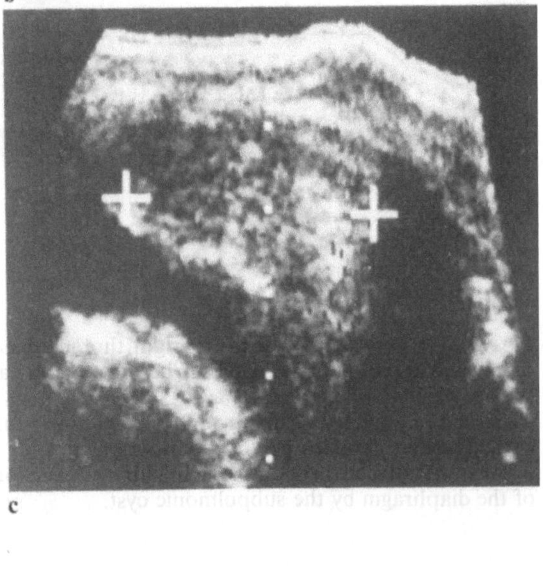

c

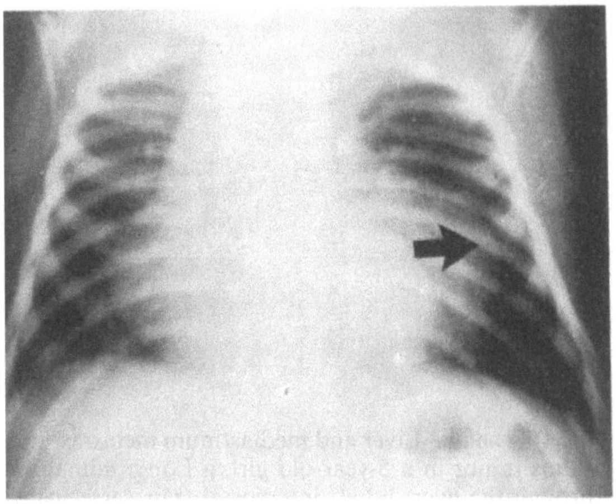

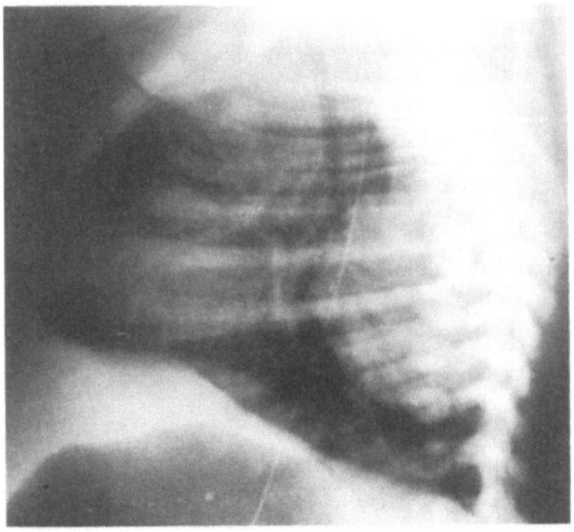

b

Fig. 13 a–c. Ten-days-old infant.
a and b Anteroposterior and lateral chest films.
c Prone longitudinal scan. The posterior mass is anechoic: neurenteric cyst.

Fig. 14 a–d. Fortuitous discovery of a mass in the posterior and inferior mediastinum in a 3-year-old girl. ▶
a Anteroposterior chest film;
b Longitudinal scan through the inferior vena cava;
c Prone transverse scan through the loin;
d Intravenous pyelogram confirms the diagnosis of intrathoracic right kidney.

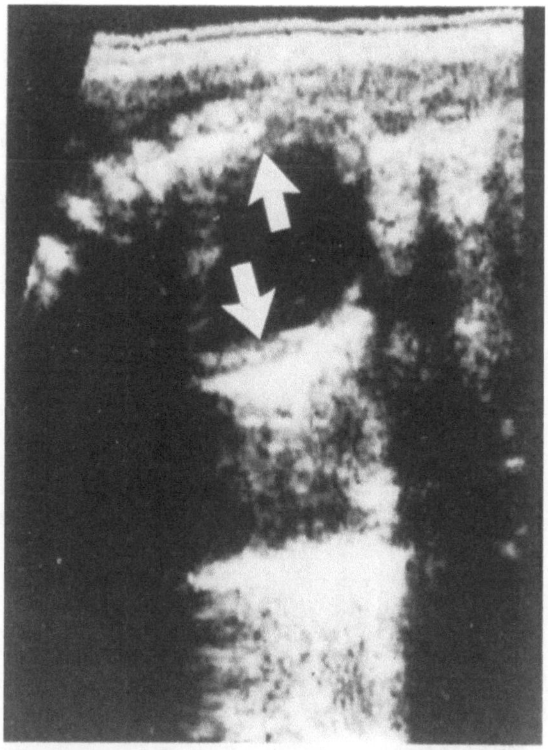

Fig. 13c

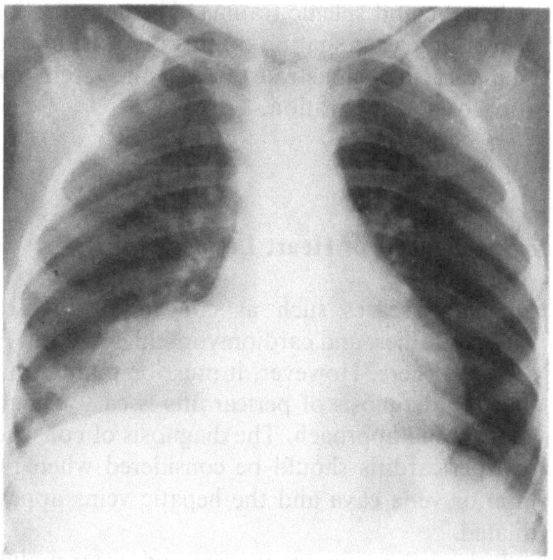

a

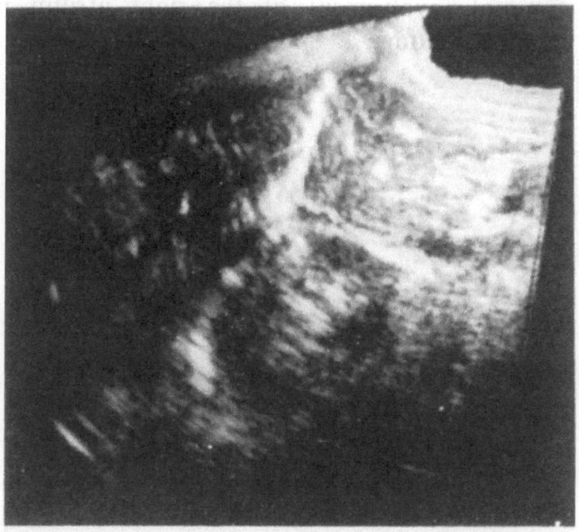

b

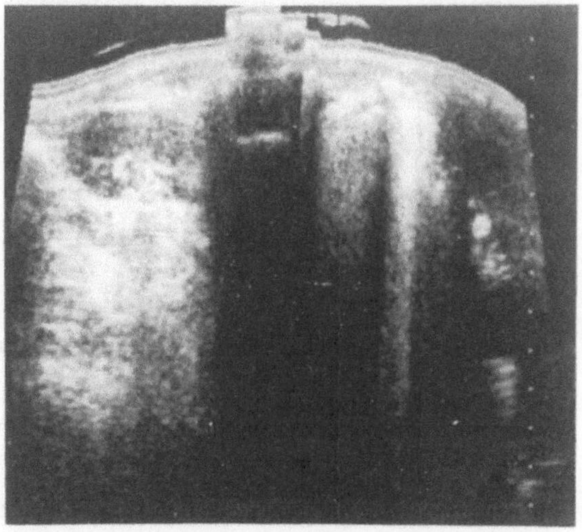

c

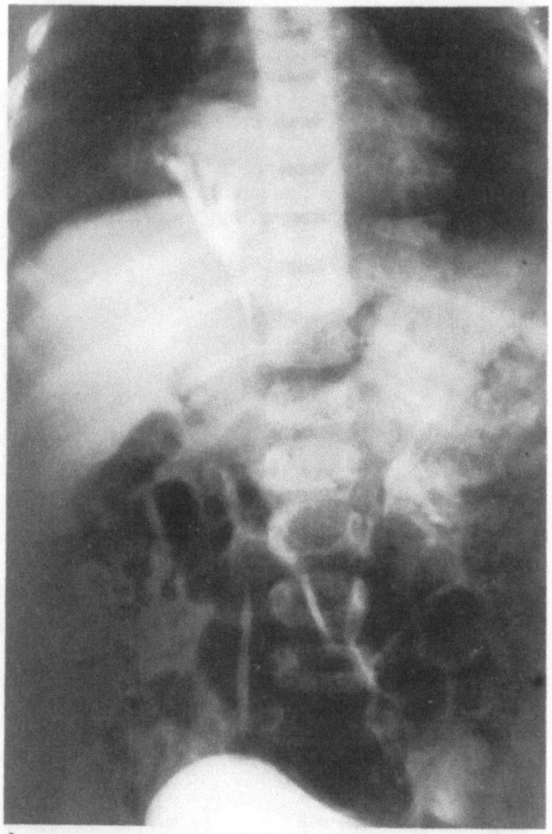

d

Fig. 14a–d

or hepatic and splenic trauma. The contribution of real-time examination on this point is unique. One can also demonstrate the systemic vascularization of a sequestration.

3.5 Diagnosis of Heart Lesions

Cardiac diseases such as congenital diseases, valvulopathies, and cardiomyopathies will not be discussed here. However, it must be pointed out that the diagnosis of pericarditis is easy using a subxyphoid approach. The diagnosis of constrictive pericarditis should be considered when the inferior vena cava and the hepatic veins appear dilated.

Intracardiac tumors are rare and occur mainly in tuberous sclerosis (Fig. 18). We have never seen tumoral involvement of the right atrium in nephroblastoma.

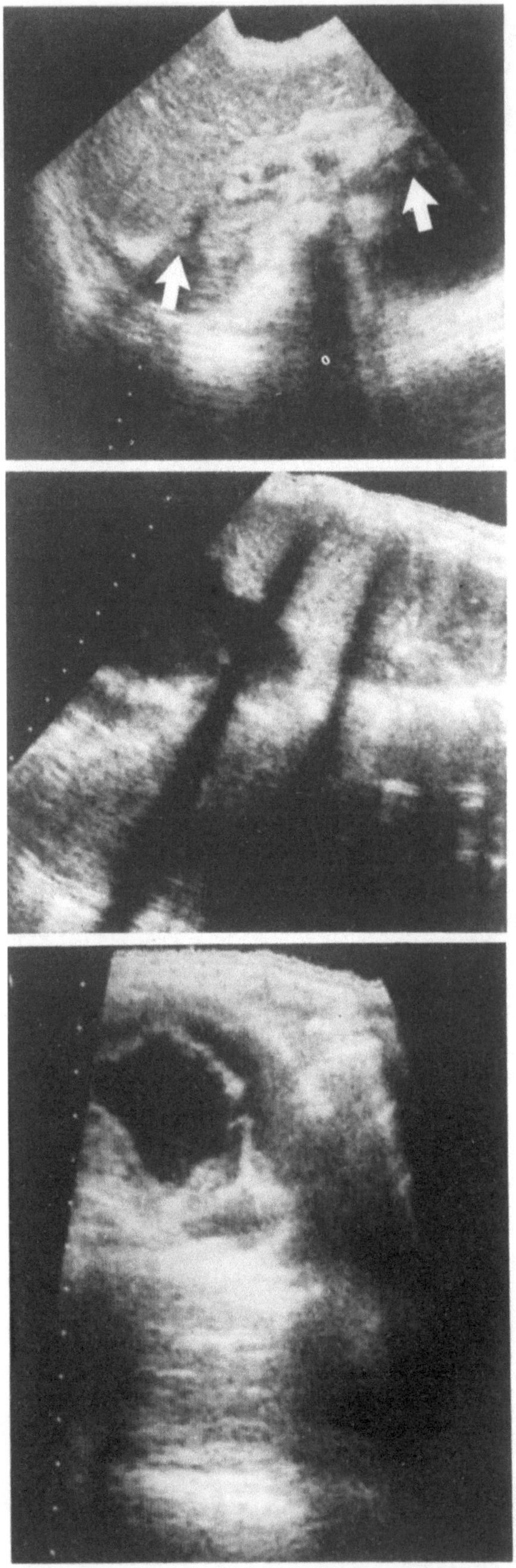

a

b

c

Fig. 15 a–c. Large meningocele without dorsal vertebra anomaly.
a Epigastric transverse scan.
b Longitudinal axillary scan through the left hemidiaphragm.
c Prone left intercostal transverse scan.
This diagnosis should be considered in view of a cystic posterior mass.

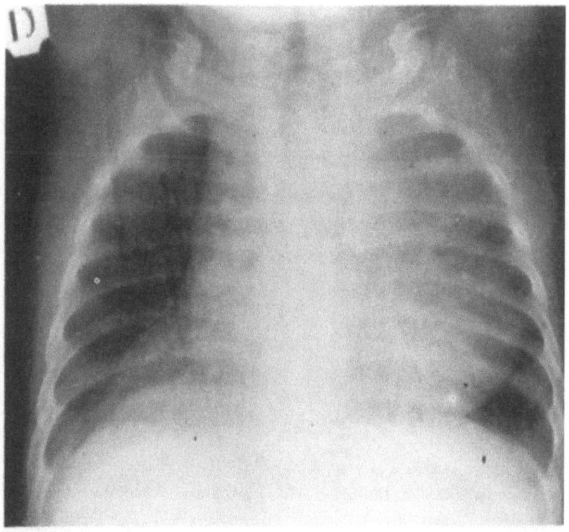

a

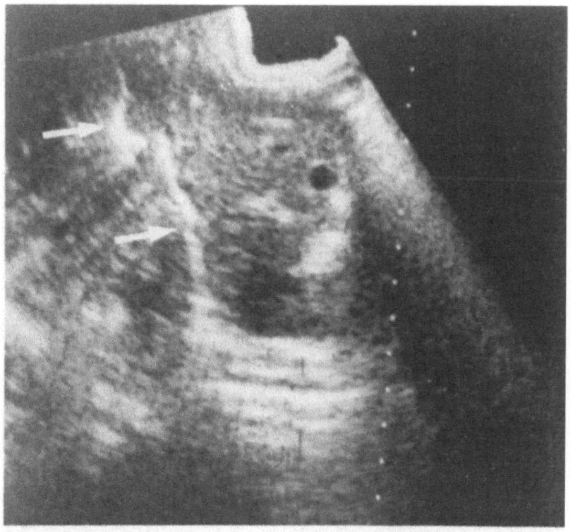

b

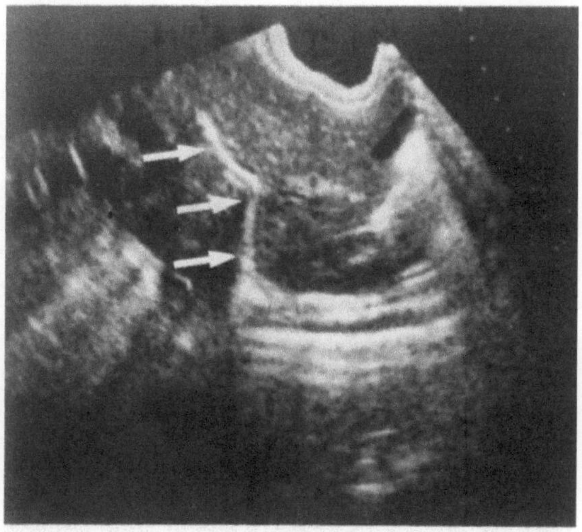

c

Fig. 16 a–c. Three-month-old infant.
a Anteroposterior chest film.
a, c Subcostal longitudinal scans through the right hemidiaphragm. The cardiophrenic anomaly represents an anteromedial diaphragmatic defect.

Conclusions

We have found that the main indications of chest sonography, besides cardiac diseases, are the analysis of the echogenicity of a superficial mass and the assessment of the diaphragm. The differentiation between normal thymus and thymic infiltration is not yet possible (Fig. 19).

Currently, real-time scanning with high frequency transducers represents a real progress. Ultrasonography is still less accurate than CT, except in the case of juxta diaphragmatic lesions. However, its contribution is significant since it is more readily available and is obtained at lower cost and with no ionizing radiation.

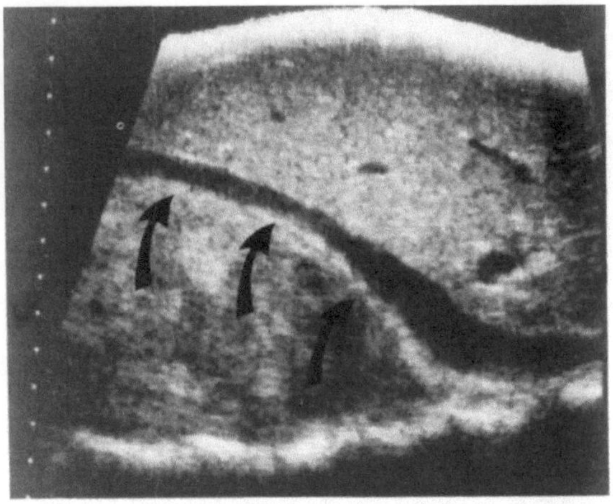

a

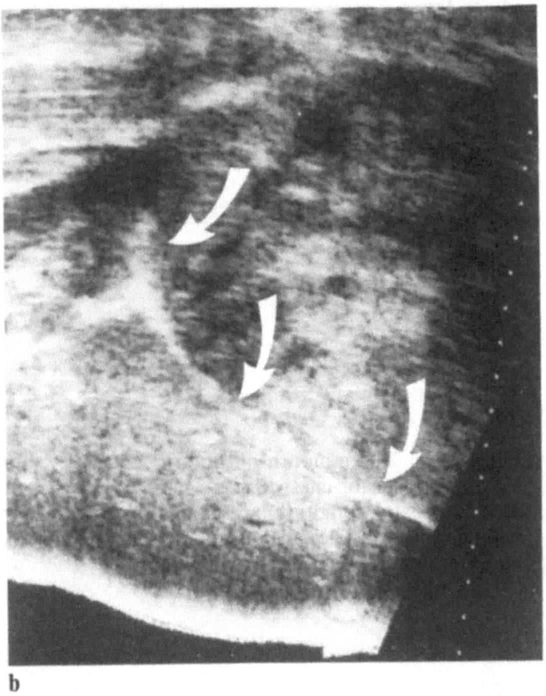

b

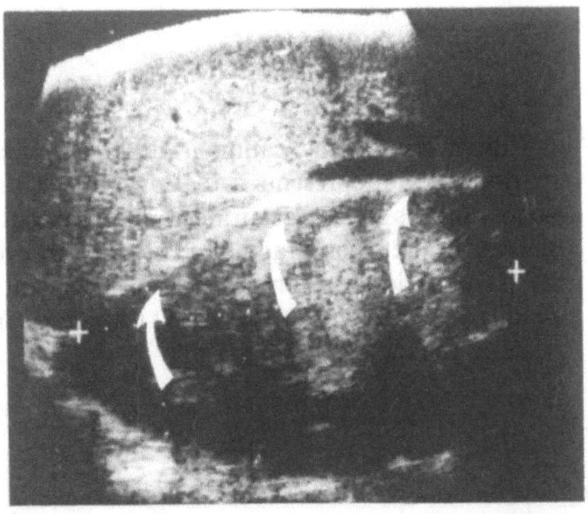

c

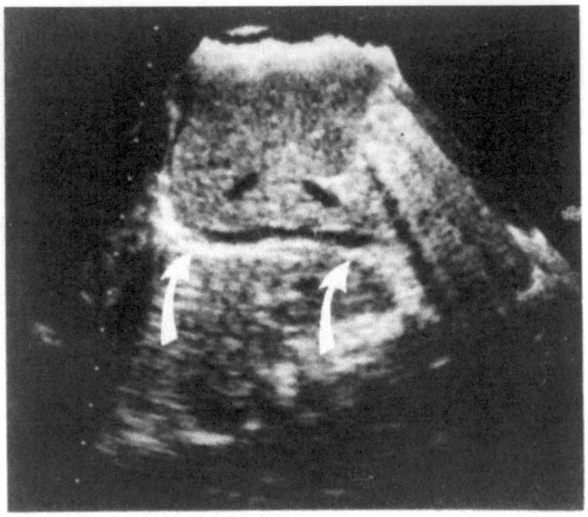

d

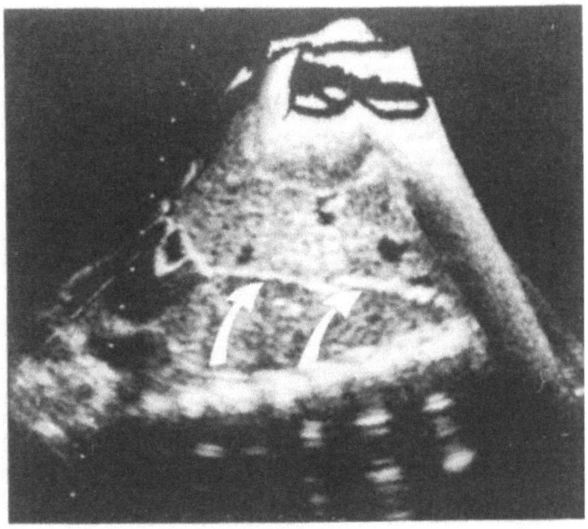

e

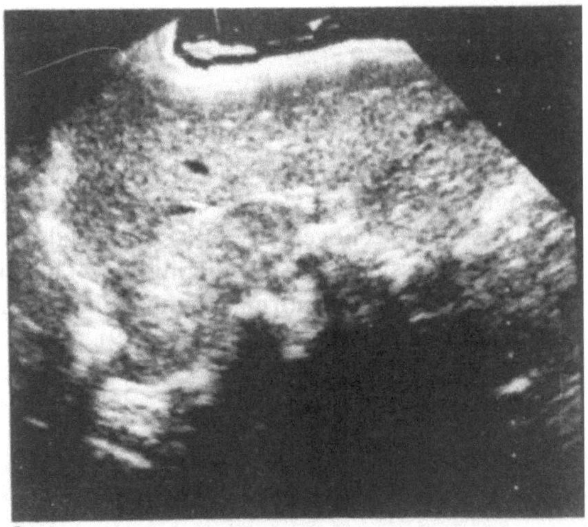

f

◀ **Fig. 17a–f.** Supradiaphragmatic tumors. **a–c** Young girl presenting with right base opacity on the chest film. Malignant embryonic tumor. **a** Longitudinal scan through the inferior vena cava; **b** Longitudinal scan through the right kidney; **c** Right subcostal transverse scan. Enormous tumor with inversion of the diaphragm, extending to the right kidney, the inferior vena cava and the right hepatic vein. **d–f** One-year-old girl with right inferior thoracic neuroblastoma. (**d** Longitudinal scan through the inferior vena cava; **e** More lateral scan; **f** Epigastric transverse scan). The diaphragm separates the tumor from the liver.

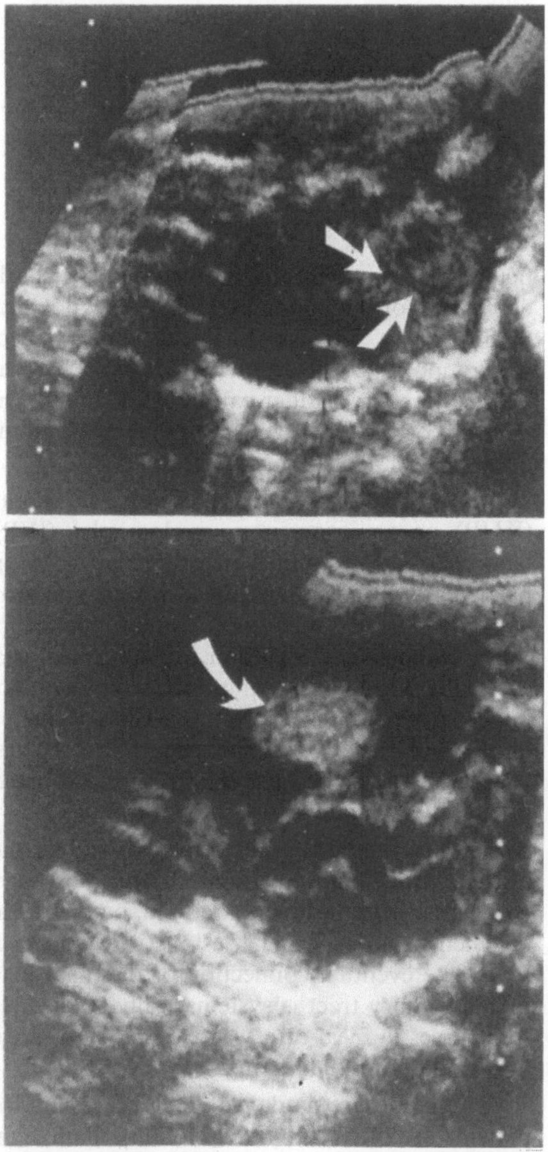

a

b

Fig. 18 a and b. Three-week-old infant with disturbances of the heart rhythm. Transverse scans through the heart showing intracardiac tumors: rhabdomyomas in a tuberous sclerosis.

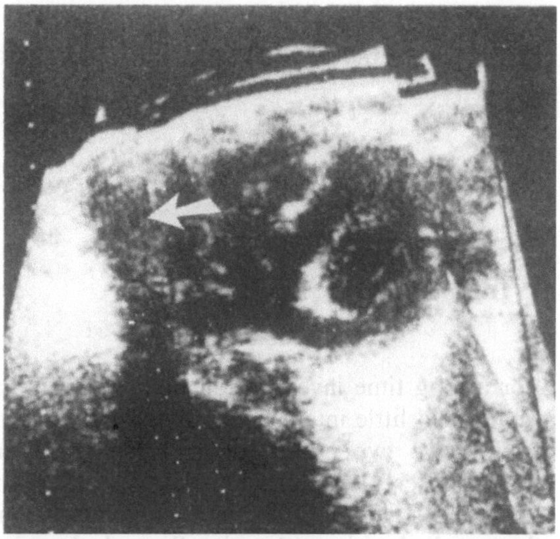

Fig. 19. Left thoracic longitudinal scan in a 1-year-old infant showing widening of the superior mediastinum. The thymus presents the same echographic aspect as a normal thymus: thymic histiocytosis.

References

1. Shkolnik A., Williams J. (1981). The Chest. In Ultrasound in Pediatrics – J.O. Haller, A. Shkolnik, ed. Churchill Livingstone (ed), 28–55
2. Haller J.-O., Schneider M., Kassner E.-G., Friedman A.-P., Waldroup L.-D. (1980). Sonographic evaluation of the chest in infants and children. A.J.R. 134:1019–1027.
3. Landay M., Harless W. (1977). Ultrasonic differentiation of right pleural effusion from subphrenic fluid on longitudinal scans of the right upper quadrant: importance of recognizing the diaphragm. Radiology 123:155–158
4. Laing F.-C., Filly R.-A. (1978). Problems in the application of ultrasonography for the evaluation of pleural opacities. Radiology 126:211–214
5. Ravin C.-E. (1977). Thoracocentesis of loculated pleural effusions using gray-scale ultrasonic guidance. Chest 71:666–668
6. Hisrch J.-H., Carter S.-J., Chikos P.-M., Colacurcio C. (1978). Ultrasonic evaluation of radiographic opacities of the chest. A.J.R. 130:1153–1156
7. Kangarloo H., Sukov R., Sample W.-F., Lipson M. (1977). Ultrasonographic evaluation of juxtadiaphragmatic masses in children. Radiology 125:785–787
8. Currarino G., Pinckney L.-E. (1981). Renal displacement caused by a supradiaphragmatic, paraspinal. Ewing-like sarcoma and simulating and adrenal mass. Radiology 139:603
9. Merten D.-F., Bowie J.-D., Kirks D.-R., Grossman H., Smith L. (1982). Anteromedial diaphragmatic defects in infancy: current approches to diagnostic imaging. Radiology 142:361–365
10. Ries T., Currarino G., Nikaidoh H., Kennedy L.(1982). Real time ultrasonography of subcarinal bronchogenic cysts in two children. Radiology 145:121–122

Chapter 5

Intraperitoneal Pathology – Abdominal Trauma

P. Le Dosseur, M. Dewald , and D. Eurin

1 Introduction

For a long time investigation of the abdominal cavity held little interest for sonographists. This could have two explanations. First, there are several different established ways to examine the entire digestive tract, the abdominal vessels, and the so-called peritoneal cavity. Second, there is a multitude of traps and normal variants in the appearance of the digestive organs. Intraintestinal air and peristaltism are the main difficulties, but they can be overcome.

The long-used practice of using contrast media to examine the alimentary tract is now taking its revenge.

We propose to demonstrate that US is an accurate and safe method of investigation in the field. It can demonstrate the intestinal walls, secretions, and contractility, without need for any external agressive agent.

The first part of this chapter will deal with general considerations concerning the investigation and preparation. Then, we will discuss the advantages of US in three frequent clinical situations: intra-abdominal masses, abdominal pain and fever, abdominal trauma. Finally, some specific indications will be illustrated, conditions in which US could replace more traditional techniques.

2 Preparation and Technique

No premedication is necessary. Drugs have little effect on intraintestinal gas excess. These difficulties can be partially surmounted by gentle depression of the abdominal wall or by postural modifications. The use of acoustic windows is of great importance. "Natural" windows such as the liver, spleen, or bladder can be used. Filling the stomach or the colon with water creates in some cases helpful acoustic windows.

All our patients undergo abdominal X-ray (KUB) or an intravenous pyelography (IVP), before the first abdominal US examination (in this particular type of pathology). X-ray examination is of great importance for the exact location of tubes, catheters, calcification, and abnormal gas, especially when considering operated patients or intensive care cases. The IVP is necessary when a mass is palpated. In our experience, IVP is the first procedure to use because it will lead to a better oriented US examination.

The examination is performed in supine but also in prone and lateral decubitus positions. Real-time sector scanners are used, but for measurements and superficial lesions we also use B scan. The eventual connection of the mass with the alimentary tract is systematically studied. In some cases, a meal or a water enema is of great help in defining the lesions.

IP abscesses are similar to other masses but the patients are often of limited mobility. Pain, contracture, bandages, and scars are important difficulties encountered during examination. Furthermore, it is usually impossible to depress the abdominal wall toward the lesion and acoustic windows are necessary.

Finally, we would like to emphasize that classic difficulties such as pneumoperitoneum or barium in the alimentary tract, seem of low importance in children as they never contradicate US studies.

3 Diagnosis of an Abdominal Mass

3.1 Assessing the Intraperitoneal Location of the Mass

The IP location can be affirmed by the combination of clinical, radiological, and echographic features. A mass that is mobile, separated from the liver and the spleen, without lumbar contact and pelvic extension is probably intraperitoneal. IVP confirms this situation when it shows that the mass is outside the kidney, psoas muscles, and ureters. An IP mass usually compresses the small and large bowels. When surrounded by an intestinal loop, the mass is usually intraparietal.

By showing the mobility of the mass in comparison with each organ US confirms the location. Deep masses, huge masses, and masses of low mobility are difficult to localize. IP masses rarely extend to the retroperitoneum but retroperitoneal masses frequently extend to the peritoneal cavity (e.g., pediculated kidney tumor). In difficult cases, CT or vascular opacification can be of great help.

3.2 Analyzing the Ultrasonic Characteristics of the Mass

The echogenicity, homogenicity, wall, size, regularity, and appearance of the adjacent intestinal loops should be studied. Based on these elements, several possibilities can be considered.

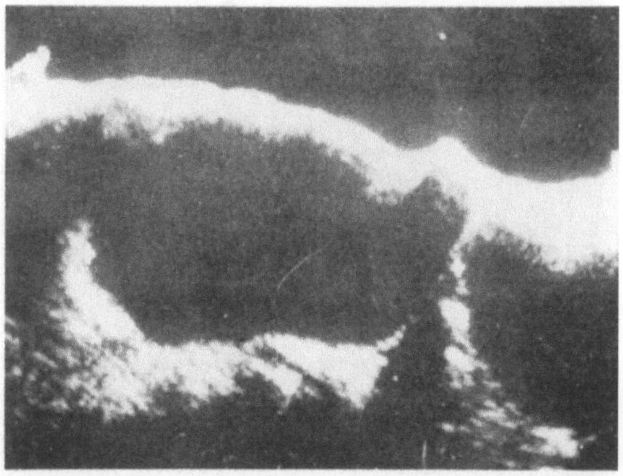

a

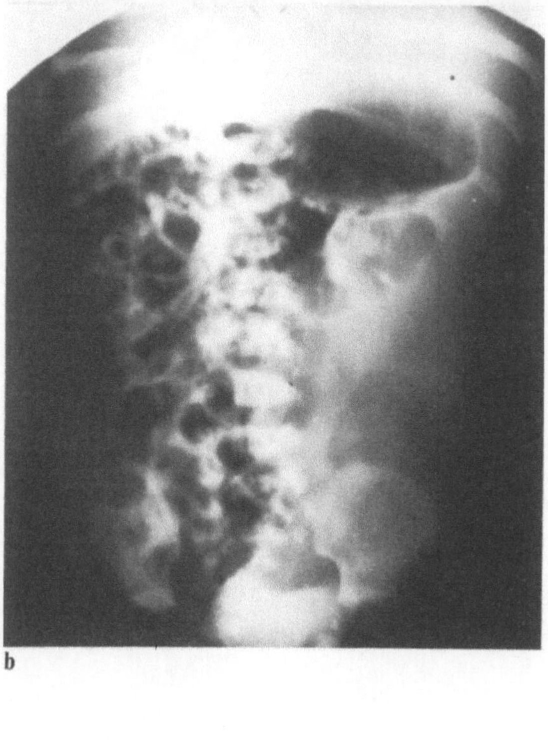

b

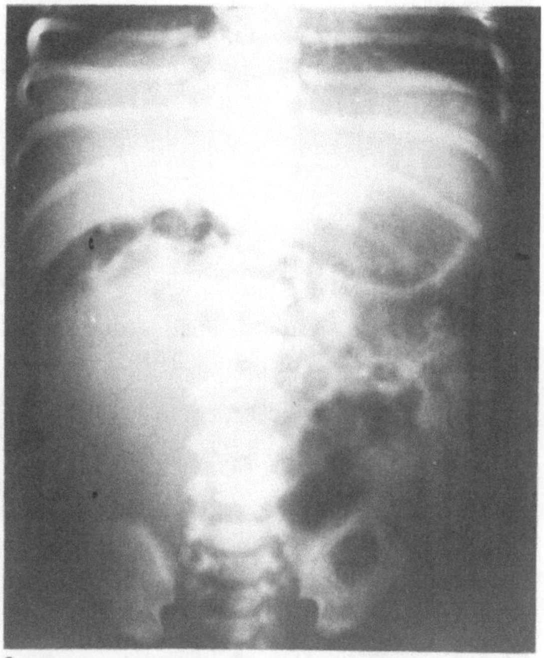

c

Fig. 1 a–c. Newborn whose antenatal US study showed an abdominal anechoic mass. **a** Postnatal US confirms the cystic mass. **b and c** Radiographs emphasize the extreme mobility of the mass which displaces the whole bowel toward the left or right part of the abdomen. At surgery a right ovarian cyst was discovered.

3.2.1 The Mass is Echogenic

The diagnosis of lymphoma should always be considered especially with a low amplitude echogenic mass. The lymphoma is often of the non-Hodgkin's type. US will show the exact extension of the mass and will measure it most precisely. The borders of the mass and its limits with the intra-abdominal organs should be studied and ascites searched for an eventual tap. The examination is completed by the search for other locations (lymph nodes, kidney, liver, or spleen).

Other diagnoses to consider are tuberculosis and yersiniosis that can involve the mesenteric lymph nodes. The examination should be completed by an intestinal barium followthrough.

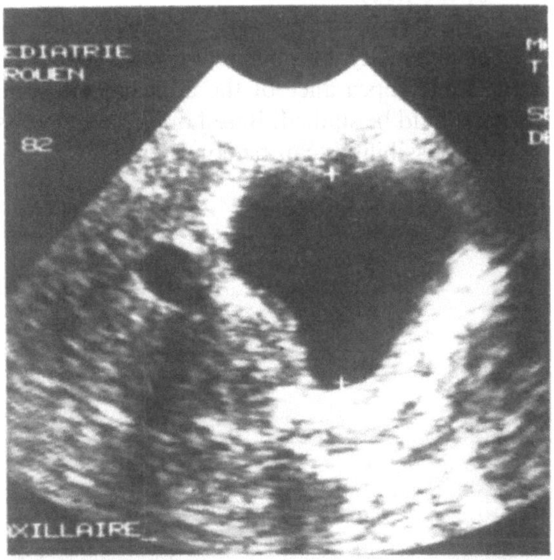

a

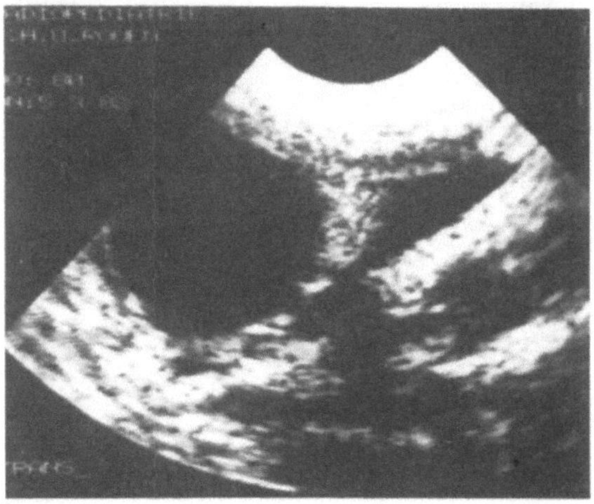

b

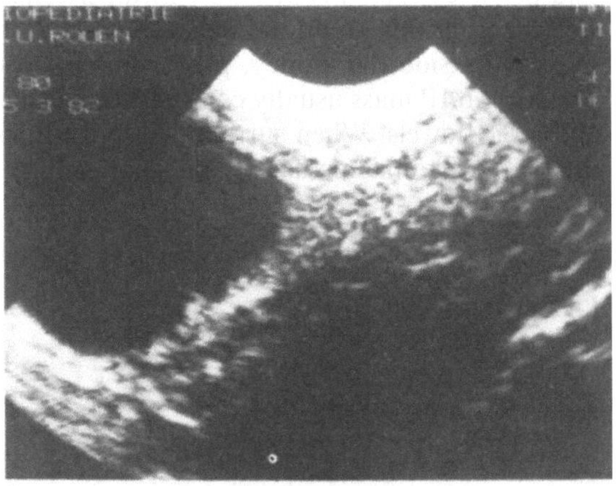

c

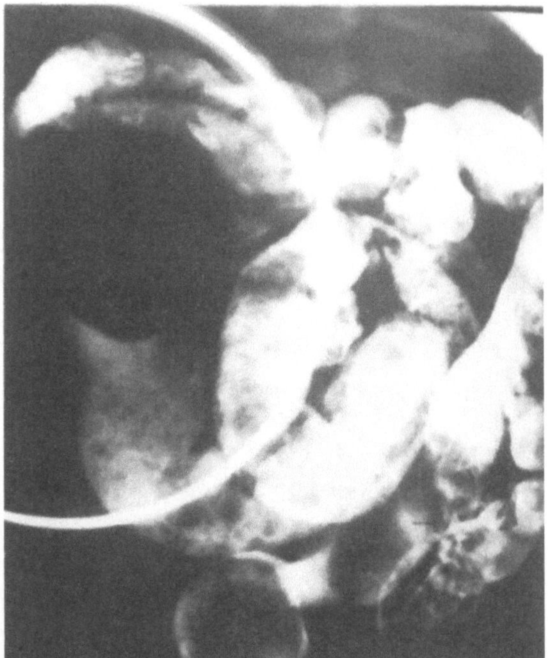

d

Fig. 2 a–d. Male infant 3 weeks old admitted for vomiting and a firm, mobile mass on the right flank. A longitudinal axillary scan **(a)** shows it to be mobile toward the hepatic border. A longitudinal anterior scan **(b, c)** shows the mass close to a small dilated bowel loop which surrounds its upper pole. Peristaltic contractions were observed. The barium enema confirms the obstruction of terminal small bowel by a mass. At surgery, ileal duplication was found 10 cm above the ileocecal junction.

3.2.2 The Mass is Anechoic or Hypoechoic but Homogeneous

If a regular wall presents acoustic enhancement, the mass is cystic (Fig. 1). An ovarian cyst should be considered in the case of a very mobile mass in an infant girl. The cysts are usually multilocular in older girls and correspond to mucinous cysts.

In cases of a mesenteric cyst or cystic lymphangioma, the mass is mobile but its topography does not change from one examination to another. With these masses, the intestinal compression is milder. Thick and incomplete septa can be seen within the cyst. Ascitic fluid can be an associated finding. A hydatic cyst should not be forgotten as differential diagnosis, especially with thin incomplete intracystic septa.

Intestinal duplication (Fig. 2). Any location on the alimentary tract is possible but the right iliac fossa is the most usual. In some cases the continuity with the digestive tract is obvious. Postprandial stasis can be observed close to the mass. A hypoechoic halo surrounds the mass, confirming its digestive origin. Choledocal cysts and pancreatic cysts are usually more posterior and less mobile. If there is no definite wall, an IP collection of fluid, abscess, hematoma, or septated ascites should be considered. One again the diagnosis of lymphoma should not be ignored.

3.2.3 The Mass has Characteristics of a Modified Digestive Structure (Fig. 3)

The usual aspect is the "cockade" or "target" sign when a transverse scan is performed, the "sandwich" or "pseudokidney" sign when a longitudinal scan is performed. A normal digestive cockade is formed by an echogenic centrum and an anechoic wall. The central echoes correspond to the lumen and its content (aliments and/or mucus); its diameter varies from 0.3 to 1.5 cm. The thickness of the wall varies from 0.3 to 0.8 mm, varying with the digestive segment but little with age.

The image, round or oval, should well centered, should have regular borders, should have the described size, and should present under real-time examination peristaltic waves. A digestive image should be considered anormal if the central echoes is excentred, the hypoechoic wall measures more than 10 mm, the structure does not present any peristalsis, or if the external or internal limits are irregular. Various processes can induce these modifications: inflammatory diseases such as

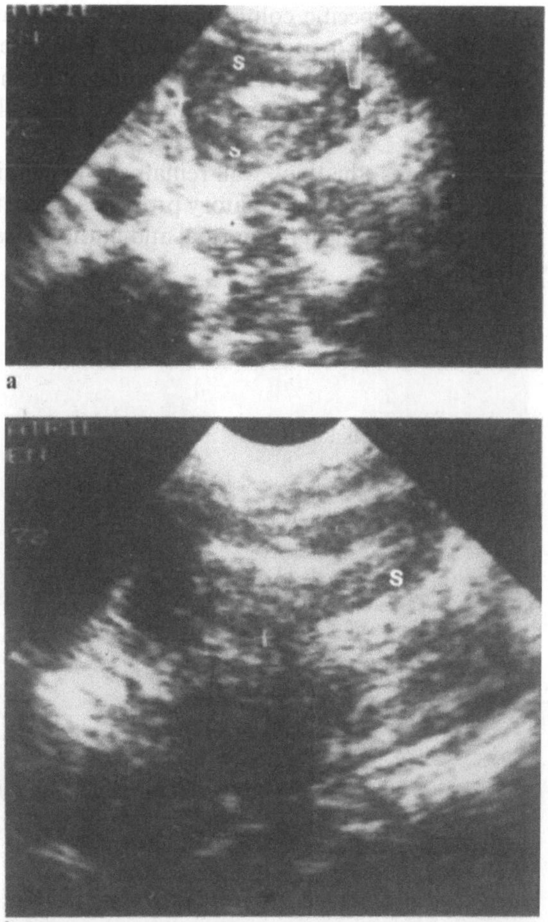

Fig. 3 a and b. Submucosal hematoma *(S)* described as "Sandwich sign" affecting the colon. Transverse **(a)** and longitudinal **(b)** scans.

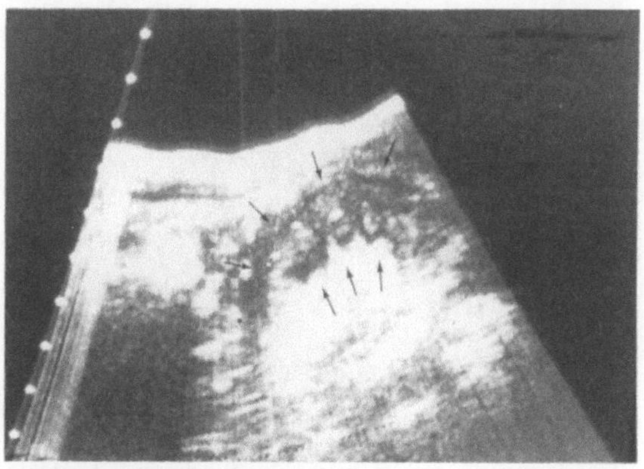

Fig. 4. Girl aged 12 years with acute diarrhea, fever, and abdominal distension. Left flank transversal scan: thickened anterior wall of left colon with scalloping of mucous membrane. Diagnosis: bacterial colitis.

ileitis or nonspecific colitis, Crohn's disease, ulcerative colitis; parietal hematoma associated with an Schönlein-Henoch, hemolytic, and uremic syndrome or trauma; tumor, usually lymphoma.

In all cases, the thick wall remains hypoechoic (Fig. 4 and 5). In inflammatory processes, there is no interface between the normal and pathological tissue.

This alteration in the digestive wall can be associated with a distension of the proximal intestinal loops by a mechanical or functional obstacle. In such cases, the digestive lumen measures more than 20 mm in diameter and the intestinal loops are usually parallel, giving alternating echogenic and anechogenic images.

In conclusion, the object of US examination is to orient toward a cystic mass, an abscess, or a

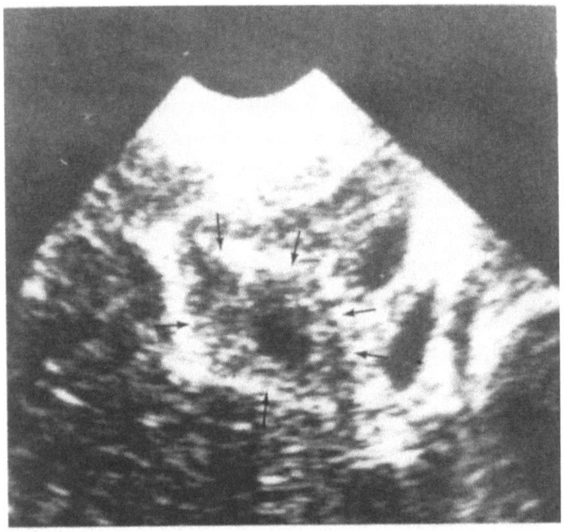

a

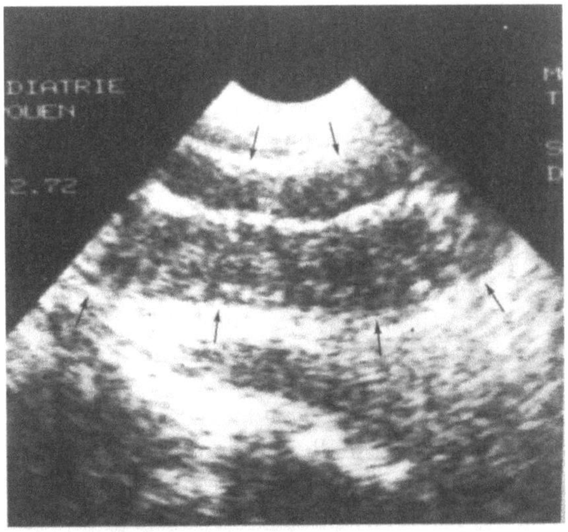

c

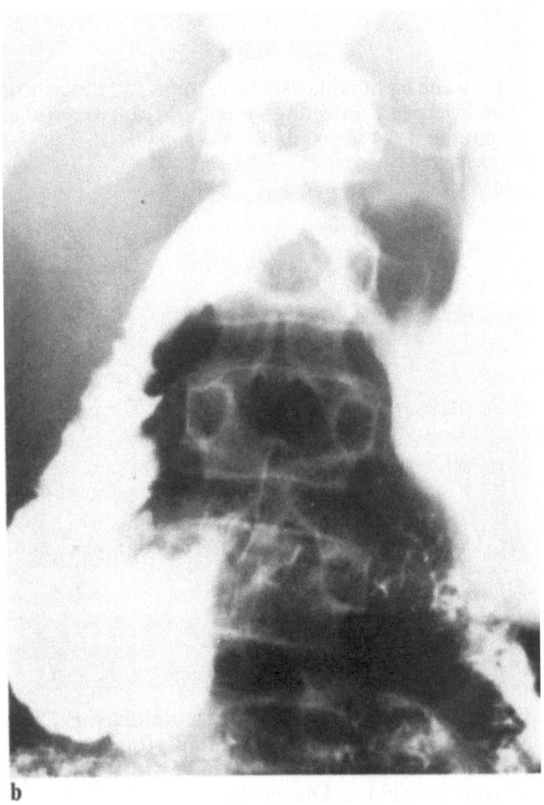

b

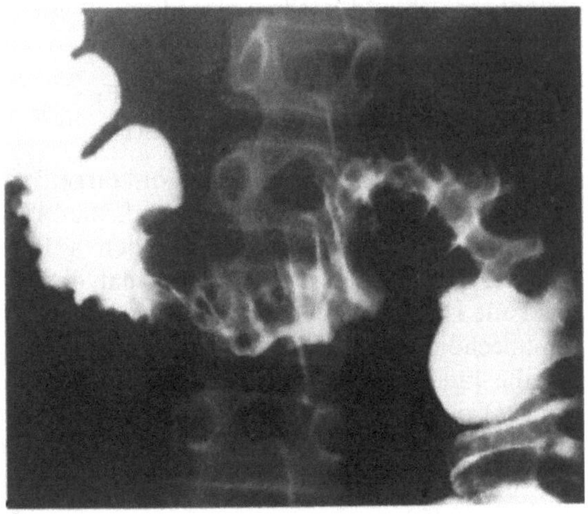

d

Fig. 5 a–d. Girl aged 9 years with abdominal pain and ecchymotic lesions of lower limbs suggesting Schönlein-Henoch purpura. **a** Epigastric transverse scan showing thickening of the duodenal wall with persistent lumen. **b** Barium meal confirms parietal infiltration and stasis caused by duodenal submucosal hematoma. Similar lesions affect the colon with correlation between the Sandwich sign at US **(c)** and the narrowing of lumen at barium enema **(d)**.

hematoma (it constitutes then a superficial preoperative work-up) or toward a malignant infiltration lesion. In this case, it will be followed by histological examination, and unnecessary surgery will sometimes be avoided. The evolution and the effect of treatment will be followed by repeated examinations.

4 Acute Abdominal Pain with High Temperature

4.1 When to Look for an Abscess

Abdominal pain and fever in children older than 2 years should indicate a simple or complicated appendicular infection. In the majority of cases, the clinical symptoms are obvious and sufficient for the diagnosis. US is useful in atypical or complicated appendicitis.

Other etiologies are more rare. Peritoneal nonappendicular infections should suggest a digestive perforation. The KUB can show a stercolith, a pneumoperitoneum or signs of obstruction. It can orient toward another origin (acute cholecystis, infected hematoma or necrotic tumor). US is most helpful in postoperative survey. It helps in the case of febrile rebound to differentiate between a real complication or a less pathological fifth-day syndrome.

4.2 What to Look for

An abscess is characterized by an hypoechoic area without peripheral halo, nonlimited, nonmobile, without peristaltic waves, and nondeformable. An heterogeneous mixed appearance is less frequent, corresponding probably to incarcerated digestive loops or to necrotic debris. When acoustic shadowing is also present, one should consider air or fecaliths. In some cases, sedimentation of liquids of different densities can be demonstrated (Fig. 6).

Indirect signs that can be observed close to the abscess are: (a) digestive loops agglutinated, with thickened walls and filled with liquid; (b) widening of the underperitoneal space with disappearance of the lamellar structure close to the abscess; (c) IP noncollected effusion.

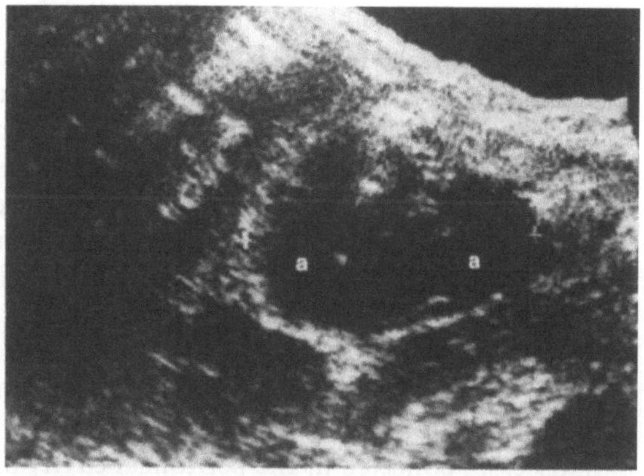

Fig. 6. Boy aged 12 years with fever 38.5 °C 8 days after surgery of appendicular peritonitis. Right iliac fossa transverse scan showing residual abscess in front of the upper pole of kidney with mixed echostructure.
a, abscess.

4.3 Where to Look for an Abscess (Fig. 7)

The examination is noteasy in the postoperative period. The accuracy of the examination relies upon a rigorous technique. Generally, the ab-

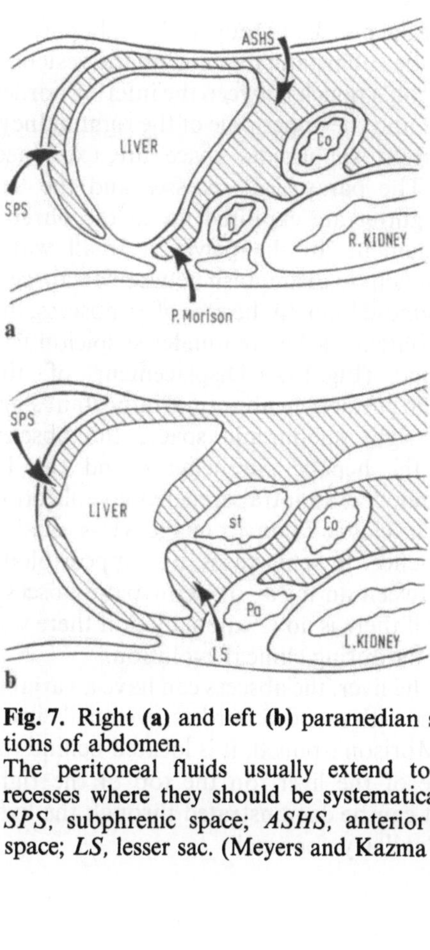

Fig. 7. Right **(a)** and left **(b)** paramedian sagittal sections of abdomen.
The peritoneal fluids usually extend to peritoneal recesses where they should be systematically sought. *SPS*, subphrenic space; *ASHS*, anterior subhepatic space; *LS*, lesser sac. (Meyers and Kazma [5]).

scesses are easier to demonstrate lateral than medial to the large bowel. The migration of pus, especially from the appendix has been particulary well studied by Morton Meyer. His conclusions can be particularly well applied to children whose peritoneal cavity is free of adherences. Abscesses usually collect in the more declive areas which are fortunately accessible to US examination. In those cases, the accuracy of the examination is sufficient. Elsewhere, the images obtained are less easy to interpret and risk of errors higher and conclusions should therefore be cautious.

Abscesses collected in the peritoneal cavity are usually located in the right iliac fossa and should be sought where the clinical and radiological signs are most evident. The transducer, depressing the abdominal wall, will help to localize the pain and hence the area under suspicion. These can be subhepatic, hypogastric, or pelvic areas.

A particular form is the pseudotumoral appendicitis developing in the pouch of Douglas between the rectum and the bladder with a chronic evolution. It should be considered in the presence of a prerectal pelvic mass.

One should be aware of the possibility of multiple locations as also described by Morton Meyer (Figs. 8–11).

1. After the pouch of Douglas the right paracolic gutter, the subhepatic region with the vesicular bed, Morison's pouch between the inferior border of the liver and the upper pole of the right kidney, and the right subphrenic space are examined (Fig. 12). The paravesical recesses and the left paracolic gutter are explored up to the phrenicocolic ligament. In the pelvis, a small water enema will help to distinguish between an abscess and the sigmoid loop. In the case of an abscess, the size and content of the area under suspicion will not change (Fig. 13). Displacement of the parietocolic gutter is an abnormal important sign.

In the right subphrenic space, the abscess displaces the hepatic parenchyma and can be misinterpreted as an intraparenchymal collection of fluid. The classic biconvex image is less usual in our experience. In some cases, it is impossible to decide between an intra- or perihepatic abscess, especially if there is no IP anomaly or if there was a septicemia during clinical evolution.

Under the liver, the abscess can have a variable appearance with rounded borders, eventually irregular. In Morison's pouch, it is located behind the right lobe of the liver, on the top of the right kidney. It can be demonstrated through the liver or by an axillary approach.

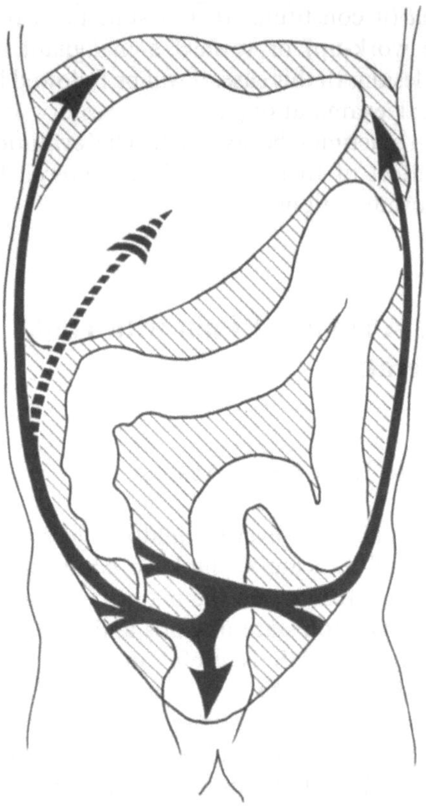

Fig. 8. The flow of pus from appendicular region to peritoneum in recumbent patients: pouch of Douglas, right and left paracolic gutters, Morison's pouch, and subhepatic space (Meyers and Kazma [5]).

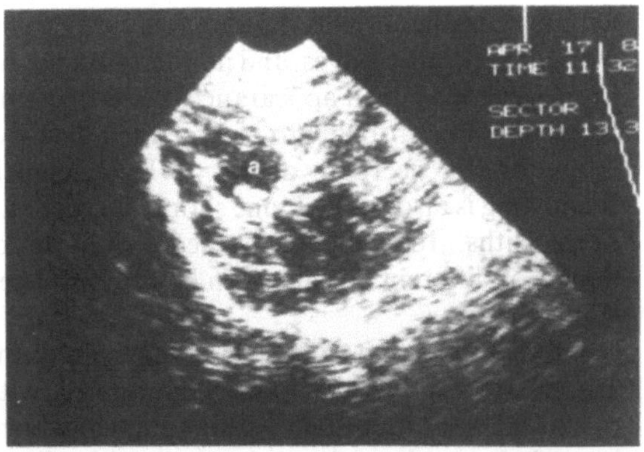

Fig. 9. Girl aged 8 years with right iliac fossa pain for several weeks and fever. Transverse scan of the painful region shows a small fluid collection with an echoic declive stercolith. Surgery confirmed an appendicular abscess *(a)*.

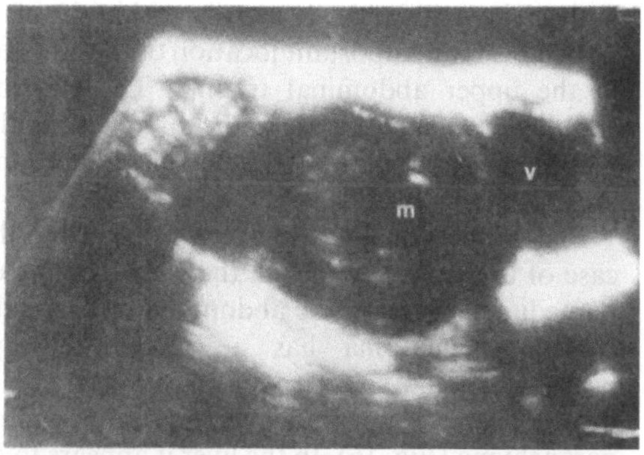

Fig. 10. Huge fixed pelviabdominal mass. Median sagittal scan shows heterogeneous mass (*m*) of low echogenicity, well limited, close to the bladder (*v*). At surgery, chronic pseudotumoral appendicitis was discovered.

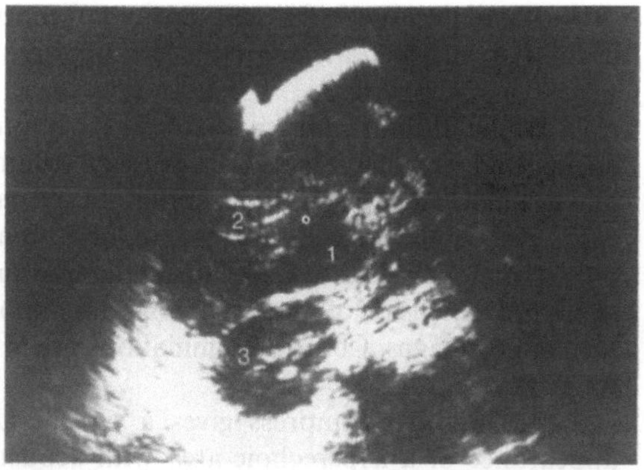

Fig. 12. Acute appendicitis and peritonitis. Transverse scan of right flank revealing abscess of Morison's pouch *(1)*, liver *(2)*, right kidney *(3)*.

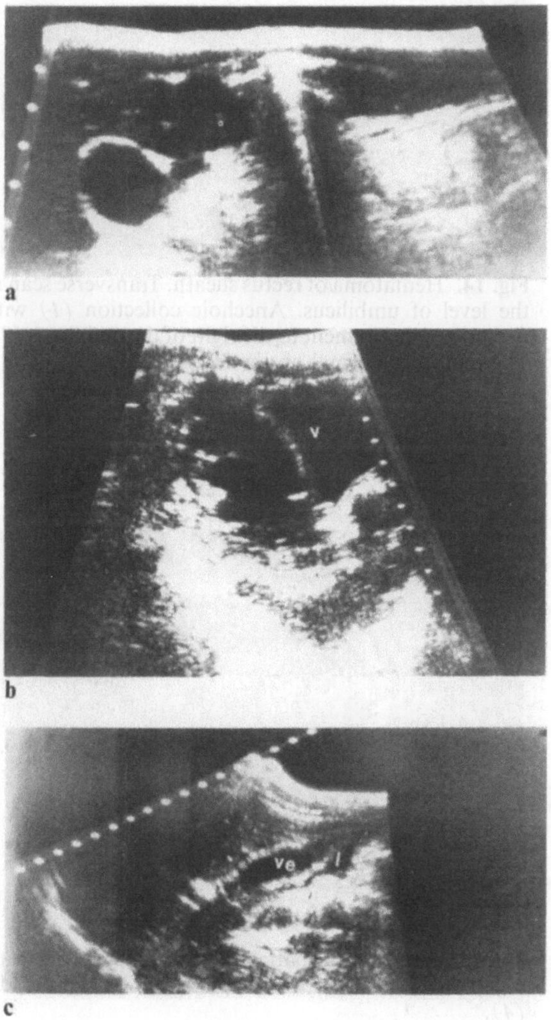

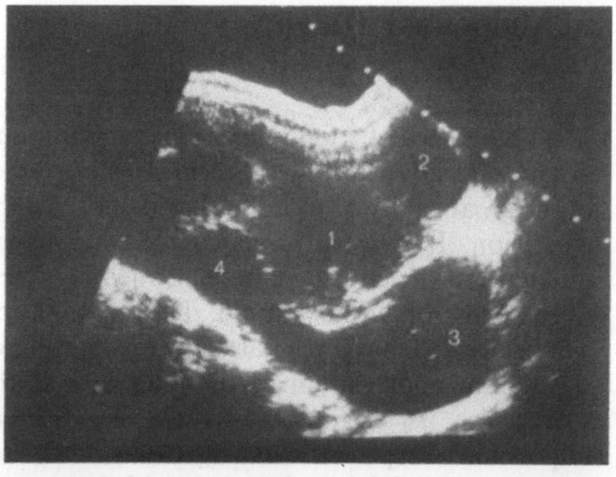

Fig. 13. Postoperative abscess of the pouch of Douglas *(1)* behind the bladder *(2)* . The rectum *(3)* and sigmoid loop *(4)* are filled by a water enema. Longitudinal oblique scan.

◀ **Fig. 11 a–c.** Boy aged 5 years with fever. Painful pelvic mass with tensing of the right flank at palpation.
a Transverse epigastric scan: total absorption of the US beneath the abdominal wall, suggesting presence of air.
b Sagittal pelvic scan; hypoechogenic collection of fluid above the bladder, distinct from sigmoid loop and rectum filled by water enema.
c Sagittal scan of left flank: intraperitoneal fluid, below the gallbladder. At surgery, appendicular peritonitis with multiple abscesses and pneumoperitoneum was discovered.

We have not observed a suppurative collection of fluid in the lesser sac, nor in the left subphrenic space.

2. Within the infracolic space, the abscesses are difficult to demonstrate except if their volume makes them evident. Small collections of fluid can easily be misinterpreted as a digestive loop, sigmoid or small bowel, or even cecum. Inflammatory signs and distension of intestinal loops are important indirect signs. Control examinations are also important.

3. A forgotten compress gives a typical US appearance of a hyperechoic area with acoustic shadowing surrounded by an hypoechoic ring corresponding to the abscess.

5 Abdominal Trauma

The occurrence of a lesion in an intra-abdominal organ can lead to a free peritoneal effusion, either in the great cavity or more localized, close to the contusion. It is usually related to a hemoperitoneum but the effusion can be formed by digestive, biliary or urinary liquid. The examination can be divided into three parts: the recognition of the lesion, appreciation of its volume, and the search for its origin. This study is of great importance in pediatric emergencies, since not every case of abdominal trauma with hemoperitoneum leads to surgery. When hemodynamics are controlled, even with important parenchymal lesions, a clinical and ultrasonic followed-up is usually sufficient. US shows the evolution of the lesion and of the peritoneal effusion, confirming or not the favorable evolution.

5.1 Where to Look for a Hematoma

The examination is oriented by superficial signs of contusion and the search for painful areas. The effusion can be localized in the proximity of the lesion, it can extend, or it can remain free in the peritoneal cavity. The hematoma can be retroperitoneal with lesion of the kidney or of its vessels. Finally, the hematoma can be located in the abdominal wall (rectus sheet) (Fig. 14).

A free effusion can be located under the anterior border of the liver where an anechoic area can be seen, limited by the inferior border of the liver (upper limit) and by the digestive loops (lower limit). The gallbladder is usually within the effusion. This is an important location of the effusion in the upper abdominal trauma. The effusion should be sought between the organs and the diaphragm and in the parietocolic gutter and around the gallbladder (Fig. 15).

Pneumoperitoneum should be suspected in the case of areflective echoes in the epigastric areas, immediately beneath the abdominal wall. A subcapsular hematoma has a crescent-like appearance in the spleen. It is associated with a heterogeneous appearance of the surrounding parenchyma (Fig. 16). In the liver it appears to be oval with irregular limits on the hepatic side (Fig. 17). A septated hematoma can be located

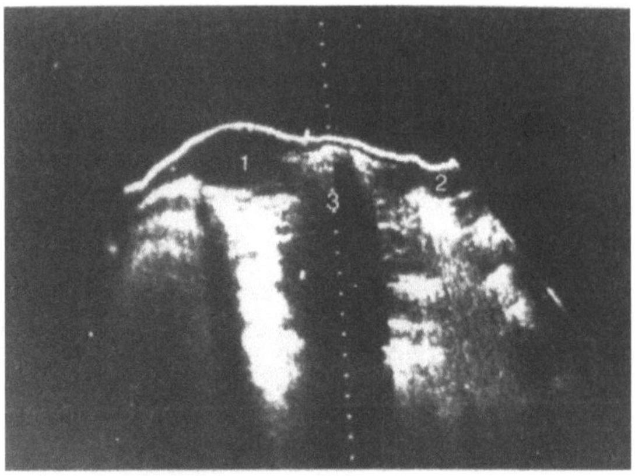

Fig. 14. Hematoma of rectus sheath. Transverse scan at the level of umbilicus. Anechoic collection *(1)* with posterior enhancement to the right of the umbilicus *(3)*. The muscle is normal on the left side *(2)*.

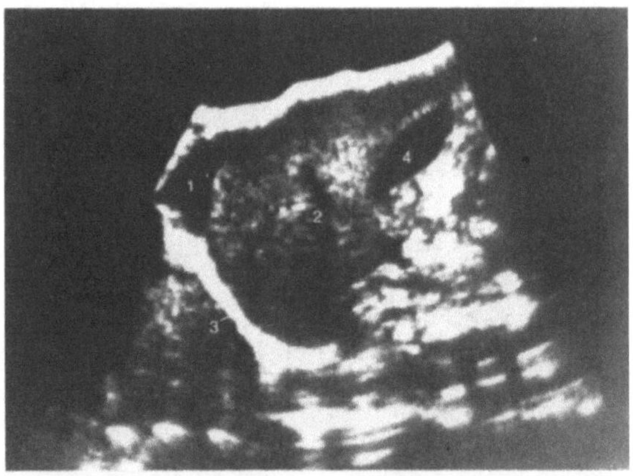

Fig. 15. Acute subhepatic anterior hemoperitoneum *(1)* between liver *(2)* and diaphragm *(3)*. Gallbladder *(4)*.

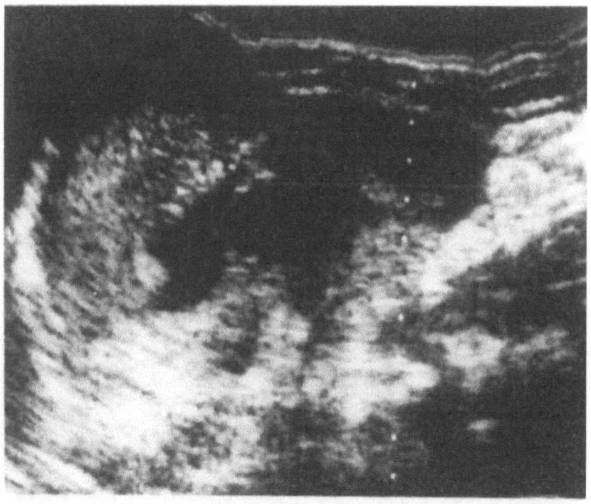
a

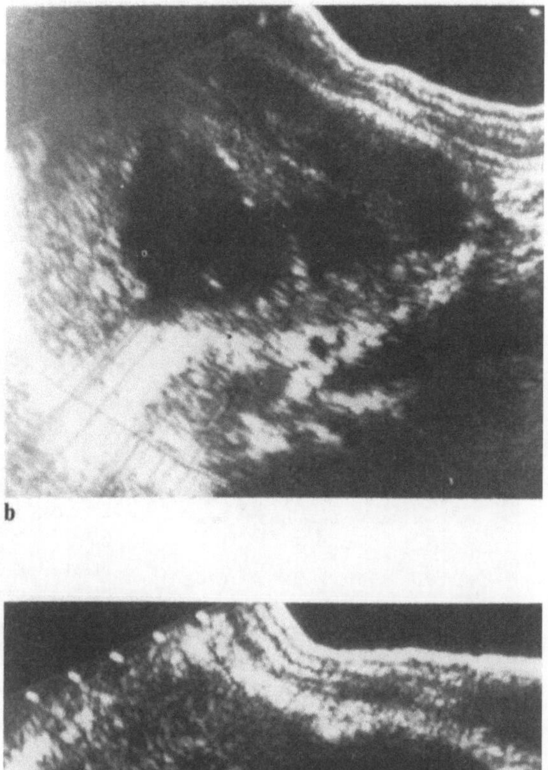
b

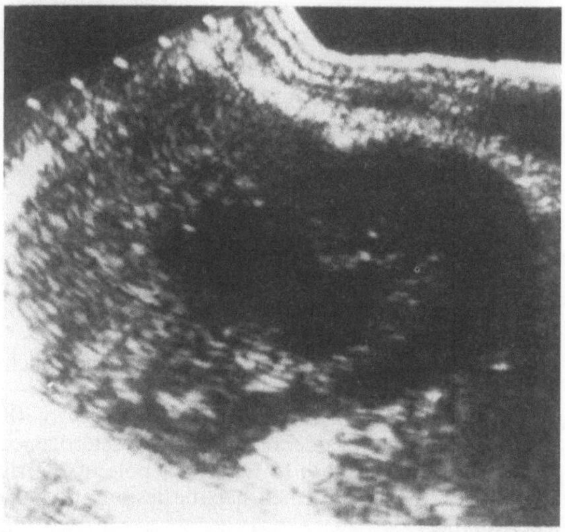
c

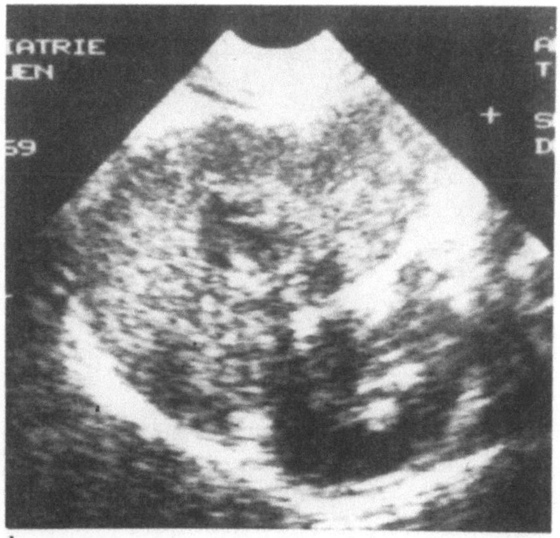
d

Fig. 16 a–d. Boy, 11 years old, who fell from 3 m on his left flank. Immediate anemia of low importance, well controlled by transfusion. Initial splenic US study **(a)**, 8 days later **(b)**, 1 month later **(c)**, 1 year later **(d)**. Evolution of intrasplenic hematoma and subcapsular hematoma. The borders of the hematoma become less regular, the center of hematoma less anechoic, and surrounding parenchyma more echogenic.

any where in the peritoneal cavity, close to an intestinal loop or to a remaniated parenchyma. Its form and content are less variable.

A retroperitoneal hematoma can be located in the renal fossa. Usually, at one pole or on the posterior face of the kidney, a biconcave image can be obtained. If the hematoma lies outside the capsule it should be distinguished from the psoas muscle which has a similar echogenicity but which is closer to the spine and has a controlateral symmetrical correspondent. When extracapsular, the hematoma is usually retrorenal or intrarenal. It can extend up to the iliac crest. When a renal lesion exists, the normal US appearance disappears. The shape of the kidney usually remains but there is localized disappearance of the sinusal echoes and of the cortical medullary differentiation. More anarchic appearance with anechoic areas can be seen (Figs. 18–21).

5.2 Evolution of the Hematoma (Fig. 16)

The US appearance of the hematic mass varies with time. It remains globally hypoechoic but usually goes through three phases.

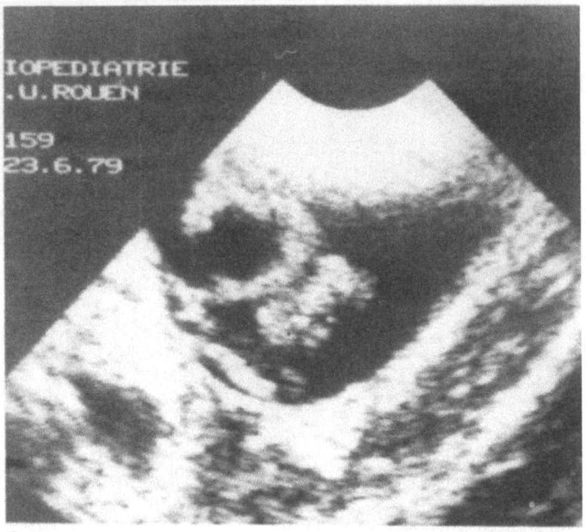

a

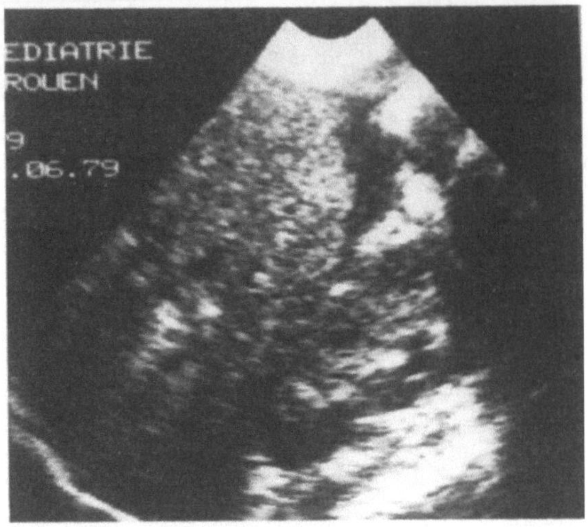

c

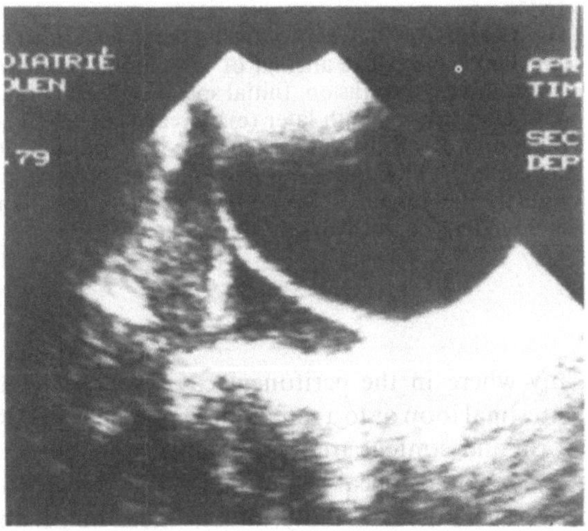

b

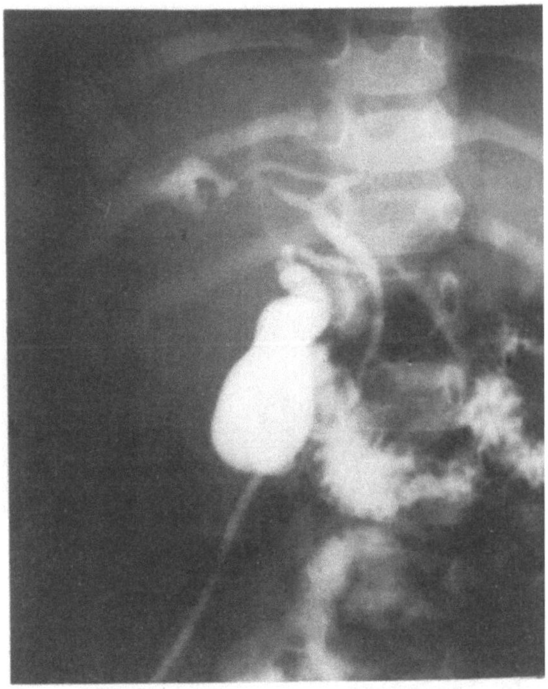

d

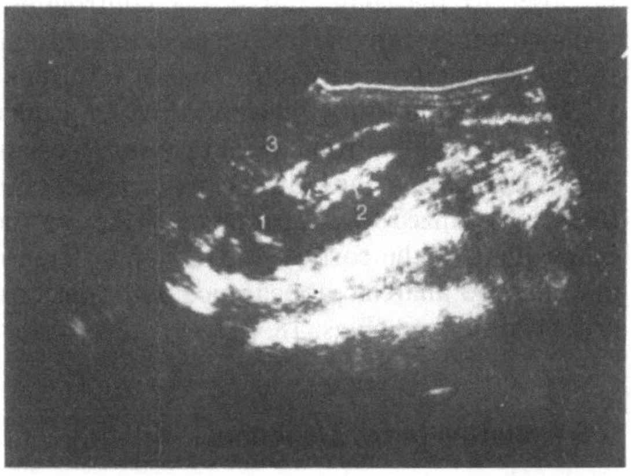

Fig. 18. Hematoma of the upper pole of right kidney. Hypoechogenicity of upper pole and disappearance of central echoes of the kidney *(1)*, normal patterns of lower pole *(2)*, liver *(3)*.

Fig. 17 a–d. Boy aged 3 years with severe trauma of right flank. Initial hemodynamic situation was good 2 days later fever and abdominal distension occurred.
a Transverse scan of left iliac fossa: distension of a bowel loop surrounded by peritoneal fluid.
b Medial sagittal scan: presence of fluid in the pouch of Douglas.
c Longitudinal scan in right flank: presence of fluid below the anterior border of the liver and heterogeneous liver parenchyma close to the upper pole of the right kidney. Surgery confirmed hepatic lesion and biliary peritonitis.
d Opacification through the cholecystostomy drain.

1. Initial Phase. The content is homogeneous, slinghtly echogenic, but less so than the surrounding parenchyma. This stage is not constant and can be seen during the first hours of a neonatal adrenal hematoma. In these circumstances, it is difficult to differentiate from a neonatal neuroblastoma. The evolution, biology, and clinical evaluation will help in the differentiation.

2. Collection phase. The content is frankly anechoic with acoustic enhancement. At this stage, sedimentation can show a liquid level.

3. Organization phase. The size of the hematoma gradually diminishes. Its borders become more echogenic while the central anechoic area disappears.

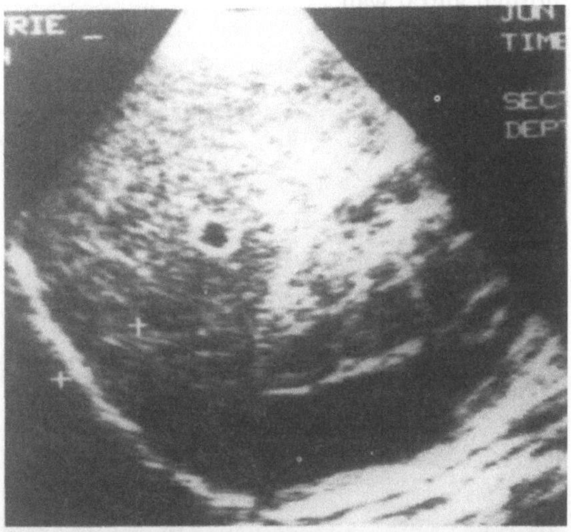

a

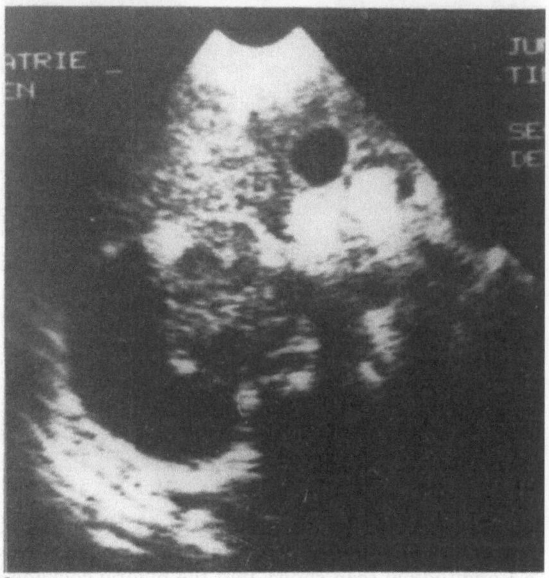

b

Fig. 19 a and b. Right lumbar trauma in a 7-year-old boy. Longitudinal scan of right flank **(a)** and transverse scan **(b)**: absence of renal lesion but voluminous hematoma of the perirenal space, posterior to the kidney.

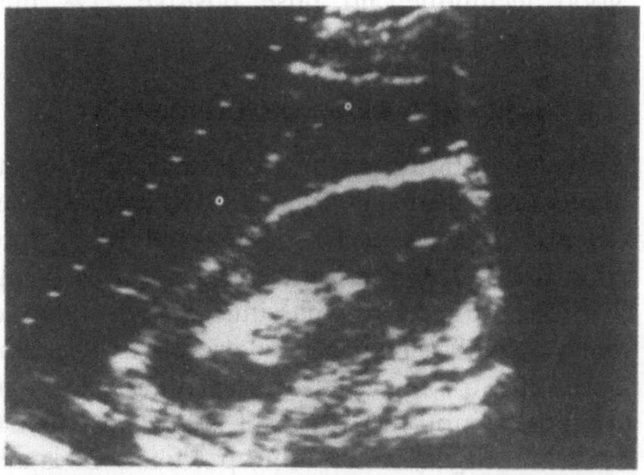

Fig. 20. Boy aged 10 years with contusion of lower pole of right kidney. Longitudinal scan: central echoes of the kidney have quite disappeared and surrounding parenchyma is of decreased echogenicity.

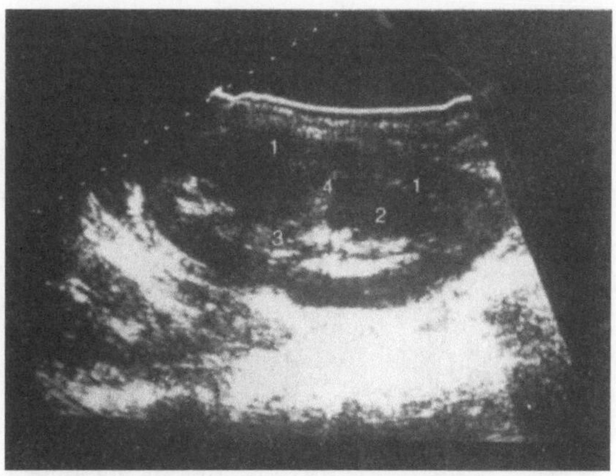

Fig. 21. Trauma of right kidney. Longitudinal posterior scan shows posterior hematoma of the perirenal space *(1)*, parenchymal contusion *(2)*, central echoes displaced forward *(3)*, possibility of a fracture *(4)*.

6 Some Specific Indications

6.1 Hypertrophic Pyloric Stenosis (HPS)

US cannot replace all the indications of a barium follow-through when HPS is suspected, but it has the advantage of providing inexpensively and without irradiation a documented proof of the hypertrophy of the pyloric muscle and of the gastric stasis, elements which are usually sufficient for the surgeon. Its accuracy is excellent with a good technique: no false positive, 5% false negative.

6.1.1 When to Look for the Pyloric Olive

US examination is performed systematically every time the clinical symptoms are typical, i.e. when vomiting occurs in a neonate aged 10–60 days along with an important stasis between meals, with peristaltic waves passing beyond midabdomen, or with a palpable pyloric olive. This concerns 80% of the cases. In the other cases, with atypical symptoms, US itself is not sufficient to indicate surgery. A barium opacifications is necessary and is performed first.

6.1.2 What to Look for

On perpendicular scans, a cockade image will be obtained. Normally, the peripheral hypoechoic halo measures less than 5 mm. The diameter of the olive should not exceed 15 mm. Beyond these measurements, HPS is ascertained (Fig. 22). A parallel scan to the long axes will sometimes show the antropyloric canal surrounded by the hypertrophied muscle (Fig.23).

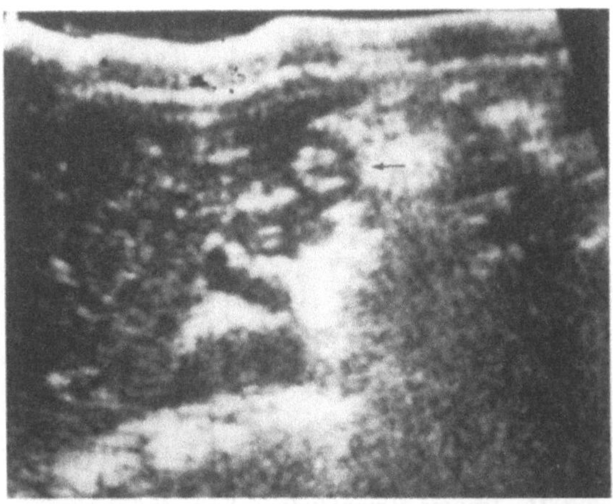

Fig. 22. Normal pattern of pyloric cockade on a longitudinal subhepatic scan. The olive measures 8 mm in diameter and the anechoic wall 3 mm (*arrow*).

6.1.3 Where to Look for the Olive

The pyloric muscle is elongated anteroposteriorly under the lower side of the liver, medially to the gallbladder. Serial sagittal scans should be performed from left to right in the epigastric area. The dilated gastric antrum is localized, and in continuity with it, the cockade image is seen with the hypertrophic muscle appearing thicker than the normal antral wall.

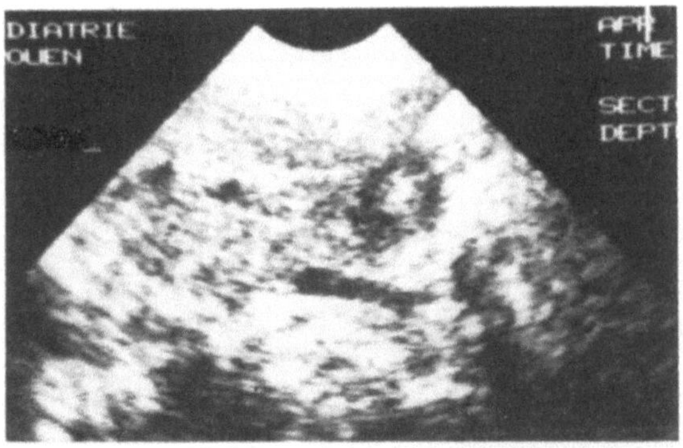

a

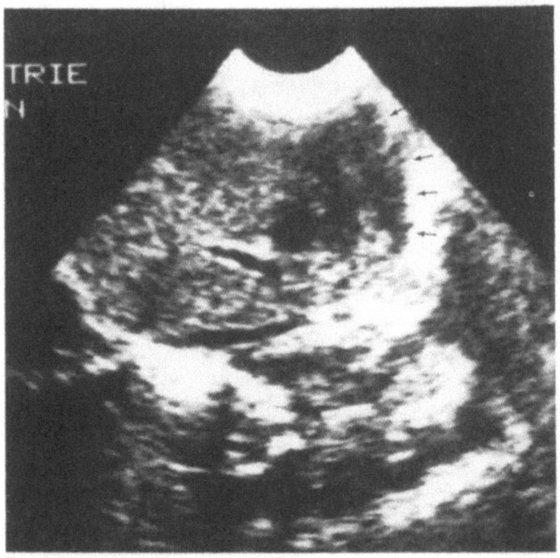

b

Fig. 23 a and b. Infant aged 10 days. Postprandial alimentary vomiting and peristaltic abdominal waves. **a** Longitudinal scan shows that the pyloric cockade is increased in size (16 mm) and its wall is thickened (6 mm). **b** Transverse epigastric scan: inside the gallbladder, the pyloric muscle is scanned by its long axis. The elongated pyloric canal is surrounded by a thickened muscular wall.

6.2 Acute Intestinal Intussusception (Fig. 24)

Barium enema is still the diagnostic and therapeutic obligatory procedure in every case of suspected intussusception. Two atypical circumstances lead us to perform a US examination in addition to the enema.

1. Some chronic intussusception forms occur as an abdominal mass with no pain. US will recognize the digestive nature of the mass and orient to a barium opacification.
2. The recurrence of an abdominal mass after reduction of an intussusception can result from a favorable etiology. US will demonstrate a simple hypertrophy of the ileocolic valve or a mass as a lymphoma, duplication cyst, or lipoma.

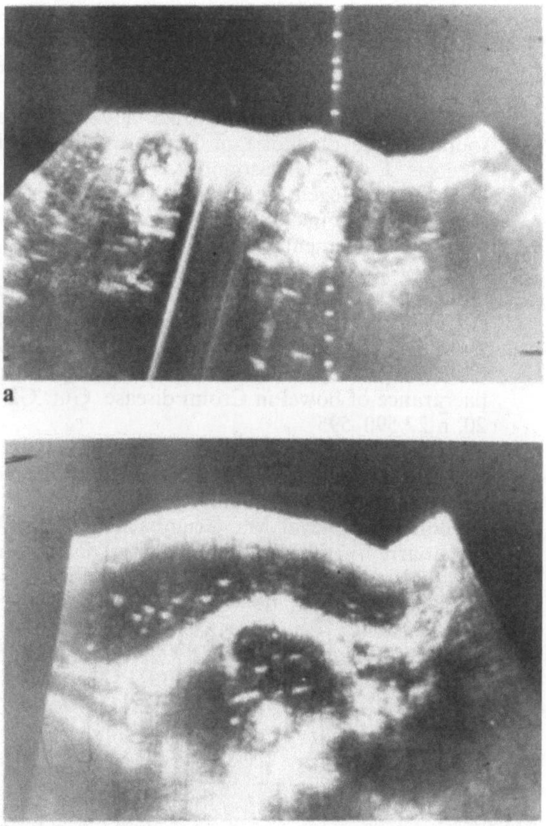

Fig. 24 a and b. Boy aged 3 years. Weak irregular mass of the left flank. **a** Longitudinal scan: the appearance of the mass suggests highly dilated digestive structures with heterogeneous contents. Barium enema: chronic ileocolic intussusception. **b** Transverse scan of low abdomen after intussusception treatment: disappearance of abnormalstructures and pattern of fluid-filled colon.

6.3 Survey of Ventriculoperitoneal Shunts

In these patients US examination shows a small amount of peritoneal effusion, which should not be considered abnormal. The extremity of the catheter is preciously localized by a KUB and can be seen free between the loops and the abdominal wall or next to the liver.

In cases of misfunctioning, or misresorption, a large ascitic or septated collection of fluid can be seen. In cases of a pseudocyst collection of fluid, an anechoic pouch can be distinguished from intestinal loops. It appears centered by an echoic structure corresponding to the catheter (Fig. 25). US examination is justified when abdominal or neurological symptoms occur; numerous changes of catheter or cerebromeningeal infection are also indications for systematic evaluation.

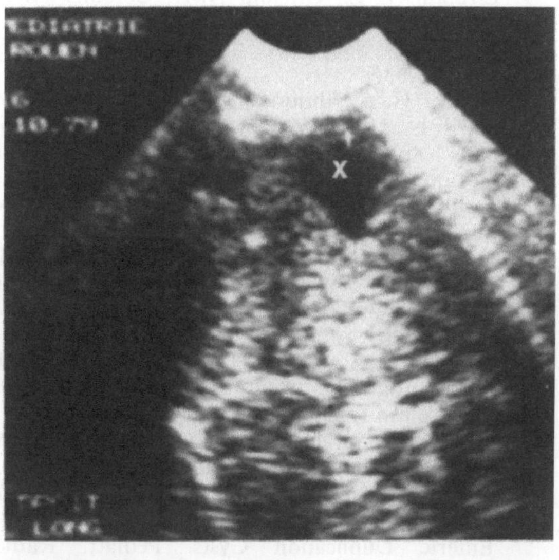

Fig. 25. Male infant aged 2.5 years. Ventriculoperitoneal shunt for hydrocephalus. Recent increase in head size. Axillary right transverse scan: well defined collection of fluid confirms the bad resorption of CSF.

References

General References

1. Fleischer, A.-C., Muhletaler C.-A., Everette James A. (1980). Sonographic patterns arising from normal and abnormal bowel. Rad. Clin. North. America 18:(1)
2. Garel L., Kalifa G. (1979). Confrontations anatomiques et échographiques dans le diagnostic des masses abdominales de l'enfant. Journées Parisiennes de Pédiatrie

3. Garel L., Lallemand D. (novembre 1981). Exploration radiologique des masses abdominales de l'enfant. Journées Nationales de Radiologie, Paris
4. Kangarloo H., Sample W.-F. (1979). Ultrasound of the pediatric abdomen and pelvis. Year book medical publishers, inc. Chicago–London
5. Meyers M.-A., Kazma E. (1976). Dynamic radiology of the abdomen. Springer Verlag. New York Heidelberg Berlin
6. Morgan C.-L., Trought W.-S., Oddson T.-A., Clark W.-M., Ricef R.-P. (1980). Ultrasound patterns of disorders affecting the gastrointestinal tract. Radiology 135:129–135
7. Thurber L.-A., Cooperberg P.-L., Clement J.-G., Lyons E.-A., Gramiak R., Cunningham J. (1979). Echogenic Fluid: A pitfall in the Ultrasonographic diagnosis of cystic lesions. J. Clin. Ultrasound 7:273–278
8. Weighall S.-L., Wolfman N.-T., Watson N. (1979). The Fluid-Filled Stomach: a new sonic window. J. Clin. Ultrasound 7:353–356

Intraperitoneal Masses

9. Effmann E.-L., Grislom N.-T., Colodny A.-H., Wawter G.-F. (1980). Neonatal Gastrointestinal Masses Arising Late in Gestation. A.J.R. 135:681–686
10. Gharbi H.-A., Brauner M.-W., Hassine M.-W., Saied H. (1982). Apport de l'échotomographie dans l̃exploration des masses abdominales palpables de l'enfant. J.E.M.U., 3, ñ 2:5–11
11. Goldberg B.-B. (1975). Ultrasonic Evaluation of Superficail Masses. J. Clin. Ultrasound 3:91–94
12. Haller J.-O., Schnider M., Kassner E.-G., Slovis T.-L., Perl L.-J. (1978). Sonographic Evaluation of Mesenteric and Omental Masses in Children. A.J.R 130:269–274
13. Moccia, W.-A., Astacio J.-E., Kaude J.-V (1981). Ultrasonographic Demonstration of Gastric Duplication in Infancy. Pediatr. Radiol. 11:52–54
14. Nicolas P., Ciprich G., Meck J.-M. (1981). Malformations de l'Ouraque. J. Radiol. 62, ñ 10:531–535
15. Teele R.-L., Henschke C.-I., Tapper D. (1980). The radiographic and Ultrasonographic Evaluation of Enteric Duplication Cysts. Pediatr. Radiol. 10:9–14
16. Wicks J.-D., Silver T.-M., Bree R.-L. (1978). Giant Cystic Abdominal Masses in Children and Adolescents: Ultrasonic Differential Diagnostic. A.J.R. 130:853–857

Peritonitis and Abscesses

17. Baudain Ph., Coupris L., Revillon Y., Sauve-Grain J. (1977). Forme pseudo-tumorale d'abcès appendiculaire chez le petit enfant. J. Radiol. Electrol. 58, ñ 6–7:445–449
18. Doust B.-D., Quiroz F., Stewart J.-M. (1977). Ultrasonic distinction of abscesses from other intraabdominal fluid collections. Radiology 125:213–218
19. Korobkin M., Callen P.-W., Filly R.-A., Hoffer P.-B., Shim Shak R.-R., Kressel H.-Y. (1978). Comparison of Computed Tomography, Ultrasonography, and Gallium 67 Scanning in the Evaluation of Suspected Abdominal Abscess. Radiology 129:89–93
20. Kressel H.-Y., Filly R.-A. (1978). Ultrasonographic Appearance of Gas-containing Abscesses in the Abdomen. A.J.R. 130:71–73
21. Sekiba K., Akamatsu N., Niva K. (1979). Ultrasound Characteristics of Abdominal Abscesses involving Foreign Bodies (Gauze). J. Clin. Ultrasound. USA, 7, ñ 4:284–286

Miscellaneous

22. Baudain Ph., Chaix D., Crouzet A. Les épanchements abdominaux de liquide céphalo-rachidien dans les dérivations ventriculo-péritonéales: intérêt de l'échographie. E.M.C. Radiodiagnostic
23. Blumhagen J.-D., Coombs J.-B. (1981). Ultrasound in the diagnosis of hypertrophic Pyloric Stenosis. J. Clin. Ultrasound 9:289–292
24. Delgoffe C., Regent D., Chaulieu C., Theheux A. (1981). Hématome duodénal spontané géant au cours d̃un traitement fibrinolytique. J. Radiol. 62, ñ 3:189–197
25. Goldfine J.-L., Turetz F., Beck A.-R., Eiger M. (1978). Cerebrospinal Fluid Intraperitoneal Cyst: an unusuall abdominal mass. A.J.R. 130:568–569
26. Golt S., Samuel E. (1979). Ultrasonographic appaerarance of bowel in Crohn disease. Gut. GER 20, ñ 27:590–595
27. Parienty R.-A., Lepreux J.-F., Gruson B. (1981). Sonographic and CT Features of Ileocolic Intussusception. A.J.R. 136:608–610
28. Remond A., Dieval M., Grumbach Y., Petit J., Delamarre J., Trinez G. (1979). Apport de l'échotomographie en urgence dans les traumatismes rénaux. A propos de 12 cas. Ann. Radiol. 22:7:579–584
29. Yeh H.-C., Wolf B.-S. (1977). Ultrasonography in Ascites. Radiology 124:783–790

Chapter 6

Liver, Biliary Tract, and Spleen

F. Brunelle and J.-Y. Cohen

1 Normal Anatomy on US

Hepatic US in children should be focused on hepatic vascularization. Real-time US makes such a study much easier. Five scans are mandatory: a longitudinal scan through the long axis of aorta, a longitudinal scan through the inferior vena cava (IVC), a subcostal oblique scan-through the confluence of the hepatic veins, a subcostal oblique scan through the portal vein bifurcation, and a longitudinal oblique scan through the long axis of the portal trunk.

1.1 Longitudinal Scan Through the Aorta

On such a scan (Fig. 1), one must look for the abdominal esophagus, the crus of the diaphragm, the aorta, the celiac trunk, and the superior mesenteric artery (SMA). The splenic vein is seen anterior to the SMA. The anatomic space between the aorta and the posterior end of the left lobe of the liver at the level of the celiac trunk is the lesser omentum. Its normal thickness in a control group of patients is inferior to one diameter of the aorta.

The examination can be impeded by a medially located stomach in cases of huge splenomegaly or hepatic atrophy. The left lateral decubitus or the right lateral decubitus, using the spleen as an acoustic window, allows good visualization of the abdominal aorta.

It is mandatory to measure the diameter of the aorta above and below the celiac trunk, which is generelly nearly identical; the diameters of the celiac trunk and the SMA are also identical.

It is sometimes possible to demonstrate a right hepatic artery branching off the SMA. This hepatic artery is located posterior to the portal trunk, while a normal hepatic artery is anterior to the portal trunk (Fig. 2a, b).

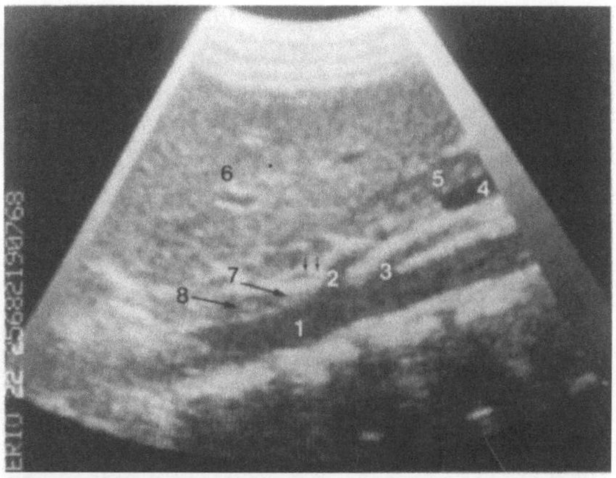

Fig. 1. Longitudinal scan through the aorta. *1*, Aorta; *2*, Celiac trunk; *3*, Superior mesenteric artery; *4*, Superior meseteric vein; *5*, Pancreas; *6*, Liver; *7*, Diaphragmatic crus; *8*, Esophagus. This scan demonstrates well that the caliber of the celiac trunk and the superior mesenteric artery is identical. The lesser omentum is measured at the level of the crus of the diaphragm above the celiac trunk, between the anterior wall of the aorta and the inferior side of the liver. In a healthy child, its thickness is less than the diameter of the aorta. In this case, the left gastric artery is visible (*arrow*).

1.2 Longitudinal Scan Through the IVC

The patency of the IVC is a very important diagnostic and prognostic factor in the evaluation of portal hypertension in children (Fig. 3). The

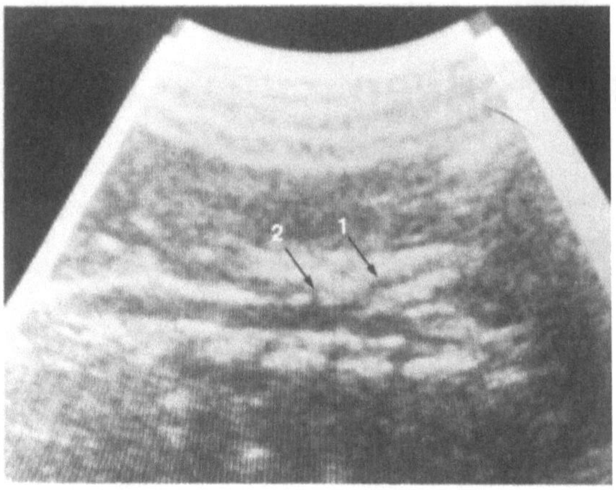

a

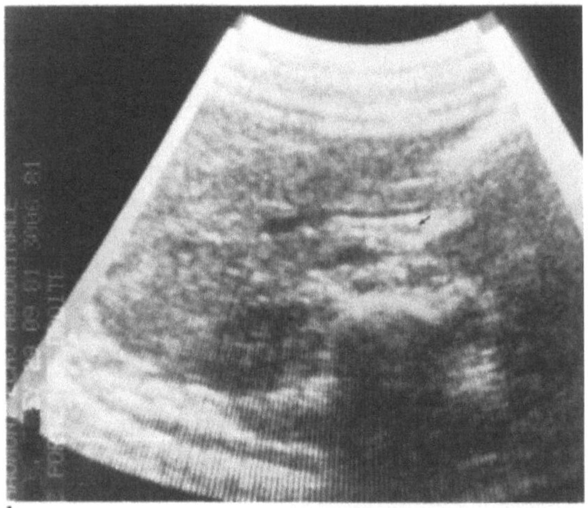

b

Fig. 2 a and b. Angioma of the right lobe of the liver in a 1-year-old child. Right hepatic artery from the superior mesenteric artery. **a** Longitudinal scan through the aorta showing the large superior mesenteric artery *(1)* whose diameter is twice that of the celiac trunk *(2)*. **b** A transverse scan through the superior mesenteric artery origin demonstrates well a large artery branching off the superior mesenteric artery (*arrow*) located behind the portal vein trunk and in front of the IVC. This anatomical state is characteristic of a right hepatic artery coming from the superior mesenteric artery. In this case, the diagnosis had been made easier by real-time examination.

diameter of the IVC should be measured in younger children during crying or, in older children, at the begining of expiration after a Valsalva maneuver. Indeed, during the Valsalva maneuver, the IVC is compressed anteriorly by the liver. The maximum diameter of the IVC is then observed at the begining of expiration. The diameter of the IVC should be measured at the level of the portal trunk on a longitudinal scan. When the IVC is not seen, one must look for a vascular structure

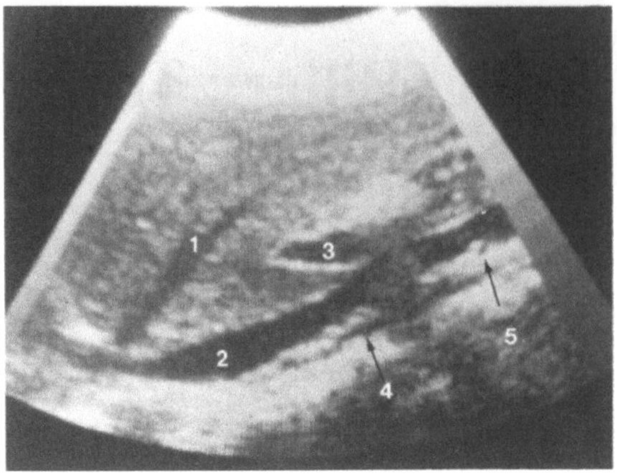

Fig. 3 Longitudinal scan through the IVC. On this scan, the medial hepatic vein *(1)*, IVC *(2)*, the portal trunk *(3)*, right crus of the diaphragm *(4)* and the left renal artery *(5)* are clearly seen.

behind the crus of diaphragm on the left or right of the aorta, which is an azygos continuation of the IVC.

1.3 Subcostal Oblique Scan Through the Confluence of the Hepatic Vein

The diameter, direction, and ostia of the hepatic veins (HV) should be examined (Fig. 4). The wall of the HV is usually not echogenic except that of the right HV which is perpendicular to the ultrasonic beam. The HV converge toward the IVC. The left and medial HV often have a common trunk. Their diameter increases from the periphery to the right auricle and their diameter presents variations during the respiratory cycles, synchronized to those of the IVC. Their ostia are well analyzed only by real-time US.

1.4 Subcostal Oblique Scan Through the Portal Bifurcation

The orientation of the portal bifurcation is variable, from a horizontal to a vertical plane (Fig. 5). Its walls are normally slightly echogenic. It is possible to follow the portal vein to the subsegmental branches.

The right portal vein has two branches: the anterior branch is horizontal, the posterior branch is vertical. The left portal branch has a characteristic posteroanterior course and ends in the umbilical recess in a branch of the quadrate

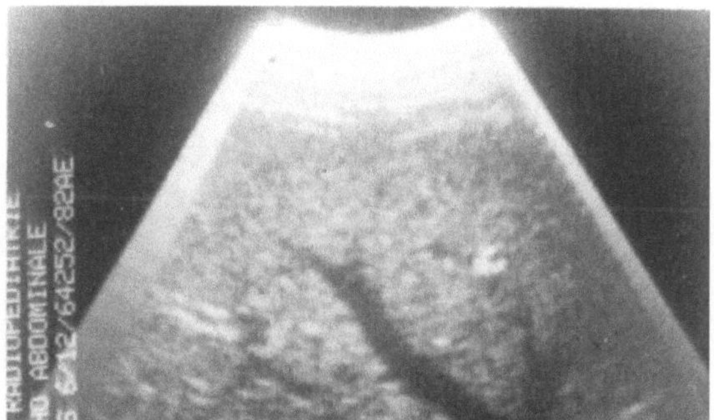

Fig. 4. a Subcostal oblique scan through the confluence of the hepatic veins. The origin of the right hepatic vein is visible *(1)*, the medial and the left hepatic veins have a common trunk before the confluence with the IVC. The anterior branch of the right portal vein is visible between the right and medial hepatic veins. A subsegmental portal branch is also seen between the medial and left hepatic veins. **b** The three hepatic veins are seen, converging toward the IVC. The medial and left hepatic veins have a common trunk.

lobe. The second and third subsegmental branches of the left portal vein are often visible.

In the newborn, the umbilical vein is normally patent during the first month of life (Fig. 6). It can be seen on a right longitudinal para-aortic scan. On a subcostal oblique scan the left portal vein often appears dilated. The umbilical vein is visible as a thin vascular structure with very echogenic walls leading from the left portal branch toward the umbilicus.

In children below 10 years of age, the intrahepatic biliary ducts are not normally visible with

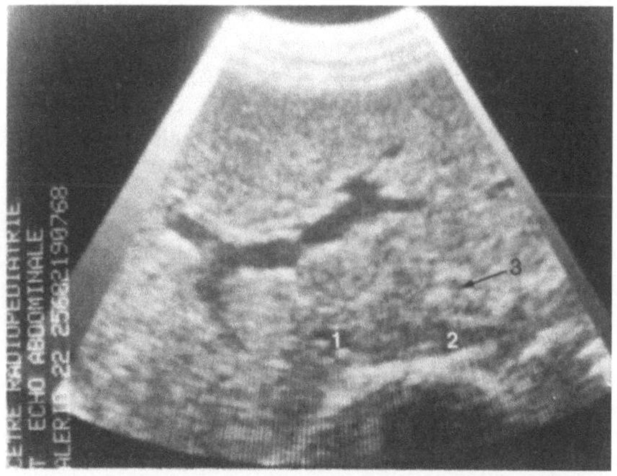

Fig. 5. Subcostal oblique scan through the portal bifurcation. This scan demonstrates well the portal bifurcation, the origin of the anterior branch of the right portal vein and the posterior branch. The left branch of the portal vein presents its characteristic posteroanterior direction and the subsegmental branches of the left lobe of the liver are clearly visible. The hepatic artery is seen in front of the portal bifurcation. *1*, IVC; *2*, Aorta; *3*, Esophagus.

transducers with a frequency inferior or equal to 5 MHz. Exceptionally, the hepatic artery may also be visible at this level.

1.5 Scan Along the Portal Trunk Axis (Fig. 7a–c)

Like the portal bifurcation, the orientation of the portal trunk is variable. It appears as a vascular structure with slightly echogenic walls. Its caliber varies with the age of the patient (Table 1).

The hepatic artery is constantly seen anterior to the portal vein slightly to the left. Normally, it has a more horizontal course than the portal trunk itself.

The main biliary duct is normally invisible in children less than 10 years of age. When visible, its diameter should be compared with normal values established by US (Table 1). It should be looked for not only anterior to the portal vein, but slightly to the right of it. The portal vein is indeed more horizontal than the main biliary duct which is almost constantly vertical.

1.6 Gallbladder (Fig. 8)

The gallbladder should be looked for by taking the right portal vein as a reference because the

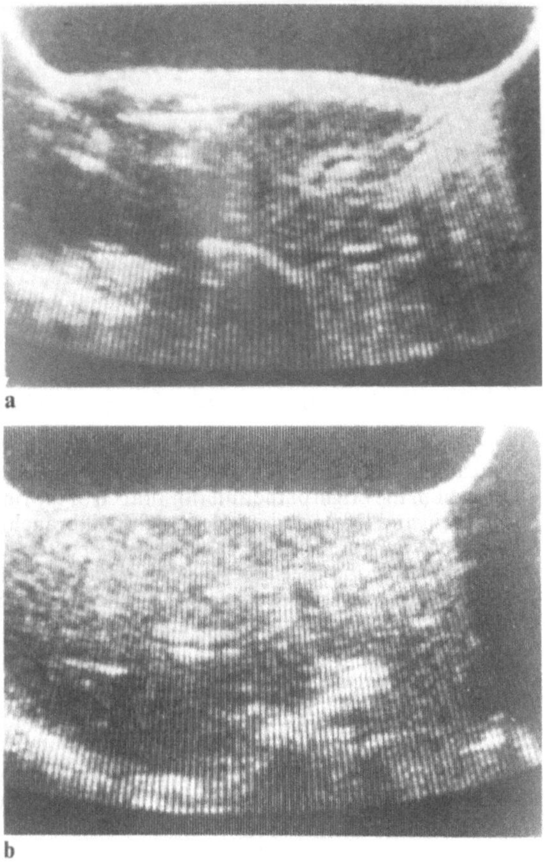

Fig. 6 a and b. Oblique scans in a 9-day-old child. **a** The umbilical vein is visible from the left portal branch and leaving the hepatic parenchyma. A patent umbilical vein must be suspected everytime that the left portal branch is dilated as it is visible in the same patient on a subcostal oblique scan **(b)**.
In our experience, a patent umbilical vein is a normal phenomenon in the first month of life and must not be considered as an indication of portal hypertension.

right portal vein has a constant anatomical relationship with the infundibulum of the gallbladder. The fundus of the gallbladder can be extremely mobile. The gallbladder is an oblong anechogenic structure, whose walls are slightly echogenic. It is normally sightly oblique to the right and downwards and is anterior to the portal vein before its bifurcation in anterior and posterior branches.

1.7 Hepatic Parenchyma

The hepatic parenchyma is normally homogeneous, scattered with thin hypoechogenic structures representing the peripheral portal branches. Its echogenicity is normally slightly higher compared to that of the (right) kidney.

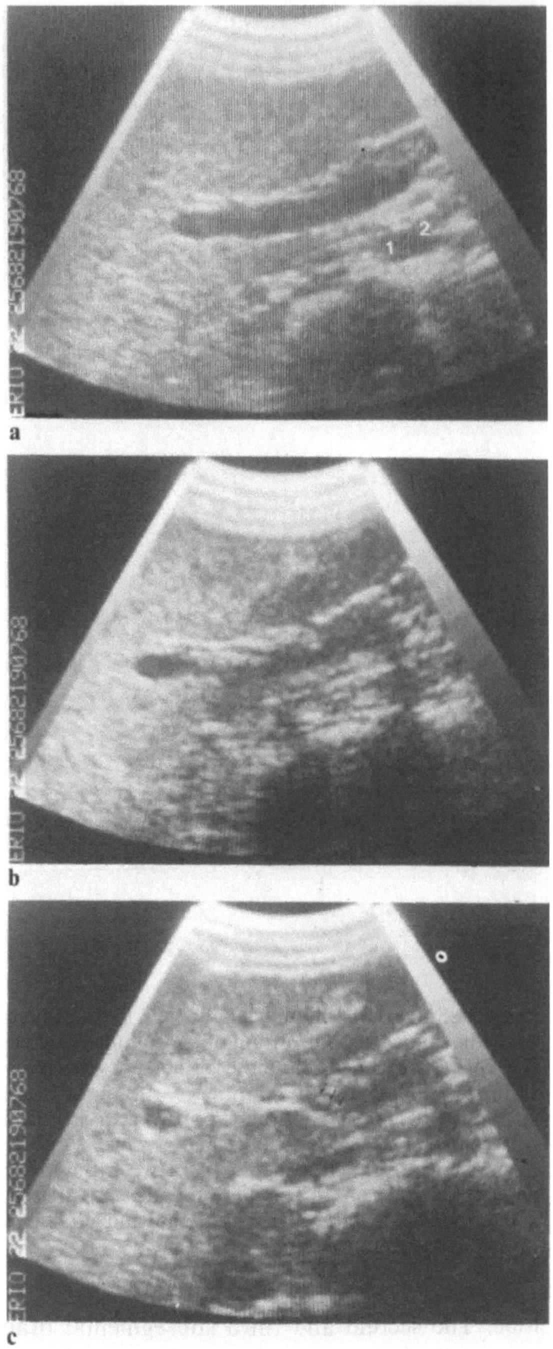

Fig. 7 a–c. Scans in a 16-year-old boy, hence the common bile duct is visible.
a Oblique scan through the long axis of the portal vein. The portal trunk is clearly visible. A vascular structure is seen in front of the portal vein, representing the hepatic artery. *1,* Aorta; *2,* Celiac trunk origin. The biliary ducts are rarely seen in front of the portal trunk and are more often seen on the right anterolateral wall of the portal vein.
b The common bile duct is visible slightly to the right of the portal trunk crossing the portal vein axis in a "X".
c On a scan slightly more to the right, the terminal portion of the common bile duct (*arrows*) is seen.

Table 1. Sonographic measurements of the normal pediatric gallbladder and biliary tract [14].

Age range (years)	AP diameter (cm)		Coronal diameter (cm)		Length (cm)		Wall thickness (mm)		Common hepatic duct size (mm)		Right portal vein size (mm)	
	Mean	Range	Mean	Range	Mean	Range	Mean	Range	Mean	Range	Mean	Range
0– 1 (8 patients)	0.9	0.5–1.2	0.9	0.7–1.4	2.5	1.3–3.4	1.7	1.0–3.0	1.3	1.0–2.0	3.8	3.0– 5.0
2– 5 (10 patients)	1.7	1.4–2.3	1.8	1.0–3.9	4.2	2.9–5.2	2.0	None	1.7	1.0–3.0	4.8	3.0– 7.0
6– 8 (11 patients)	1.8	1.0–2.4	2.0	1.2–3.0	5.6	4.4–7.4	2.2	2.0–3.0	2.0	None	5.7	6.0– 9.0
9–11 (12 patients)	1.9	1.2–3.2	2.0	1.0–3.6	5.5	3.4–6.5	2.0	1.0–3.0	1.8	1.0–3.0	6.8	4.0– 9.0
12–16 (10 patients)	2.0	1.3–2.8	2.1	1.6–3.0	6.1	3.8–8.0	2.0	1.0–3.0	2.2	1.0–4.0	7.8	6.0–10.0

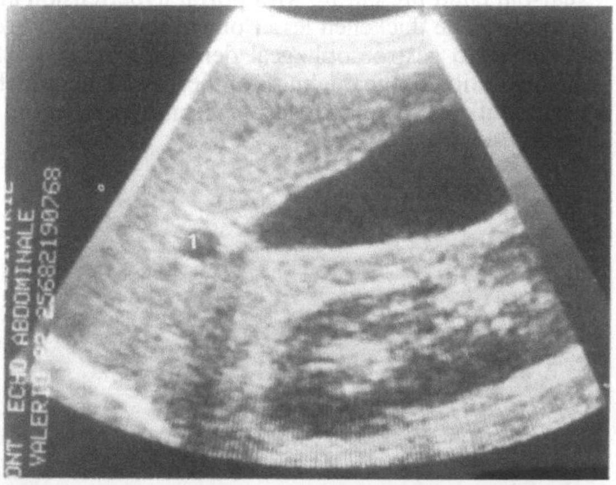

Fig. 8. Longitudinal scan through the gallbladder and right kidney clearly showing the gallbladder. It is a completely sonolucent structure with a thin wall. The infundibulum of the gallbladder presents a constant anatomical relationship with the right portal vein *(1)*. An acoustic shadow is often seen at the level of the infundibulum. This shadow is due to the refraction of the ultrasonic beam. This shadow can be distinguished from a lithiasis by making the patient change position.

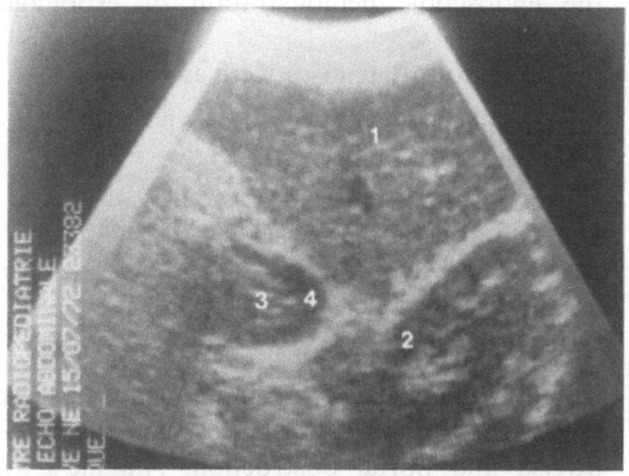

Fig. 9. Left subcostal oblique scan clearly showing the initial splenic vein. From the splenic hilum, the vein has an anteroposterior course around the tail of the pancreas. *1*, Spleen; *2*, kidney; *3*, Pancreas; *4*, Splenic vein

1.8 Spleen

The spleen is usually visible only when using intercostal scans or during deep inspiration. In general its echogenicity is homogeneous, equal to that of the liver. The splenic vein is visible behind the tail of the pancreas with a characteristic course: first, a downward portion from the splenic hilum and then a tranverse course which slightly ascends, hooking the tail of pancreas (Fig. 9). It joins the superior mesenteric vein (SMV) to form the portal trunk. The splenic artery can be seen at the level of the celiac trunk and on a longitudinal left para-aortic scan, cephalad to the splenic vein.

1.9 Extrahepatic Portal System

We have just mentioned that the splenic vein is usually visible behind the pancreas. The SMV is difficult to see because of the overlying abdominal gas. It is indeed located behind the transverse colon and the first jejunal loops. In children, the left gastric vein and the inferior mesenteric vein (IMV) are usually invisible.

2 Portal Hypertension

Portal hypertension is defined by an elevation of the corrected portal pressure (direct portal pressure minus IVC pressure above 20 cm of water).

The major consequence is the development of hepatofugal portosystemic derivations of which the most important are the esophageal varices fed by the right, left, and posterior gastric veins.

2.1 Material

These results are based on the echographic analysis of 125 children with portal hypertension. The diagnosis of portal hypertension has been made either by direct measurement of the portal pressure (splenoportography, transhepatic portography, or measurement during surgery) or by the endoscopic demonstration of esophageal varices.

The various diagnoses were as follows:

Portal obstruction	51
Cirrhosis	27
Biliary atresia	24
Congenital hepatic fibrosis	10
Budd Chiari Syndrome	8
α_1-antitrypsin deficiency	5
Others	3

Three patients had two simultaneous diseases: Budd-Chiari and portal obstruction, biliary atresia and portal obstruction, Alagille's syndrome and portal obstruction.

A total of 58 children underwent US examination after a portocaval shunt; 38 had pre- and postoperative US examinations.

2.2 US Diagnosis of Portal Hypertension (Fig. 10)

In the case of portal hypertension, the lesser omentum is, in our experience, constanly thickened. This surgical finding is due to the presence of gastroesophageal derivations and to the lymphatic stasis at this level.

On a longitudinal scan through the aorta, the lesser omentum is seen as a very echogenic structure between the posterior aspect of the liver and the crus of the diaphragm. In the case of portal hypertension, its thickness is superior to the diameter of the aorta. The lesser omentum can be seen on a subcostal scan through the portal vein bifurcation as an echogenic line running from the left portal vein to the abdominal esophagus (Fig. 11). This line, having been described as the ligamentum venosum, represents in fact the hepatic insertion of the lesser omentum. The ligamentum venosum is only one of the anatomical structures within the lesser omentum. In a control group of children, this line was never seen, except in cases of pathologic obesity.

It is mandatory to look for gastroesophageal derivations within the lesser omentum: They are visible as vascular structures running from the splenic vein to the abdominal esophagus (Fig. 12).

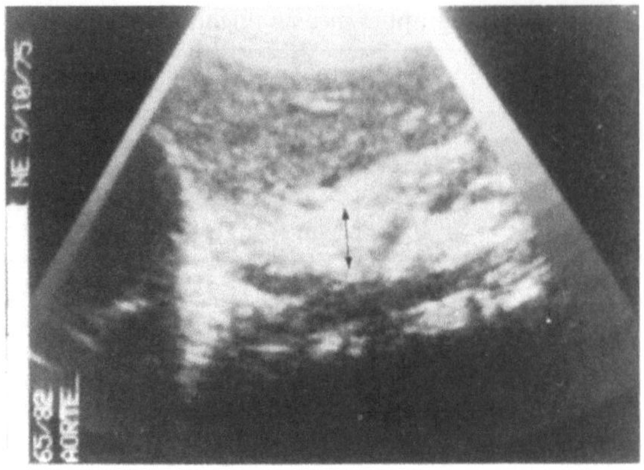

Fig. 10. Longitudinal scan through the aorta in a 9-year-old child presenting with portal hypertension and cirrhosis. The thickened lesser omentum is clearly seen (*arrow*). No gastroesophageal derivation is seen. The augmentation of the thickness of the lesser omentum by itself confirms the diagnosis of portal hypertension.

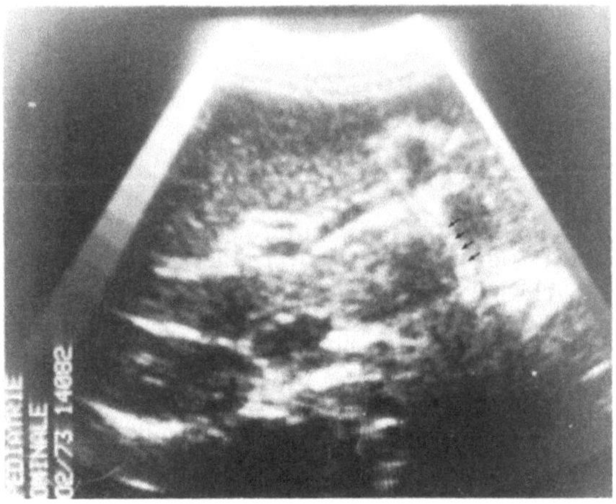

Fig. 11. Congenital hepatic fibrosis and portal hypertension. Subcostal oblique scan through the portal bifurcation. The lesser omentum is visible as a dense line from the left portal vein to the abdominal esophagus.

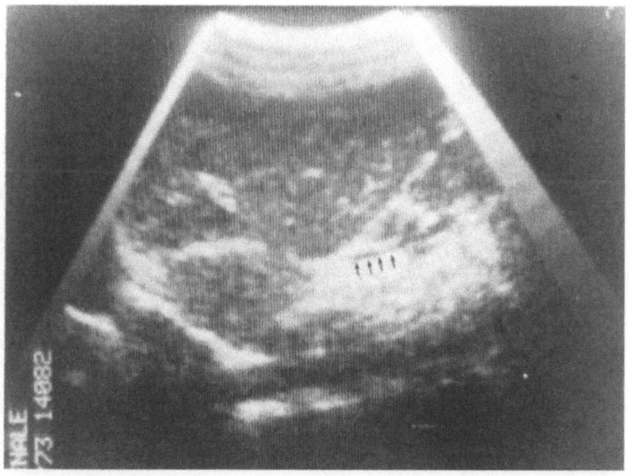

Fig. 12. Same patient as Fig. 11. Longitudinal scan through the aorta showing a vascular structure in the lesser omentum coming from the splenic vein and corresponding to a dilated left gastric vein.

2.3 Echographic and Fibroscopic Correlations

Six of the 125 examinations were inconclusive because of abdominal gas. Among the other 119 patients, US demonstrated gastroesophageal derivations as well as endoscopy in 85 patients (71% true positives). In 26 cases of 119 (22%), there were no gastroesophageal derivations demonstrated by either US or endoscopy (true negatives). In 6 cases (5%) US demonstrated gastroesophageal varices although no submucosal varices were demonstrated by endoscopy (false positives). In 2 cases (2%) although no gastroesophageal derivations were demonstrated by US there were submucosal esophageal varices demonstrated by endoscopy (false negatives). The overall diagnostic accuracy of US in showing esophageal varices is 93%.

2.4 Discussion

The true negative group mainly consists of patients with portal hypertension and a patent surgical portosystemic shunt. The false positive group is composed of very young patients (less than 2 years of age) with gastroesophageal derivations seen by US without submucosal esophageal varices. It is reasonable to assume that the submucosal esophageal varices develop with age.

The vascular structures demonstrated by US and those demonstrated by endoscopy are not exactly the same. US shows intra-abdominal derivations, although endoscopy indicates submucosal esophageal varices.

When the diagnosis of portal hypertension is made, it is essential to establish its origin.

2.5 Etiologic Diagnoses

2.5.1 Portal Obstruction or Cavernous Transformation of the Portal Vein

The portal bifurcation is replaced by a very echogenic structure in which multiple vascular tortuous structures are seen. They are particularly visible at the level of the infundibulum of the gallbladder. They represent the hepatopetal derivations draining the mesenteric venous blood toward the liver (Figs. 13 and 14).

The trunk of the portal vein, normally visible on a longitudinal oblique scan, has disappeared and is replaced by an echogenic structure. The hepatopetal derivations (pancreaticoduodenal veins) can sometimes be misdiagnosed as a normal portal trunk (Fig. 15). Careful analysis of their direction can establish their anatomical nature. The normal portal trunk is indeed retropancreatic although the pancreaticoduodenal derivations are more often anterior to the pancreas (Fig. 16).

2.5.2 Budd Chiari Syndrome

The Budd-Chiari syndrome is defined by the existence of an obstruction of the hepatic vein whatever its location or origin. In contrast, the Budd-Chiari *disease* is defined by ostial stenosis of the hepatic veins involved in a very precise chronological order, the left medial, and then the

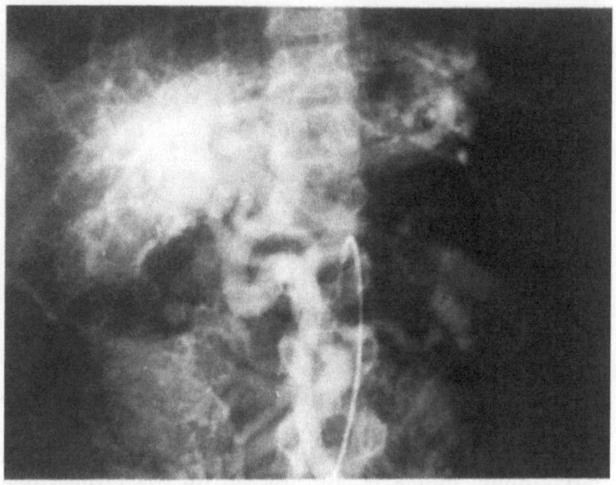

Fig. 13. Portal vein obstruction. Venous phase of a superior mesenteric artery injection. Many hepatopetal derivations are seen converging toward the hepatic hilum.

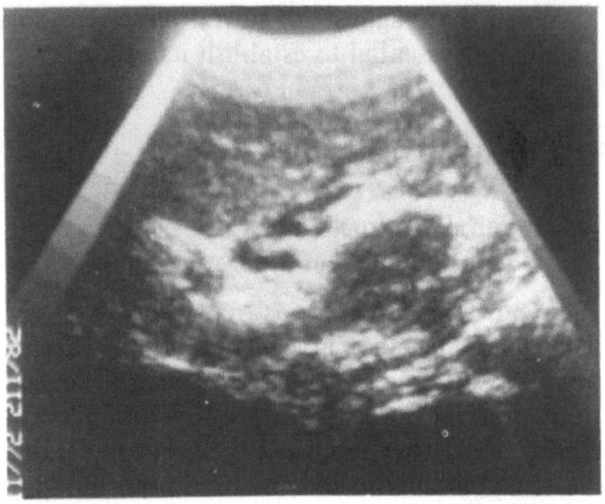

a

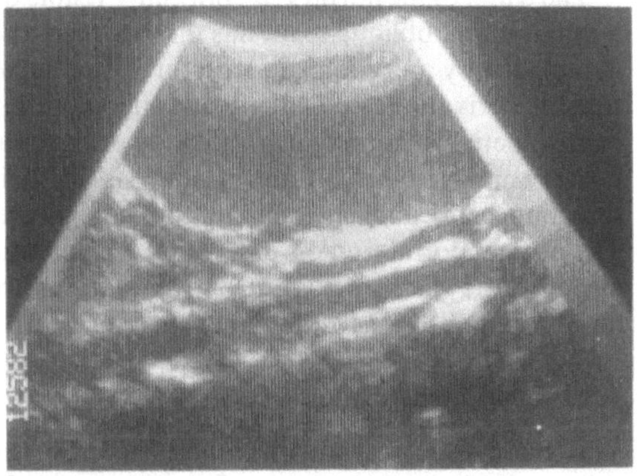

b

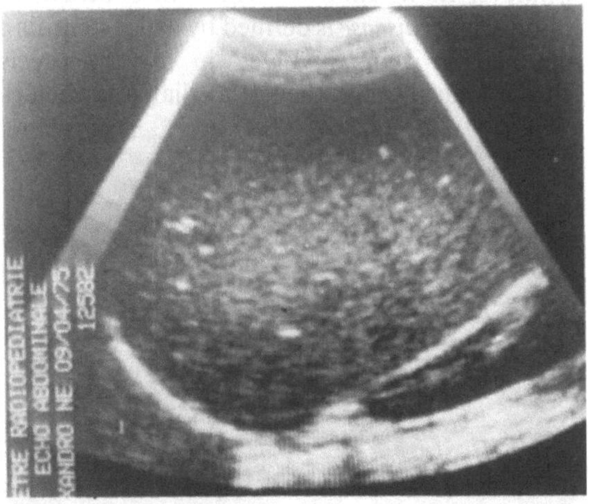

c

Fig. 14a–c. Portal vein obstruction in a 7-year-old. **a** The hepatic hilum is occupied by a very hypoechogenic zone inside which the numerous hepatopetal derivations are visible. **b** Longitudinal scan through the left kidney, which is compressed by the large spleen. **c** The diagnosis of portal hypertension can be made because of the presence of a dilated left gastric vein, clearly visible in front of the aorta in this longitudinal scan.

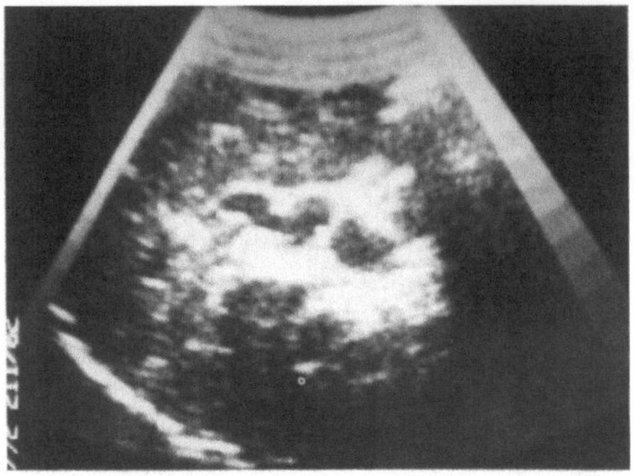

a

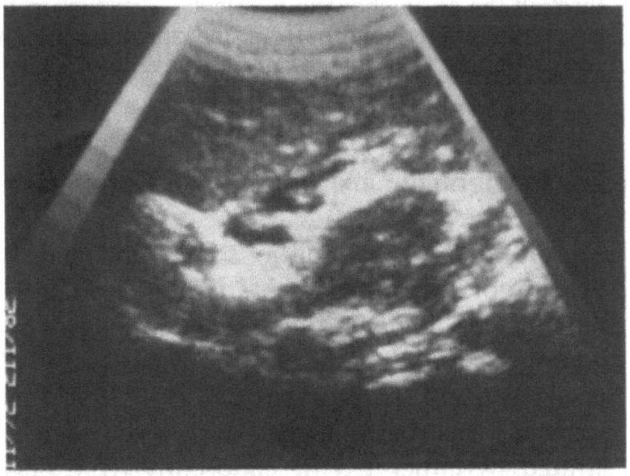

b

Fig. 15. a Portal vein thrombosis. Longitudinal scan along the long axis of the portal vein. Multiple hepatopetal collaterals are seen as tortuous vascular structures in the gastrohepatic ligament.
b On this subcostal oblique scan, multiple vascular structures are seen within the porta hepatis, representing the hepatopetal collaterals.

right hepatic veins and finally the vein of the caudate lobe.

The analysis of the hepatic veins allows three types of anomalies to be demonstrated: the hepatic veins are dilated, their direction is abnormal, and the junction with the IVC is invisible or presents a stenosis (Fig. 17 and 18).

It is mandatory to study carefully the IVC to look for an associated thrombosis or diaphragm.

The veno-occlusive disease is defined by an obliterating endophlebitis of the small centrolobular veins. In this case, the hepatic veins are either invisible or very small. Their junction with the IVC is normal.

The echographic signs of portal hypertension are usually discrete. The gastroesophageal derivations appear later (Fig. 19). On the other hand,

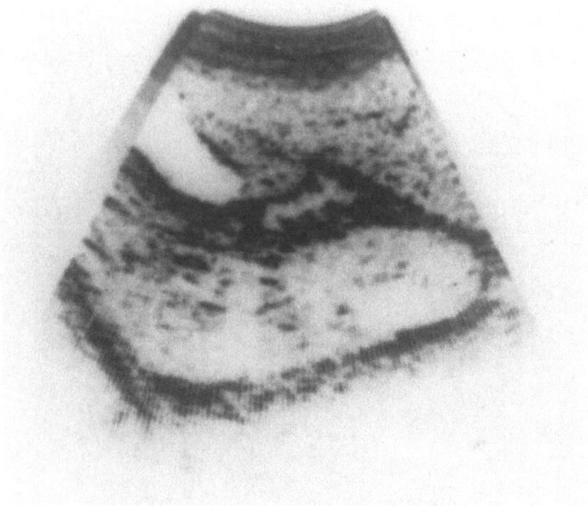

a

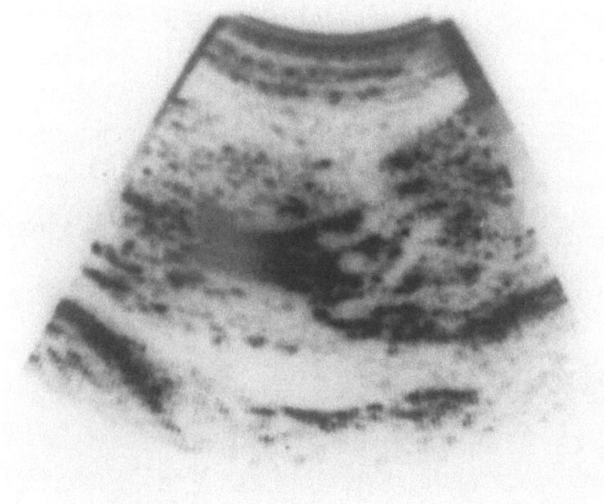

b

Fig. 16a and b. Other example of hepatopetal derivations in an 11-year-old. **a** Tortuous vascular structure seen within a very dense hepatic hilum. The lesser omentum is seen as a dense line.
b Longitudinal scan through the IVC. Numerous vascular structures are seen within the gastrohepatic ligament. One of these vascular structures has a prepancreatic course, corresponding to an anterior pancreaticoduodenal derivation.

the presence of ascites is frequently demonstrated (Fig. 20).

2.5.3 Intrahepatic Blocks

The echographic signs of intrahepatic blocks are essentially negative. The hepatic veins and the portal bifurcation are patent and normal. However, the portal vein walls are hyperechogenic (Fig. 21). The presence of portal hypertension signs allows diagnosis of an intrahepatic block.

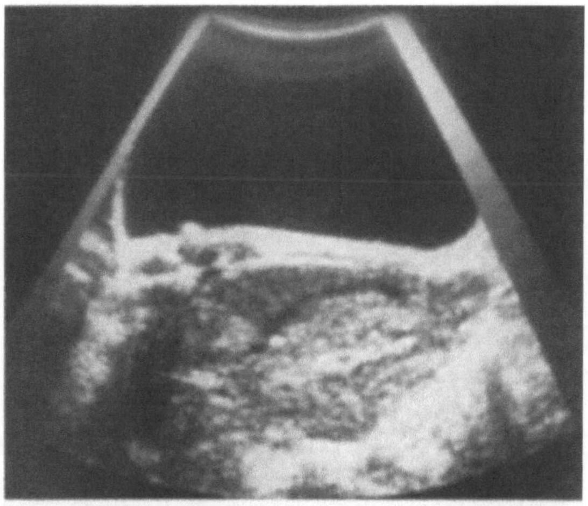

a

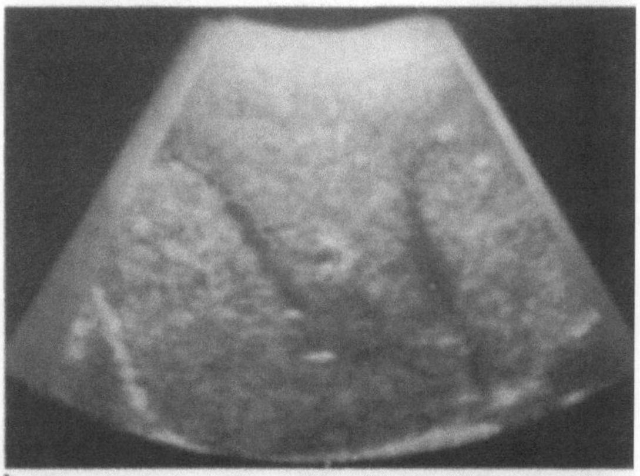

b

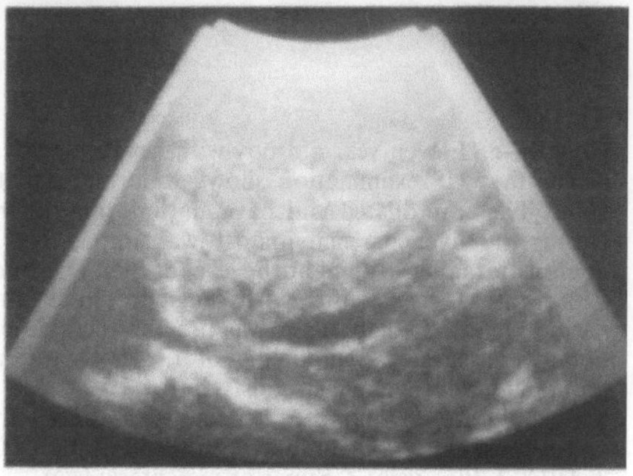

c

Fig. 17a–c. Budd Chiari disease. **a** Longitudinal scan that demonstrates well a dilatation of the medial hepatic vein. **b** Subcostal oblique scan that demonstrates well the abnormal course of the hepatic veins. **c** Same patient. Longitudinal scan through the IVC demonstrating thrombosis of the retrohepatic portion of the IVC. This thrombosis was confirmed by angiography.

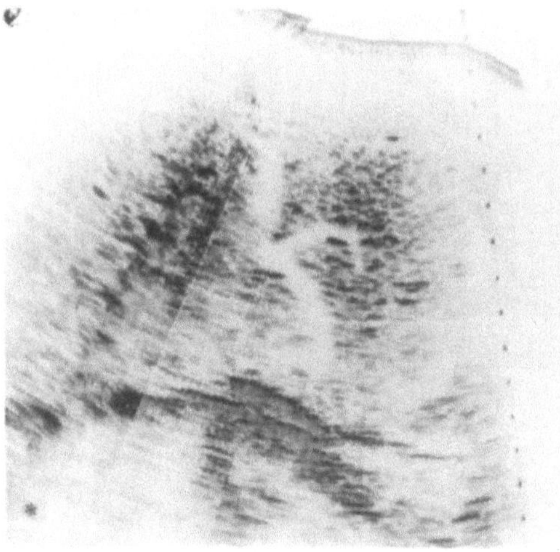

a

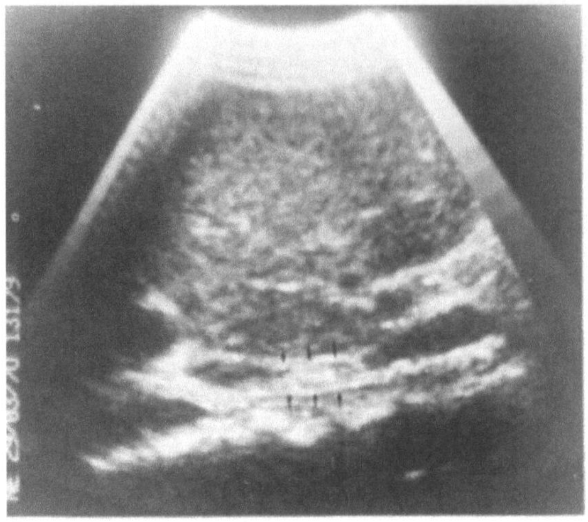

c

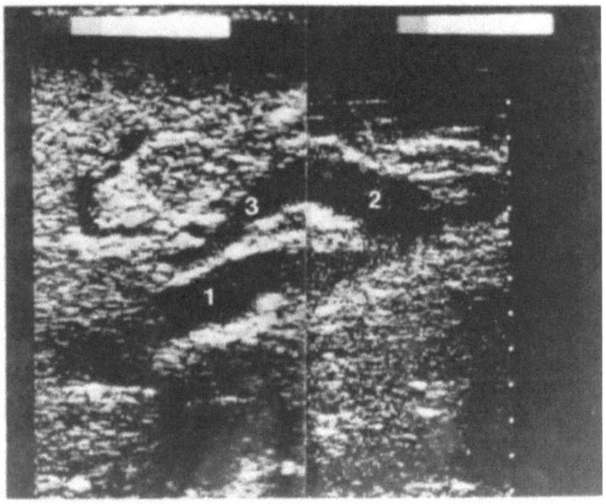

b

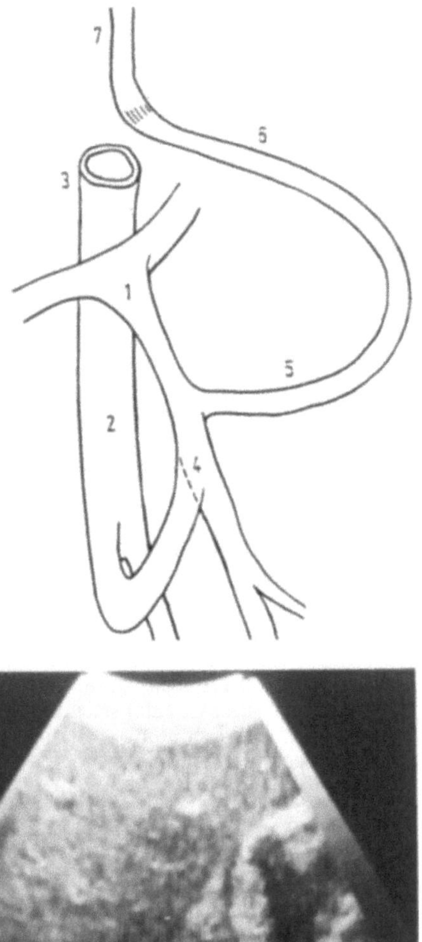

d

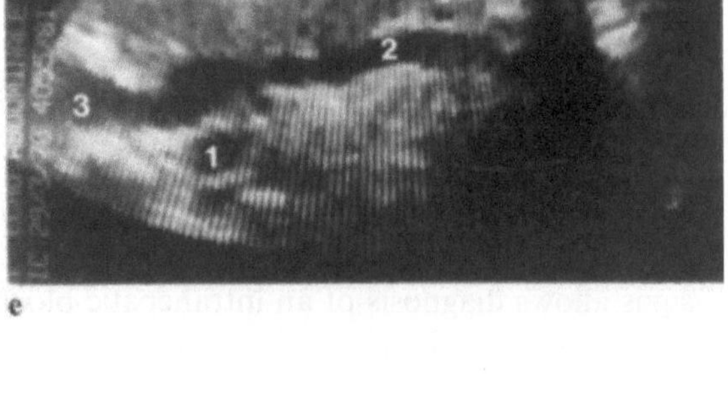

e

Fig. 18a–e. Eleven-year-old boy with hepatomegaly.
a The first US examination shows abnormal hepatic veins. They are dilated and have an abnormal course within the liver parenchyma. It was impossible to demonstrate their ostium at the level of the IVC. Budd Chiari disease was confirmed by angiographic examination. The IVC diaphragm was present. The patient underwent surgical remodeling of the IVC and an iliomesentericocaval anastomosis.
b Postoperatively, ultrasound demonstrates well this anastomosis on a longitudinal scan through the IVC. *1*, IVC; *2*, Iliac vein; *3*, Superior mesenteric vein.
c Postoperatively, a thrombosis of the IVC developed, which is clearly demonstrated on a longitudinal scan through the IVC (*arrows*).
d Because of the IVC thrombosis, a spleno-azygos anastomosis with interposition of the jugular graft was performed after splenectomy.
1, Portal vein; *2*, IVC; *3*, IVC thrombosis; *4*, Mesentericocaval anastomosis; *5*, Splenic vein; *6*, Tugular graft; *7*, Azygos vein.
e On a left subcostal oblique scan, the jugular graft is clearly seen in front of the aorta, merging with the right azygos vein. *1*, Aorta; *2*, Graft; *3*, Azygos vein.

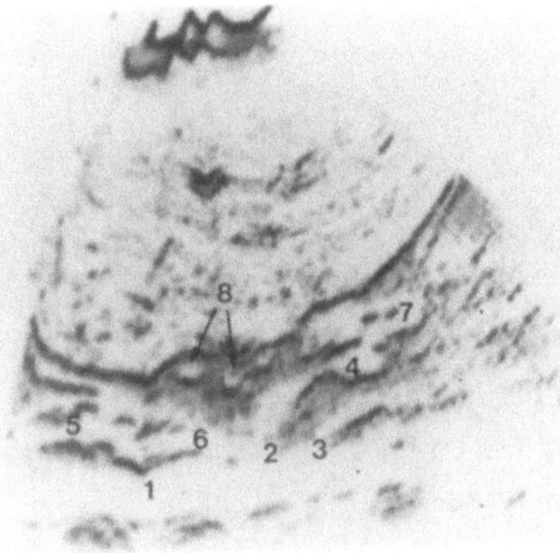

Fig. 19. Longitudinal oblique scan through the aorta in a 2-year-old girl with Budd Chiari disease. The scan clearly demonstrates the second lesser omentum and the gastroesophageal derivations within it. *1*, Aorta; *2*, Celiac trunk; *3*, Superior mesenteric artery; *4*, Splenic vein; *5*, Abdominal esophagus; *6*, Diaphragmatic crus; *7*, Gastric antrum; *8*, Gastroesophageal derivations.

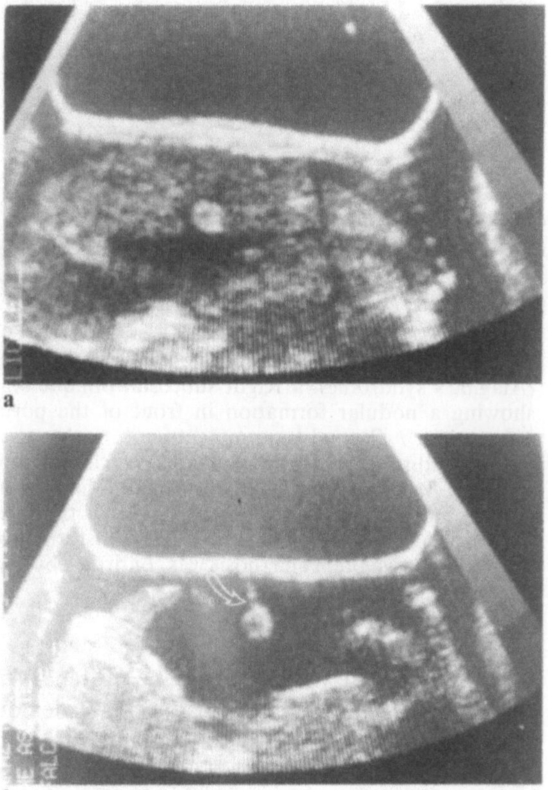

Fig. 20 a and b. Three-year-old with Budd Chiari disease, ascites, and portal hypertension. **a** Transverse scan. The umbilical ligament is seen between the right and left lobes of the liver within a small hypoechogenic central zone, corresponding to a patent umbilical vein. **b** Falciform ligament (*arrow*) is visible on a scan performed at a slightly lower level.

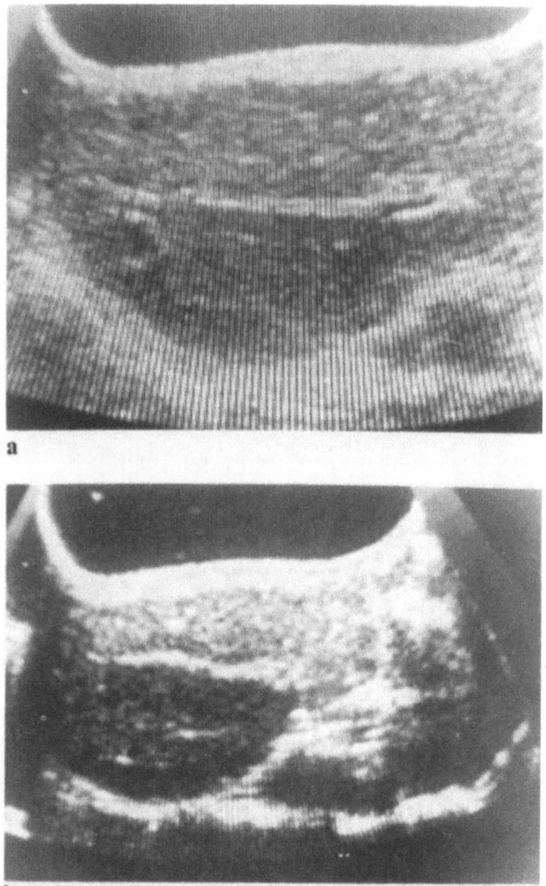

Fig. 21 a and b. Two-year-old child with corrected biliary atresia.
a A right subcostal oblique scan clearly demonstrates the portal bifurcation with hyperechogenic walls. **b** A nodular mass is demonstrated in the right lobe of the liver, probably corresponding to a nodular transformation of the liver. Liver biopsy revealed signs of biliary cirrhosis.

2.5.4 Cirrhoses

There is no specific modification of the echostructure of a liver affected by cirrhosis. However, there are sometimes some morphological modifications. In posthepatitis cirrhosis, there is an atrophy of the right lobe of the liver. This atrophy can be suspected because the axis of the liver has shifted and the bifurcation or the portal vein is more vertical than usual. The gallbladder is laterally located in the right hypochondrium (Fig. 22).

Some macronodular cirrhoses, in particular in biliary atresia, can have some echographic manifestation. The whole liver is scattered with ill-defined nodular formations and the intrahepatic

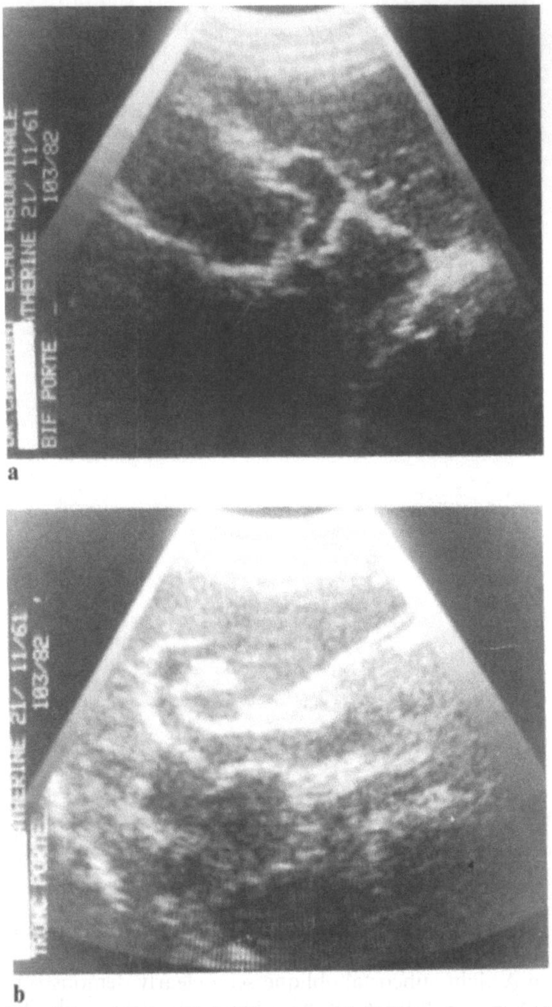

Fig. 22 a and b. Girl, 17 years old, followed up for 10 years because of a chronic hepatitis with cirrhosis. **a** The right subcostal scan demonstrates atrophy of the right lobe of the liver with verticalization of the portal bifurcation. The right portal branch is seen as a dense line with no lumen visible. Left portal branch is dilated. The dense line between the left portal vein and the abdominal esophagus confirm the portal hypertension. This dilatation of the left portal vein is confirmed by a longitudinal scan through the portal trunk **(b)**, showing the continuity between the portal trunk and the left portal branch.

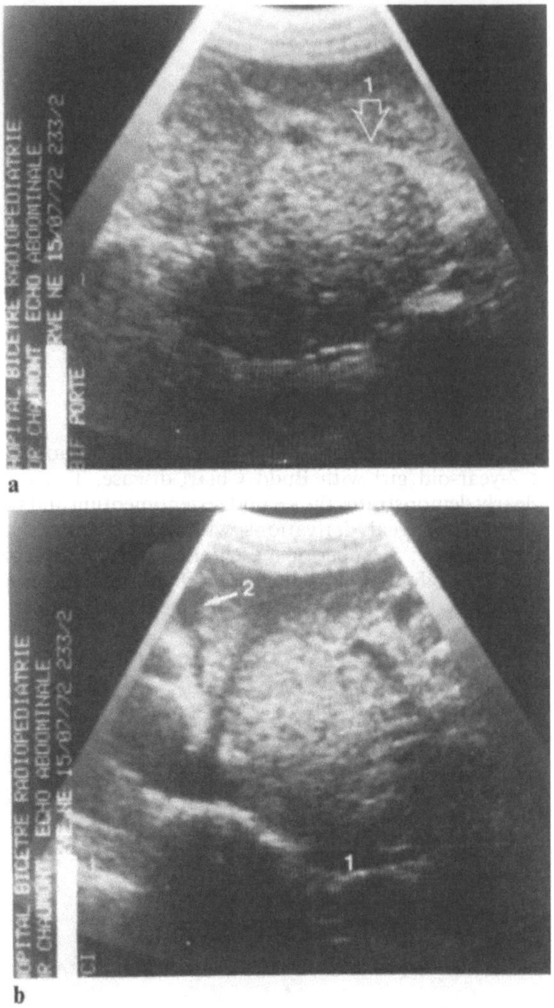

Fig. 23 a and b. Child with intrahepatic biliary atresia (Alagille's syndrome). **a** Right subcostal oblique scan showing a nodular formation in front of the portal bifurcation. *1*, Second lesser omentum.
b Longitudinal scan. This nodular mass is compressing the IVC. α-fetoprotein level is normal. There is no clinical indication of a malignant tumor of the liver. This aspect is characteristic of nodular transformation during cirrhosis. Biliary cirrhosis was confirmed by liver biopsy. *1*, IVC; *2*, Ascites.

portal system can be distorted by those nodules. The portal veins are, however, patent (Fig. 23).

When the positive and etiological diagnosis of portal hypertension is made, it is mandatory to make a complete examination including the IVC and the extrahepatic portal system.

2.6 Natural Splenorenal Anastomosis

The analysis of the left renal vein allowed us, in some patients, to demonstrate a natural splenorenal anastomosis (Fig. 24a–c). The left renal vein in a child with portal hypertension can be demonstrated be demonstrated by a left subcostal oblique scan. It has an oblique direction, medial and cephalad. It crosses the anterior wall of the aorta behind the superior mesenteric artery to join the IVC. Its diameter never exceeds 5 mm in a healthy child. Dilatation of the left renal vein and demonstration of perirenal vein are highly indicative of natural splenorenal anatomosis.

In some selected cases, it is possible to dem-

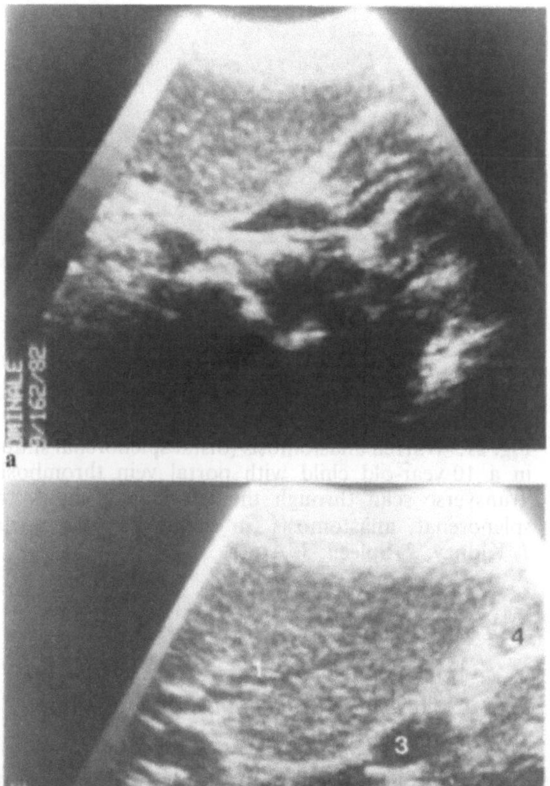

Fig. 24a–c. Portal vein thrombosis in a 13-year-old boy.
a Transverse scan through the left kidney demonstrating dilatation of the left renal vein. This finding suggests the possibility of a natural splenorenal shunt. **b** This natural splenorenal shunt is demonstrated on a longitudinal scan through the spleen. *1*, Spleen; *2*, Splenic vein; *3*, Renal vein; *4*, Inferior pole of the left kidney. Natural splenorenal shunts are usually insufficient to cure the portal hypertension. **c** Splenoportogram.

onstrate direct communication between the splenic and left renal veins (Fig. 24b). Such a natural splenorenal anastomosis is not sufficient by itself for the signs of portal hypertension to be ignored.

It is necessary to emphasize that US itself is not sufficient if surgery is planned particularly, for example, in cases of digestive hemorrhage.

A complete angiographic examination (SMA injection or splenoportography) is the only way for the surgeon to obtain adequate detailed information necessary to choose the type of surgery best suited to the patient.

2.7 Postoperative US Examination

In the case of portal hypertension, postoperative US must affirm the patency of the shunt.

2.7.1 Technique

The technique to demonstrate the portocaval anastomoses varies with the different types of shunt because of their various anatomical locations (Fig. 25).

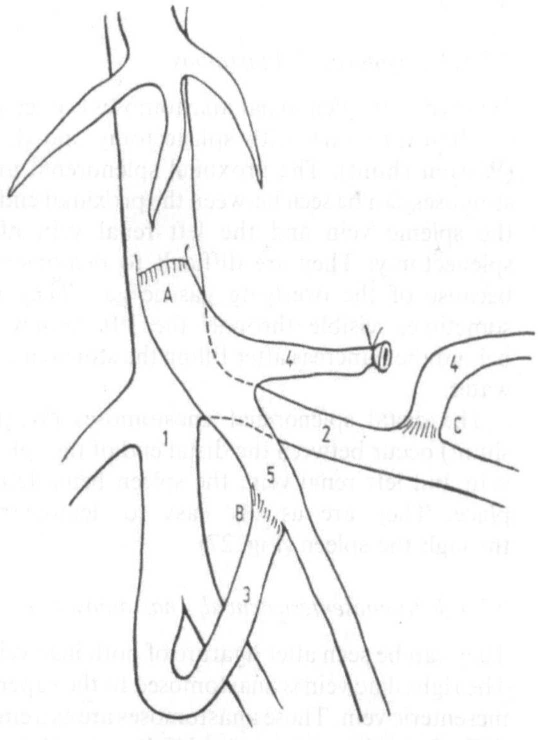

Fig. 25. Various portocaval anastomoses in children. *1*, IVC; *2*, Left renal vein; *3*, Right iliac vein; *4*, Splenic vein; *5*, Superior mesenteric vein; *A*, Terminolateral portocaval anastomosis; *B*, Iliomesentericocaval anastomosis; *C*, Distal splenorenal (Warren) shunt. Mesentericocaval anastomoses with jugular graft interposed between the IVC and the superior mesenteric vein are not shown in this drawing.

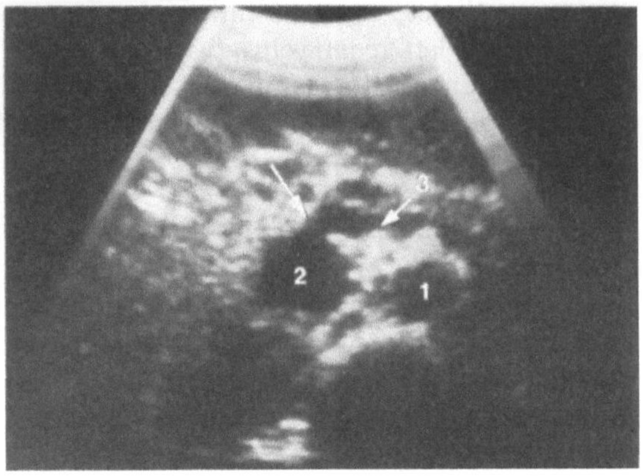

Fig. 26. Transverse scan of the abdomen in a 15-year-old boy with a portocaval anastomosis (*arrows*) in the case of glycogen storage disease. *1*, Aorta; *2*, IVC; *3*, Portal vein

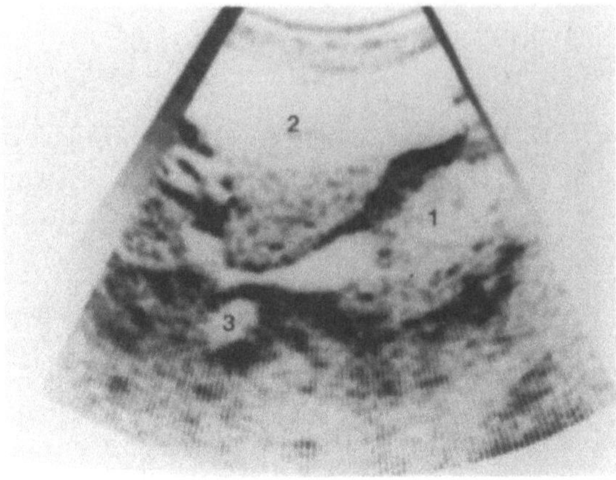

Fig. 27. Warren anastomosis (distal splenorenal shunt) in a 10-year-old child with portal vein thrombosis. Transverse scan through the left kidney shows the splenorenal anastomosis in front of the aorta. *1*, Kidney; *2*, Spleen; *3*, Aorta

2.7.1.1 Terminolateral Portocaval Anastomoses

They are usually very easy to demonstrate because they are located immediately behind the liver (Fig. 26).

2.7.1.2 Splenorenal Anastomoses

Two types of splenorenal anastomoses are seen in children, proximal with splenectomy and distal (Warren shunt). The proximal splenorenal anastomoses can be seen between the proximal end of the splenic vein and the left renal vein after splenectomy. They are difficult to demonstrate because of the overlying gastric gas. They are sometimes visible through the left kidney or behind the pancreas after filling the stomach with water.

The distal splenorenal anastomoses (Warren shunt) occur between the distal end of the splenic vein and left renal vein, the spleen being left in place. They are usually easy to demonstrate through the spleen (Fig. 27).

2.7.1.3 Iliomesentericocaval Anastomoses

They can be seen after ligature of both iliac veins. The right iliac vein is anastomosed to the superior mesenteric vein. Those anastomoses are extremely difficult to demonstrate by US because they are usually obscured by the abdominal gas. They can be demonstrated by a posterior approach through the right kidney (Fig. 30). It is sometimes possible to see a gap in the IVC wall which represents the ostium of the anastomosis. It is exceptional to see the iliac vein itself (Fig. 18b).

2.7.1.4 Mesentericocaval Anastomoses with Jugular Vein Graft

They are visualized with a jugular vein graft interposed between the superior mesenteric vein and the IVC. Their demonstration requires the same techniques as the former anastomoses (Fig. 28).

2.7.2 Patent Portosystemic Anastomoses

Of 14 splenorenal anastomoses 11 have been demonstrated (78%), of 37 mesentericocaval anastomoses 17 (46%) and 2 of 3 portocaval anastomoses. The patency of the shunt can be evaluated along to four indirect criteria. It is necessary in this situation to compare the preoperative and postoperative US.

2.7.2.1 Thickness of the Lesser Omentum

The thickness of the lesser omentum postoperatively, in the case of patent anastomosis, is less than preoperatively. This diminution of the thickness of the lesser omentum has been demonstrated in all except 2 of the 37 patients with patent anastomosis.

2.7.2.2 Gastroesophageal Collaterals

In all cases of patent anastomoses, the gastroesophageal collaterals disappeared or diminished in size.

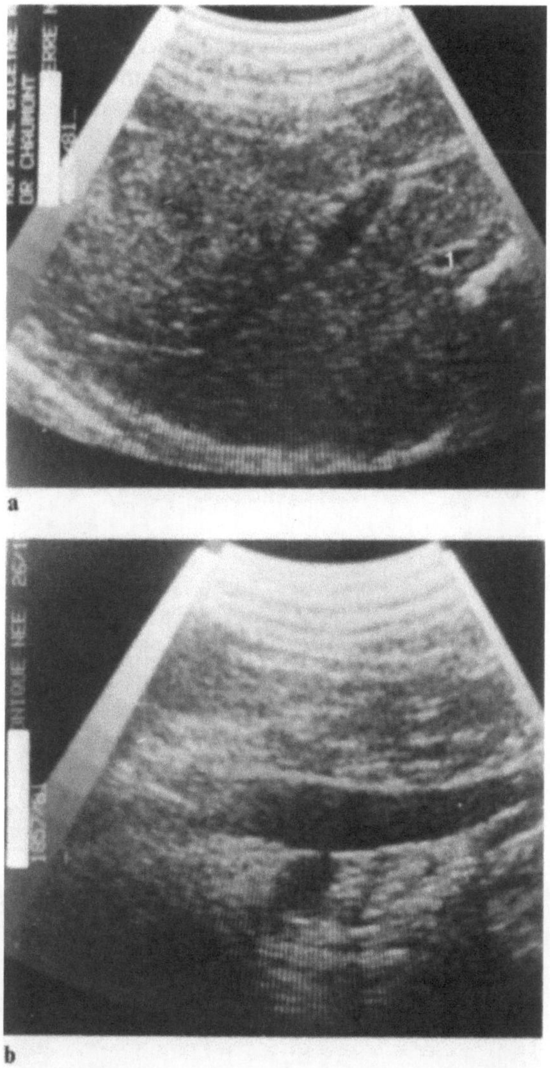

Fig. 28 a and b. Portal vein thrombosis in a 9-year-old girl. Mesentericocaval anastomosis with interposed jugular graft. **a** Posterior longitudinal scan through the right kidney. The IVC and the jugular graft are clearly seen. The anastomosis appears slighly stenosed. However, despite this stenosis (angiographically confirmed), the anastomosis is functional, as no hepatopetal derivation is seen at the level of the porta hepatitis. **b** Subcostal oblique scan. The portal bifurcation is barely visible because of the disappearance of the hepatopetal derivation. *1*, IVC

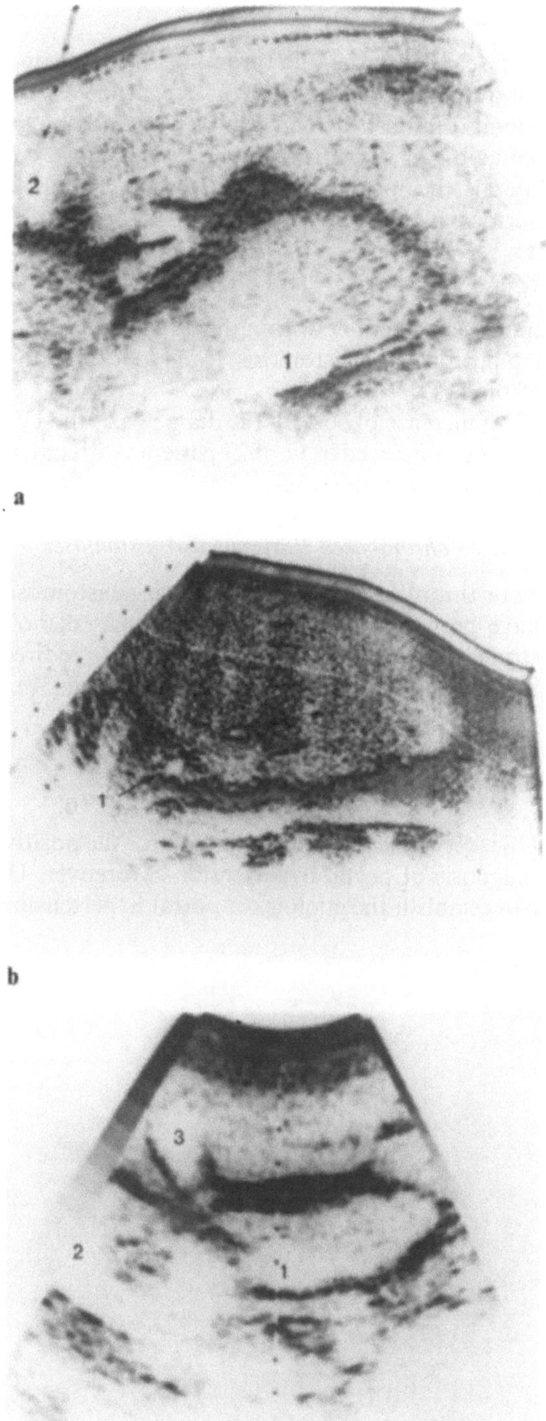

Fig. 29 a–c. Twelve-year-old girl with portal vein thrombosis. **a** Subcostal oblique scan demonstrates a hyperechogenic hilus with hepatopetal derivations within it clearly seen around the gallbladder. *1*, IVC; *2*, Gallbladder. The dense line between the liver hilus and abdominal esophagus is visible. In the case of portal vein thrombosis, the aorta is sometimes difficult to see because of the interposition of the stomach due to liver atrophy and splenomegaly. **b** The right lateral decubitus deplaces the spleen in front of the aorta and allows posterior gastric derivations (*arrows*) to be seen. **c** This child underwent a mesentericocaval anastomosis. The subcostal oblique scan shows the disappearance of hepatopetal derivations at the level of the liver hilus, proving that the anastomosis is functional. *1*, IVC; *2*, Right kidney; *3*, Gallbladder.

2.7.2.3 Hepatopetal Collaterals

In the case of portal vein thrombosis with a patent anastomosis, the size of the hepatopetal collaterals diminished. This can be explained by the reduction in the portal flow through those collaterals, the portal flow being diverted through the portocaval anastomosis (Fig. 29).

2.7.2.4 Diameter of the IVC

Increase in the flow within the IVC as a result of the portocaval anastomosis, leads to a dilatation of the IVC.

An increase of 50% in the diameter of the IVC has been observed in 17 of 27 patients with patent portocaval anastomoses.

2.7.2.5 Thrombosed Portocaval Anastomoses

Four thrombosed mesentericocaval anastomoses have been examined by Us. None was demonstrated directly by US and none of the indirect signs were seen in these four patients (Fig. 30).

2.8 Conclusion

US is a very accurate examination for the positive diagnosis of portal hypertension. Moreover, US can establish the etiology of portal hypertension.

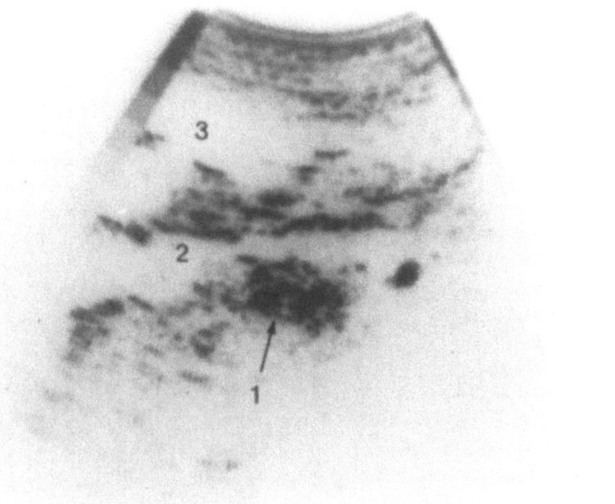

Fig. 30. Portal vein thrombosis. After mesentericocaval anastomosis with synthetic graft, the portal hypertension signs are still present. On this posterior longitudinal scan through the right kidney a very echogenic structure (*1*) is seen in front of the IVC, representing the thrombosed Dacron graft. No indirect sign of patency of the anastomosis was seen in this patient. *2*, IVC; *3*, Right kidney. Thrombosis of the graft was confirmed angiographycally.

Postoperatively, US can demonstrate the patency of shunt. The very high accuracy and noninvasiveness of US make it the first examination in children where portal hypertension is suspected.

3 Hepatic Tumors

A hepatic tumor is usually clinically suspected. However, in some cases abdominal physical examination cannot directly determine the tumor if it is deeply located.

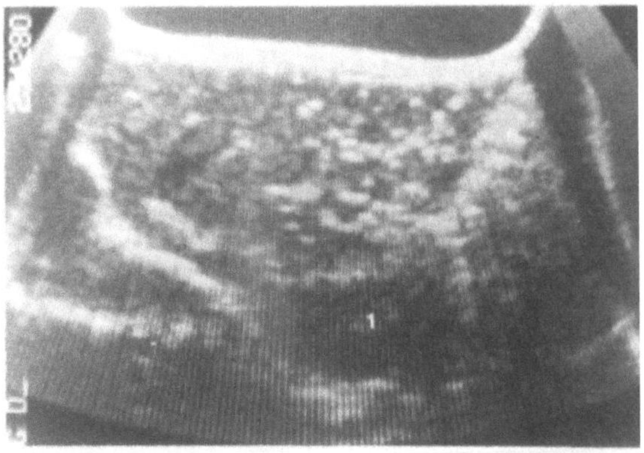

a

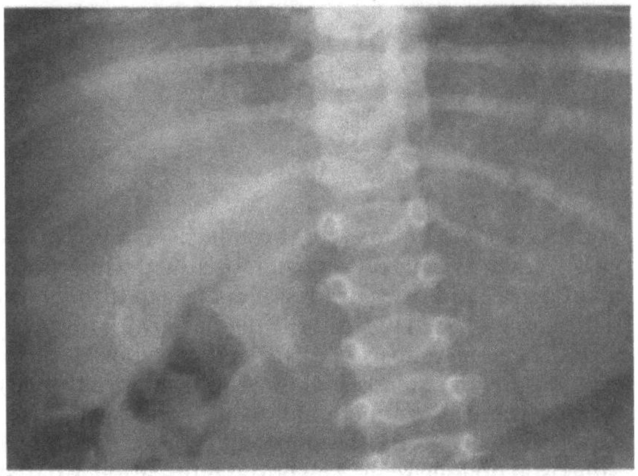

b

Fig. 31 a and b. Boy, 18 months old, with hepatomegaly. The first US examination demonstrated two nodules in the right lobe of the liver and one in the left. **a** Follow-up US demonstrated a mass with very small echogenic echoes in the right lobe of the liver (longitudinal scan through the right lobe of the liver). *1*, Right kidney. **b** Those hypoechogenic formations correspond to multiple calcifications clearly visible on the plain film of the abdomen. Calcifications usually occur during the spontaneous evolution of the hepatic angiomas. The calcifications are usually too small to create acoustic shadowing and are then visible as multiple small hypoechogenic dots scattered throughout the hepatic parenchyma.

US must, as a first step, prove that the tumor is within the liver. Careful analysis of the intrahepatic vascular structures can usually confirm the diagnosis. The analysis of the limits of the tumor is indeed sometimes very difficult in the case of huge tumors. Sometimes the limits of a big renal or adrenal tumor can not be seen within the hepatic parenchyma. On the other hand, some intrahepatic tumors can exhibit a hypoechogenic rim and can compress the kidney and mimic an adrenal tumor. But only an intrahepatic tumor can modify the intrahepatic vascularization!

3.1 Benign Tumors

3.1.1 Angiomas

Hepatic angiomas are often encountered in newborns and infants. These tumors can be unique or scattered throughout the parenchyma.

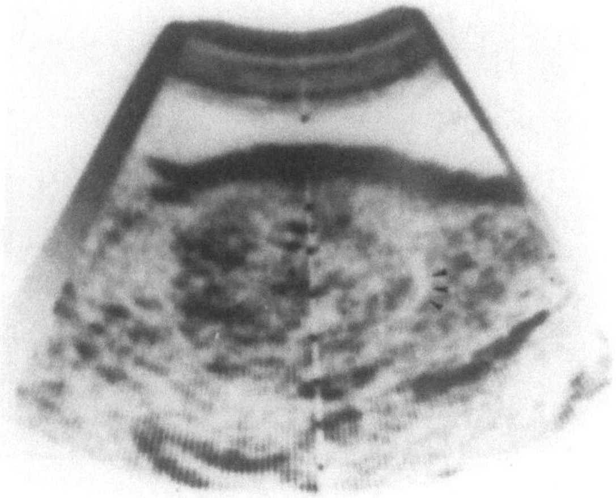

a

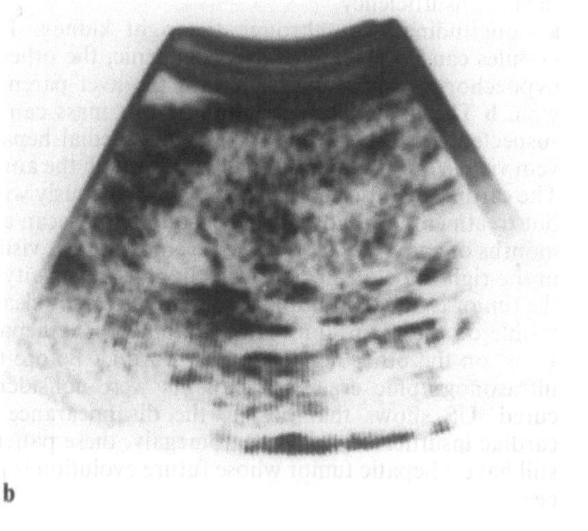

b

3.1.1.1 Localized Tumors

The echogenicity of angiomas is highly variable and more often isoechogenic with the liver. It is sometimes possible to demonstrate intratumoral calcifications (Fig. 31). Those tumors can be

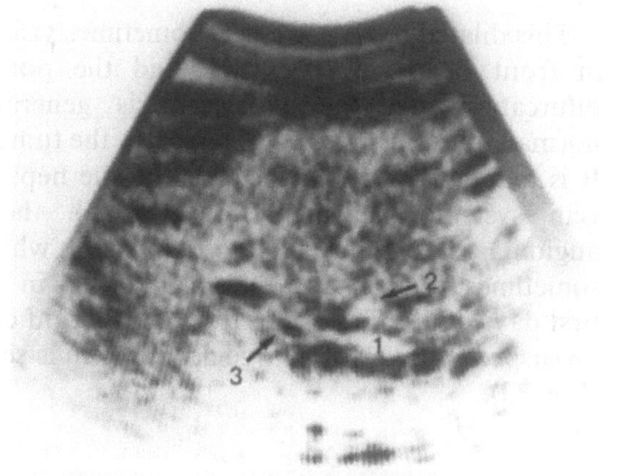

c

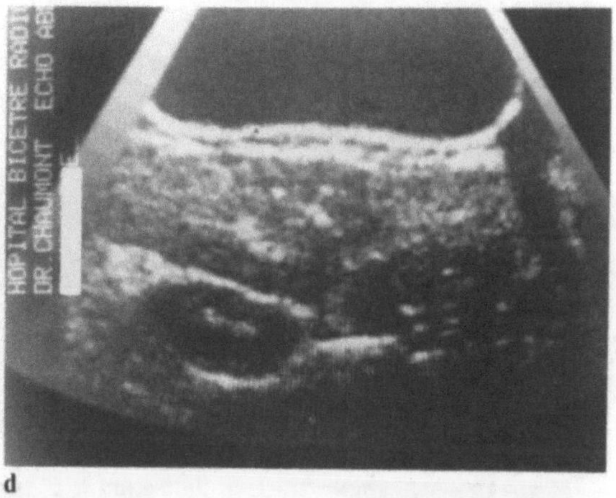

d

Fig. 32a–d. Ten-day-old girl with hepatomegaly and cardiac insufficiency.
a Subcostal oblique scan demonstrating an heterogeneous mass filled with multiple vascular structures. A dilated hepatic vein is visible along the internal edge of the tumor (*arrows*). **b** Longitudinal scan through the aorta demonstrating the conspicuous difference in diameter between the thoracic and abdominal aortas. This difference in caliber is due to dilatation of the celiac trunk which is visible on the left paramedial scan. **c** Left paramedial longitudinal scan. *(1)* Aorta; *(2)* Celiac trunk; *(3)* Esophagus. It is mandatory in the examination of hepatic tumors in children to look for their vascular characteristics. An indirect sign of hypervascularization is the discrepanscy in the diameter of the thoracic and abdominal aortas. A direct sign is the visualization of a dilated hepatic artery. **d** Transverse scan at the level of the right kidney after radiotherapy. The mass is smaller and a calcification can be seen within it with acoustic shadowing.

heterogeneous because of the presence of venous lakes. The diagnosis relies on careful analysis of the vascularization of the tumor. On a longitudinal scan through the aorta, there is very often a conspicuous difference in caliber between the aorta and the abdominal aorta below the celiac trunk (Fig. 32). This difference is due to a large hepatic artery shunting the aortic flow toward the liver.

This dilated hepatic artery is sometimes visible in front of the portal trunk and the portal bifurcation. The portal system is generally normal, but sometimes compressed by the tumor. It is mandatory to analyze carefully the hepatic vein system. The high flow through those angiomas is caused by a left to right shunt, which sometimes results in a cardiac insufficiency in the first days of life. This shunt from left to right can be suspected by US if a large hepatic vein is seen (Fig. 33).

3.1.1.2 Multinodular Angiomas (Fig. 34)

Multinodular angiomas are difficult to see, because the echostructure of the liver is sometimes homogeneous without any tumoral mass. Sometimes it is possible to demonstrate multiple intrahepatic nodules as their echogenicity is variable and sometimes identical to that of the normal liver. After radiation therapy, those tumors exhibit a peculiar evolution. Multiple hypoechogenic nodules can be seen, probably because of intranodular hemorrhage. After embolization in two cases, hypoechogenic stripes were seen outlining the intrahepatic nodules.

3.1.2 Hamartomas

The term "hamartoma" describes a group of benign hepatic tumors with one or several components of the normal liver parenchyma. Hepatocy-

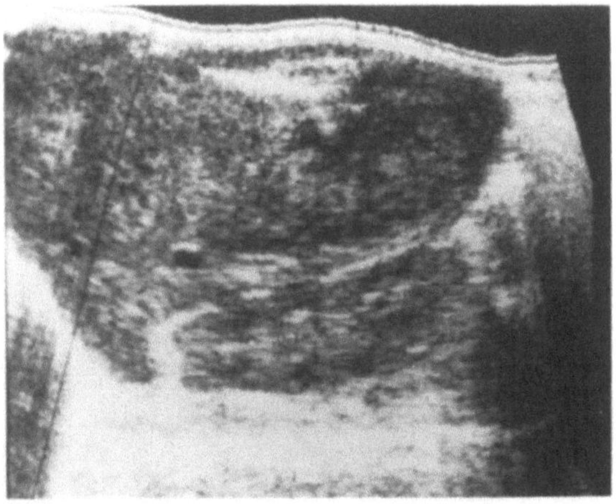

a

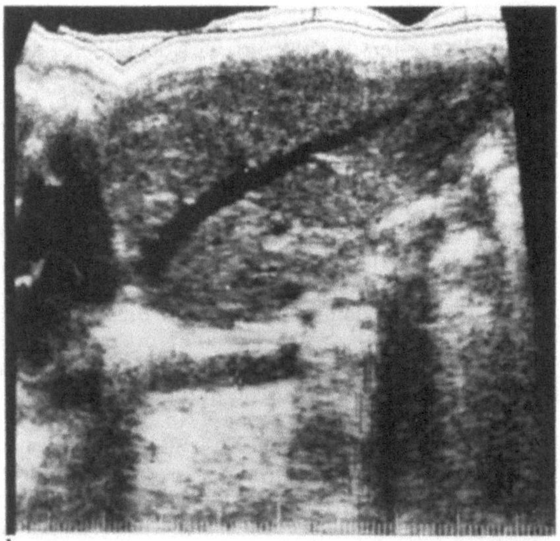

b

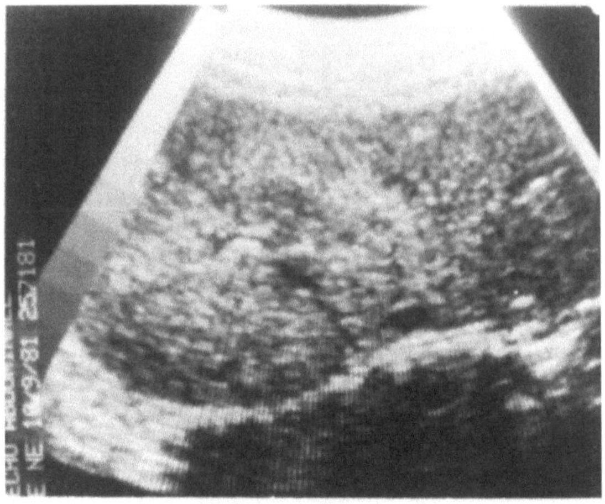

c

Fig. 33 a–c. Two-day-old boy with hepatomegaly and cardiac insufficiency.
a Longitudinal scan through the right kidney. Two nodules can be seen. One is isoechogenic, the other is hypoechogenic in comparison with the liver parenchyma. **b** The hypervascularization of this mass can be suspected because of dilatation of the medial hepatic vein visible on this longitudinal scan through the aorta. The cardiac insufficiency regresses spontaneously without treatment. **c** Follow-up subcostal oblique scan at 6 months of age. A large hyperechogenic tumor is visible in the right lobe of the liver. The hyperechogenicity of the tumor is due to multiple micro-calcifications clearly visible on the plain film of the abdomen. The hepatic veins, on the other hand, are now normal. Before the ultrasonographic era, such patients were considered cured. US shows that despite the disappearance of cardiac insufficiency and hepatomegaly, these patients still have a hepatic tumor whose future evolution is not clear.

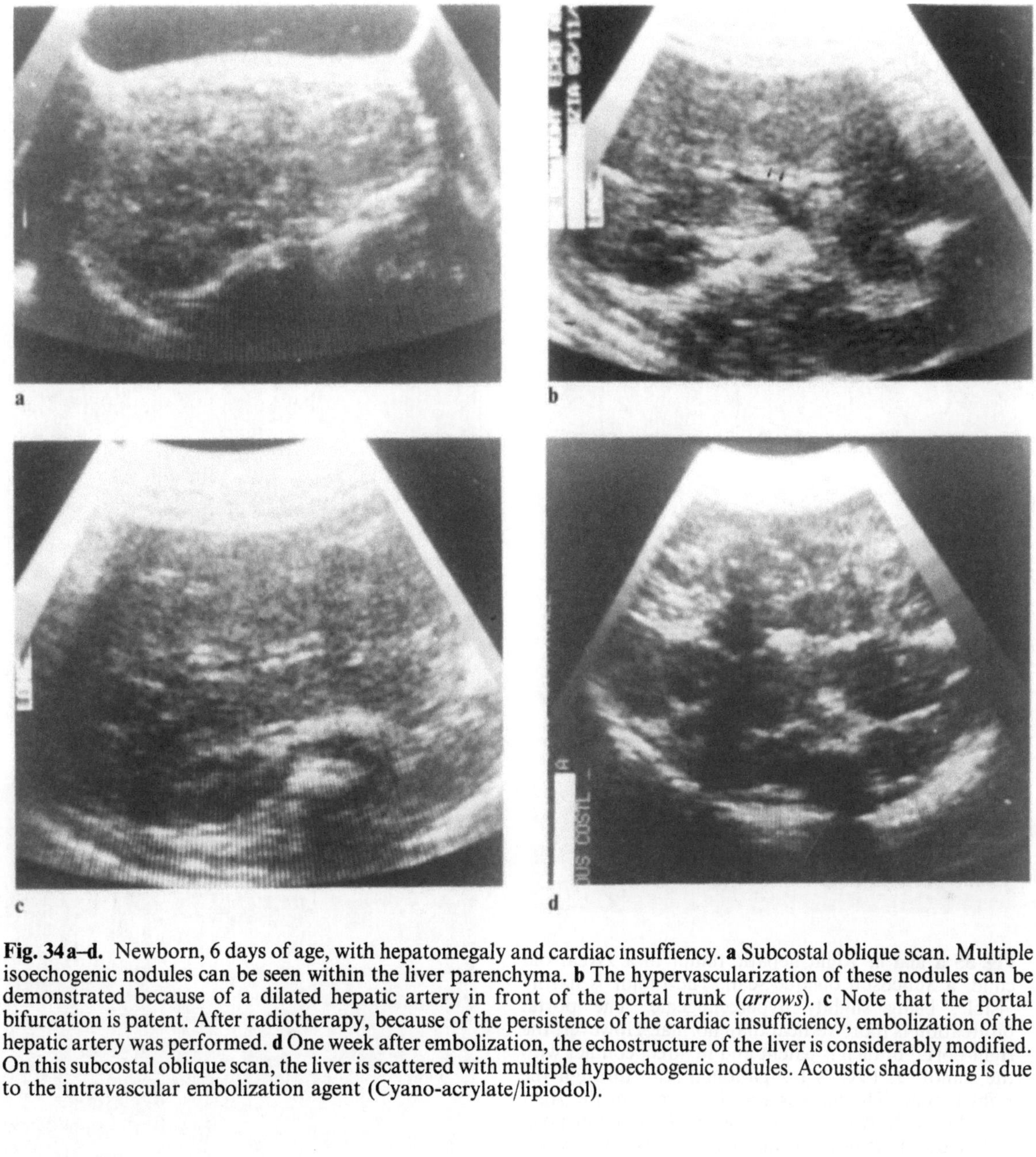

Fig. 34a–d. Newborn, 6 days of age, with hepatomegaly and cardiac insuffiency. **a** Subcostal oblique scan. Multiple isoechogenic nodules can be seen within the liver parenchyma. **b** The hypervascularization of these nodules can be demonstrated because of a dilated hepatic artery in front of the portal trunk (*arrows*). **c** Note that the portal bifurcation is patent. After radiotherapy, because of the persistence of the cardiac insufficiency, embolization of the hepatic artery was performed. **d** One week after embolization, the echostructure of the liver is considerably modified. On this subcostal oblique scan, the liver is scattered with multiple hypoechogenic nodules. Acoustic shadowing is due to the intravascular embolization agent (Cyano-acrylate/lipiodol).

tic, biliary, or mesenchymal hamartomas can be distinguished. The vascularization of the hamartomas is variable, depending on the importance of the vascular component.

The echogenicity of those tumors is extremely variable (Fig. 35). They can be hypo-, iso-, or hyperechogenic. A hypoechogenic rim is sometimes seen, the signification of which is disputed. Some of these hypoechogenic rims are artefactual, similar to the refraction shadow seen at the gallbladder level (Fig. 36b).

3.1.3 Hepatic Adenomas

We have seen seven patients with glycogen storage disease type I with intrahepatic adenomas. These adenomas vary in echonicity, a hypoechogenic rim is often seen and they behave as a benign tumor (Fig. 36). Adenomas are far rarer in other types of glycogen disease.

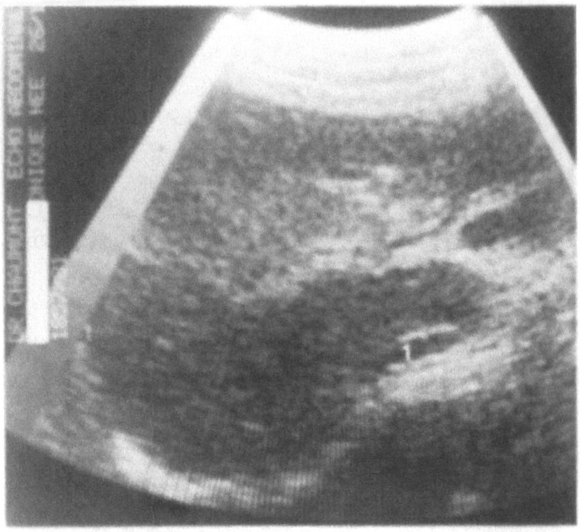

a

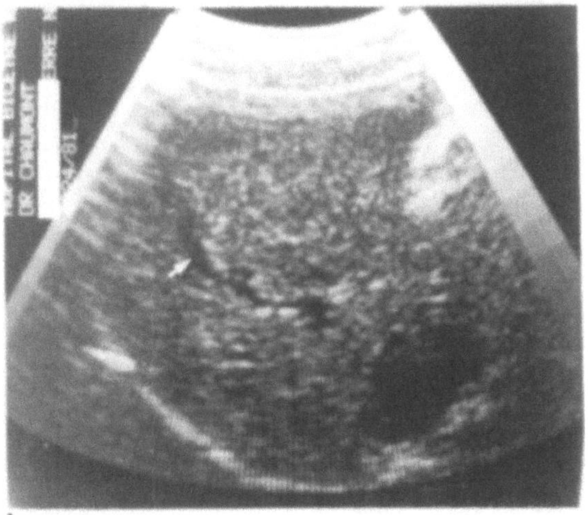

b

Fig. 35 a and b. Right hepatic tumor in a 2-year-old child. **a** Subcostal oblique scan. The tumor is hardly visible, being slightly hyperechogenic. The portal bifurcation is more vertical than normal. However, the right portal branch is patent and in direct contact with the tumor. *1*, IVC. **b** Longitudinal scan through the right kidney. The mass is visible in front of the right portal branch. A vessel is seen around the tumor pole-setting during real-time examination. This vessel corresponds to a dilated segmental hepatic artery (*arrow*). The histologic diagnosis after embolization and surgery was that of a hypervascular hepatocitic hamartoma.

3.1.4 Cystic Tumors

We have seen three cystic intrahepatic tumors which proved to be intrahepatic cystic lymphangiomas. In our experience, a true cystic component inside a hepatic tumor is a strong criterion for the benignity of the tumor (Fig. 37).

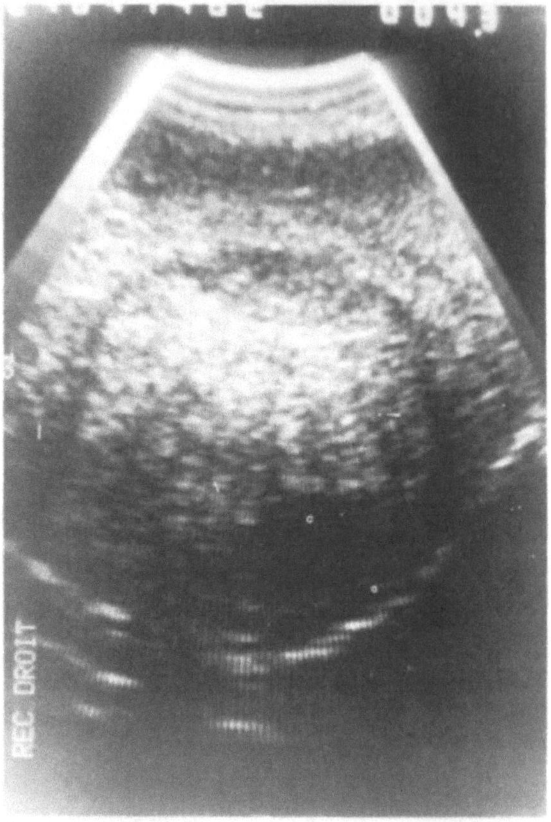

a

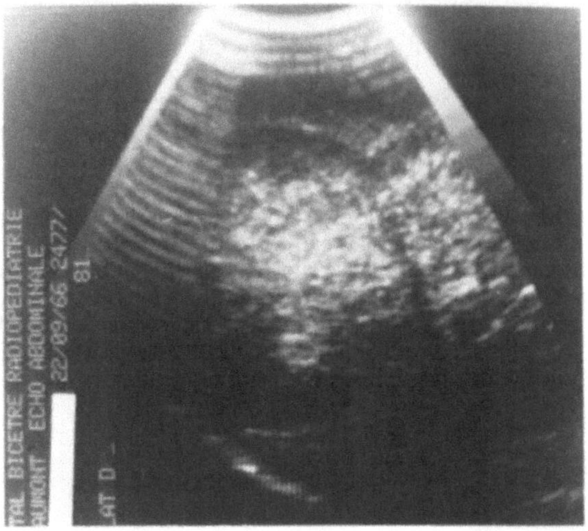

b

Fig. 36 a and b. Glycogen storage disease type I in a 14-year-old child.
a Right subcostal oblique scan demonstrating a hypoechogenic rim around an isoechogenic mass within the right lobe of the liver. The liver is very echogenic and a high absorption of the US beam is seen although the correct technique was used. **b** Longitudinal scan through the adenoma. Acoustic shadowing is seen tangential to the adenoma, which is probably due to refraction of the ultrasonic beam.

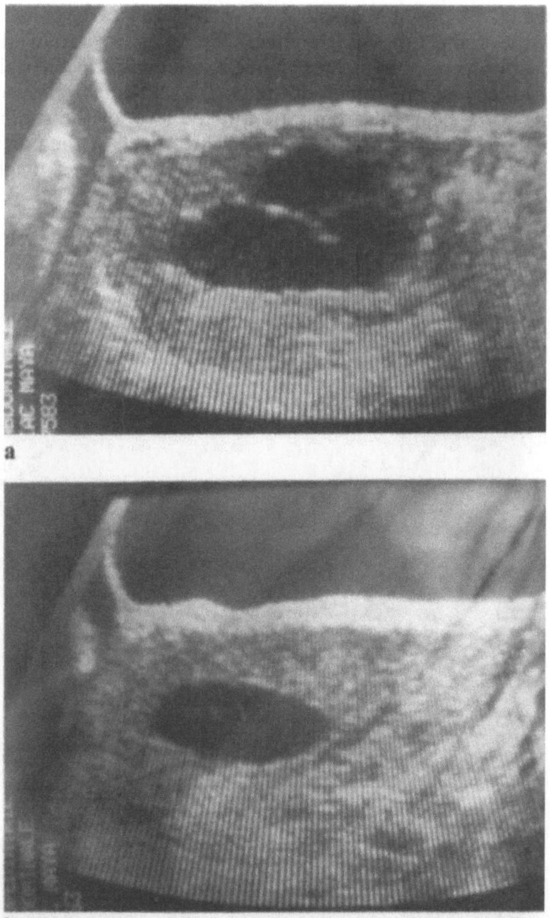

Fig. 37 a and b. Six-day-old boy with hepatomegaly. The umbilical aortogram and umbilical portogram demonstrated a hypovascular mass of the right lobe of the liver. **a** Transverse scan of the liver demonstrates cystic masses within right lobe of the liver with well defined walls. **b** Subcostal oblique scan demonstrating a cystic mass of the right lobe of the liver. Note the patency of the portal vein bifurcation. This patient was operated upon and diagnosis of a cystic lymphangioma of the liver was confirmed by pathologic examination.

3.1.5 Hydatid Cysts (Fig. 38)

Hydatid cysts are easy to diagnose by US. They can be seen as multiple cystic cavities with well-defined walls. It is sometimes possible to demonstrate a detachment of the proligerous membrane and a liquid-liquid level inside the cysts due to the presence of hydatid sand.

A practical problem is the visualization of residual hydatid cysts after surgery. Some of these cysts are indeed very small and can be overlooked during a partial US examination. US examination must be comprehensive in looking for the localizations in spleen and kidney.

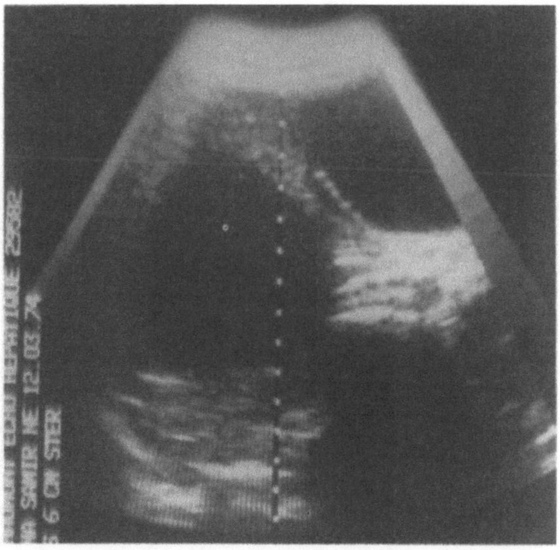

Fig. 38. Boy, 14 years old, with hydatid cyst. Two cystic masses are seen on this transverse scan of the liver.

3.2 Malignant Tumors

3.2.1 Hepatoblastoma

Hepatoblastoma is the most frequent malignant tumor of the liver in children. It is seen in children before 3 years of age. The α-fetoproteins are elevated in 85%–90% of the cases.

The diagnosis is generally suspected clinically and biologically. The US examination must establish the extent of the mass and the surgical possibility.

These tumors are generally heterogeneous, slightly more echogenic than the normal liver parenchyma. Analysis of the intrahepatic vascular structure is mandatory. These tumors have a high growth rate and compress and invade the portal vein branches and the hepatic veins. The portal bifurcation is usually shifted toward the healthy side. The invasion of the portal vein is sometimes directly visible when a neoplastic thrombus is seen within the portal vein. More often, it is the absence of visibility of a portal branch in the vicinity of the tumor that indicates this thrombosis (Fig. 39).

In all except one of the nine cases of malignant tumors US demonstrated such an invasion in the vicinity of the tumor. The data were confirmed in all cases by angiography (Fig. 40).

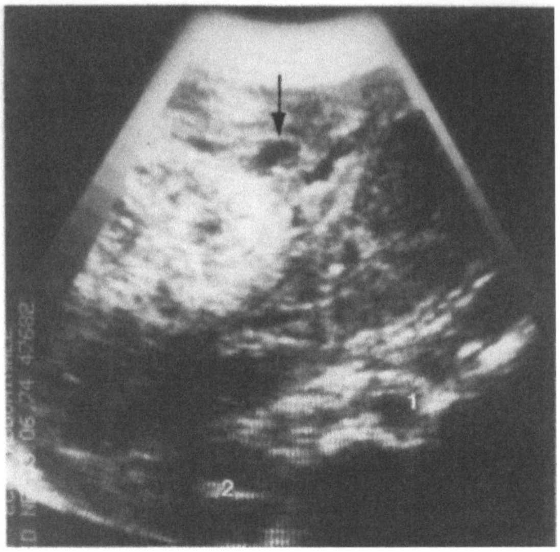

◀ **Fig. 39.** Eight-year-old boy with hepatocarcinoma of the right lobe of the liver. Transverse scan of the abdomen showing an hyperechogenic mass in the right lobe. The left branch of the portal vein is seen (*arrow*), with a clear-cut amputation at the level of the tumor. Complete amputation of the right branch of the portal vein was confirmed by angiography. *1*, Aorta; *2*, Right kidney

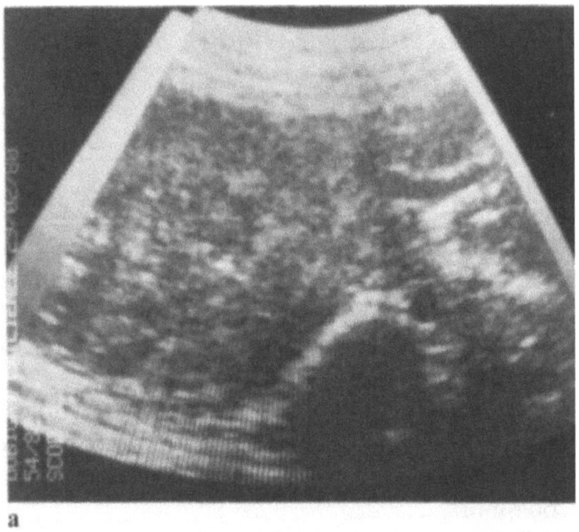

a

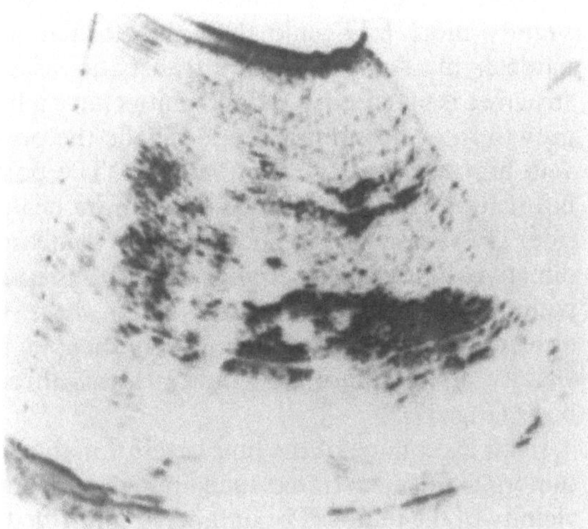

b

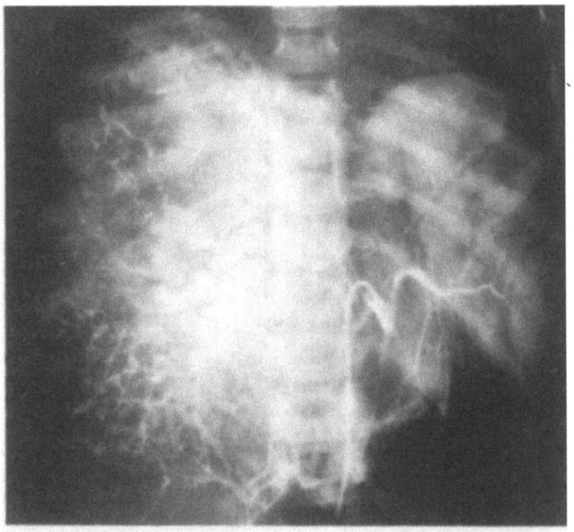

c

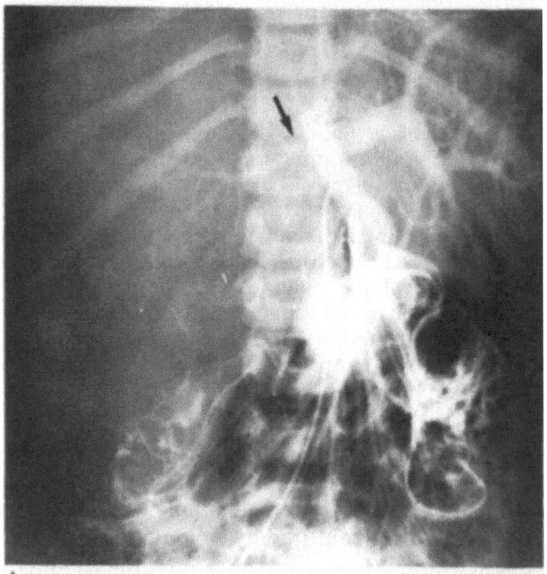

d

Fig. 40 a–c. Three-year-old girl with hepatomegaly. The α-fetoprotein levels are elevated. **a** Subcostal oblique scan clearly demonstrating a right hepatic tumor. The left branch of the portal vein is visible. No right portal vein was found in this patient. **b** Selective hepatic arteriogram showing a right hypervascular mass within the right lobe of the liver. **c** Venous phase of a superior mesenteric artery injection. The left branch of the portal vein is clearly seen and there is a clear-cut amputation of the right branch.

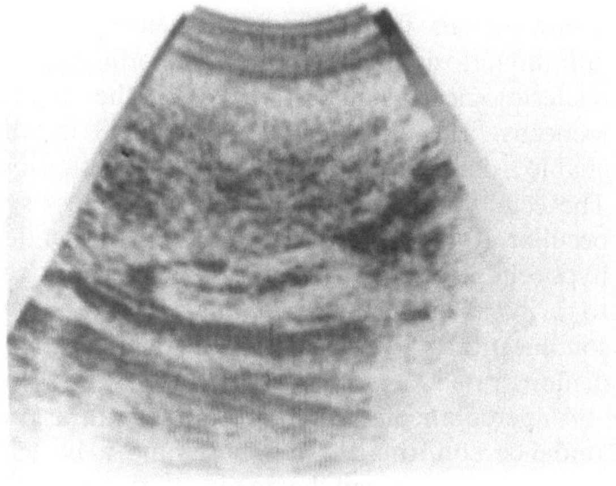

a

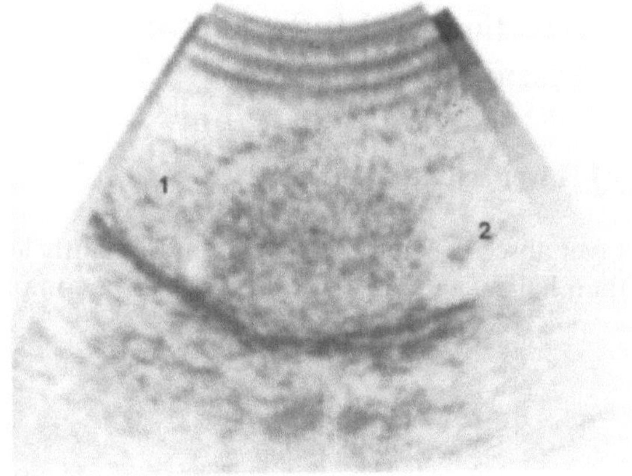

c

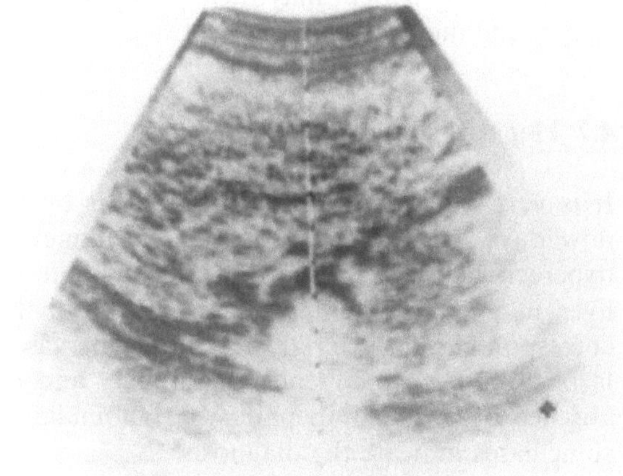

b

Fig. 41 a–c. Hepatomegaly in a 15-day-old newborn. **a** Longitudinal scan through the right lobe of the liver. The liver is heterogeneous, scattered with small hypoechogenic ill-defined nodules. **b** Transverse scan. A hyperechogenic mass is seen on the left side of the spine. **c** Left longitudinal scan through the left kidney. The tumor is located between the spleen *(1)* and the superior pole of the left kidney *(2)*. The diagnosis of Pepper syndrome was confirmed by the elevation of urinary catecholamines.

3.2.2 Hepatocarcinoma

There is no possibility of showing the difference between hepatocarcinoma and hepatoblastoma by US alone. However, hepatocarcinoma is often a complication of a pathologic liver: cirrhosis or metabolic disorder. The presence of portal hypertension and the age of the patient can make the diagnosis of hepatocarcinoma more likely.

The echographic examination of this tumor must include an analysis of the hepatic veins and the IVC and look for a neoplastic thrombus within the IVC or the right auricle.

3.2.3 Pepper Syndrome

Pepper syndrome is defined by the association of a neuroblastoma and primary intrahepatic metastases in newborn infants. The liver is diffusely heterogeneous. Multiple small hypoechogenic nodules, a few millimeters in diameter, give the liver a very peculiar granular aspect (Fig. 41). The edges of the liver appear convex. The intrahepatic portal system is generally patent. There is no sign of hepatic hypervascularization. Diagnosis is made only on the demonstration of the primary tumor (Fig. 41c).

3.2.4 Hepatic Metastases

Metastases of the liver are exceptional in children. They can be secondary to a nephroblastoma or occur in cases of very rare pancreas cancers. They should be systematically looked for in the examination of a nephroblastoma. They are usually hypoechogenic, scattered throughout the liver parenchyma. But in rare cases they can be hyperechogenic.

4 Infectious and Inflammatory Diseases

4.1 Liver Abscesses (Fig. 42)

Liver abscesses are rare in children. In slightly less than half of the cases, they are seen as a complication of an immunologic defficiency (septic granulomatosis). When they are primary, the bacteriological agent is more often the staphylococcus. The clinical context and US usually enable a diagnosis to be made without hesitation. The echographic evolution of liver abscesses is peculiar. Initially, the appear as an ill-defined hypoechogenic zone which probably corresponds to a localized septic hepatitis. Later, a true sonolucent cavity with necrotic debris can be demonstrated.

A percutaneous puncture under ultrasonic guidance confirms the diagnosis and a bacteriological analysis can be made of the pus and sometimes the patient may then be cured thanks to a percutaneous drainage.

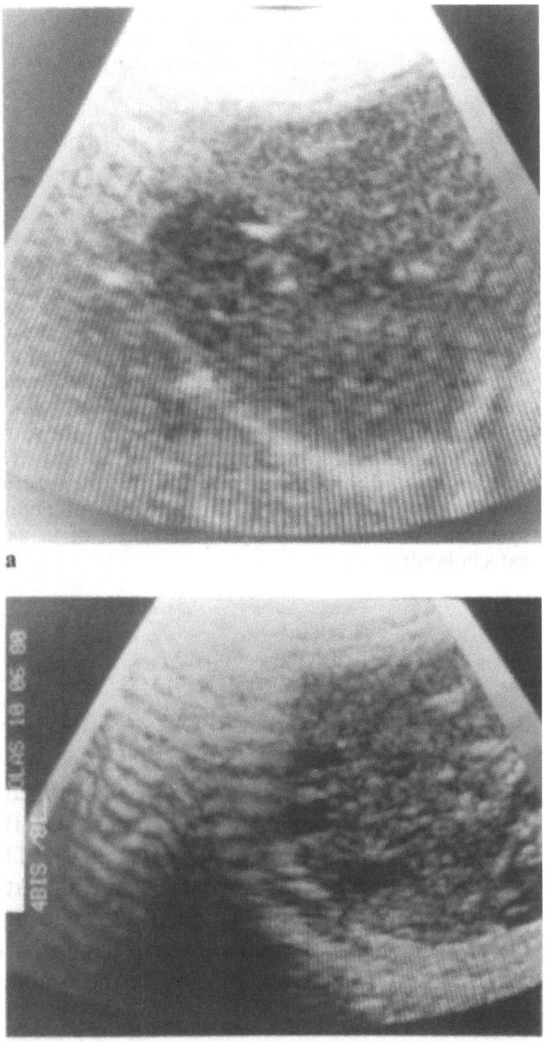

a

b

Fig. 42 a and b. Chronic granulomatous disease in an 18-month-old child. US examination was performed because of hepatomegaly and fever.
a Transverse scan through the right flank demonstrating a hypoechogenic ill-defined zone in the right lobe of the liver. **b** The same view 10 days later.
Multiple abscesses are seen in the right lobe of the liver. This observation is typical of the evolution of hepatic abscesses. They are usually ill-defined and hypoechogenic during the initial period and then become hyperechogenic and sonolucent.

4.2 Hepatitis

It is very difficult to diagnose hepatitis by US nowadays. However, in some cases, numerous hyperechogenic spots scattered throughout the liver parenchyma can be seen. They probably correspond to an arterial or portal hypervascularization. The homogenity of the liver and the absence of portal or hepatic vein anomalies in some cases indicate the diagnosis.

5 Metabolic Diseases

5.1 Glycogen Storage Disease

Apart from the demonstration of intrahepatic adenomas, there is no specific echostructural modification in glycogen storage disease. The only anomaly is the high absorption of the ultrasonic beam by the liver. The liver appears bright in comparison with the renal parenchyma; the latter is very hypoechogenic because of the high absorption of the ultrasonic beam by the liver. The kidneys are usually large in glycogen storage disease type I.

5.2 Other Metabolic Disorders

In Niemann-Pick disease, there is usually an hepatosplenomegaly. As in glycogen storage disease, the liver and spleen are very echogenic (Fig. 43).

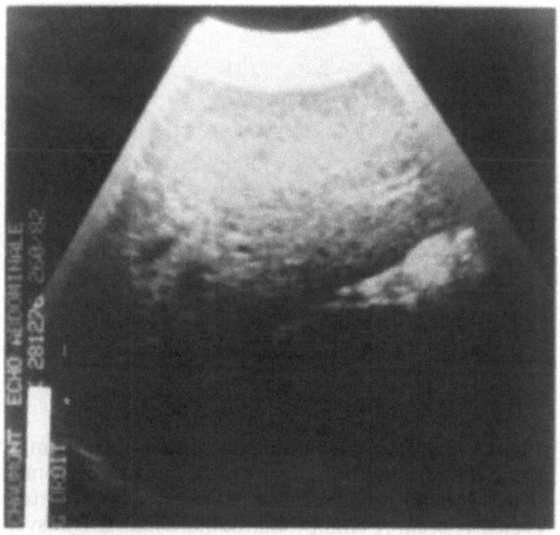

a

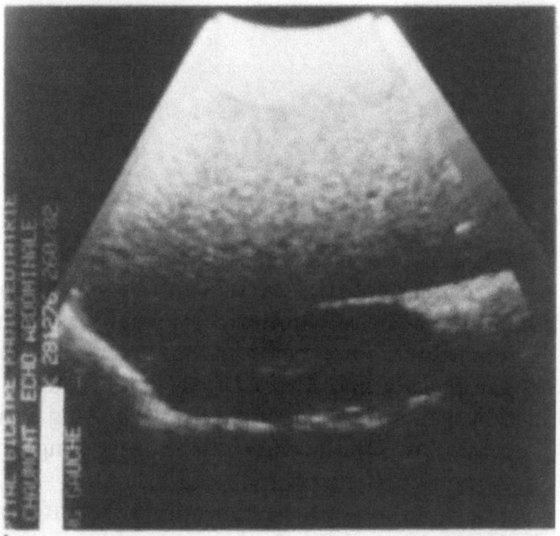

b

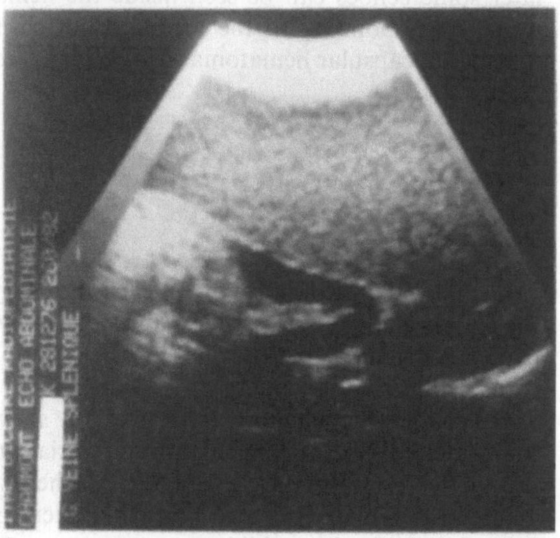

c

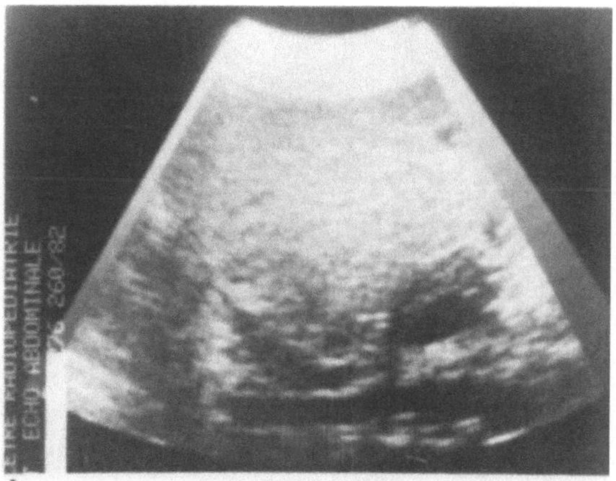

d

Fig. 43 a–d. Niemann-Pick disease type B and hepatosplenomegaly in a 6-year-old child. **a** Longitudinal scan through the right kidney. The right kidney is barely seen due to high absorption of the ultrasonic beam by the liver, which is hyperechogenic. **b** Same finding on a longitudinal scan through the spleen. The spleen is hyperechogenic, the left kidney is hypoechogenic, despite a correct setting. **c** Left subcostal oblique scan. The splenic vein is dilated with a characteristic course, initially sagittal, then transverse, around the tail of the pancreas. **d** Despite dilatation of the portal system, there is no sign of portal hypertension. The longitudinal scan through the aorta demonstrates a lesser omentum of normal, thickness, with no gastroesophageal derivation. In children, a dilatation of the portal system is not sufficient to diagnose portal hypertension. Any splenomegaly, whatever the cause, leads to dilatation of the portal system due to an augmentation of the splenic flow.

6 Abdominal Traumatism

The liver is particularly exposed in abdominal trauma because of its superficial location. US can demonstrate a subcapsular hematoma (Fig. 44) or sometimes modifications of the intrahepatic echostructure due to contusion of the liver. The contused zones appear hyperechogenic. Dilatation of the hepatic artery together with dilatation of the intra- or extrahepatic bile ducts can be seen in the case of posttraumatic hemobilia. The US examination must be comprehensive in the search for associated lesions such as pancreatic, duodenal, or splenic.

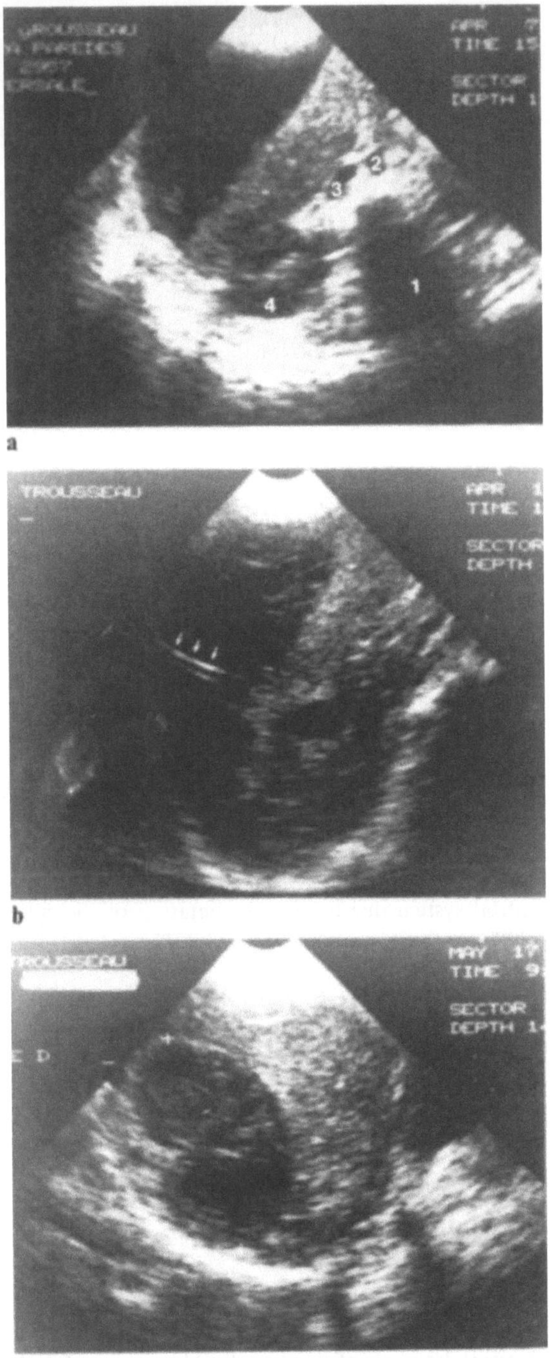

Fig. 44 a–c. Abdominal traumatism with hepatomegaly and anemia in a 15-month-old child. **a** Transverse scan of the right flank demonstrating a subcapsular hematoma of the liver compressing the liver parenchyma. *1*, Spine; *2*, Aorta; *3*, IVC; *4*, Right kidney.
b The subcapsular hematoma has been percutaneously drained. This scan demonstrates the catheter within the hematoma (*arrows*).
c One month later the hematoma is forming clearly seen on this right subcostal oblique scan. This hematoma is well defined, scattered with small echoes due to blood clots.

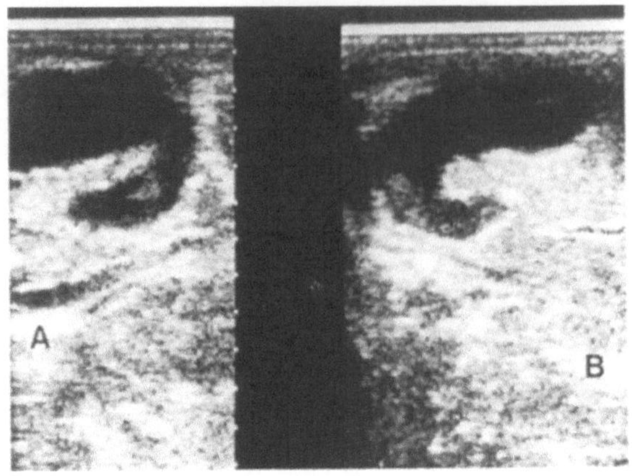

Fig. 45 A and B. Neonatal subcapsular hematoma of the liver. Traumatic delivery with Shock, abdominal distension, and anemia. A large subcapsular hematoma is clearly seen. **A** Right longitudinal scan; **B** Transverse scan.

A peculiar entity is the subcapsular hematoma seen in newborns with hemorrhagic disease. The traumatism is obstetrical and the clinical signs are hepatomegaly and anemia (Fig. 45). US examination makes the diagnosis easy by showing a big subcapsular sonolucent mass compressing the underlying hepatic parenchyma.

The evolution of these subcapsular hematomas is characteristic. Initially they are sonolucent, and later some echoes can be seen inside the hematoma, corresponding to the formation of clots. Splenic subcapsular hematomas can be observed.

7 Cardiac Liver

In a child with a surgically corrected cardiopathy, the presence of an enlarged liver can be due to two causes: chronic hepatitis due to the multiple transfusions during surgery or a cardiac liver.

US enables the diagnosis to be made by showing a dilated IVC lacking its normal variations during the respiratory cycle (Fig. 46). The hepatic veins are also dilated or "set". Portal hypertension is rarely seen in these children.

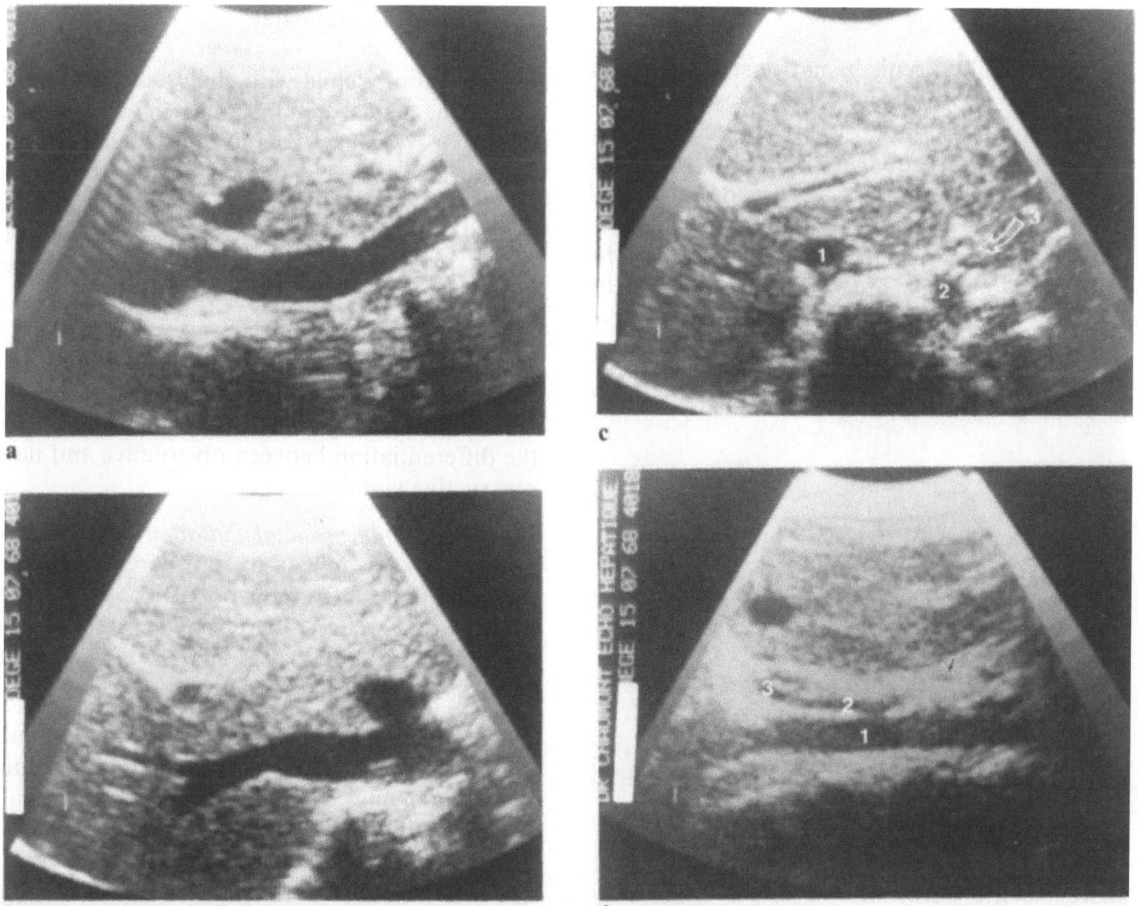

Fig. 46 a–d. Cardiac cirrhosis with congenital mitral insufficiency. **a** Longitudinal scan through the IVC. The IVC is dilated and has lost the normal variations of its diameter during the respiratory cycle. **b** Subcostal oblique scan demonstrating a very large dilatation of the right hepatic vein and of the origin of the medial hepatic vein. **c** Right subcostal oblique scan through the portal bifurcation demonstrates the hyperechogenicity of the walls of the portal vein and a slightly visible line between the left portal branch and the abdominal esophagus proving the presence of portal hypertension. *1*, IVC; *2*, Aorta; *3*, Abdominal esophagus. **d** Longitudinal scan through the aorta. The lesser omentum is thickened and a small gastroesophageal derivation is visible within it *(arrow)*. *1*, Aorta; *2*, Diaphragmatic crus; *3*, Esophagus.

8 Splenomegaly

8.1 Isolated Splenomegaly

Under this terminology, we group all the non-tumoral splenomegalies observed apart from portal hypertension. The etiologies are variable: hemolitic anemia, viral diseases (measles, infectious mononecleosis), and idiopathic.

These splenomegalies are homogeneous and hypervascular. Their hypervascular nature is seen because of a dilated splenic vein and a large extra- and intrahepatic portal system. This dilatation of the portal system is probably the consequence of the augmentation of the blood flow through the spleen. None of those patients had portal hypertension (Fig. 43).

8.2 Splenic Tumors

Splenic tumors are rare in children.

8.2.1 Benign Tumors

They are usually splenic hamartomas or dermoid cysts. Ultrasonographically, they present a cystic mass with a liquid-liquid level. The echogenicity of the underlying liquid is probably due to the presence of cholesterol crystals or desquamated keratin (Fig. 47).

An intrasplenic hematoma can have exactly the same ultrasonic appearance. The diagnosis will be made at surgery.

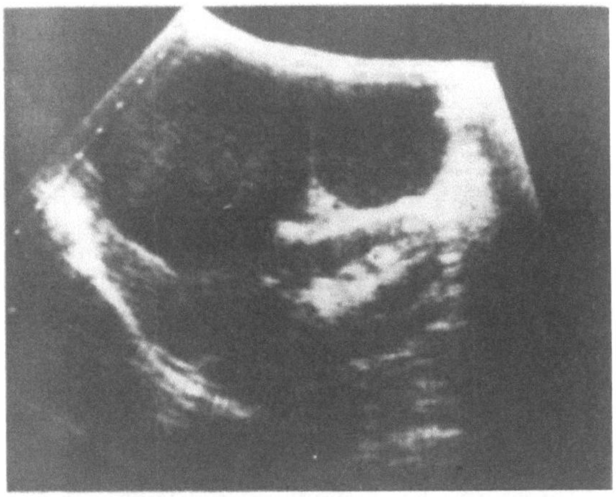

Fig. 47. Left longitudinal scan in an 11-year-old child with splenomegaly. Two cystic formations are visible within the spleen. The splenic parenchyma is visible above the left kidney. During surgery a lobulated epidermoid cyst of the spleen was discovered. The small echoes within the cyst are due to cholesterol crystals and/or keratin fragments.

8.2.2 Malignant Tumors

Primary malignant tumors of the spleen are exceptional in children. On the other hand, in non-Hodgkin lymphomas, the spleen can be infiltrated by multiple hypoechogenic nodules. The complete US examination will indicate the diagnosis by showing all the localizations: kidney, pancreas, and paraaortic adenopathies.

9 Biliary Tract

Ultrasonography of the biliary system in children is now able to establish anomalies which used to be first diagnosed in adolescents or even adults (e.g., choledochal cyst). This noninvasive and widely used technique documents biliary abnormalities that are not as rare as it was believed.

9.1 Cholestatic Jaundice

Evaluation of a child with cholestatic jaundice is the main clinical circumstance in which a US study is performed. Therapy may be either surgical or medical depending on whether the cholestasis is extra- or intrahepatic. Cholestasis raises the problem of the integrity and patency of the extrahepatio biliary system since surgical management is necessary in extrahepatic cholestasis.

Clinical findings and laboratory data are associated means of studying and classifying these patients, while the US examination assesses the status of the biliary system and is of great value in the differentiation between obstructive and nonobstructive jaundice.

Intrahepatic biliary ductal dilatation. The enlarged biliary radicles appear to have a characteristic radiating pattern from the porta hepatis. In cases of mild obstruction, there may be difficulty in distinguishing minimally dilated biliary ducts from the portal venous radicles.

Dilatation at level of the porta hepatis. On subcostal oblique scans, there is a "parallel channel sign" involving enlarged right and left main hepatic ducts which are located immediately anterior to the corresponding main portal vein branch.

Dilatation of the common bile duct. On sagittal scans of the portal vein, when dilatation occurs, the diameter of the common bile duct tends to become equal to the portal vein. These two tubular parallel structure have been described as the shot "gun sign".

The dilated common bile duct may compress the portal vein so that the former has a larger diameter than the latter (Fig. 48).

9.1.1 Cholestasis in Newborns and Infants

Intrahepatic cholestasis with normal extrahepatic bile duct is more common than extrahepatic cholestasis and the main cause is neonatal hepatitis. US study only provides negative criteria: there is no dilatation of the intra- and extrahepatic bile duct.

Extrahepatic cholestasis. Most cases of extrahepatic biliary atresia are discovered in the first weeks of life with a complete and constant cholestasis. The extent of the obstruction of the bile ducts replaced by fibrous cord is extremely variable. It may be associated with intrahepatic bile duct abnormalities. The gallbladder is involved in this

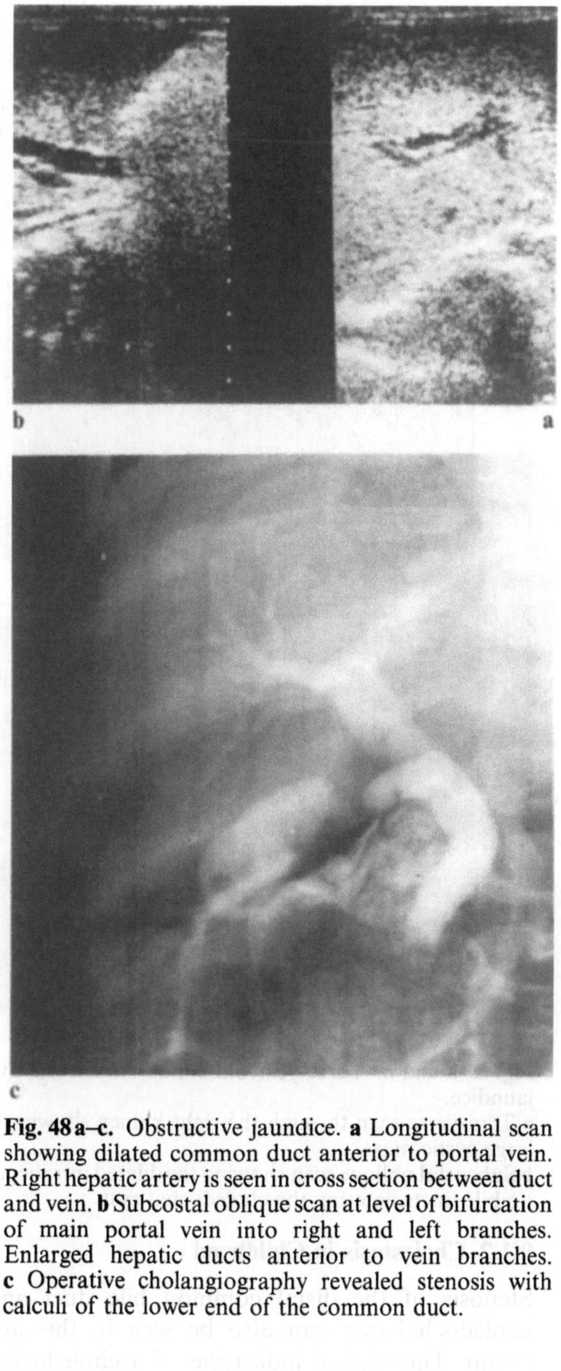

Fig. 48a–c. Obstructive jaundice. **a** Longitudinal scan showing dilated common duct anterior to portal vein. Right hepatic artery is seen in cross section between duct and vein. **b** Subcostal oblique scan at level of bifurcation of main portal vein into right and left branches. Enlarged hepatic ducts anterior to vein branches. **c** Operative cholangiography revealed stenosis with calculi of the lower end of the common duct.

fibrous process in 80% of the cases. These points explain the US findings of no bile duct dilatation and the gallbladder visualized in only 20% of the cases.

Biliary atresia is sometimes associated with the congenital polysplenia syndrome and US examination can discover interrupted vena cava, situs inversus, and horizontal liver.

Visualization of a normal gallbladder is important for prognosis as it allows hope for the patency of the common bile duct with the possibility of an anastomosis between gallbladder and the porta hepatis.

Choledochal cysts are congenital dilatations of the extrahepatic part of the biliary tree. The most common clinical indication in this age group is an obstructive jaundice without palpable mass. The cysts are due to an anomalous junction between the common bile duct and the pancreatic duct, allowing reflux of the pancreatic juice into the biliary ductal system leading to cholangitis and dilatation of the biliary tract.

The cystic mass in the porta hepatis is easily identified by US as a rounded anechoic mass with a thin wall, separate from the gallbladder. Demonstration of the distended common bile duct or hepatic duct directly entering the cystic mass confirms the diagnosis. There is often an associated dilatation of the intrahepatic biliary system (Figs. 50 and 51). The anomalous relation between the common bile duct and the pancreatic duct is sometimes demonstrated together with a pancreatic duct dilatation (Fig. 49).

The surgical procedure is a complete excision of the choledochal cyst with choledocojejunostomy and needs a detailed study of the anatomic lesions, which is often obtained by percutaneous transhepatic cholangiography.

Intrinsic obstruction of the distal common bile duct is an uncommon entity in infancy. US study shows an intra- and extrahepatic biliary dilatation. The lower portion of the common bile duct is often obscured by bowel gas; however, in some cases a stone can be visualized at this level by US.

Percutaneous transhepatic or operative cholangiography demonstrates the obstruction by stones at the lower end of the common duct. These calculi can be eventually aspirated by a side-hole catheter. There is rarely a true stenosis of the distal common bile duct which then requires a surgical diversion of the biliary-system.

Spontaneous perforation of the extrahepatic bile duct is a rare entity discovered within the first 3 months of life, usually after a silent period. Obstructive jaundice and biliary ascites are prominent clinical findings.

US shows extra- and intrahepatic biliary dilatation. Cholangiography visualizes a stenosis at the junction between cystic and common duct, in some cases with calculi.

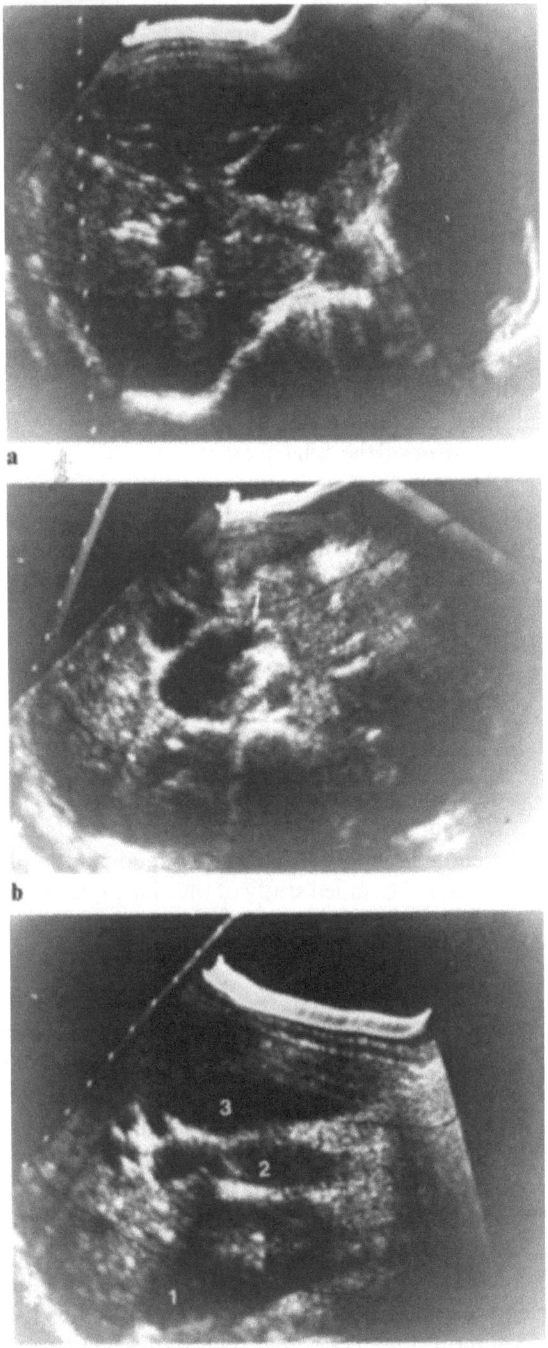

a b c

Fig. 49 a–c. Six-year-old child, referred for "chronic hepatitis."
a Subcostal oblique scan showing markedly intrahepatic biliary dilatation. It is difficult to distinguish between portal venous elements and biliary structures because of the importance of the bile duct dilatation. **b** Longitudinal section showing important dilatation of the common duct. Portal vein is not visualized. *1*, Right kidney; *2*, Common duct; *3*, Gallbladder.
c Transverse section through choledochal cyst. Dilated pancreatic duct is seen as a tubular structure at the medial border of the choledochal cyst (*arrow*).

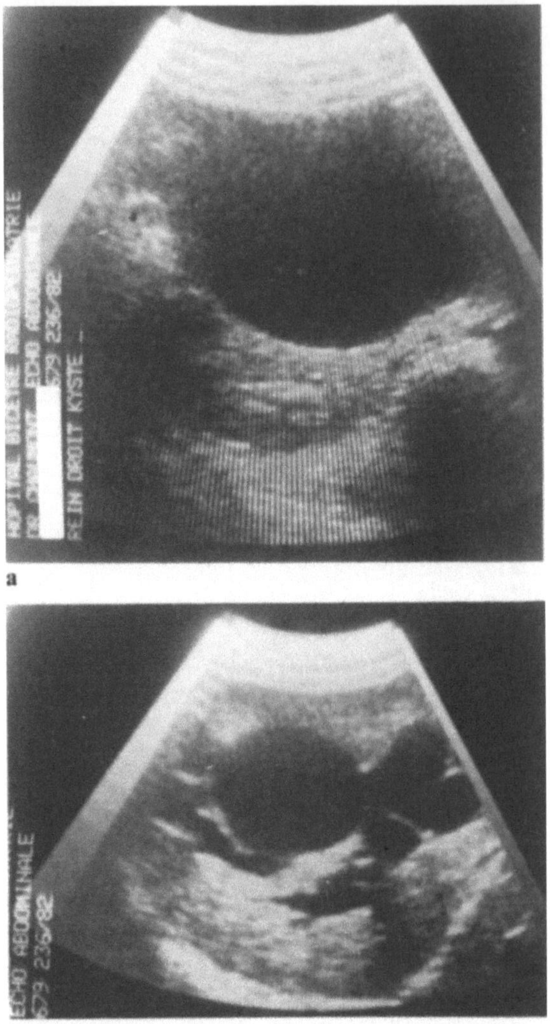

a b

Fig. 50 a and b. Three-year-old child with obstructive jaundice.
a Transverse scan through the right kidney showing a large cystic mass.
b Subcostal oblique scan showing the dilated intrahepatic bile ducts entering the choledochal cyst.

9.1.2 Cholestasis in Childhood

Stenosis of the distal common bile duct and choledochal cyst can also be seen in this age group. The clinical indication of a choledochal cyst is a palpable mass with intermittent jaundice.

Other rare causes of extrahepatic cholestasis can be demonstrated by US. These include pancreatic disease and neoplasms. The latter group consists of histiocytosis X, lymphoma (lymph nodes in the porta hepatis appear as nodular masses with regular margins, less echogenic than hepatic tissue; associated with intrahepatic biliary dilatation) (Fig. 52), and rhabdomyosarcoma of the bile ducts.

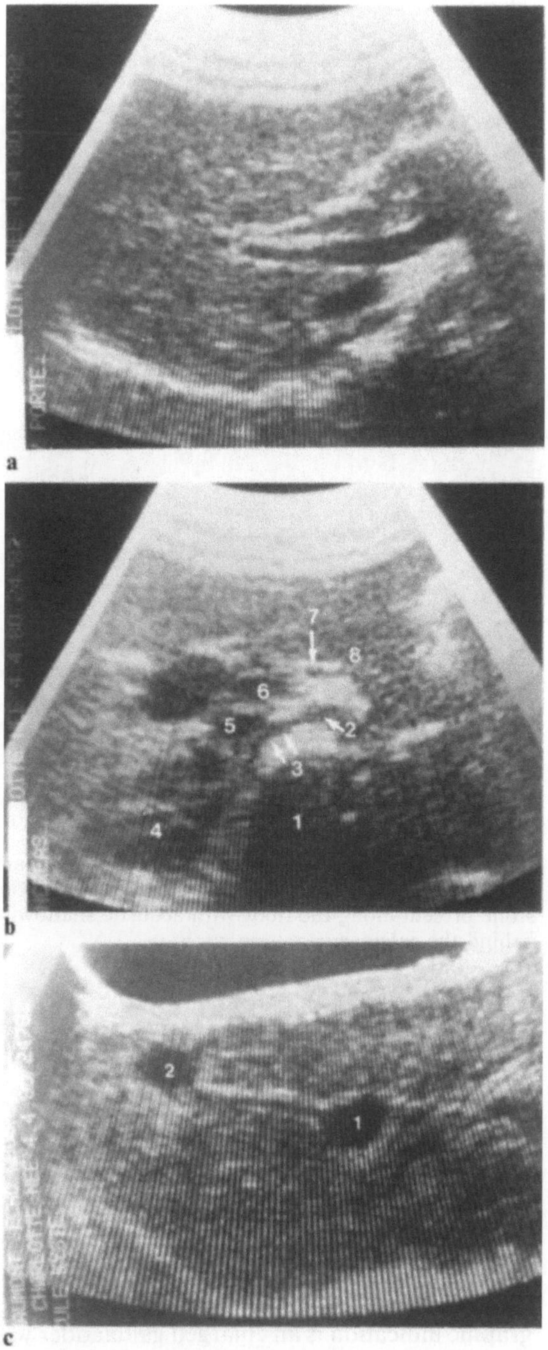

Fig. 51 a–c. Two-year-old-child with relapsing jaundice.
a Longitudinal scan showing anechoic tubular structure anterior to portal vein.
b Transverse scan. The lesion is lateral to the superior mesenteric vein. There is no dilatation of the intrahepatic bile ducts.
1, Spine; *2*, Aorta; *3*, Diaphragm; *4*, Right kidney; *5*, Inferior vena cava; *6*, Mesenteric superior vein; *7*, Mesenteric superior artery; *8*, Pancreas. **c** Subcostal oblique scan. The channel between the gallbladder and the choledochal duct *(2)* establishes the diagnosis of choledochal cyst *(1)*.

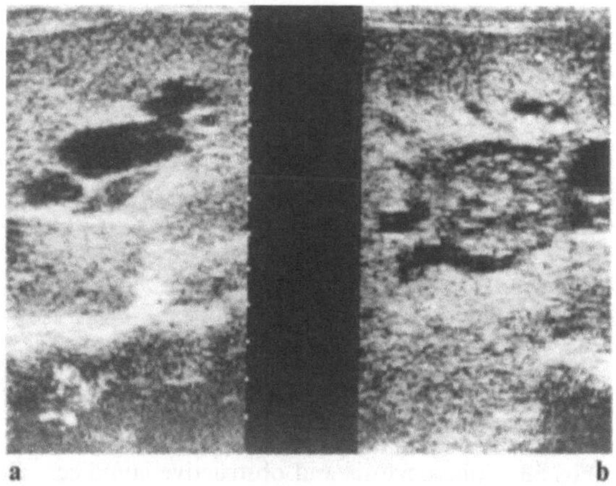

Fig. 52 a and b. Lymphoma in an 8-year-old boy with obstructive jaundice and right upper quadrant mass.
a Subcostal oblique section at level of porta hepatis showing important bile duct dilatation anterior to portal bifurcation.
b Subcostal oblique scan showing dilatation of the biliary tract associated with a mass lateral to the portal vein.

9.2 Gallbladder Disease

9.2.1 Cholelithiasis

Cholelithiasis is usually seen in adolescence but cases in infancy are sometimes reported. The etiological factors are dehydration and total parenteral nutrition.

Gallstones in children were usually opaque calculi visualized on plain films in approximately 60% of the cases, but this percentage is from a series of cases before the discovery of US which now leads to an earlier diagnosis of nonopaque cholelithiasis.

The main causes are:

1. Hemolytic anemias [sickle cell disease, spherocytosis (Fig. 53), thalassemia]. Cholelithiasis should be systematically searched for before splenectomy.
2. Liver diseases favoring biliary stasis: Cystic fibrosis where the gallbladder is often small with irregular walls and the pancreas is more echogenic than normal and small; Byler disease in which case US often shows an enlarged gallbladder; Malformations of the biliary tract causing biliary stasis.
3. Interruption of the enterohepatic circulation of bile salts: extensive ileal resection and regional enteritis.
4. Total parenteral nutrition.

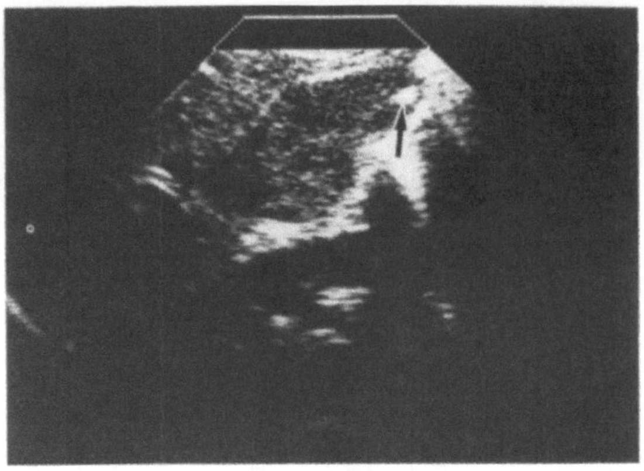

Fig. 53. Spherocytosis and obstructive jaundice. Longitudinal scan showing enlarged gallbladder with a stone (*arrow*). The bile sludge is related to the fact that US examination was performed the day after a hemolytic crisis. The obstructive jaundice is explained by the severity of the crisis.

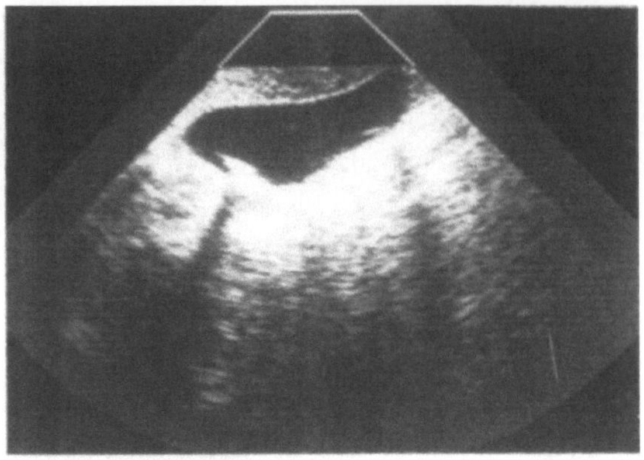

a

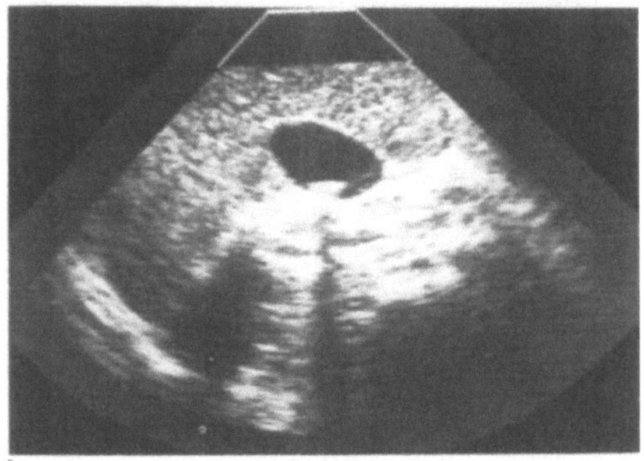

b

Fig. 54 a and b. Sickle cell anemia. Longitudinal **(a)** and transverse **(b)** scans through the gallbladder showing stone present along the floor with acoustic shadowing behind the calculus.

However, in more than 50% of the cases, cholelithiasis is idiopathic. Symptoms are usually abdominal pain, but cholelithiasis can be a fortuitous discovery during US examination.

Diagnosis of cholelithiasis is usually easy: gallstones are identified as round echogenic areas within the gallbladder (Fig. 54) that demonstrate acoustic shadowing and move with changes in the patient's position. The gallbladder is rarely totally filled with stones, in which case it would be more difficult to recognize (Fig. 55).

9.2.2 Acute Hydrops of the Gallbladder

Several cases of acute hydrops of the gallbladder without cholelithiasis have been reported. An anomaly of the cystic duct is rarely found. This entity appears more often in mucocutaneous lymph node syndrome. Hydrops has been also reported in other diseases such as scarlet fever, leptospiroris, and viral hepatitis. However, sometimes no etiologic factor is found and this entity has even been described in the neonate.

Abdominal pain and a palpable mass in the right upper quadrant are prevalent findings. US demonstrates an enlarged gallbladder with a well defined, thin wall, and a bile sludge is often present and produces a "fluid/fluid level" image (Fig. 56).

Diagnosis is confirmed by the benign course with follow-up US revealing the return of the gallbladder to normal size in 1–2 weeks.

9.2.3 Acute Cholecystitis

Unlike adult cases of cholecystitis, most childhood cases do not have associated cholelithiasis.

The usual symptoms of acalculous cholecystitis are abdominal tenderness, vomiting, and slight fever. Often secondary to infection, they are seen in association with generalized sepsis or gastrointestinal inflammatory process. The ultrasonographic indication is an enlarged gallbladder with a markedly thickened sonolucent wall, which is sometimes ill-defined, irregular, and hyperreflective (Fig. 57). These signs may be associated with the presence of stagnant bile or sludge within the gallbladder. Another important indication is severe tenderness on palpation of the gallbladder.

Some patients have sonographically demonstrable thickening of the gallbladder wall without intrinsic gallbladder disease. These cases include right-sided heart failure, hypoalbuminemia, ascites, and viral hepatitis (Fig. 58).

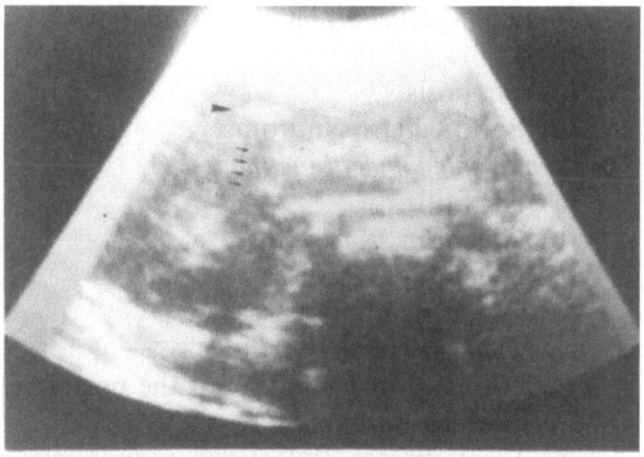

a

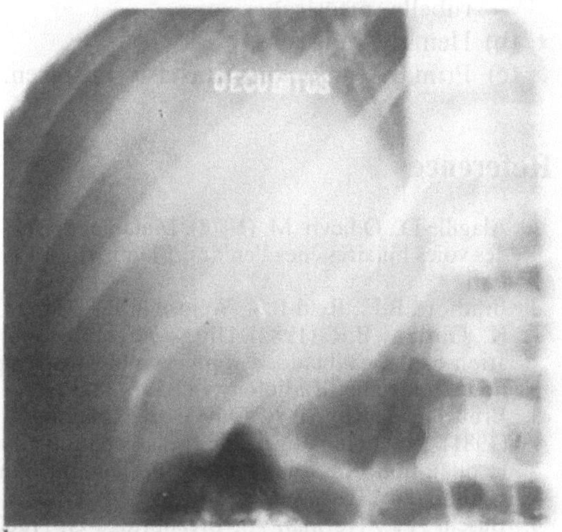

b

Fig. 55 a and b. Four-year-old child with gallstones. **a** Transverse scan through the right kidney. Hyperechogenic area (;) with acoustic shadowing (→) at the level of porta hepatis. The gallbladder is not visualized. **b** Oral cholecystogram showing a stone in a small, contracted gallbladder. The recognition of gallstones is sometimes difficult when the gallbladder is contracted because of disease.

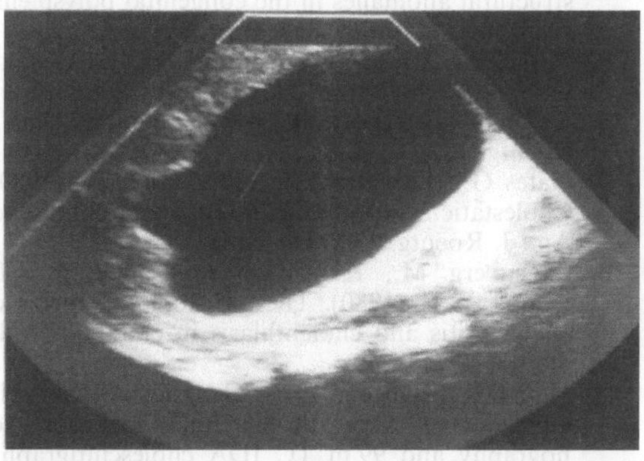

Fig. 56. Viral hepatitis with a right upper quadrant mass. Longitudinal scan showing markedly emlarged gallbladder with no extra hepatic biliary dilatation. Acute hydrops of the gallbladder.

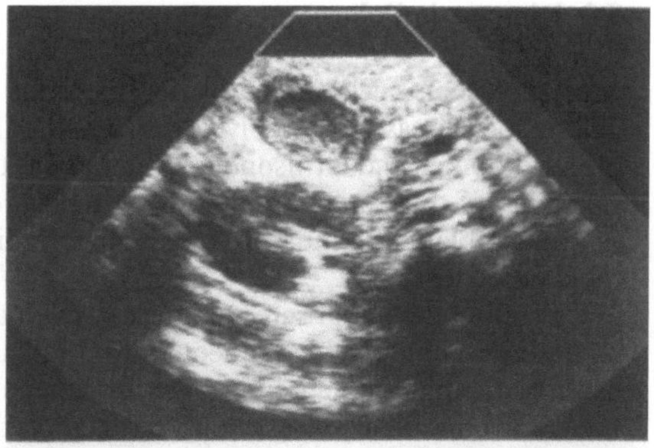

a

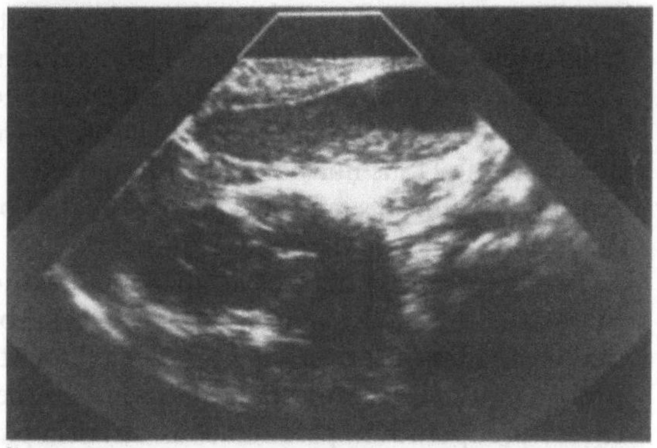

b

Fig. 57 a and b. Generalized sepsis. Abdominal pain in the right upper quadrant. Transverse **(a)** and longitudinal **(b)** scans of gallbladder showing increased gallbladder wall thickness with "fluid level" image. Diagnosis of acute acalculous cholecystitis was made.

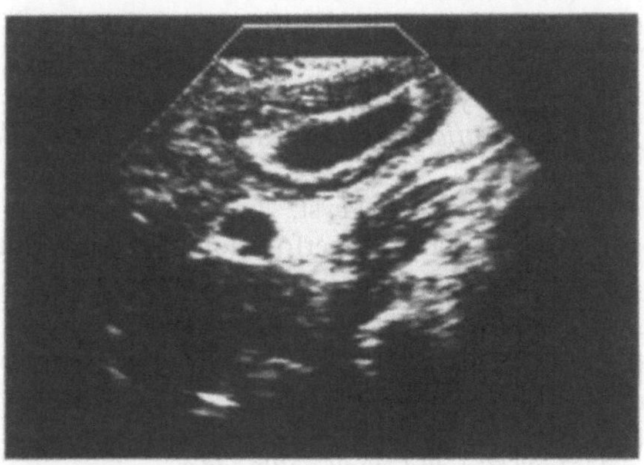

Fig. 58. Six-year-old boy with abdominal pain in the right upper quadrant without jaundice. The gallbladder wall was thickened and there was neither sludge nor stone. Jaundice appeared 2 days later. Diagnosis of viral hepatitis was made.

9.3 Diagnostic Policy

Most problems encountered in the diagnosis of gallbladder diseases are resolved with a plain film of the abdomen and ultrasonography. In fact, the reliability of this examination in the visualization of the gallbladder almost excludes other radiologic procedures.

Us is now the initial screening test to evaluate cholestatic jaundice. In the neonatal period US cannot distinguish hepatitis from extrahepatic biliary atresia. Biliary atresia must be diagnosed if timely surgery is to be carried out, in which case clinical findings and biological data with hepatobiliary scintigraphy are the means of diagnosis.

Intrahepatic or extrahepatic bile duct dilatation can be detected by US in all cases. In some cases, however, the US is normal and it should then be repeated if clinical symptoms persist because bile duct dilatation can take weeks to form.

Two points may not be clear: the exact location of obstruction (nonvisualization of the distal bile duct because of the overlying bowel gas) and the precise nature of the anatomical lesions. In these cases preoperative percutaneous transhepatic cholangiography has to be performed (IV cholangiography is usually unsuccessful in jaundiced patients).

Diagnostic plan for hepatobiliary diseases in children

1. *Cholestatic jaundice without biliary tract dilatation in infants*
   (a) Nonvisualization of the gallbladder: extrahepatic biliary atresia
   (b) Gallbladder visualized:
       Neonatal hepatitis;
       Extrahepatic biliary atresia;
       Cystic fibrosis.
2. *Cholestatic jaundices with biliary tract dilatation*
   (a) Choledochal cyst;
   (b) Spontaneous perforation of the bile duct;
   (c) Primary lithiasis of the common duct.
3. *Jaundice and enlarged gallbladder*
   (a) Acute hydrops;
   (b) Byler's disease;
   (c) Congenital hepatic fibrosis.
4. *Jaundice and small gallbladder*
   (a) Cystic fibrosis;
   (b) Cirrhosis;
   (c) Cholelithiasis;
   (d) Cholestatic hepatitis.
5. *Hepatoplenomegaly with portal hypertension* (PH)
   (a) Cirrhosis
   (b) Budd Chiari syndrome.
6. *Hepatosplenomegaly without PH*
   (a) Hepatitis;
   (b) Glycogen storage disease;
   (c) Niemann-Pick disease;
   (d) Other metabolic diseases.
7. *Splenomegaly with PH*
   Cavernous transformation of the portal vein.
8. *Splenomegaly without PH*
   (a) Viral disease (infectious mononucleosis, rubella, measles);
   (b) Hemolytic disease;
   (c) Primary tumor or metastases in spleen.

References

1. Alagille D., Odievre M. (1978). Maladies du foie et des voies biliaires chez l'enfant. Flammarion Edit., Paris
2. Bradford B.F., Reid B.S., Weinstein B.J., Sang Oh K., Girdany B.R. (1982). Ultrasonographic evaluation of the gallbladder in mucocutaneous lymph node syndrome. Radiology 142:381–384
3. Brunelle F., Riou J.Y., Douilet P., Chaumont P. (1981). La cholangiographie trans-hépatique dans la dilatation des voies biliaires de l'enfant. Ann. Radiol., 24:131–139
4. Buschi A.J., Norman A., Breenbridge G. (1980). Sonographic diagnosis of cholelithiasis in childhood. Am. J. Dis. Child 134:575–576
5. Cadier L., Broussin B., Bucco P., Diard F. (1980). Intérêt de l'échographie des voies biliaires dans la surveillance des enfants en nutrition parentérale exclusive. Ann. Radiol. 23:428–429
6. Carroll B.A., Oppenheimer D.A., Muller H.H. (1982).High frequency real-time ultrasound of the neonatal biliary system. Radiology 145:437–440
7. Chandra R.S. (1974). Biliary atresia and other structural anomalies in the congenital polysplenia syndrome. J. Pediat. 85:649–653
8. Franck J.L., Hill M.C., Chirathivat S., Sfakirnakis G.N., Marchildon M. (1981). Antenatal observation of a choledochal cyst by sonography. Am. J. Roentg. 137:166–168
9. Gates G.F., Sinatra F.R., Thomas D.W. (1980). Cholestatic syndromes in infancy and childhood. Am. J. Roentg. 134:1141–1148
10. Greenberg M., Kangarloo H., Cochran S.T., Sample W.F. (1980). The ultrasonic diagnosis of cholecystitis and cholelithiasis in children. Radiology 137:745–749
11. Han B.K., Babcock D.S., Gelfand M.H. (1981). Choledochal cyst with bile duct dilatation: sonography and 99 m TC IDA cholescintigraphy. Am. J. Roentg. 136:1075–1079
12. Kangarloo H., Sarti D.A., Sample W.F., Amunson G. (1980). Ultrasonographic spectrum of choledochal cysts in children. Pediatr. Radiol. 9:15–18.

13. Kirks D.R. (1979). Lithiasis due to interruption of the enterohepatic circulation of bile salts. Am. J. Roentg. 133:383–388
14. McGahan J.P., Phillips H.E., Cox K.L. (1982). Sonography of the normal pediatric gallbladder and biliary tract. Radiology 144:873–875
15. Ralls P.W., Quinn M.F., Juttner H.U., Halls J.M., Boswell W.D. (1981). Gallbladder wall thickening: patients without intrinsic gallbladder disease. Am. J. Roentg. 137:65–68
16. Schrumpf J.D., Handmaker H. (1982). Hydrops of gallbladder in a premature neonate. Am. J. Dis. Child. 136:172–173
17. Ternberg L.J., Keating J.P. (1975). Acute acalculous cholecystitis. Complications of other illnesses in childhood. Arch. Surg. 110:543–547
18. Witcombe J.B., Cremin B.J. (1978). The width of the common bile duct in childhood. Pediatr. Radiol. 7:147–149

Chapter 7

Pancreas

M. Spehl-Robberecht, L. Garel, and D. Lallemand

1 Introduction

US examination has shown that the pancreas in children is abnormal more often than previously thought. The examination technique is similar to that of adults and the pancreas is usually easy to demonstrate in children. Patients with pancreatitis (chemical, trauma, familial disease) are a group with a clinical and biological presentation that can be unclear; pancreatic lesions of cystic fibrosis, varying with the patient's age, represents a second group in this pediatric pancreatic pathology; a third group consists of pancreatic tumors that are represented by pancreatic involvement of lymphomas and neuroblastomas rather than by true pancreatic tumors. We shall not discuss variations of the vascular pancreatic markers since portal hypertension is dealt with in Chap. 6.

2 Measurements

US examination allows the size of the pancreas to be measured. Tables giving normal diameters of the head, body, and tail of the pancreas have been used for a long time in adults and were recently proposed for children by Rosenberg et al. (see [5]) during the 19th ESPR Congress; the figures they gave were

Head	10–20 cm
Body	4–10 cm
Tail	8–18 cm

Another way of measuring pancreatic size consists of calculating its largest surface on a transverse scan using the splenic vein as vascular marker (Fig. 1): this method of measurement takes the variation of the pancreatic form into account but the normal curves have not yet been completed. The use of pancreatic measurements has been of benefit in the characterization of attacks of acute pancreatitis in oncology. Acute pancreatitis is a frequent complication of asparaginase treatment in children with acute lymphoblastic leukemia. Its early diagnosis is made possible if US is performed before treatment and its findings used as personal normal standard values when control checks are made in the case of acute abdominal pain during the course of treatment (Figs. 2–4).

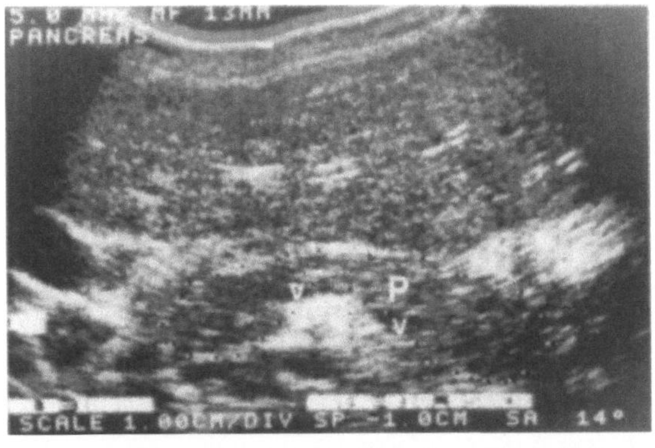

Fig. 1. Direct measurement of pancreatic surface on transverse scan along the splenic vein axis by means of an echo computer (the calculated surface appears on the bottom right corner of the screen).
Here area = 10.0 cm². *P*, pancreas; *V*, splenic vein.

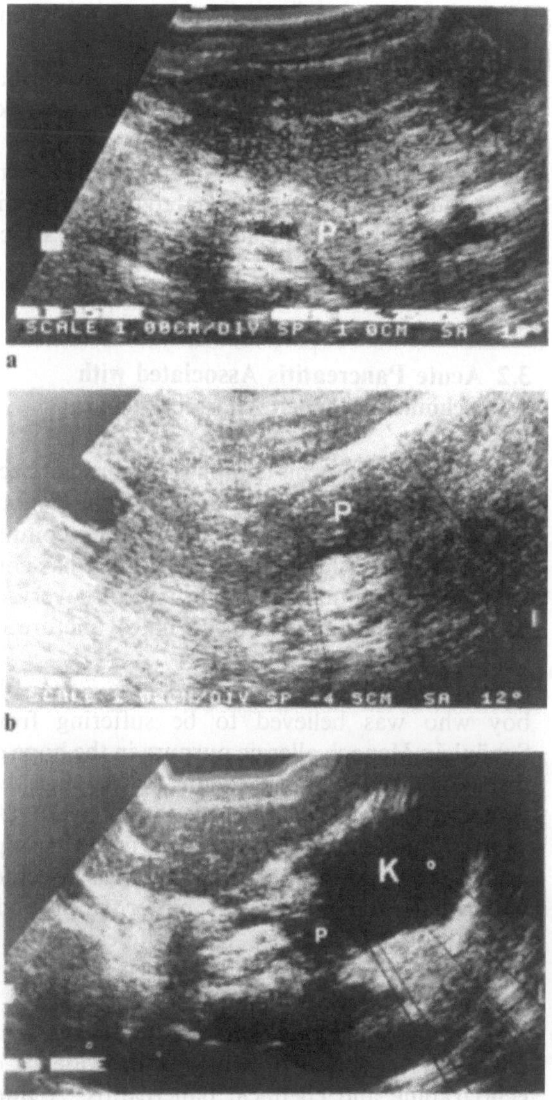

◀ **Fig. 2a–c.** Two-year-old girl with acute lymphocytic leukemia. Asparaginase treatment was given.
a Normal echopattern of pancreas *(P)* before treatment.
b One week after beginning of treatment: acute pancreatitis with enlarged hypoechogenic pancreas *(P)*.
c Six weeks after **b**, pseudocyst *(K)* of 6 cm diameter at the pancreatic tail *(P)* and hyperechogenic pancreatic body.

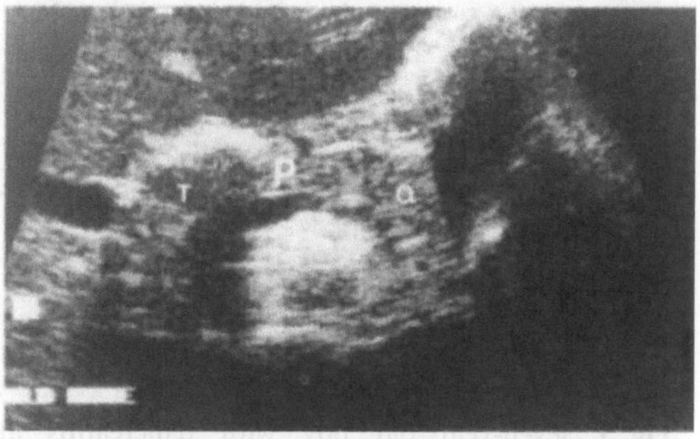

Fig. 3. Asparaginase treatment in a 5-year-old girl with clinical and biological acute pancreatitis. Pancreas *(P)* appears patchy except for its head *(T)*, which appears hypoechogenic. *Q*, Tail.

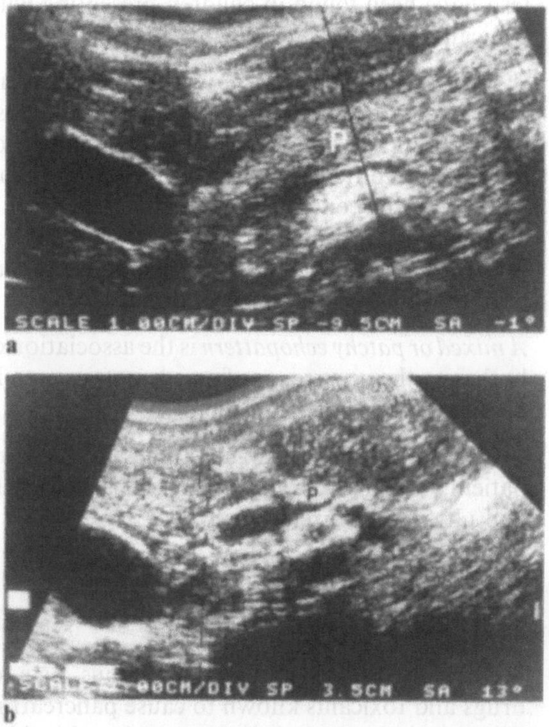

Fig. 4a and b. 15-year-old girl presented with pancreatitis while undergoing asparaginase treatment 2 years presviously. Relapse of abdominal pain. **a** Acute pancreatitis occurring in an already hyperechogenic pancreas. Patchy appearance and swelling of pancreas *(P)*. **b** The patient is asymptomatic 16 months later. Pancreas *(P)* is small and hyperechogenic.

3 Pancreatitis

Even though there are numerous well-known causes of pancreatitis, echographic examination of the pancreas has made pancreatic pathology an everyday clinical preoccupation because of its easy diagnostic imaging in comparison with the somewhat more difficult biological investigation (seric lipase is difficult to measure, high amylase levels can quicklly return to normal in blood and urine and can therefore be of no help). It seems difficult, and even incorrect, to separate acute and chronic pancreatitis in view of pancreatic US results as there are three types of structure that can be found: (a) hypoechogenic together with an increased pancreatic volume; (b) hyperechogenic, either localized or generalized, without evident volume change; (c) mixed, patchy echopattern.

In our experience these three types of echopattern have been found in children presenting with clinically evident acute pancreatitis.

A hyperechogenic pattern is due to different phenomena that can be present alone or in close association: (a) an increase in the number of interfaces of different acoustic impedance; (b) an increase in the contents of the pancreatic tissue – collagen, fat, or calcium.

A hypoechogenic pattern corresponds to an edema, which is usually generalized.

A mixed or patchy echopattern is the association of both, i.e., the occurrence of an edematous area in an already hyperechoic pancreas.

Only long-term follow-up studies in the same patients will allow accurate clinical, pathological, and ultrasonic correlations.

3.1 Iatrogenic Medical Pancreatitis

Medical literature contains numerous lists of drugs and toxicants known to cause pancreatitis; These include alcohol, borates, chlorothiazides, oral contraceptives, steroids, asparaginase, salicylazosulfapyridine, and tetracyclines. However, the mechanisms leading to pancreatitis are not always known.

3.1.1 Asparaginase (Figs. 2–4)

We examined four children presenting with biologically proven acute pancreatic complications due to asparaginase treatment in a series of 19 children with acute lymphoblastic leukemia. Asparaginase, while causing a decrease in fibrinogen, V, VII, VIII, and IX factors, and plasminogen, leads to disseminated intravascular coagulation and therefore pancreatitis.

US findings were similar in our four patients:

1. Hypoechogenic pattern and pancreatic volume increase (either localized or generalized) during the acute phase;
2. Patchy hyperechogenic pattern and volume increase in cases of acute relapse;
3. Mixed or variable echostructure with normal or slightly decreased volume after a few weeks (1–4 weeks in our series);
4. In one child there was development of a 6 cm diameter pseudocyst external to the pancreatic tail 6 weeks after the acute pancreatitis attack (Fig. 1).

3.2 Acute Pancreatitis Associated with Schönlein-Henoch Allergic Purpura

As far as we know, this complication has not been described in association with Schönlein-Henoch allergic purpura. The presence of this complication illustrates how much echography has contributed to our understanding and discovery of pancreatic participation in a clinical picture of abdominal pain.

Abdominal US was performed in a 7-year-old boy who was believed to be suffering from Schönlein-Henoch allergic purpura in the hope of displaying hemorrhagic edema of the digestive wall (corticosteroids had not yet been given). US showed duodenal thickening that could be separated from the head of the pancreas together with a marked hypoechogenic pattern of the body and tail of the pancreas. The acute echographic pancreatitis was confirmed by elevated amylasemia and amylasuria (Fig. 5).

A second child was examined under the same conditions and also presented with evidence of echographic and chemical pancreatitis. A third case of pancreatitis associated with allergic purpura is confirmed by biological findings alone.

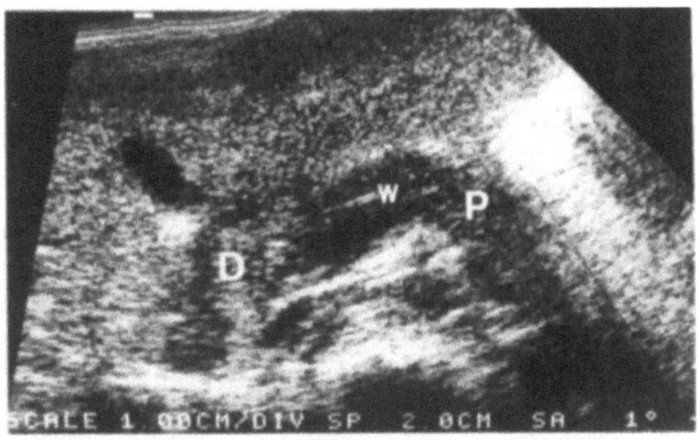

Fig. 5. Seven-years-old boy with pancreatitis and Schönlein-Henoch allergic purpura. Edema of duodenal wall *(D)* without separation from pancreatic head *(P)*. Hypoechogenic pattern of the pancreas. Pancreatic duct *(W)*.

The etiology of acute pancreatitis in the course of Schönlein-Henoch syndrome is not definite: is it due to diffuse arteriolitis with fibrinoid necrosis within the pancreas or does the pancreatitis appear secondary to a stenosis of the intramural pancreatic duct following duodenal hematoma?

Demonstration of Wirsung's canal in children with the type of equipment used is common and therefore cannot be considered as a point in favor of the second hypothesis and the question remains unanswered.

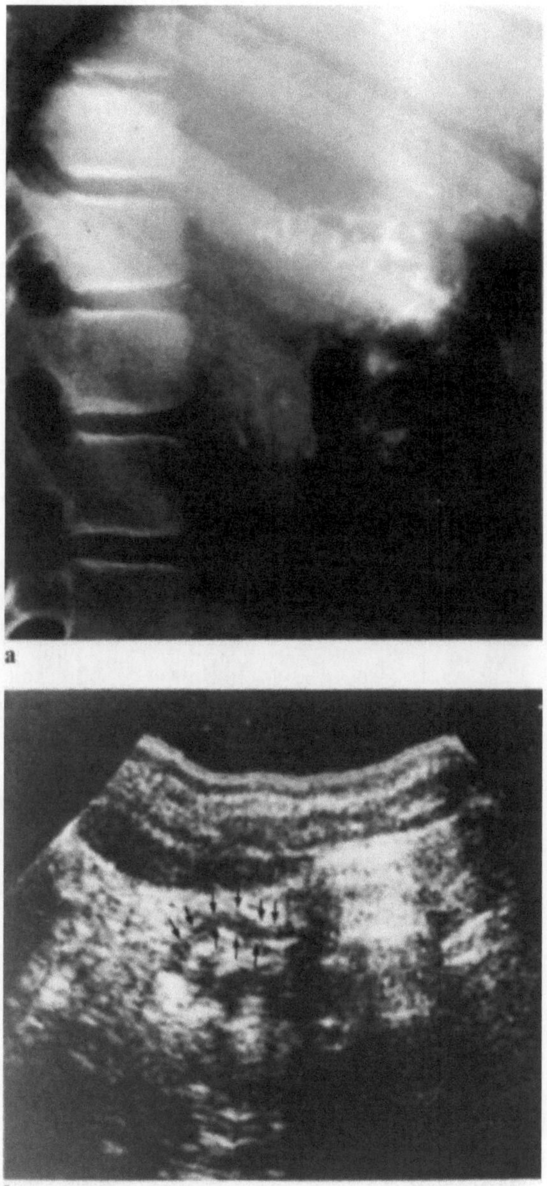

a

b

Fig. 6 a and b. Familial calcifying pancreatitis in a 12-year-old boy.
a Plain film of the abdomen showing important pancreatic calcifications.
b Transverse scan (right anterior oblique) showing hyperechogenic pancreatic area with dilatation of Wirsung's canal (confirmed by ERCP).

3.3 Familial Pancreatitis

One patient presented with extensive pancreatic calcifications (Fig. 6), making the sonographic evaluation of the duct of Wirsung difficult. Three cases occurred in the same family: two sisters and their young brother were operated upon within a year. The fifth case of our series is illustrated in Fig. 7. These last four cases have several similarities: severe clinical symptoms; progressive dilatation of the duct of Wirsung; drastic and stable improvement after surgery.

ERCP was performed in all cases as a preoperative study and the findings were parallel to those of US. US was especially valuable in following closely these patients during the acute episodes of pancreatitis and after surgery.

An example of rapid pancreatic changes is shown in Fig. 8 in a case of a recurrent pancreatitis related to drugs.

The possibility exists of segmental portal hypertension (2 cases) in those children with recurrent pancreatitis by trapping the splenic vein in the peripancreatic fibrosis. The usual features of portal hypertension along the lesser sac are then lacking and a careful study of the splenic hilums must be made to look for posterior gastric collaterals in order to make the surgeon aware of the preoperative vascular difficulties.

4 Exocrine Pancreas Insufficiency

4.1 Cystic Fibrosis

Within our series of 52 children, 45 presented with clinical and biological pancreatic insufficiency and 6 had essentially respiratory disease without pancreatic signs. All these children were examined by US once a year for liver, pancreas, and biliary check-up.

Where pancreatic examination is an easy technical task in a fasting healthy child, the same examination can become very difficult in children with cystic fibrosis, and in 10% of our cases the pancreas could not be displayed. That technical difficulty is not linked with age but seems dependent on the abdominal topographic changes following pulmonary overdistension.

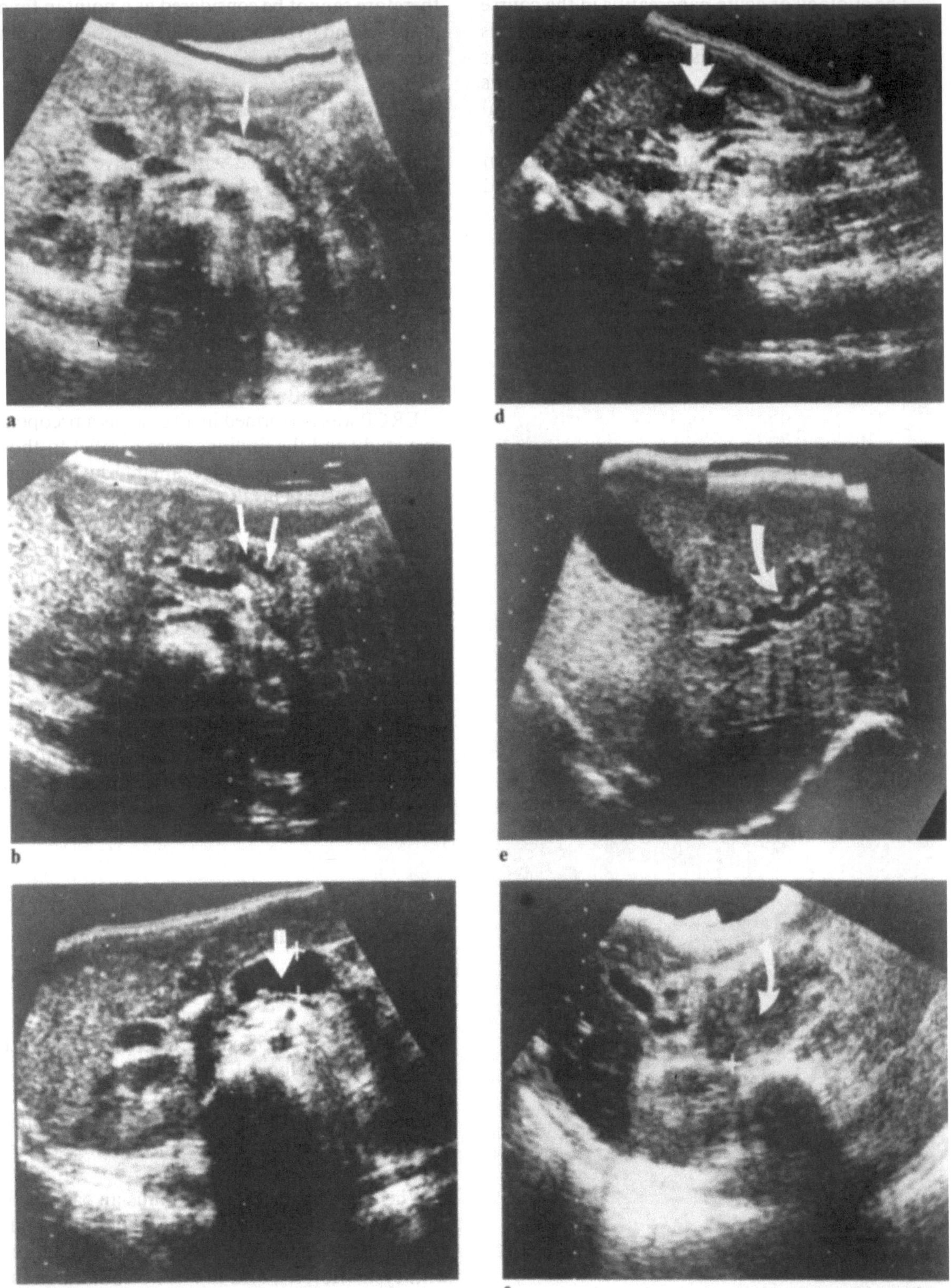

Fig. 7 a–f

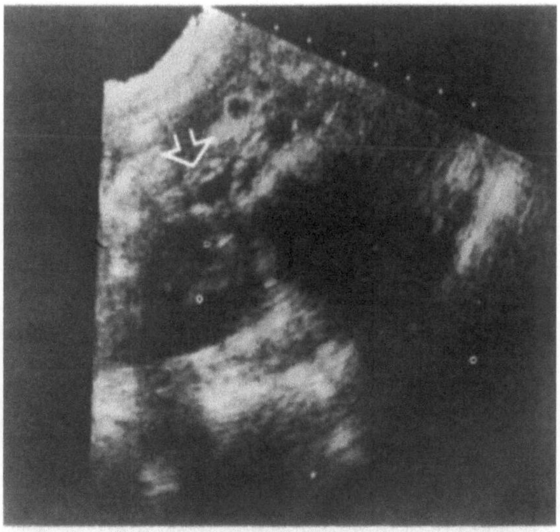

g

Fig. 7a–g. Familial calcifying pancreatitis in a 5-year-old girl (the father and one uncle have been operated for pseudocyst) at an acute stage of the illness. **a and b** Transverse scans showing the beginning of dilatation of Wirsung's canal and its branches. **c** Transverse epigastric scan; **d** Sagittal aortic scan. **e** Oblique scan 3 weeks later. Dilatation of Wirsung's canal is very important (15 mm): the main biliary duct is also dilated. Pancreatectomy (body and tail) was performed with two digestive anastomoses (Wirsung and gallbladder) sparing the splenic vessels. **f** Transverse scan on pancreatic head 1 month after operation: acute pancreatitis (head measures 39 mm) that disappeared with medical treatment. **g** One year later the condition is stable.

◄

Fig. 8a–g. Total colectomy for a 9-year-old boy with Crohn's disease. Relapse in the ileorectal anastomosis. Corticoid and azathiopine therapy. Acute abdominal symptoms. **a** Sagittal scan through right kidney. Ascitis with floating digestive loops. **b and c** Epigastric transverse scans: large homogenous pancreas. **d** Epigastric transverse scan 5 days later: decrease in the size of the pancreas but the gland has become heterogeneous. **e** Transverse scan 15 days later, evident pathology of pancreas body. **f** Ten days later. **g** Transverse scan 1 month later: 2 cm pseudocyst in the pancreas body. The child has become asymptomatic.

d–g see p. 134

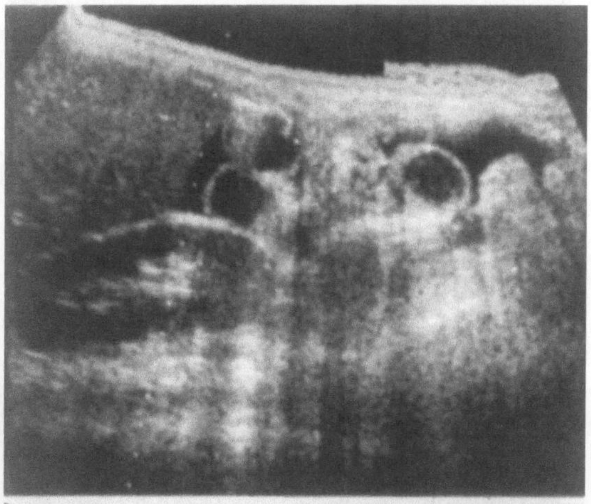

b

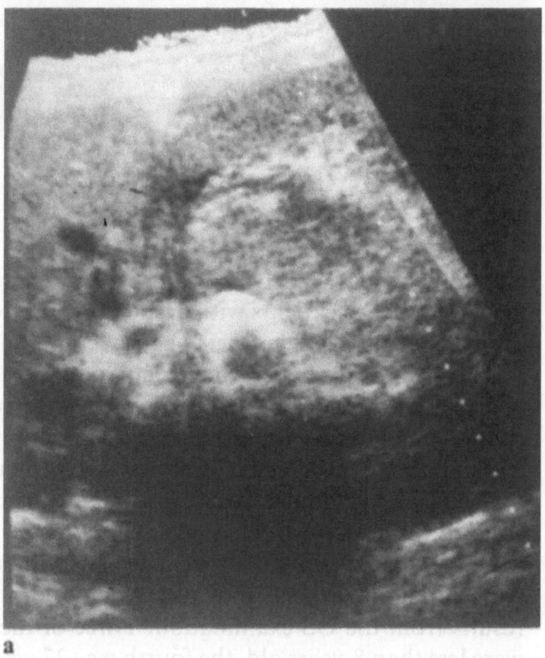

a

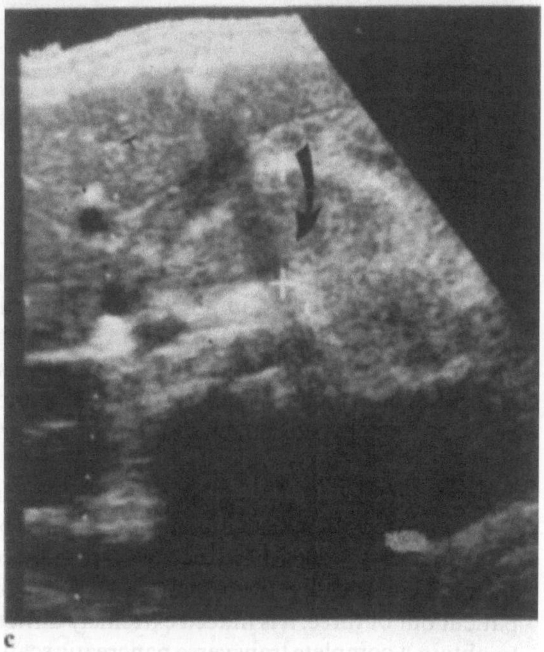

c

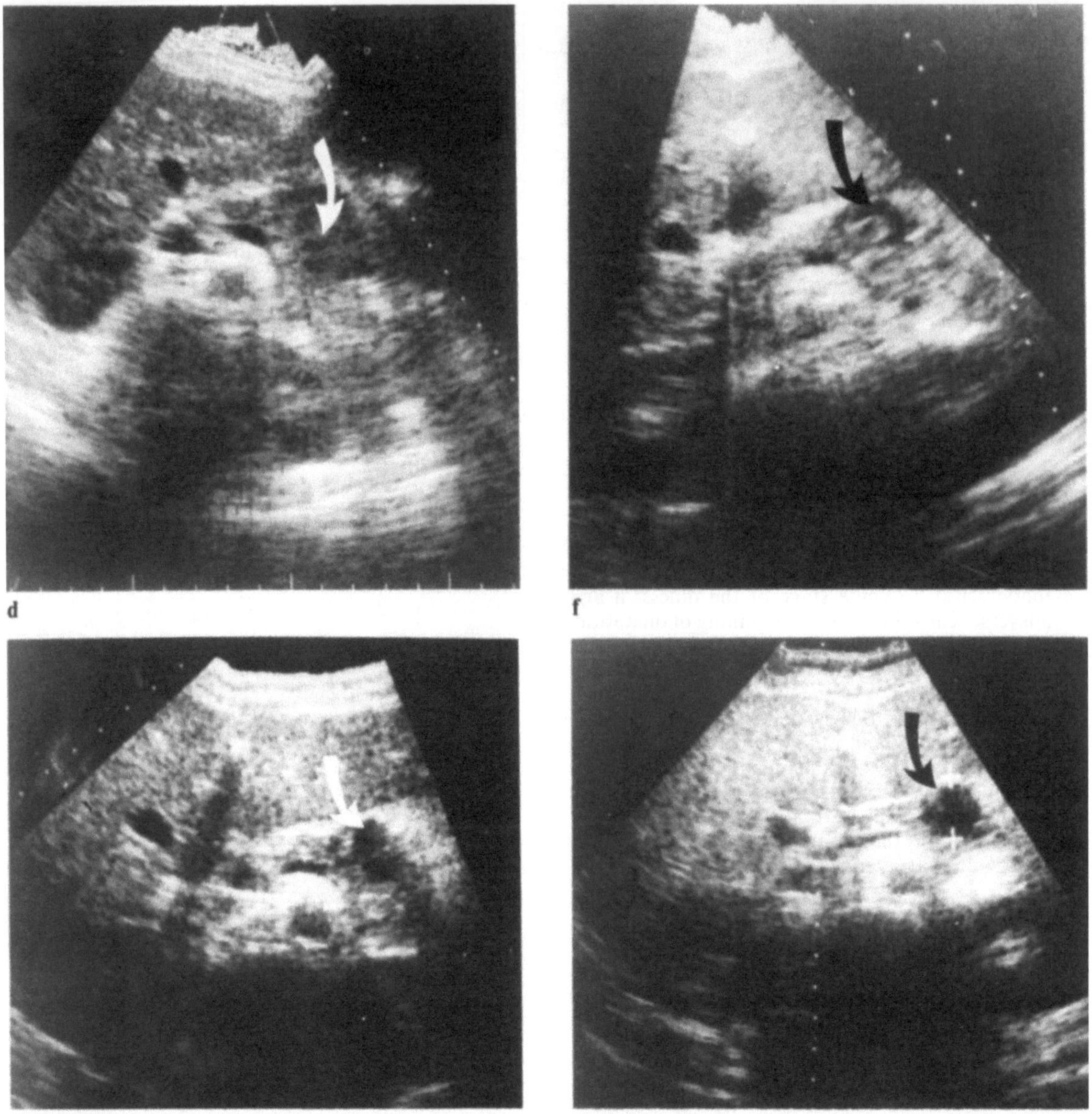

d f e g

Fig. 8d–g

Under the age of 2 years, the pancreas appeared echographically normal in all children with pancreatic insufficiency (Fig. 9). After 8 years of age, the pancreas appeared hyperechogenic in all cases of insufficiency (Figs. 10 and 11). Between 2 and 8 years, normal, hyperechogenic, or patchy patterns were observed and evolution from normal to hyperechogenic has twice taken less than 2 years.

Pancreatic volume also diminishes with age but measurements other than the distance between splenic vein and liver were only possible in one patient out of three: it is indeed extremely difficult to obtain a complete transverse pancreatic scan in patients with cystic fibrosis. In any case, measurements show that patients with cystic fibrosis have a smaller pancreas than their healthy controls.

The progressive hyperechogenicity of pancreas in cystic fibrosis is probably due to different causes: small cysts within the pancreas multiplying interfaces, progressive fibrosis, fatty tissue replacing the glandular tissue, and high calcium concentration in obstructed pancreatic ducts.

Of six patients with cystic fibrosis without pancreatic impairment, four had strictly normal results from the US examination. Three of them were less than 8 years old, the fourth was 27 years

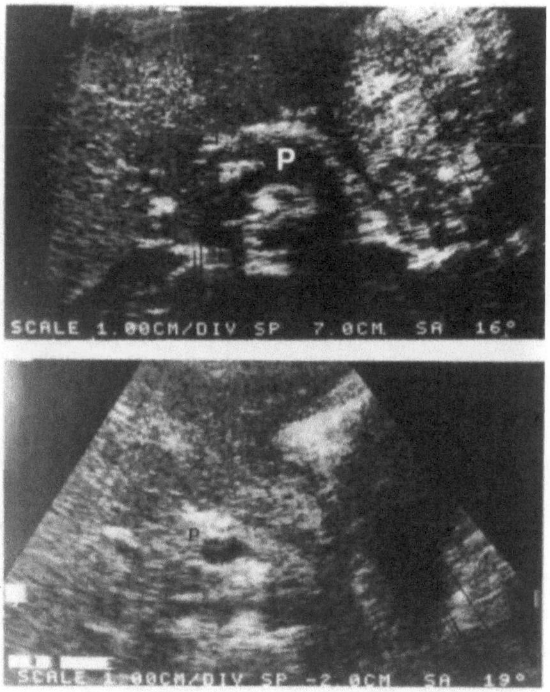

a

b

Fig. 9. a Two-year-old girl with cystic fibrosis and obvious pancreatic insufficiency. Normal pancreas echopattern *(P)*.
b Same child after 22 months of palliative enzyme treatment. Hyperechogenic pancreas *(P)*.

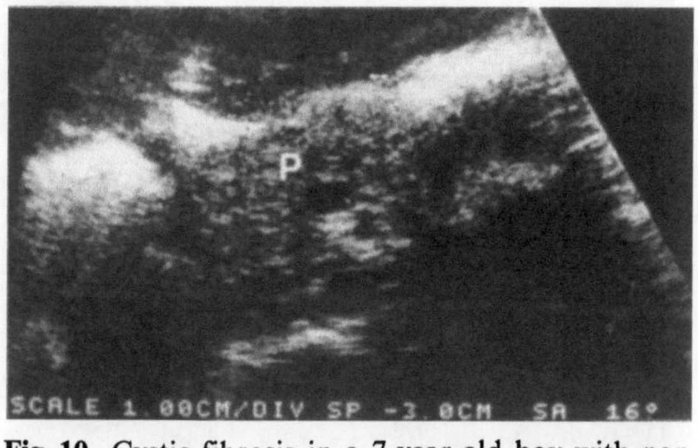

Fig. 10. Cystic fibrosis in a 7-year-old boy with pancreas insufficiency. Patchy intermediary echopattern of the pancreas *(P)*.

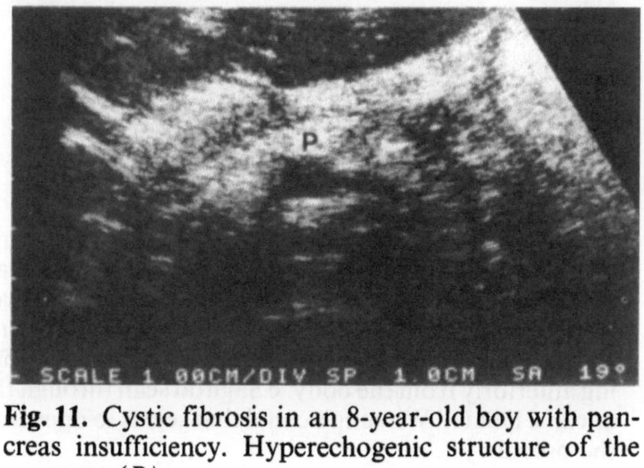

Fig. 11. Cystic fibrosis in an 8-year-old boy with pancreas insufficiency. Hyperechogenic structure of the pancreas *(P)*.

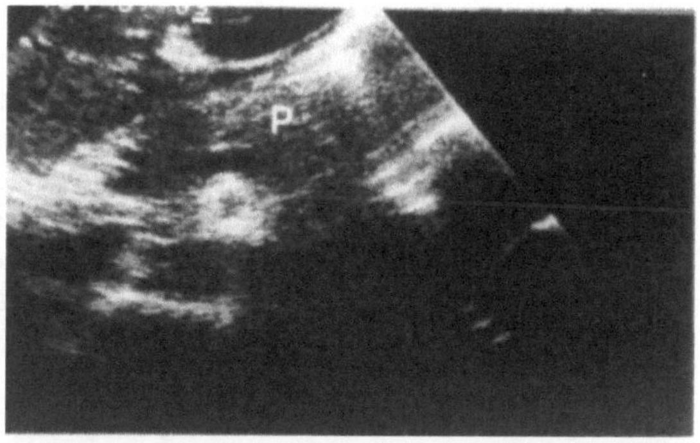

Fig. 12. Cystic fibrosis in a 26-year-old patient without pancreatic insufficiency. Normal pancreas *(P)*.

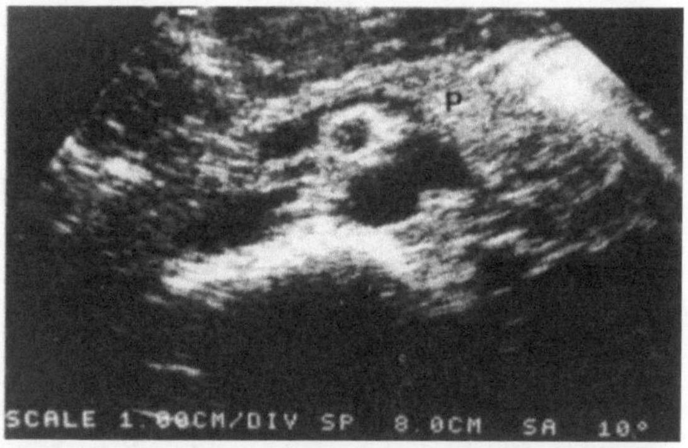

Fig. 13. Brother of patient in Fig. 12, 19 years old. Cystic fibrosis without pancreatic insufficiency. Diffuse hyperechogenic pattern of the pancreas *(P)*.

old. Two showed a patchy pattern which could be due to localized, quantitatively unimportant, pancreatic lesions (Figs. 12 and 13).

4.2 Schwachman-Diamond Syndrome

Schwachman-Diamond syndrome is characterized by exocrine pancreatic insufficiency mostly associated with neutropenia. It differs from cystic

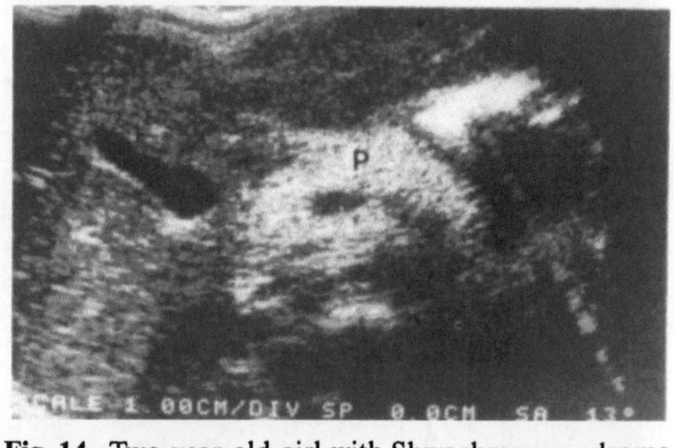

Fig. 14. Two-year-old girl with Shwachman syndrome (exocrine insufficiency). Marked hyperechogenicity of the pancreas *(P)*.

fibrosis by a normal sweat test and the absence of pulmonary lesions. Two children with Schwachman-Diamond syndrome were examined: US examination of the pancreas showed a normal volume of pancreatic space containing very hyperechogenic tissue that represents complete fat replacement of glandular tissue. Ducts and islets of Langerhans are intact as shown by pathological studies (Fig. 14).

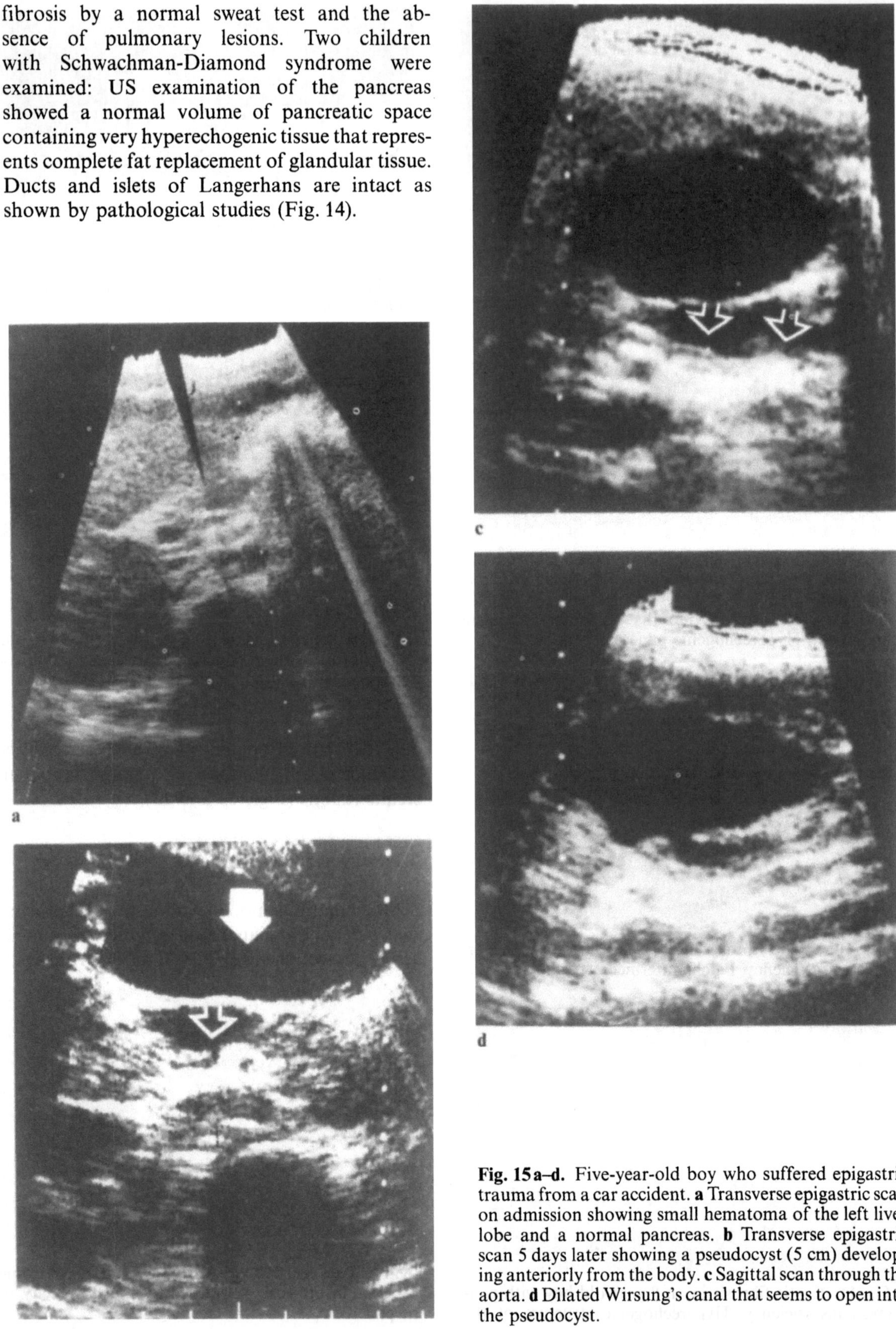

a c d

Fig. 15 a–d. Five-year-old boy who suffered epigastric trauma from a car accident. **a** Transverse epigastric scan on admission showing small hematoma of the left liver lobe and a normal pancreas. **b** Transverse epigastric scan 5 days later showing a pseudocyst (5 cm) developing anteriorly from the body. **c** Sagittal scan through the aorta. **d** Dilated Wirsung's canal that seems to open into the pseudocyst.

5 Traumatic Pseudocysts

We have observed seven cases where traumatism was caused by accidents ranging from falls from a toboggan to shooting wounds. Some points concerning the US examination have to be emphasized: repeated epigastric screenings may show a developing cyst (Fig. 15) or, on the contrary, its disappearance (Fig. 16); a pseudecyst may have a rich echopattern (Fig. 17) sometimes containing a liquid/liquid level (Fig. 18); a parenchymal fracture (Fig. 19), rupture (Fig. 20), or a dilatation (Fig. 11) of the main pancreatic ducts leads to surgical treatment, after which a relapse is still possible (Figs. 21 and 22).

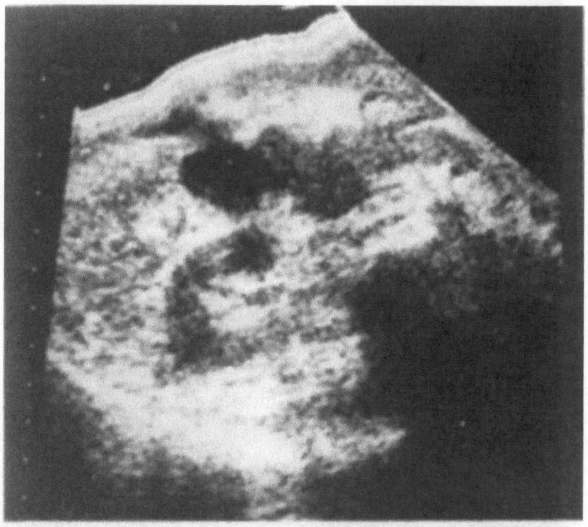
a

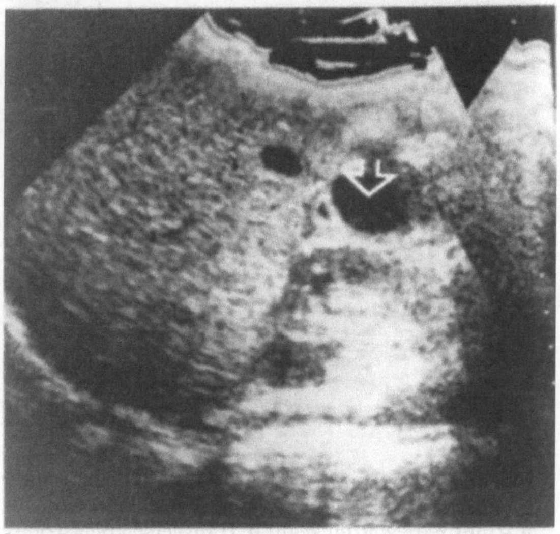
b

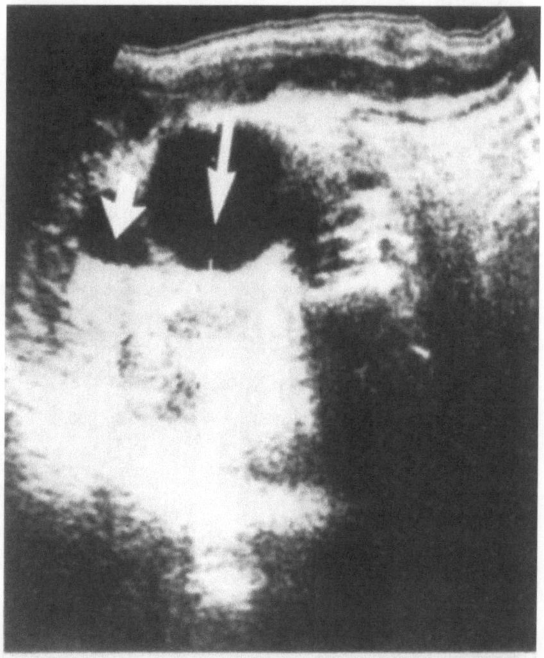
c

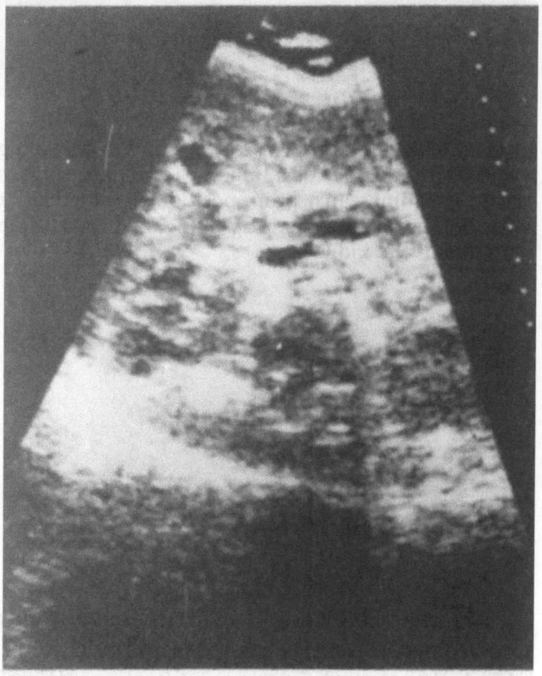
d

Fig. 16 a–d. Five-year-old boy with epigastric trauma caused by a blow when falling against a fence.
a Transverse epigastric scan showing big edematous pancreas and pseudocyst developing in the duodenal lumen.
b Sagittal scan through right kidney and gallbladder showing relationship with the pseudocyst.
c Transverse epigastric scan 1 month later showing initial pseudocyst to be three times bigger and revealing a second pseudocyst. The child's physical state was excellent and no treatment was given.
d Transverse scan 2 months later: pseudocysts have disappeared.

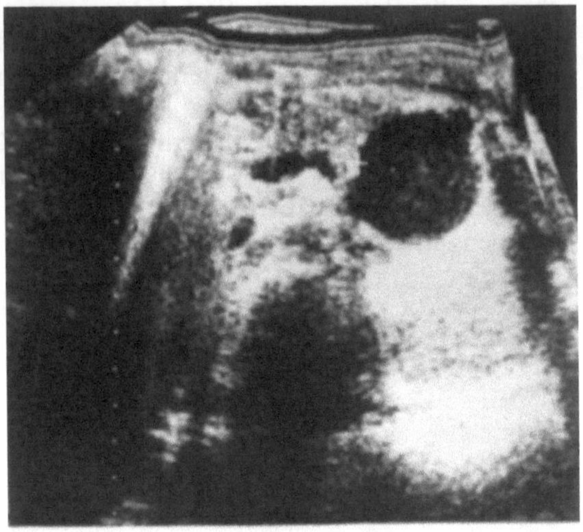

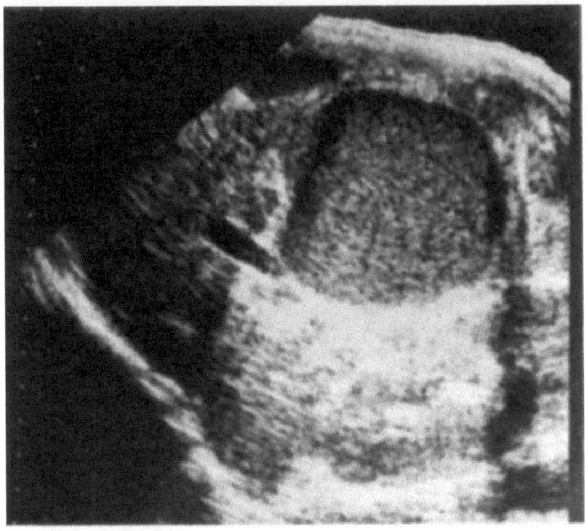

a

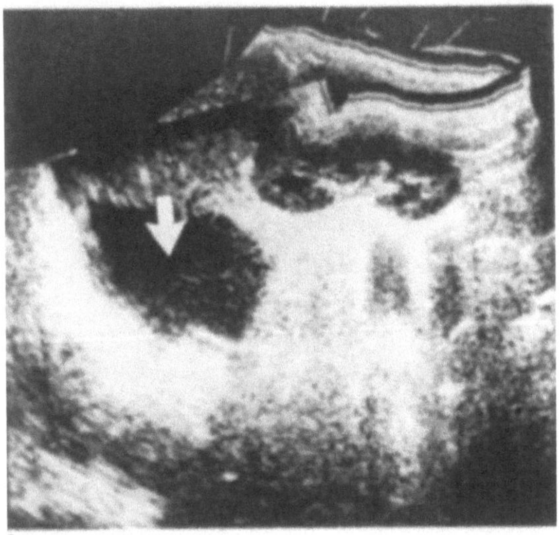

b

Fig. 17 a and b. Left epigastric mass in a 3-year-old girl who had no history of trauma. **a** Transverse epigastric scan; **b** Sagittal scan in prone position on the left kidney: pseudocyst of the pancreatic tail related to the spleen hilum and the kidney.

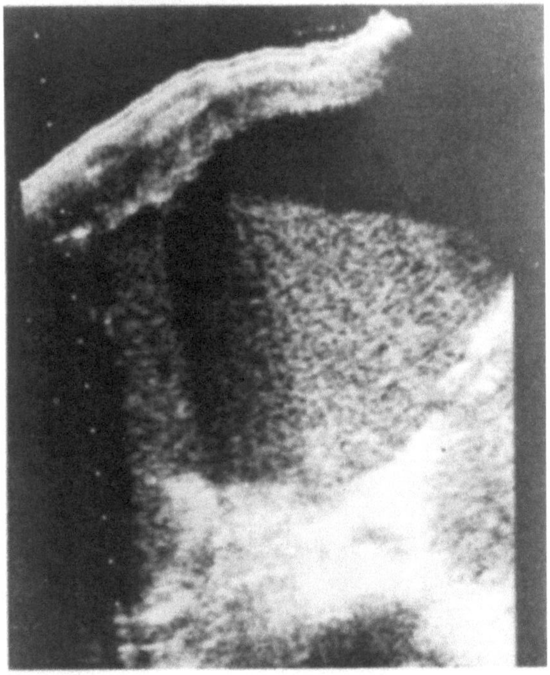

b

Fig. 18 a and b. Fourteen-year-old boy who had suffered a penetrating epigastric wound 3 weeks previously. **a** Right parasagittal scan; **b** Transverse epigastric scan showing a big liquid mass containing echoes and liquid/liquid level and an infected pseudocyst of the lesser sac.

6 Pancreatic Tumors

Cases of a "blown-up" pancreas have been reported accompanying neuroblastomas (Fig. 17 in Chap. 10), lymphomatous infiltrations (Fig. 22; see also Figs. 25–28 in Chap. 10), and pancreatic involvement of duodenal tumors, but they are rare among children. On the other hand, among the seven cases of hyperinsulinism in neonates and infants studied echographically none had any signs of pancreatic lesion. Tumors of Zollinger-Ellison syndrome or other secreting tumors have not been studied.

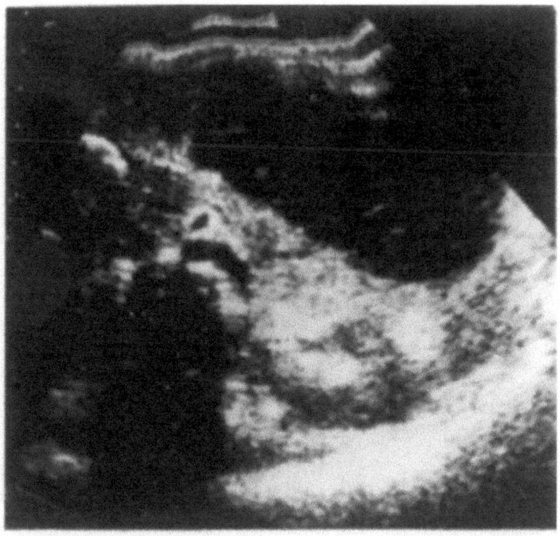

a

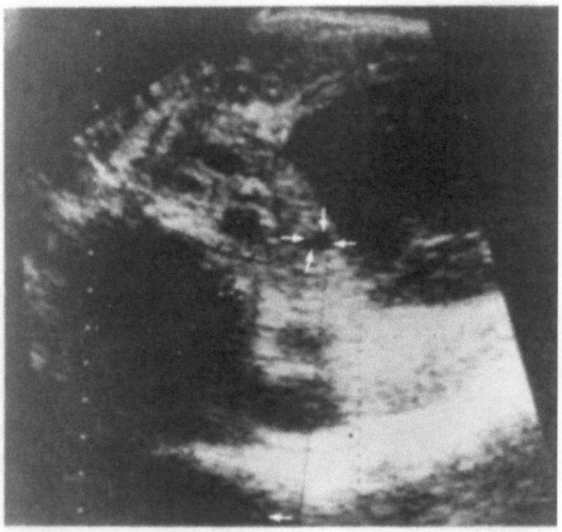

b

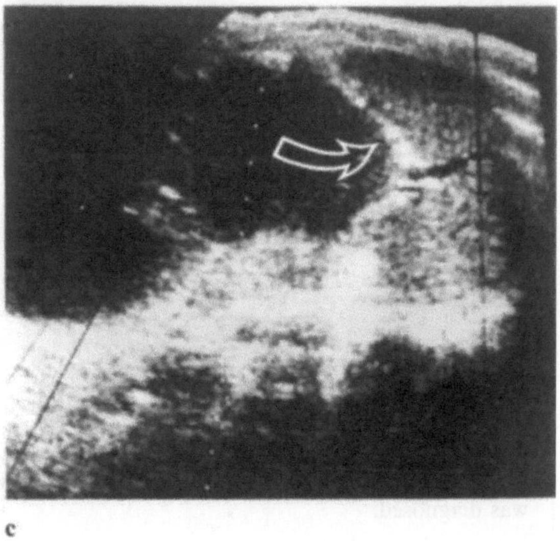

c

◀ **Fig. 19 a–c.** Six-year-old boy with a big mass at the left hypochondrium. Careful interview revealed a fall from a toboggan 1 week before.
a Epigastric scan showing pseudocyst developing in front of body and tail of the pancreas. **b** Transverse epigastric scan showing hypoechogenic area in the pancreatic tail. This fracture was very accurately demonstrated on CT. **c** Intercostal scan of the spleen showing pseudocyst in close contact with the hilum.

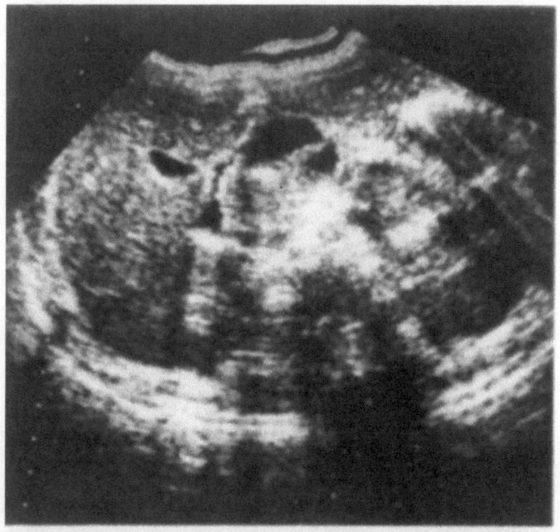

a

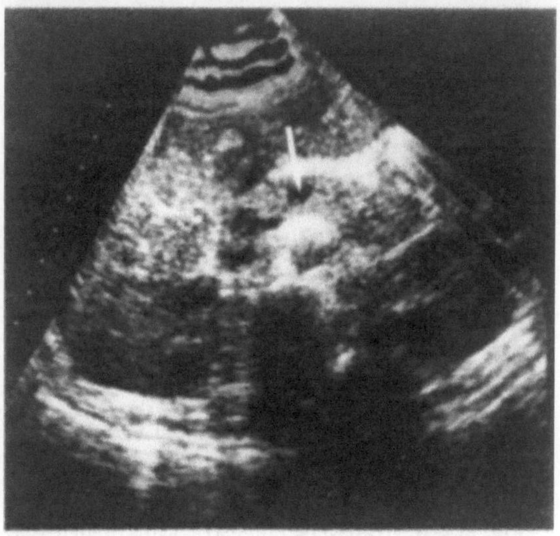

b

Fig. 20 a and b. Pancreas fracture in a 5-year-old girl after a car accident.
Transverse epigastric scans show a pseudocyst developing in front of pancreatic head **(a)** with laceration of body **(b)**.

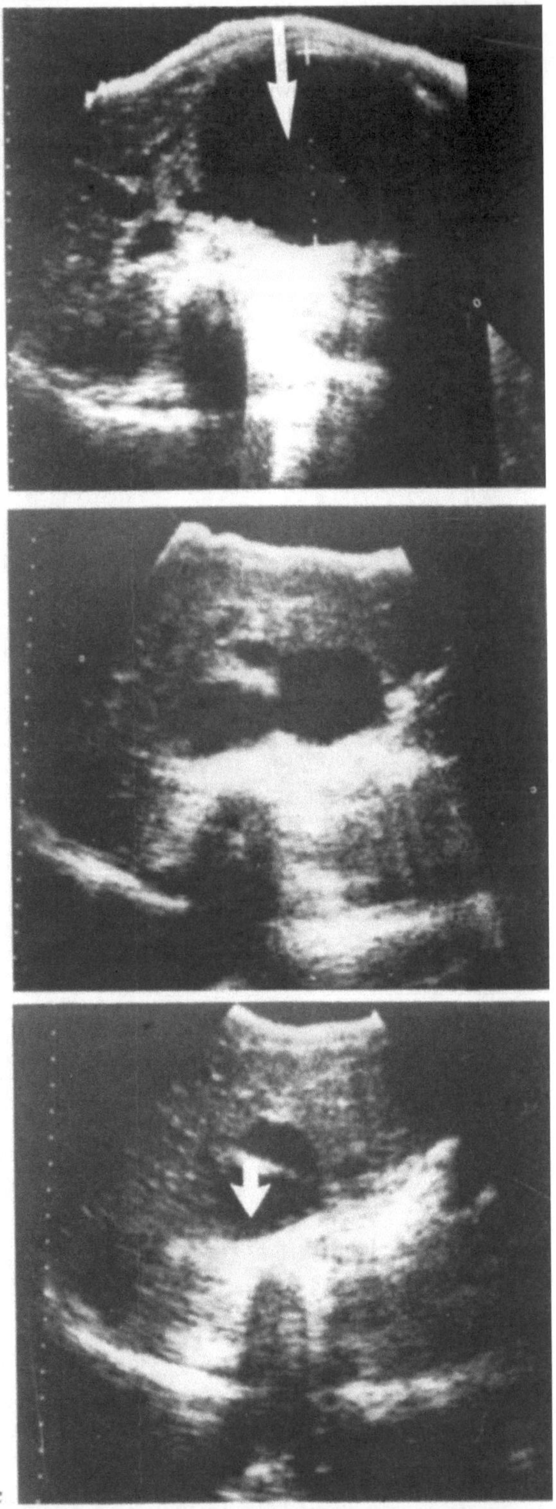

a b c

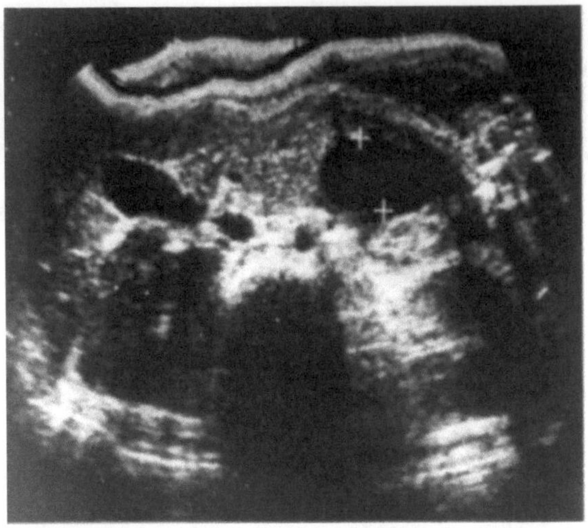

d

Fig. 21 a–d. Transverse epigastric scans of an 8-year-old girl who had been in a car accident 15 days before. **a** Pseudocyst (8 cm) of head and tail; **b** Scan a little lower than **a** showing a liquid leak toward the liver that is seen even better on **c** (transverse scan on right liver). Treated by simple cyst drainage. **d** One month later: recurrence of pseudocyst (2 cm).

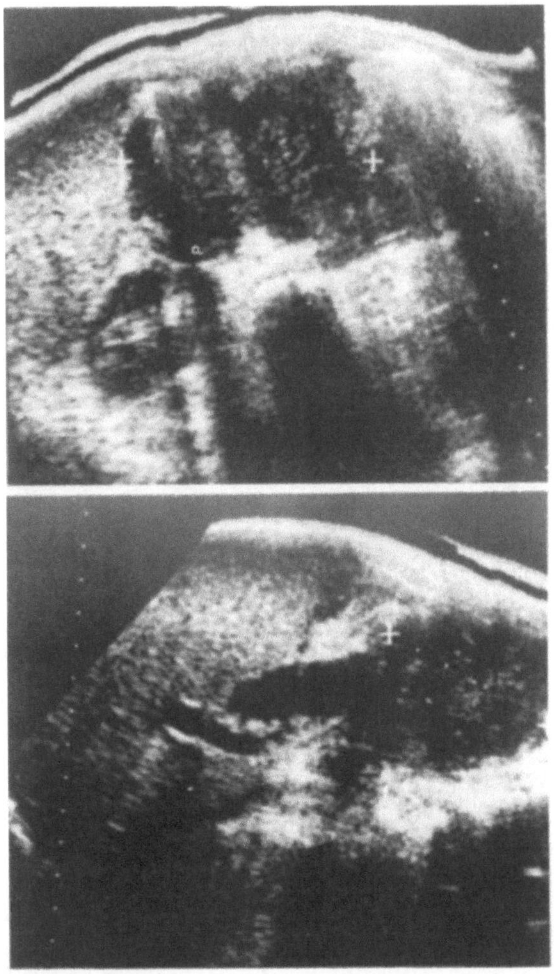

a b

Fig. 22 a and b. Thirteen-year-old boy with obstructive jaundice and poor physical condition. **a** Transverse epigastric scan. **b** Sagittal scan of portal vein. Solid mass (7 cm) containing few echoes in the pancreatic area with major dilatation of main bile duct. Burkitt's lymphoma was diagnosed.

7 Conclusion

US examination has become the number one imaging technique of the pancreas in children because of its obvious diagnostic and follow-up value.

References

General

1. de Graaff C.S., Taylor K.J.W., Simonds B.D. and Rosenfield A.J. (1978). Gray scale echography of the pancreas. Radiology 129:157–161
2. Doust B.D., Pearce J.D. (1976). Gray scale ultrasonic properties of the normal and inflamed pancreas. Radiology 120:653–657
3. Haber K., Freimanis A.K., Asler W.M. (1976). Demonstration and dimensional analysis of the normal pancreas with gray scale echography. A.J.R. 126:624–628
4. Weill F., Schraub A., Elsenscher A., Bourgoin A. (1977). Ultrasonography of the normal pancreas. Radiology 123:417–423

Pancreatitis

5. Coleman B.G., Arger P.H., Rosenberg H.K., Mulhern C.B., Ortega W., Stauffer D. (1983). Gray scale sonographic assessment of pancreatitis in children. Radiology 146:145–150
6. Fleischer A.C. and al. (1983). Sonographic findings of pancreatitis in children. Radiology 146:151
7. Nouwynck C. (1980). Complications de la chimiothérapie. Revue Méd. Brux. 1:331–336
8. Roy C.C., Silverman A., Cozzetto F.J. (1975). Pediatric clinical gastroenterology. The C.V. Mosby Company, St Louis
9. Samuels B.I., Culbert S.J., Okamura J. (1977). Early detection of chemotherapy related pancreatic enlargement in children using abdominal scintigraphy: a preliminary report. Cancer 38:1515–1523

Cystic Fibrosis

10. Spehl-Robberecht M., Baran D., Dab I., Perlmutter-Cremer N. (1981). Ultrasonic study of pancreas in cystic fibrosis. Ann. Radiol. 24:49–52
11. Willi U.V., Reddish J.M., Littlewood Teele R. (1980). Cystic fibrosis: its characteristic appearance on abdominal sonography. A.J.R. 134:1005–1010
12. Phillips H.E., Cox K.L., Reid M.H., Mc Gahan J.P. (1981). Pancreatic sonography in cystic fibrosis. A.J.R. 137:69–72

Pseudocysts

13. Garel L., Brunelle F., Lallemand D., Sauvegrain J. (1983). Pseudocysts of the pancreas in children: which cases require surgery? Pediat. Radiol. 13:120–124
14. Dahman B., Stephens C.A. (1981). Pseudocysts oof the pancreas after blunt abdominal trauma in children. J. of Pediat. Surgery 16:17–21
15. Slovis T.L., Vongerg V.J., Mikelic V. (1980). Sonography in the diagnosis and management of pancreatic pseudocysts and effusions in childhood. Radiology 135:153–155
16. Fried A.M., Selcke A.C. (1978). Pseudocyst formation in hereditary pancreatitis. J. Pediat. 135:950–953
17. Kuligowska E., Miller K., Birkett D., Burakoff R. (1981). Cystic dilatation of the pancreatic duct simulating pseudocysts on sonography. A.J.R. 136:409–410

Chapter 8

Urinary Tract Abnormalities

S. Neuenschwander and J.P. Montagne

1 Investigation of the Urinary Tract

Ultrasonography in this area consists of examination of the kidneys, the ureters, and the bladder. It is not necessary to sedate the child, a bottle given during the examination will calm the child sufficiently. A 5 Mhz transducer is used and occasionally a 3.5 Mhz transducer in the older child. The examination is started in a supine position to reasure the child.

The right kidney is first examined in a supine position via the hepatic window. Its upper pole is always visible on longitudinal and transverse sections, whereas its lower pole is often obscured by intestinal gas. The child is then placed in a prone position with, if necessary, a cushion under the abdomen to lessen the lumbar lordosis. One can then undertake transverse and sagittal sections of both kidneys. The ureteropelvic junction is studied on longitudinal sections with internal angulation of the transducer. Sections in right and left decubitus lateral positions are then carried out specifically in the search for an ureteral dilatation.

For the bladder, longitudinal and transverse sections are indispensable not only to measure the shape and size, but also to judge the appearance of the lower ureters and the ureterovesical junction. In the very young child who normally has a diminished bladder capacity, numerous spontaneous mictions take place during the examination. To obtain a sufficiently full bladder, furosemide 0.5–1 mg/kg per os may be administered. In this way sufficient filling of the bladder is achieved without diagnostic difficulties due to water-filled intestinal loops. However, the furosemide provokes a slight dilatation of the upper urinary tract which should not be considered pathological. After the examination, one must make sure that the child is sufficiently hydrated.

2 The Normal Kidney

The frontal or bivalve section of the kidney corresponds with an anatomical section of the kidney and is very similar to the image seen on IV urography. One identifies the typical "bean shape" with an internal hilus as well as the pelvis and the initial part of the ureter (Fig. 1). Transverse sections have a variable appearance depending on the level and corresponding with either the polar or the hilar region (Figs. 2 and 3). In the newborn, the renal outline has an irregularly rounded appearance corresponding with fetal lobulations (Fig. 4).

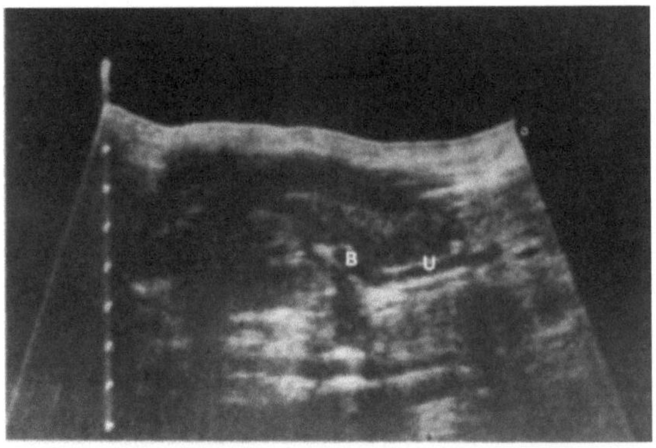

Fig. 1. Normal kidney, "bivalve" section: the pelvis *(B)* is very narrow, extended medially and below by the ureter *(U)*.

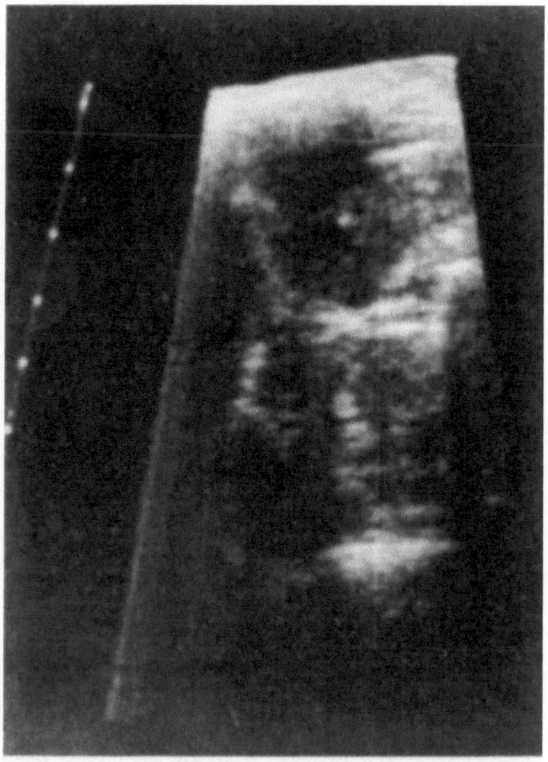

a

Ultrasonography gives an immediate and real measurement of the kidneys, although it is difficult to carry out precise measurements. In fact, the length remains difficult to determine as the section must pass through the longest axis.

The renal structure can be divided into a parenchymal region with little echogenicity and a central zone with increased echogenicity which is made up of the pelvis, the blood vessels, and fat. (Fig. 55):

1. At the level of the echogenic region called the central zone or central pyelovascular region, the pelvis is identified as an oval liquid pouch with a vertical long axis that varies in size depending on the degree of the patient's diuresis. In the very young child, the pelvis is often extrahilar and globular. One may mistake this for early hydronephrosis (Fig. 27). An excess of sinusoidal fat may render this central region very echogenic (Fig. 6).

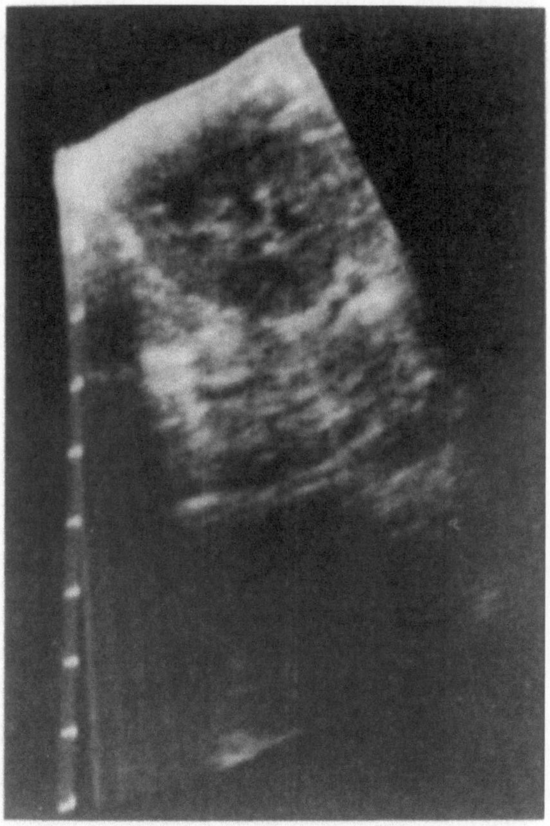

c

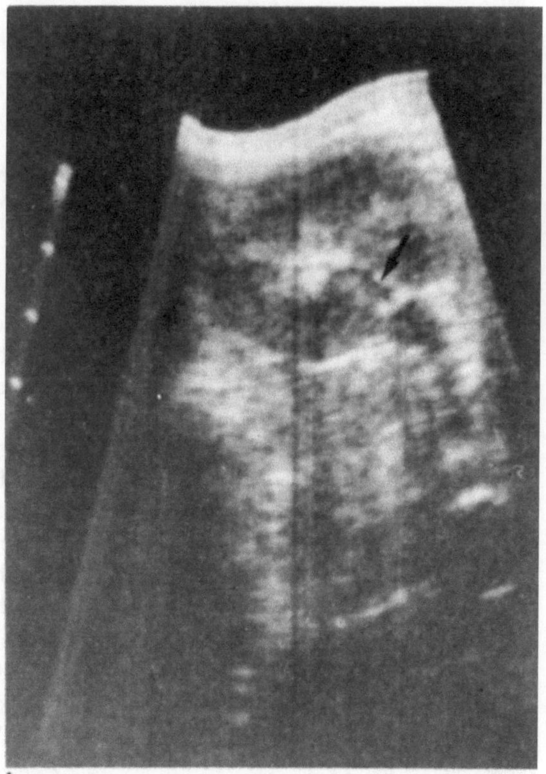

b

Fig. 2a–c. Transverse section of a left normal kidney in a prone position.
a Upper pole, partly obscured at its outer edge by the shadow of a rib.
b Middle portion with the pelvis (*arrow*).
c Inferior pole.

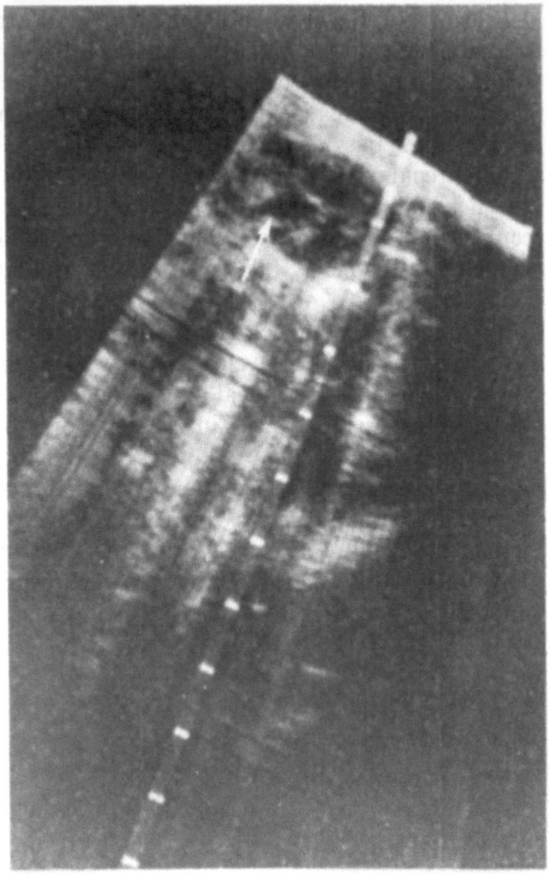

Fig. 3. Normal kidney in a 21 days old boy. Transverse section of the right kidney in prone position at the level of the pelvis (*arrow*).

2. The renal parenchyma is normally less echogenic than the hepatic parenchyma (Fig. 7). In the child, it is always possible to differentiate between the renal cortex and the medulla. The medulla is composed of the pyramids of Malpighi, which are echo-free. They are triangular, the base of the triangle being cortical and the apex in contact with the region of central echo. The renal cortex, weakly echogenic but more echogenic than the pyramids, extends between the pyramids via the septa of Bertin (Fig. 8). Bertin septal hypertrophy or pseudotumor can manifest itself as a region of weak echogenicity, globular, and in continuity with the outer cortex with sometimes a concave imprint on the pyelovascular zone (Fig. 9).

The pyramids are seen particularly clearly in the premature or term infant. As the cortex in these children is more echogenic than in older children, the echo-free pyramids should not be confused with a dilatation of the excretory system or with cysts (Figs. 7 and 8).

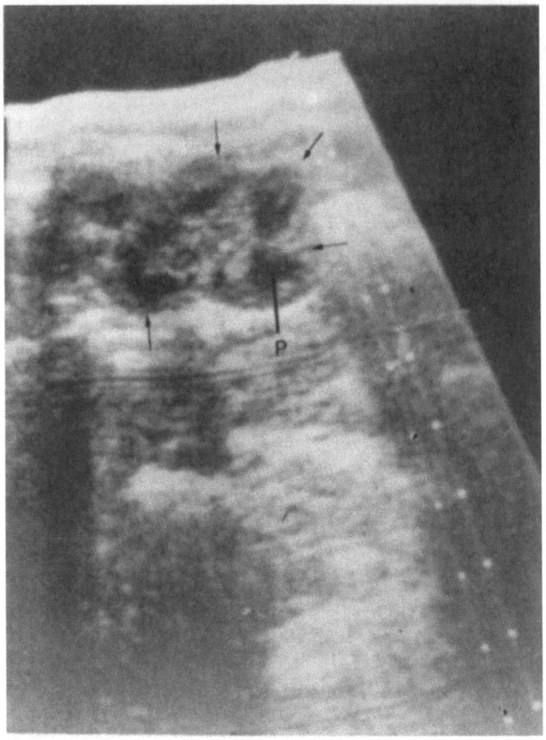

Fig. 4. Normal kidney of a 3-month-old infant. Longitudinal section of the left kidney in prone position. The regularly rounded aspect of the renal outline corresponds with fetal lobulations (*arrows*). The pyramids *(P)* are clearly visible due to the relative hyperechogenicity of the cortex seen at this age.

One should also explore the vascular elements (Fig. 10):

1. The aorta, inferior vena cava, and portal vein are easily identified.
2. The right renal artery has a retrocaval course. Use of real-time ultrasonography facilitates the differential diagnosis of the right crus of the diaphragm (Fig. 10a).
3. The left renal artery (Fig. 10b).
4. The right renal vein has a short course (Fig. 10c).
5. The left renal vein passes in front of the aorta and behind the superior mesenteric artery (Fig. 10d).

Fig. 5 a and b. Longitudinal sections of a right normal kidney in prone position. ▶
a Medial section at the level of the central pyelovascular zone (*arrow*).
b A more external section at the level of the parenchyma. The pyramids *(P)*, cortex *(c)*, and septa of Bertin *(b)*.

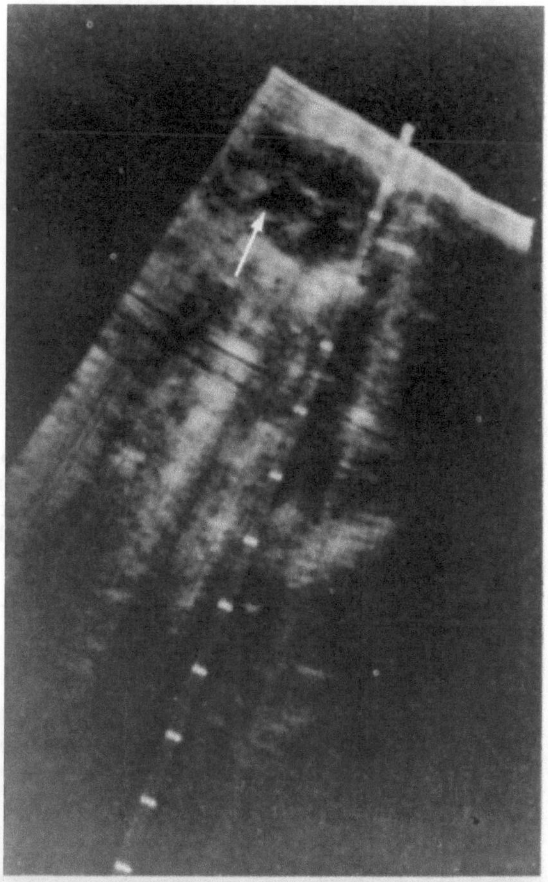

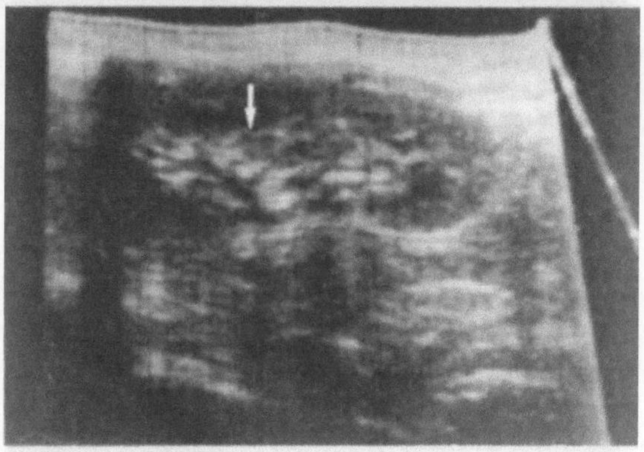

a

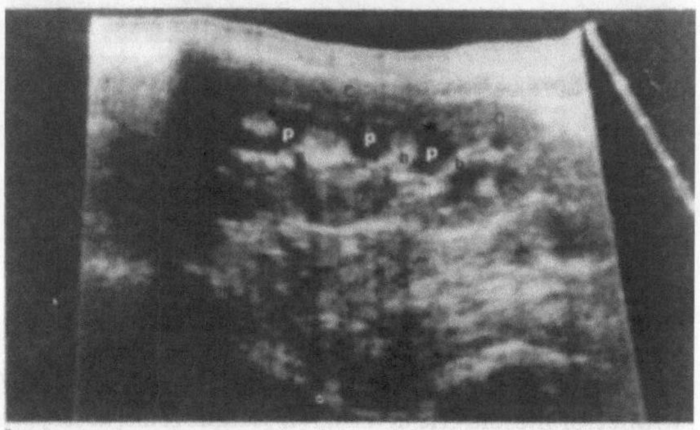

b

Fig. 5 a and b

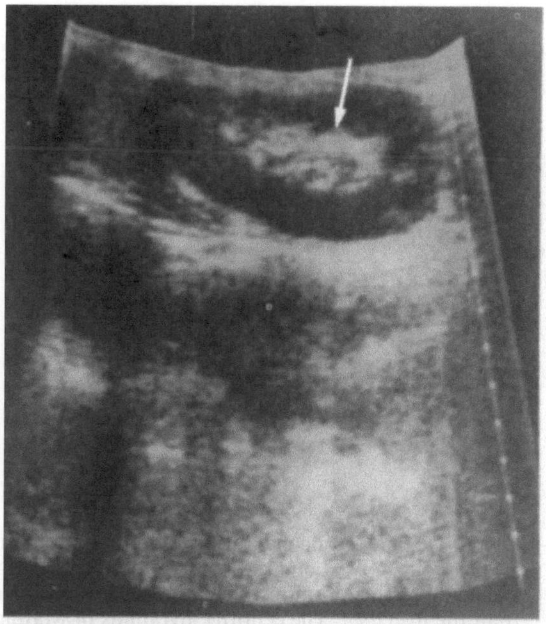

a

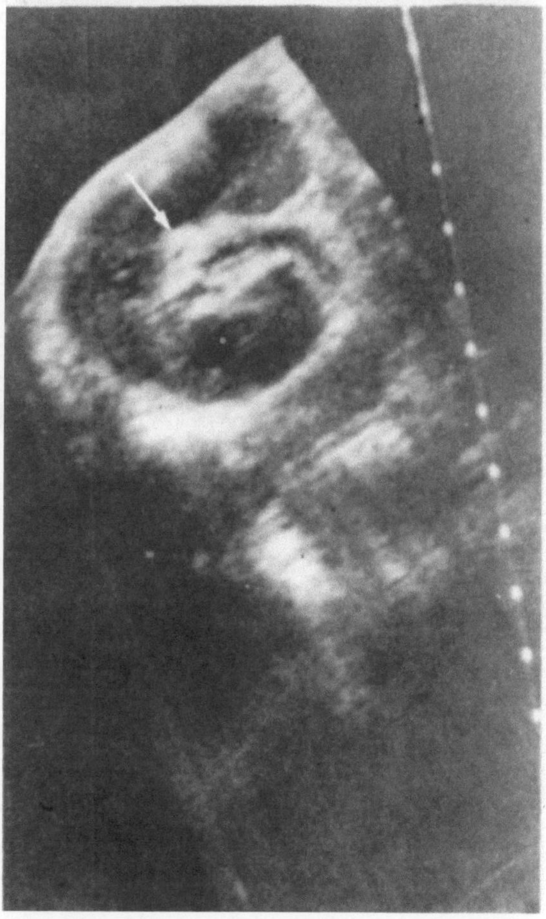

b

Fig. 6 a and b. Excess sinusoidal fat in a 7-year-old girl. **a** Longitudinal section; **b** Transverse section of the left kidney in prone position. The central echo is bulging and corresponds with an excess amount of fat at the level of the sinus (*arrows*).

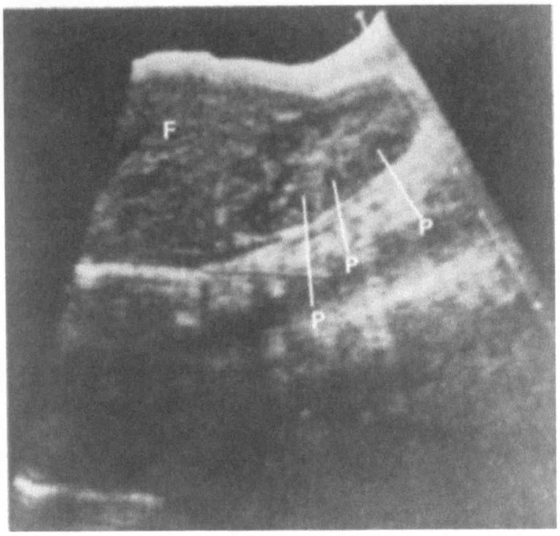

Fig. 7. Normal corticomedullary differentiation in a 5 days old boy. Longitudinal section of the right kidney in supine position. The kidney is less echogenic than the liver *(F)*. The echofree pyramids of Malpighi *(P)* are triangular, the base being cortical and the apex in contact with the central echo.

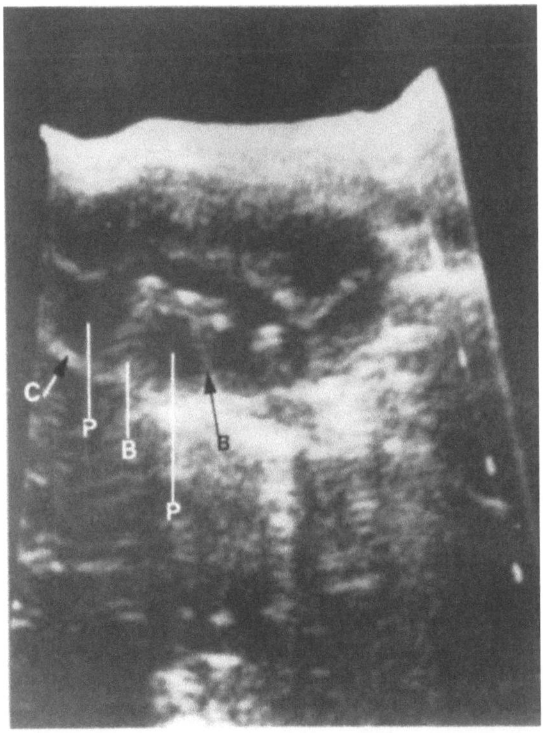

Fig. 8. Normal corticomedullary differentiation in a 6 days old girl. Longitudinal section of the right kidney in prone position. The echogenic cortex *(C)* and the septa of Bertin *(B)* outline the nonechogenic pyramids *(P)*.

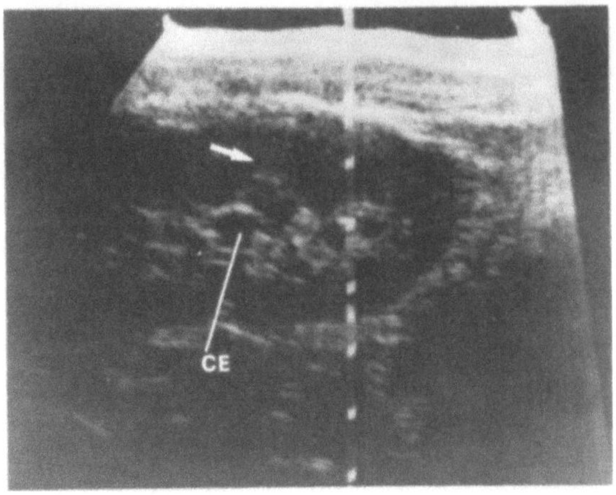

Fig. 9. Septum of Bertin hypertrophy in a 7 years old girl. Longitudinal section of the left kidney in prone position showing the hypertrophied column of Bertin (*arrow*), its internal portion bulging, in contact with the excretory cavity *(CE)*.

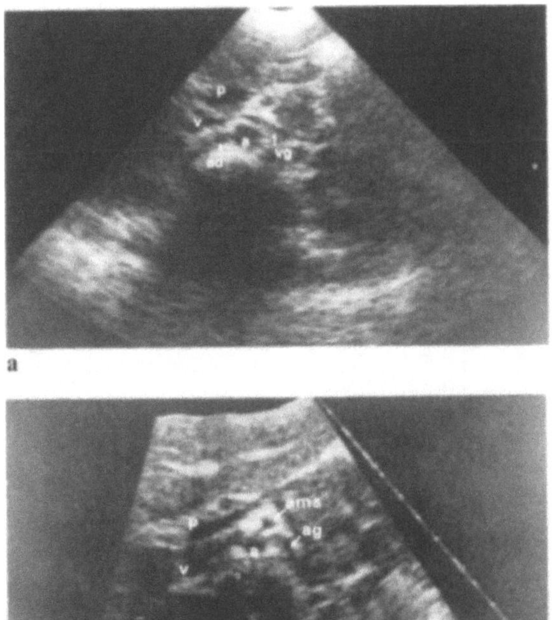

a

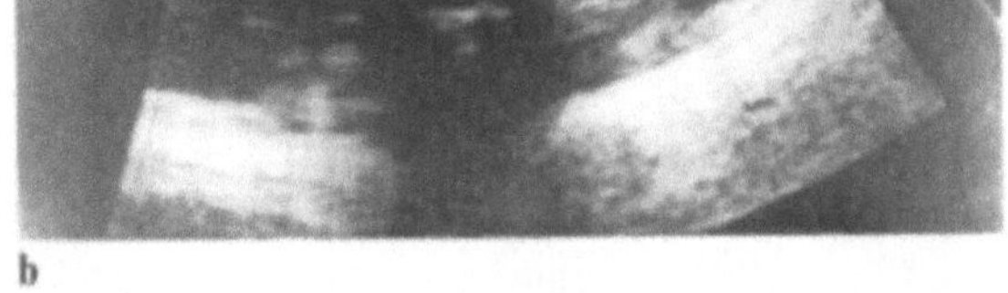

b

Fig. 10 a–d. The blood vessels (transverse sections in supine position).
A, Aorta; *V*, Inferior vena cava; *P*, Portal vein; *AMS*, Superior mesenteric artery; *AD*, Right renal artery; *AG*, Left renal artery; *VD*, Right renal vein; *Vg*, Left renal vein; *RD*, Right kidney; *RG*, Left kidney.

3 Aplasia, Ectopia, and Fused Kidneys

3.1 Aplasia and Ectopia

Congenital absence of a kidney is difficult to confirm because intestinal loops present in the lumbar fossa may be confused with a small irregularly shaped kidney. On the other hand, a small atrophic kidney flattened against the vertebral column can be missed on US examination.

If the lumbar fossa is empty, one must look for an ectopic kidney by systematic examination of the entire abdomen and pelvis (Figs. 11 and 12). The kidney may sometimes be located within the thoracic cage (Fig. 13).

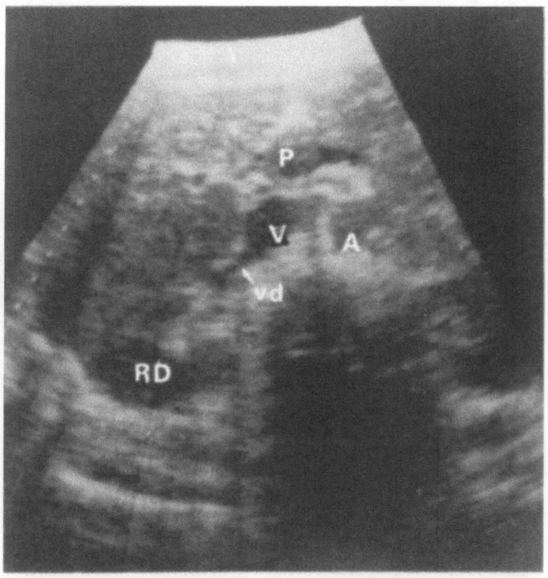

c

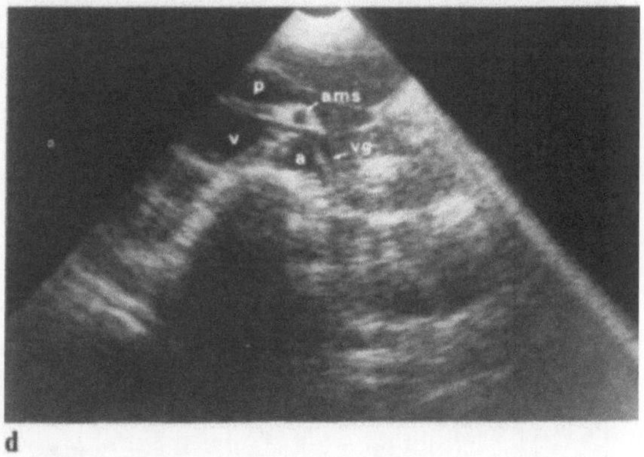

d

Fig. 10 c and d

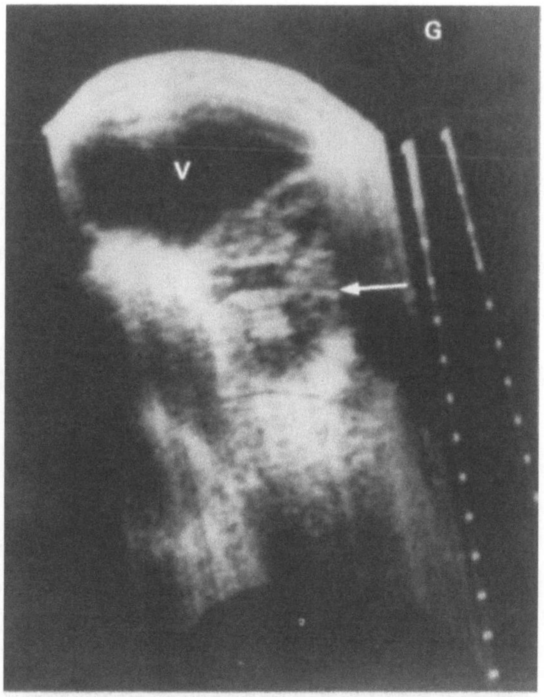

a

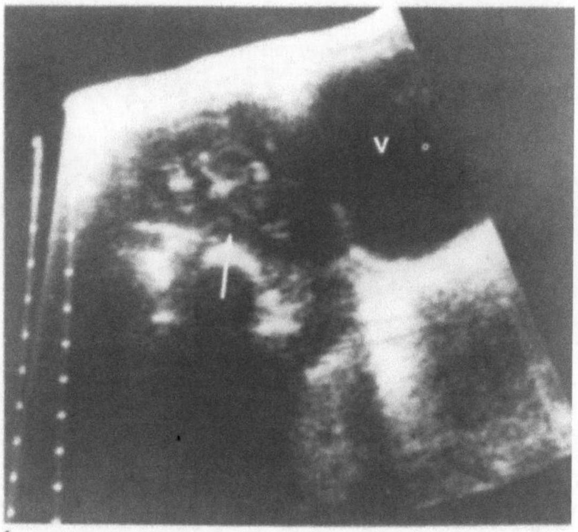

b

Fig. 11 a and b. Pelvic ectopic kidney in a 9 years old girl with a pelvic mass.
a Transverse section of the lower abdomen showing supravesical mass, lateralized to the left (*arrow*) with the form and structure of a kidney. *V*, Bladder.
b Longitudinal section.

3.2 Fused Kidneys

Fused kidneys may be revealed by an abdominal mass on palpation. Identification of a renal parenchyma, which exhibits a corticomedullary differentiation and excretory tracts on US, allows

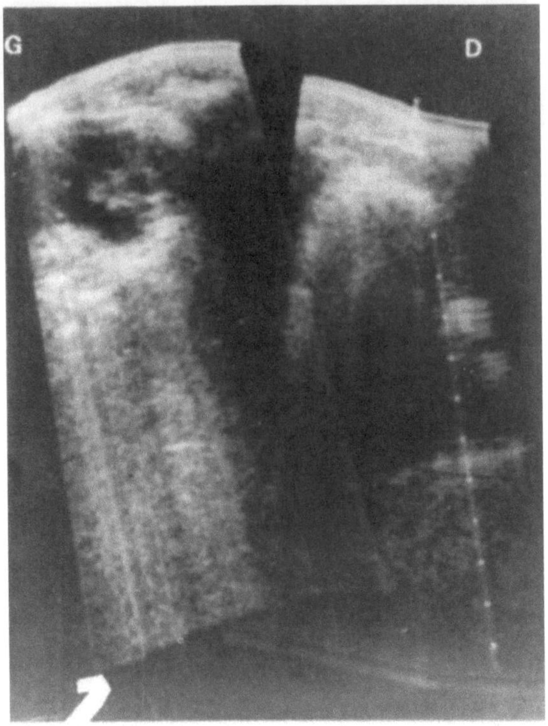

a

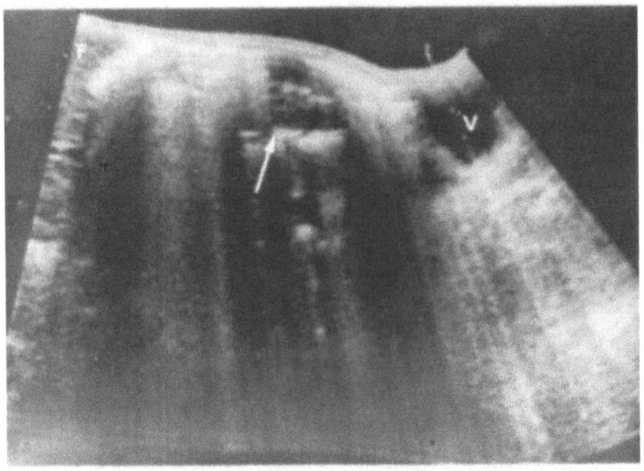

b

Fig. 12a and b. Right ectopic kidney in a 13 months old boy with an abdominal mass.
a Transverse section of the lumbar fossa in prone position. There is no kidney in the right lumbar fossa.
b Longitudinal section in supine position: at distance from the liver *(F)* and bladder *(V)* in the midst of digestive artefacts, a renal structure can be seen (*arrow*).

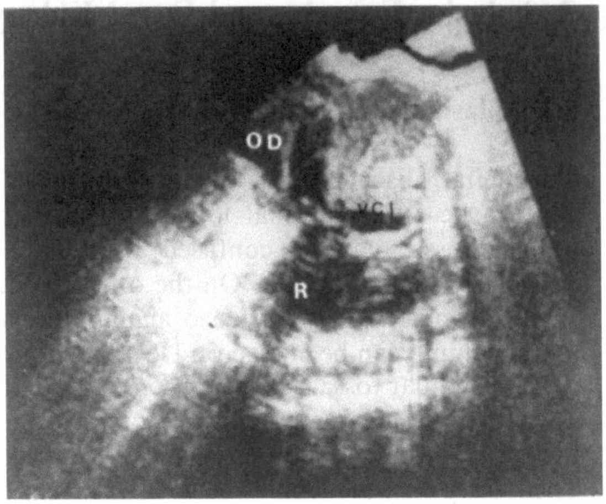

Fig. 13. Right kidney, retrocaval thoracic ectopia in a 4 months old boy.
Longitudinal section at the level of insertion or the inferior vena cava *(VCI)* into the right atrium *(OD)*. A renal structure *(R)* is situated behind the inferior vena cava and its upper pole is partially masked by the air in the right lung.

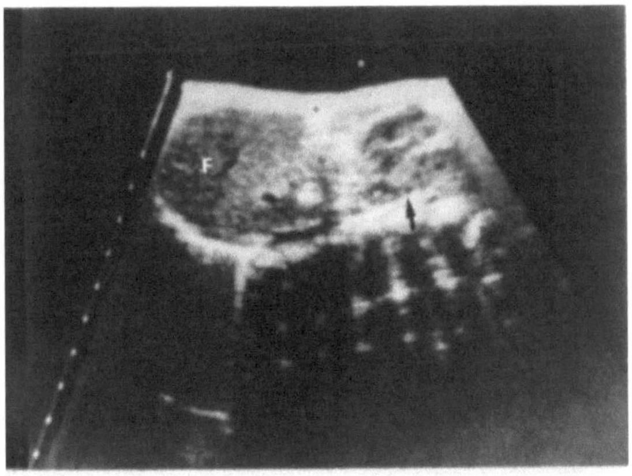

a

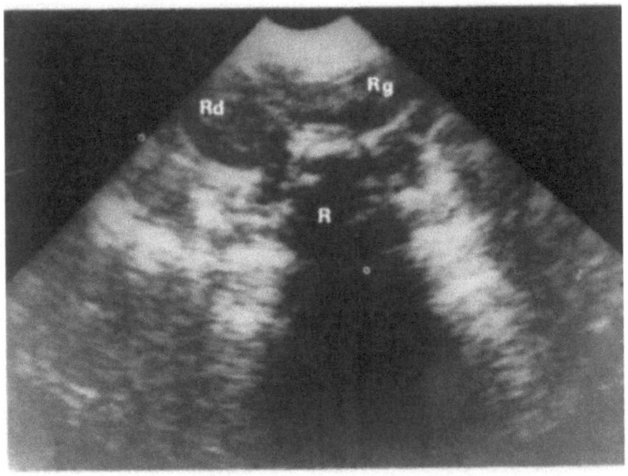

b

Fig. 14a and b. Fused ectopic kidneys in a 6 weeks old ▶ boy with a right iliac mass.
a Longitudinal laterovertebral section in supine position: the lumbar fossa is empty. A kidney is present in a low lombar position (*arrow*).
b Subumbilical longitudinal section: the left kidney *(Rg)* is situated transversally across the vertebral column and in continuity with the lower pole of the right kidney *(Rd)*. *F*, liver; *R*, spine.

the normal renal nature of the mass to be affirmed and also enables one to exclude a neoplastic formation (Fig. 14).

4 Malformative Uropathies

The circumstances of discovery are variable. The uropathy may be diagnosed during an antenatal US examination. In the neonatal period, one encounters numerous different presentations: frank mass, urinary tract infection, renal failure, unexplained pneumothorax, multiple malfarmation syndromes. In the older child one may be confronted with a lumbar mass or lumbar pain, a urinary tract infection, an isolated hematuria or a hematuria presenting after trauma.

4.1 Multicystic Dysplasia

Anatomically, the kidney is replaced by numerous cysts of varying size and number surrounding a fibrous nucleus and associated with an atresia of the excretory tract to a greater or lesser extent. Bilateral lesions are exceptional and lethal. However, in 30% of cases a malformative uropathy is found in the opposite kidney. On IV urography, the multicystic kidney is nonfunctioning. If a large amount of contrast medium is injected, the cysts appear as radiolucent zones surrounded by opaque walls ("RIM" sign).

4.1.1 Pseudotumoral Form

In our experience, this is the most common cause of a unilateral nonfunctioning kidney in the first 15 days of life and can be discovered in the neonatal period. Ultrasonography permits an easy diagnosis in typical cases which are also the most frequent. Instead of a kidney one finds a more or less voluminous mass made up of numerous liquid cavities, variable in shape and distributed haphazardly (Fig. 15). These cavities are round or oval, sometimes with an irregular outline (Fig. 16). This last characteristic may, in certain cases, be consistent with the presence of dysplastic renal tissue. There is also a small echogenic area which corresponds with the fibrous nucleus. It is important to note that, on US examination, no communication is visible between the cysts.

Sometimes there is an increased amount of echogenic tissue which may give the impression of a mass with mixed echogenicity. However, adjacent sections permit confirmation of the multicystic nature of the mass (Fig. 17). In other cases there are only a few cystic cavities (Fig. 18) or the cystic cavity may be single, in which case it is not possible on US to differentiate it from single cavity hydronephrosis.

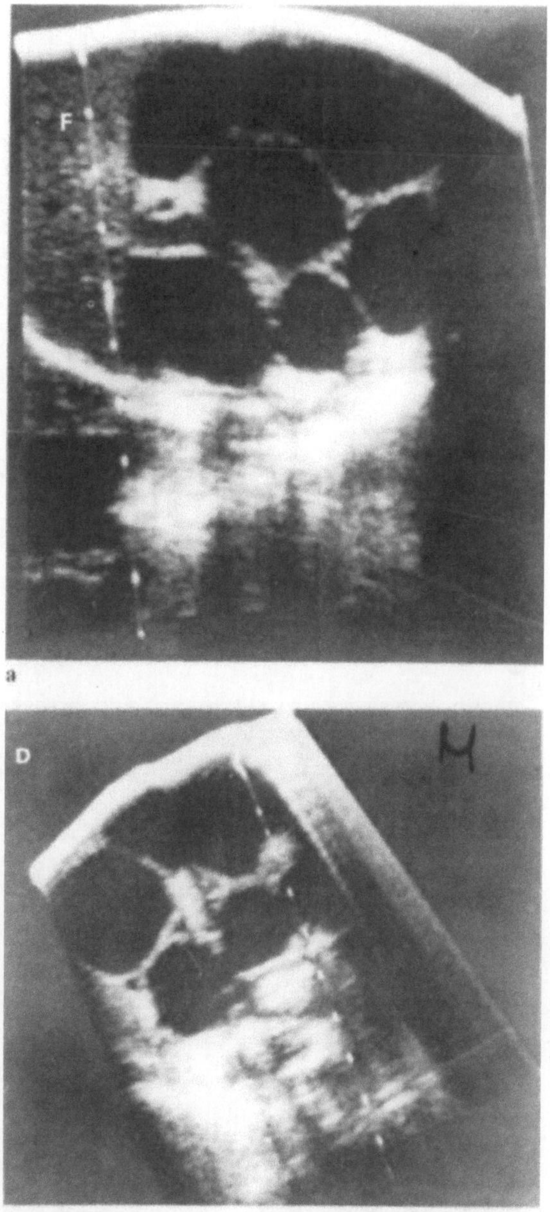

Fig. 15a and b. Typical pseudotumoral form of multicystic dysplasia in a 1 day old boy with a right flank mass.
a Longitudinal section in supine position. *F*, liver.
b Transverse section of the right flank in supine position. In place of the right kidney. There are multiple liquid cavities inequal in size, in a haphazard distribution without intercommunications.

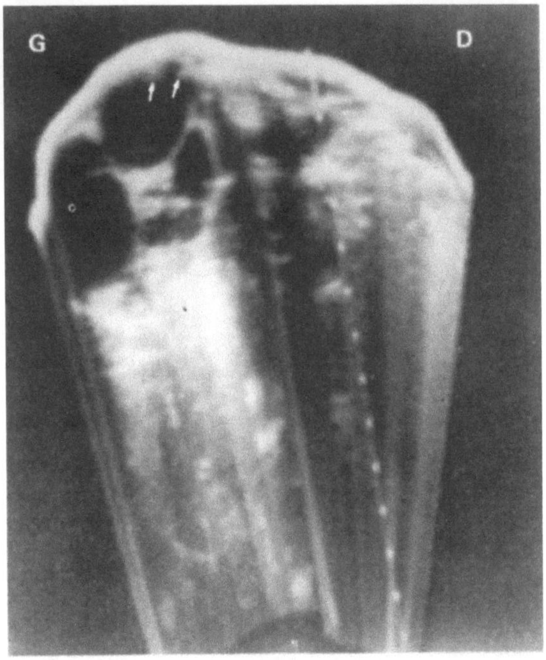

a

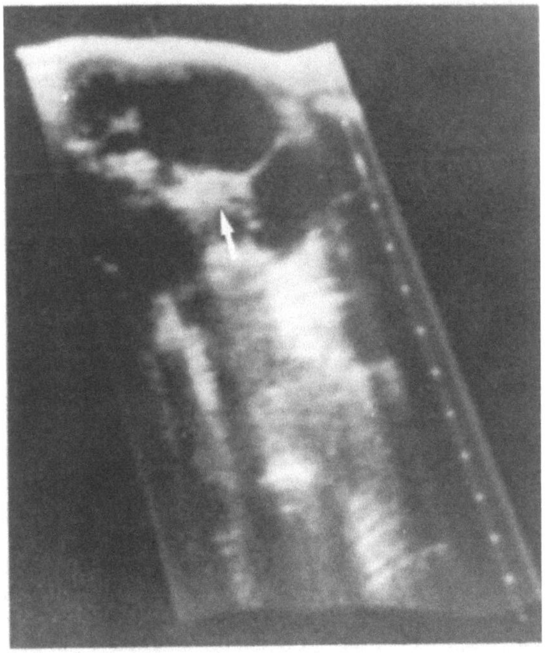

b

Fig. 16a and b. Typical form of multicystic dysplasia in a 3 days old girl with a left flank mass.
a Transverse section in prone position: the outline of the most posterior cavity is slightly irregular (*arrows*).
b Longitudinal section of the left kidney in prone position: an area of increased echogenicity between the cystic cavities corresponds with the fibrous portion (*arrow*).

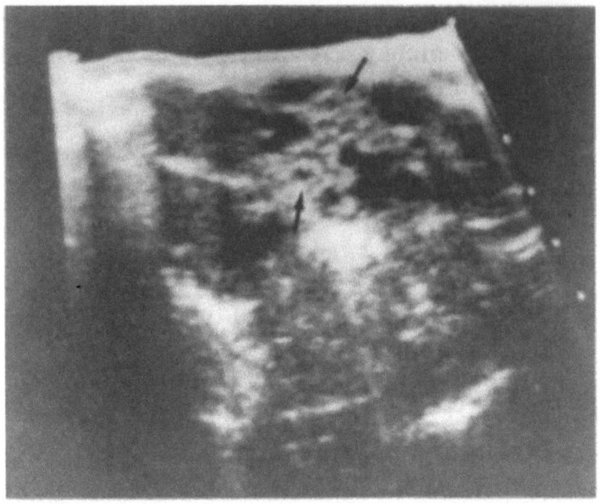

a

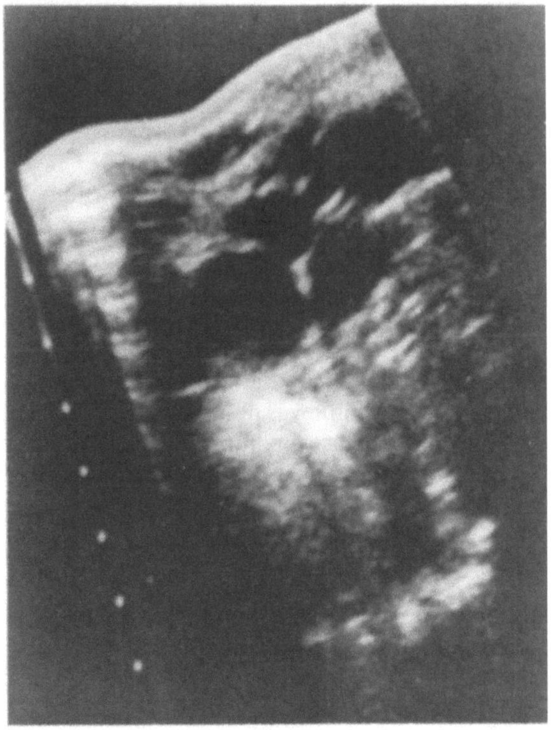

b

Fig. 17a and b. Multicystic dysplasia in a 6 days old boy with a left flank mass. Longitudinal sections of the left kidney in prone position.
a There exists an echogenic central component, heterogeneous, hollowed out by numerous cavities, millimetric in size (*arrow*).
b A slighty more external section shows larger cavities, arranged in a disorderly fashion with no visible communications between them.

The differential diagnosis between multicystic dysplasia and hydronephrosis will be considered after discussion of hydronephrosis. Let us remember that it is essential to examine carefully the opposite kidney. In fact, the prognosis depends on this. Controlateral abnormalities consist mainly of hydronephrosis or megaureter.

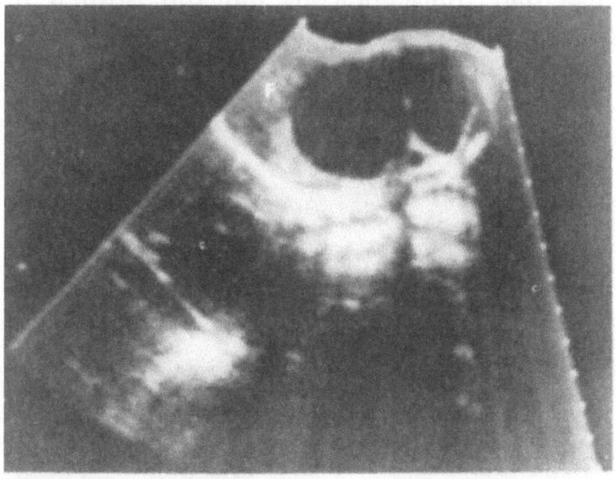

a

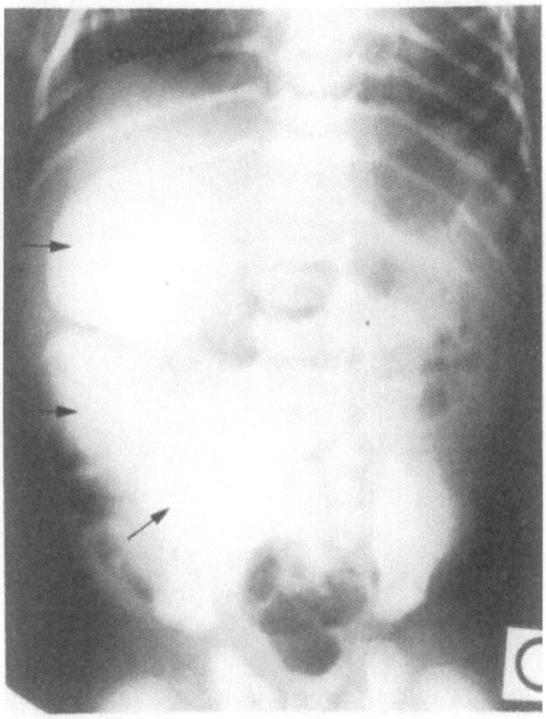

b

Fig. 18a and b. Pseudotumoral multicystic dysplasia. **a** Longitudinal section of the right flank in supine position. The kidney is replaced by two voluminous cavities extending from the right hypochondrium to the right iliac fossa. *F*, liver.
b Puncture and opacification: one can distinguish three juxtaposed cavities (*arrows*) communicating by punctiform orifices not visible on urogram. The pelvis is not opacified.

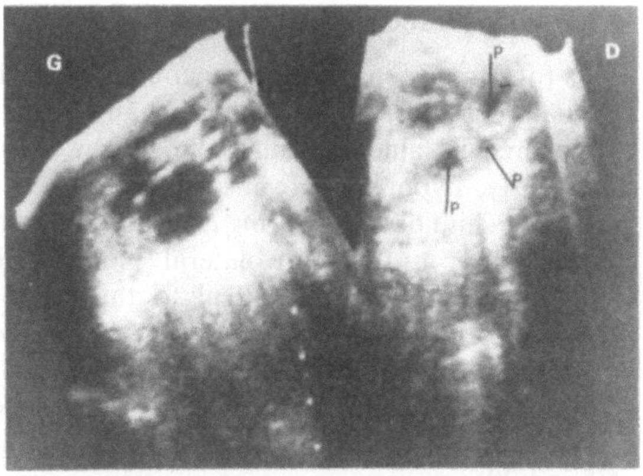

Fig. 19. Hypoplastic form of multicystic dysplasia in a 4 months old boy. Diagnosis suspected on antenatal ultrasonography. Transverse section of the two lumbar fossae in prone position. On the left there are multiple liquid cavities of unequal size and in a haphazard distribution. The size of the left kidney is approximately equal to that of the right kidney. The right kidney is normal: note the clearly visible corticomedullary differentiation and the nonechogenic triangular pyramids *(P)*.

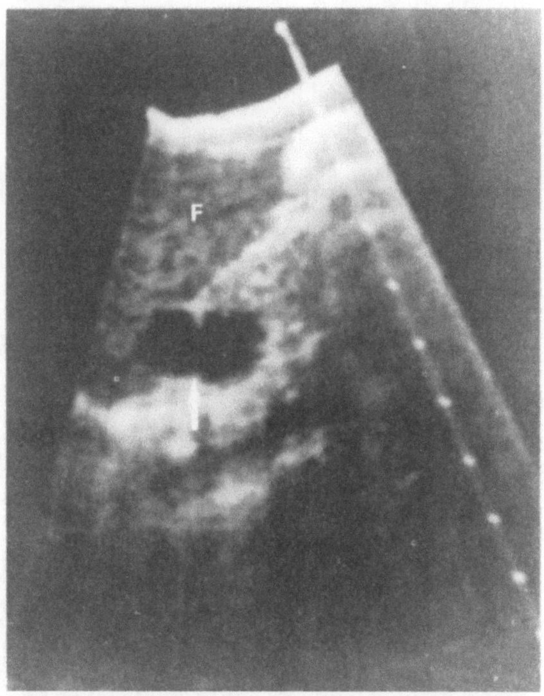

Fig. 20. Hypoplastic form of multicystic dysplasia in a 14 days old girl. A liquid renal image was seen on antenatal ultrasonography. Longitudinal section of the right flank in supine position. The right kidney is composed of two cystic cavities, each 1 cm in diameter (*arrows*). *F*, Liver

4.1.2 Hypoplastic Forms

This form may sometimes be encountered in the neonatal period and is usually an abnormality discovered by antenatal ultrasonography. More frequently, hypoplastic forms are discovered in the older child or adult during investigation of an abnormality in the controlateral kidney. The appearance on US is identical to the pseudotumoral forms: an image of cysts varying in size, distributed haphazardly with no intercommunication. However, the mass is usually small, often equal to or smaller than the opposite kidney (Figs. 19 and 20).

The most difficult diagnostic forms are:
1. Multicystic dysplasia with duplication of the excretory tract: only half of the kidney is affected.
2. Multicystic dysplasia in an ectopic position, the cystic mass not being situated in the lumbar fossa, but in an iliac or pelvic position. In this case it may be mistaken for a tortuous megaureter. We feel that transcutaneous puncture with a fine needle and opacification is a simple means of confirming the diagnosis (Fig. 21).

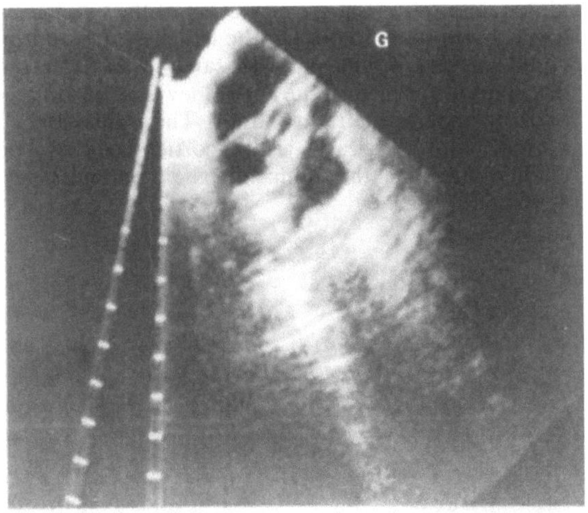

a

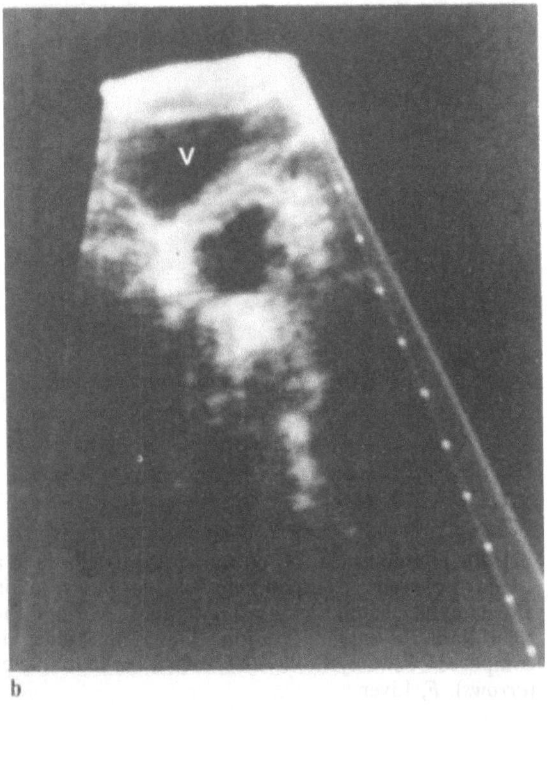

b

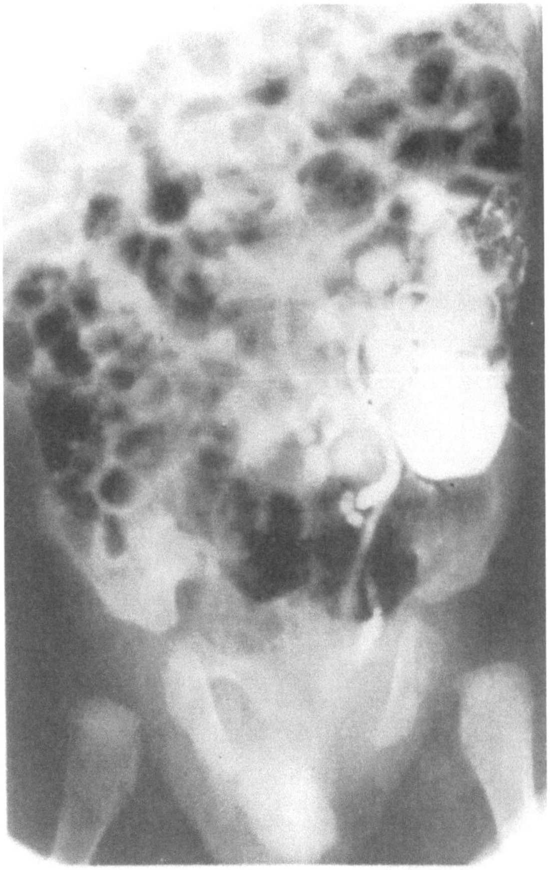

c

Fig. 21 a–c. Left ectopic multicystic dysplasia in a 2 months old boy with left iliac fossa mass.
a Transverse section in prone position just above the left iliac artery. Multiple cavities of variable size with no communications.
b Transverse section of the bladder in supine position. A liquid cavity with nodular outline is visible behind and to the left of the bladder *(V)*.
c Puncture and opacification: cavities of varying size distributed in a haphazard fashion and communicating via narrow chanels. There is no opacification of the bladder.

4.2 Hydronephrosis

The diagnosis depends on visualization of a dilated pyelocalyceal system with absence of ureteral dilatation.

4.2.1 Moderate Hydronephrosis

The pelvis appears as a liquid cavity, elliptical, situated either inferior to the kidney, replacing the normal central echo, or in an extrarenal position. The calyceal dilatation is visible and forms smaller intraparenchymal liquid sacs grouped around the pelvis and in communication with it. The outline of the pyramids of Malpighi disappears (Fig. 22).

4.2.2 More Significant Hydronephrosis

Round liquid masses with a well defined architecture can be seen: the largest cavity corresponds with the pelvis and is anteromedial. The other cavities are grouped peripherally and are in communication with it. The thickness of the renal parenchyma is diminished and the corticomedullary differentiation is no longer visible (Fig. 23). On longitudinal sections, the dilated calyceal cavities may give the kidney a multilocular aspect but on sagittal sections communications are visible between peripheral cavities and the anteromedial cavity which corresponds with the pelvis (Fig. 24).

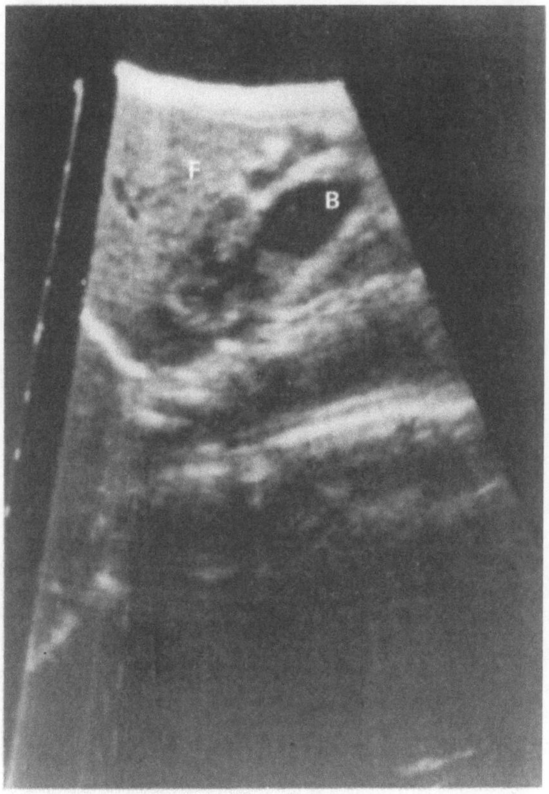

a

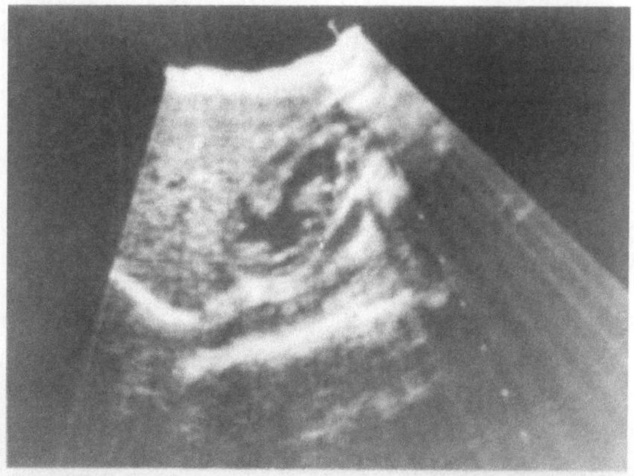

b

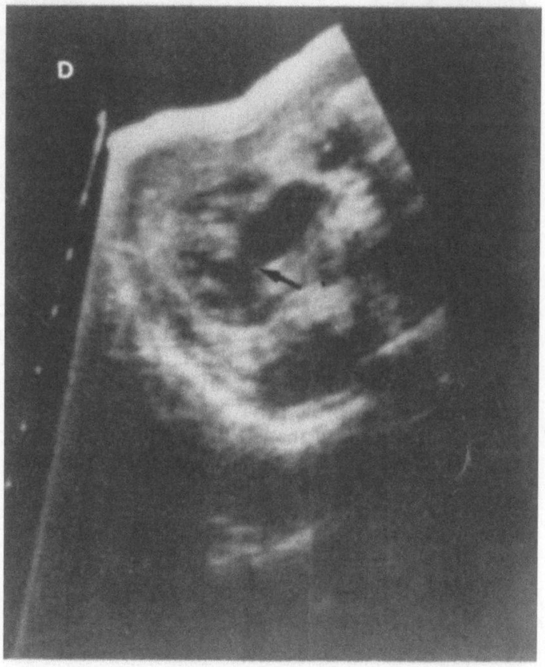

c

Fig. 22 a–c. Moderate hydronephrosis in a 3 days old boy. Right renal liquid image on US examination towards the end of pregnancy.
a Longitudinal section of the right flank in supine position. The dilated pelvis *(B)* appears as an elliptical central renal liquid image. *F*, Liver.
b A more external parallel section shows the dilated calices.
c Transverse section of the right kidney in supine position: the communication between the dilated calices and pelvis is clearly visible (*arrow*).

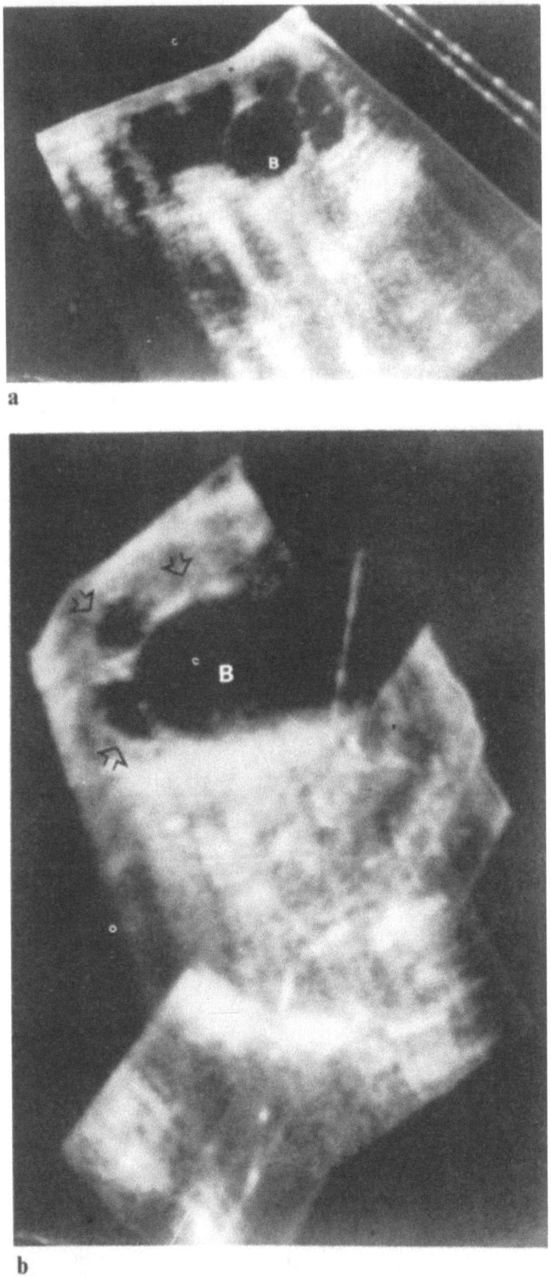

Fig. 23a and b. Frank hydronephrosis in a 10 days old boy with left flank mass. **a** Sagittal section of the left kidney in prone position; the largest cavity is the anterior pelvis *(B)*, other cavities are smaller and communicate with the pelvis.
b Sagittal section of the left kidney in prone position; the dilated pelvis *(B)* is anteromedial. The thickness of the renal parenchyma is diminished (*arrows*).

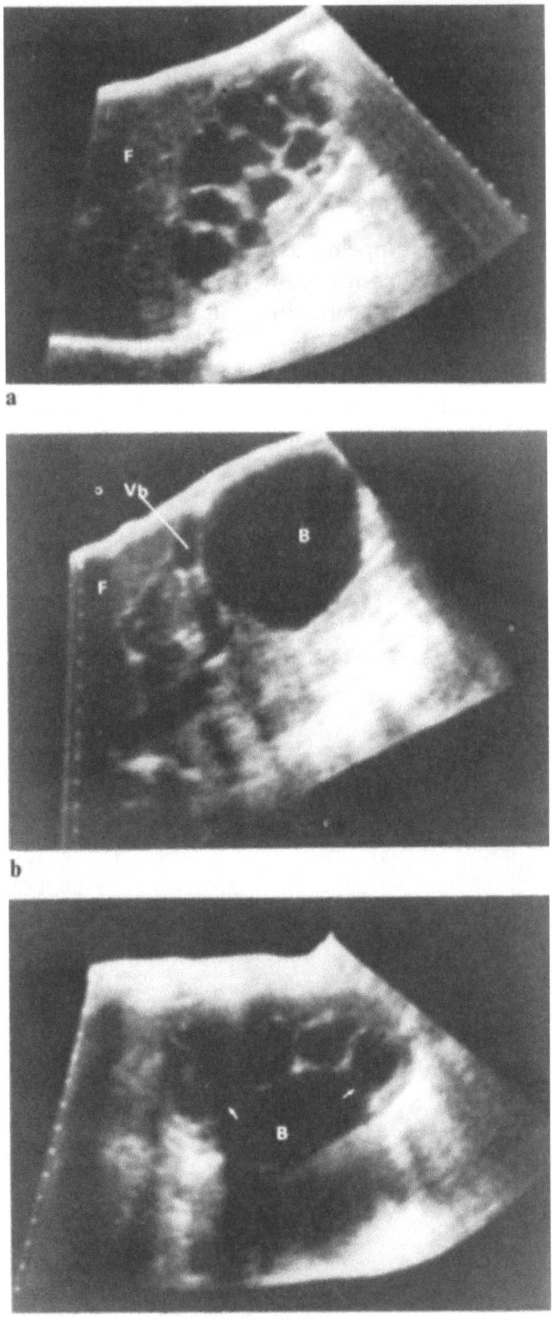

Fig. 24a–c. Frank hydronephrosis in a 13 years old boy. Severe right flank pain and tenderness.
a Longitudinal section of the right flank in supine position showing numerous thin walled cystic images. *F*, Liver.
b A more internal parallel section: a voluminous liquid cavity situated inside the above images. *B*, Pelvis; *Vb*, Gallbladder.
c Sagittal section of the kidney in prone position. The continuity between the dilated calices and pelvis *(B)* is demonstrated (*arrows*). The ureter is not visible.

4.2.3 Severe Hydronephrosis

The extremely dilated pelvis passes the midline and one can no longer identify the renal parenchyma (Fig. 25). In very severe forms there is only a single, very voluminous, liquid cavity. The absence of ureteral dilatation is checked at the level of the ureteropelvic junction by sagittal sections of the kidney and also at the level of the ureterovesical junction with sections through a well-filled bladder.

In all cases it is important to study the opposite kidney carefully in search of a bilateral anomaly. The possibility of a controlateral dysplastic kidney (Fig. 26) has been mentioned above.

4.2.4 The Differential Diagnosis

In moderate forms, diagnostic problems may arise particularly in the neonatal period. In fact, at this age, the renal pelvis is often globular and forms an elliptical anteromedial liquid image, more so during the first days of life during which time the child has an increased diuresis.

In addition, the corticomedullary differentiation, which is particularly visible at this age, should not lead to confusion between the pyramids of Malpighi which are echo-free, triangular with their apices oriented towards the hilus and the moderately dilated calyces (Fig. 27). The megacalyx is a rare diagnosis and is manifested by

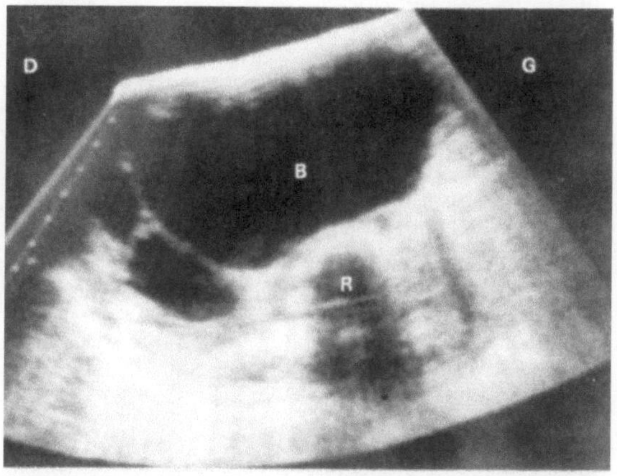

a

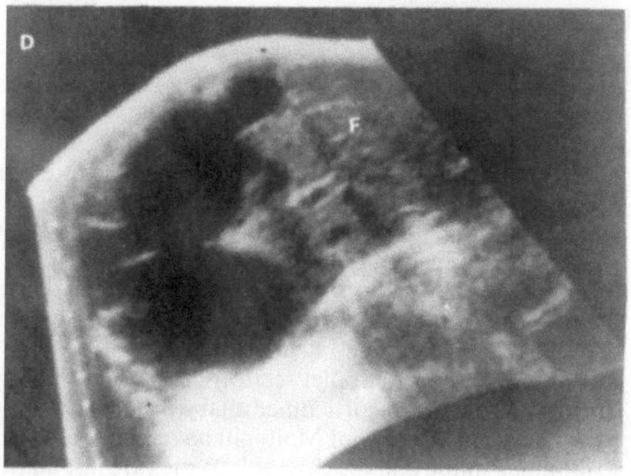

b

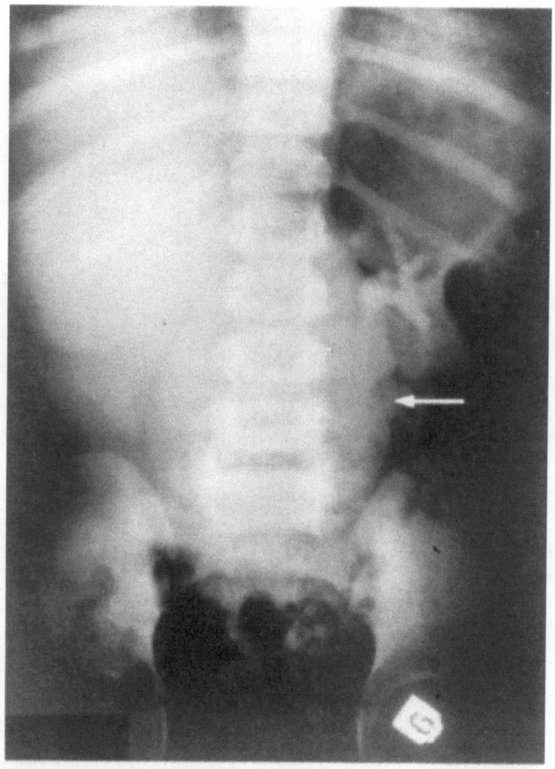

c

Fig. 25a–c. Severe hydronephrosis in a 4 years old boy with a voluminous abdominal mass.
a Subumbilical transverse section in supine position: numerous liquid cavities, of which the most voluminous *(B)* is anterior and extends beyond the midline *R*, Vertebral column.
b Communication between the cavities is demonstrated on a subcostal section.
c Film 8 h after IVP shows weak opacification of the pyelocalyceal cavities. The inner border of the very dilated pelvis extends beyond the midline (*arrow*).

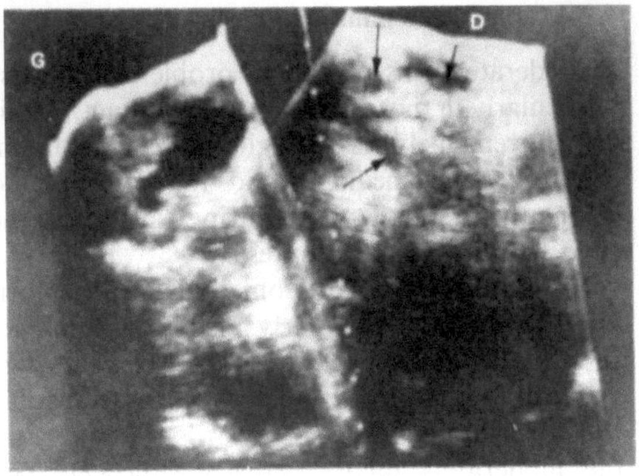

a

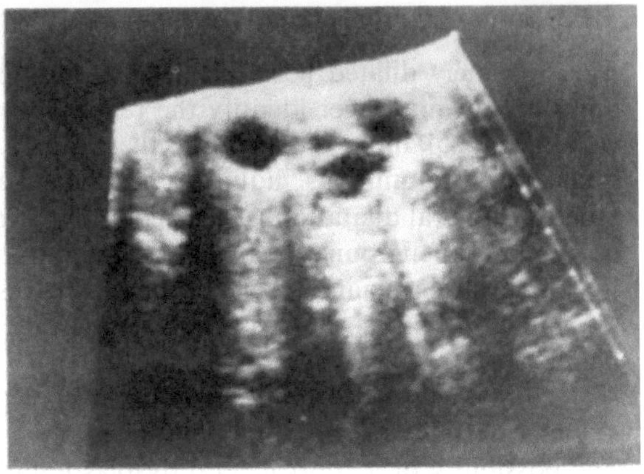

b

Fig. 26 a and b. Hydronephrosis and controlateral dysplasia in a boy aged 7 months with congenital heart disease. Systematic search for other associated abnormalities. **a** Transverse section of both lumbar fossae in prone position showing, left hydronephrosis. On the right, a few very small liquid cavities (*arrows*). **b** Longitudinal section on the right lumbar fossa in prone position: liquid cavities unequal in size, with no intercommunications. The renal size is less than 4 cm: hypoplastic form of multicystic dysplasia.

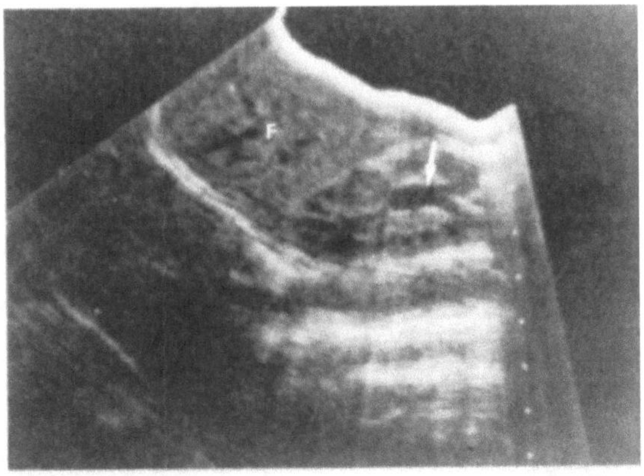

a

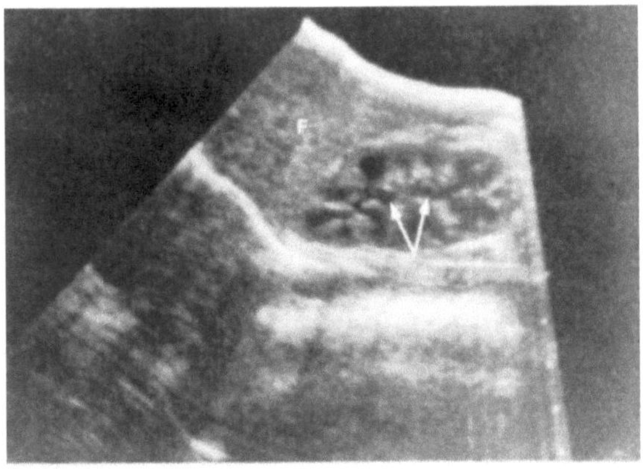

c

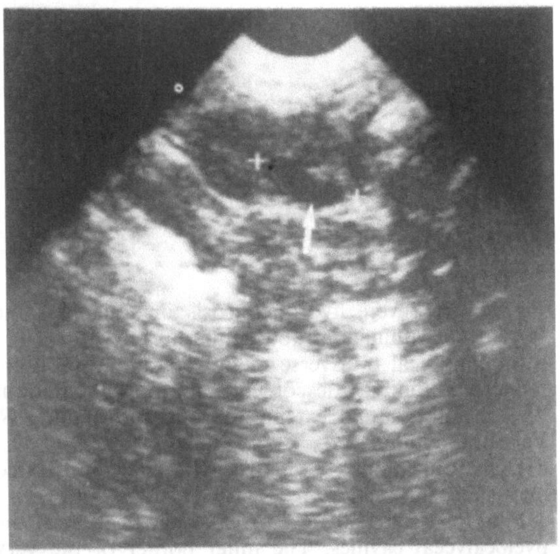

b

Fig. 27 a–c. Normal kidneys with differential diagnosis of a moderate hydronephrosis in a 15 days old boy after suspicion of dilated pelvices on antenatal ultrasonography.
a Longitudinal section of the right kidney in supine position. *F*, Liver.
b Longitudinal section of the left kidney in prone position. The pelvis appears as an oval liquid-filled cavity (*arrow*).
c A more external parallel section of the right kidney: normal kidney, the corticomedullary differentiation is distinct. The pyramids of Malpighi have a characteristic triangular shape and the calyceal cavities are not dilated (*arrow*)

a uniform dilatation of the calyces which contrats with a nondistended pelvis.

In the more significant or severe forms the diagnosis may be confused with a pseudotumoral form of multicystic dysplasia (Table 1). If the diagnosis remains unclear an IV pyelogram is of no help as the kidney is usually nonsecreting. The situation may be clarified by a transcutaneous puncture using a fine needle and opacification of the cavities.

In fact, there is no contraindication to this type of procedure because there is no risk of puncturing a malignant tumor as the US examination has confirmed the liquid nature of the lesion. If one is dealing with a multicystic dysplasia, three different images are possible: The punctured cyst is the only one opacified, there are punctiform communications between numerous cysts, or the cysts are in communication via fine channels. In all cases it is impossible to visualize a pelvis or ureter (Figs. 8 and 28). If one is dealing with a hydronephrosis, the peripheral cavities are in obvious communication with a dilated pelvis situated in an anteromedial position.

After surgical cure of the ureteropelvic junction anomaly, US examination allows a followup of renal size and measurement of the parenchymal thickness. The pyelocalycel cavities never resume a normal shape – the dilatation is unchanged or diminished. However, one can easily identify the underlying ureter (Fig. 29).

Complications may arise during the evolution

Table 1. Differential diagnosis on ultrasonography of multicyst dysplasia with hydronephrosis.

Multicystic dysplassia	Hydronephrosis
Liquid-filled cavities	
Haphazard arrangement with a fibrous nucleus Noncommunicating	Grouped around a larger anteromedial cavity Communicating

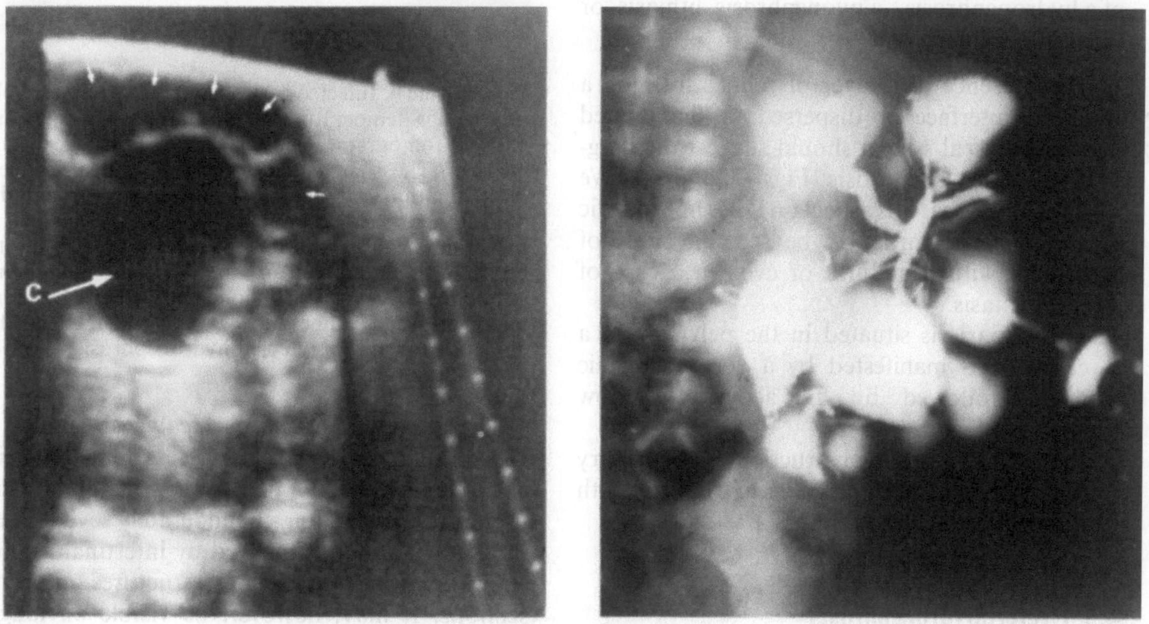

a b

Fig. 28a and b. Differential diagnosis of multicystic dysplasia with hydronephrosis in a 10 days old girl. Left flank mass. **a** Longitudinal section of the left lumbar fossa in prone position. Voluminous anterior cavity *(C)* with smaller peripheral cavities (*arrows*) but without intercommunications. **b** Percutaneous puncture and opacification: numerous cysts of variable size and haphazard disposition communicating one with another via fine chanels. Pelvis not identifiable. Diagnosis of multicystic dysplasia.

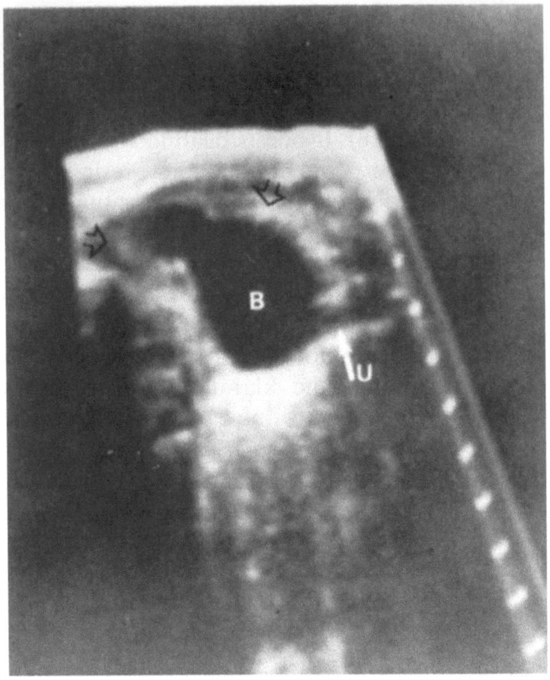

Fig. 29. Sagittal section of the kidney in prone position 3 months after surgical repair of a stenosis at the ureteropelvic junction. The pelvis *(B)* remains dilated but the underlying ureter is easily visible *(U)*. The parenchymal thickness is approximately 1 cm at the upper pole (*arrow*).

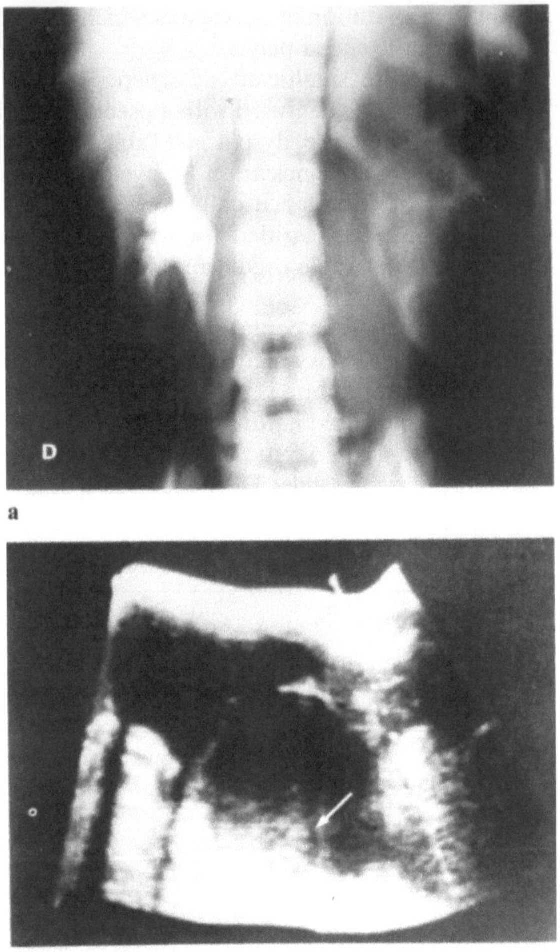

a

b

Fig. 30 a and b. Infected hydronephrosis in a 7 years old boy with a temperature 40 °C and left lumbar fossa pain. **a** Tomogram 2 h after IV injection of contrast medium. The right kidney is normal and on the left threre is a thin strip of opaque parenchyma around the dilated, nonopacified excretory cavities.
b Longitudinal section of the left kidney in prone position: numerous liquid cavities, the most voluminous anteromedial cavity corresponds with the pelvis containing a layer of echoes (*arrow*). This image orients the diagnosis toward an infected hydronephrosis.

of a hydronephrosis – a pyonephrosis, lithiasis, or calyceal rupture:

1. The presence of a layer of echoes forming a liquid interface or dispersed in the dilated pyelocalyceal system should suggest the diagnosis of a pyonephrosis (Figs. 30 and 31). We must stress that this aspect on US is not specific and may in particular be seen in cases of trauma with hematuria or even in a case of severe stasis.
2. The lithiasis is situated in the pelvis or in a calyx. It is manifested by a very echogenic image followed by an acoustic shadow (Fig. 32).
3. In the case of severe obstruction of the urinary tract there may be a calyceal rupture with urinary leaks in the renal bed.

4.3 Ureterohydronephrosis

The diagnosis of ureterohydronephrosis depends on the visualization of dilated pyelocalyceal cavities associated with a dilatation of the underlying ureter (Fig. 33).

The dilatation of the pyelocalyceal cavities is variable. However, the pelvis is less dilated than in hydronephrosis due to an obstruction at the ureteropelvis junction. In moderately severe cases the lumbar ureter is masked by intestinal gas on supine sections and by bony structures on prone sections. It may, however, be visible on longitudinal sections of the flank in a lateral decubitus position (Fig. 34). The dilated pelvic ureter may be visualized through a bladder window; in other words, one is obliged to maintain a full bladder throughout the examination. On a longitudinal or

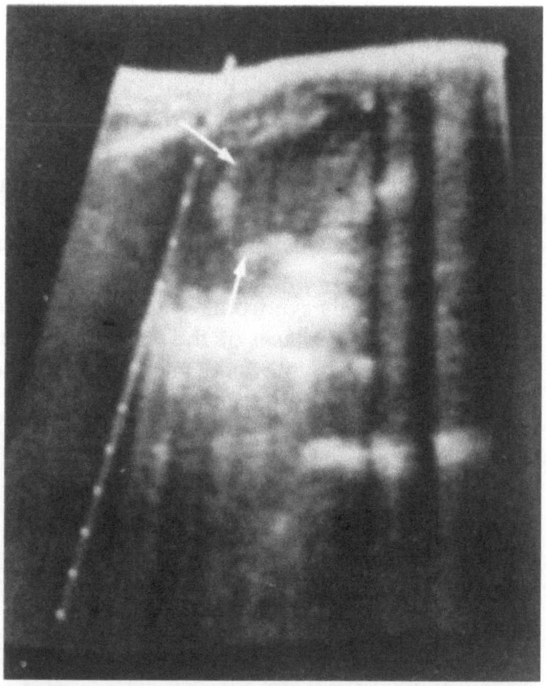

Fig. 31. Pyonephrosis in a 9 months old boy with right flank mass and temperature of 40° C. His general condition was poor. Longitudinal section of the right kidney in prone position: the pyelocalyceal cavities are dilated, filled with homogeneous echoes. The pelvic wall appears thicker than usual (*arrows*).

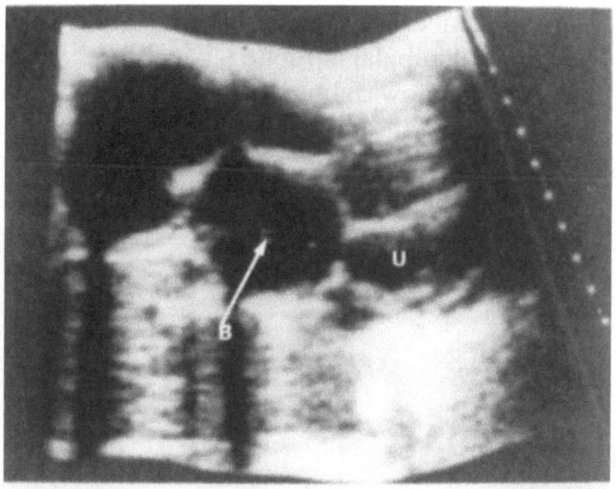

a

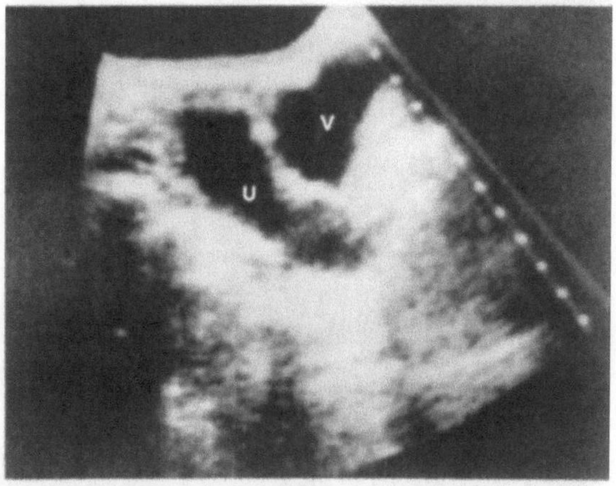

b

Fig. 33. Ureterohydronephrosis in a 6 years old boy. **a** Longitudinal section of the right kidney in prone position. Dilated pyelocalyceal cavities communicating with the pelvis *(B)*. The initial part of the ureter *(U)* extends down from the pelvis. **b** Longitudinal right paramedian section. The right dilated ureter *(U)* is identified behind the bladder *(V)*.

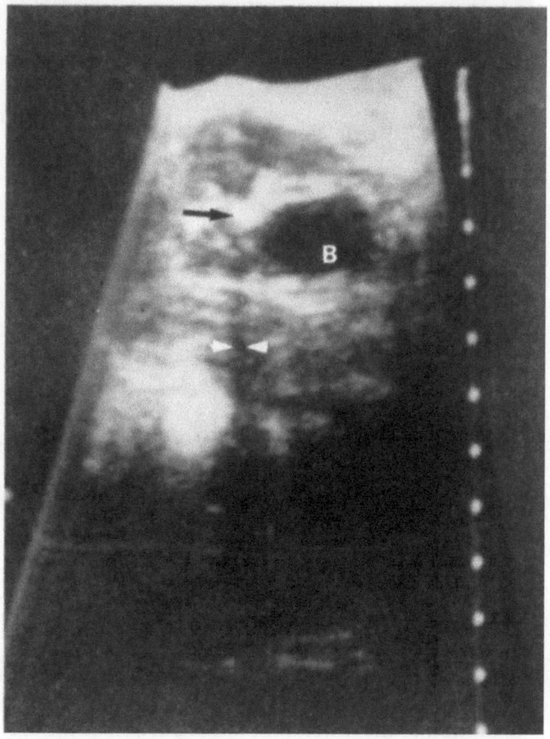

◀ **Fig. 32.** Hydronephrosis and calicial lithiasis in a 4.5 years old boy. Transverse section of the left kidney in procubitus position showing the pelvis *(B)* to be dilated. There is an echogenic image (*arrow*) followed by an acoustic shadow (*arrowheads*). This lithiasis is situated in the stem of a calyx.

oblique section, the ureteral dilatation is seen as a retrovesical tubular structure which one should attempt to follow right to its bladder insertion. In certain cases, the monstrously dilated tortuous ureter is manifested on US by the juxtaposition of thin-walled liquid images (Fig. 35).

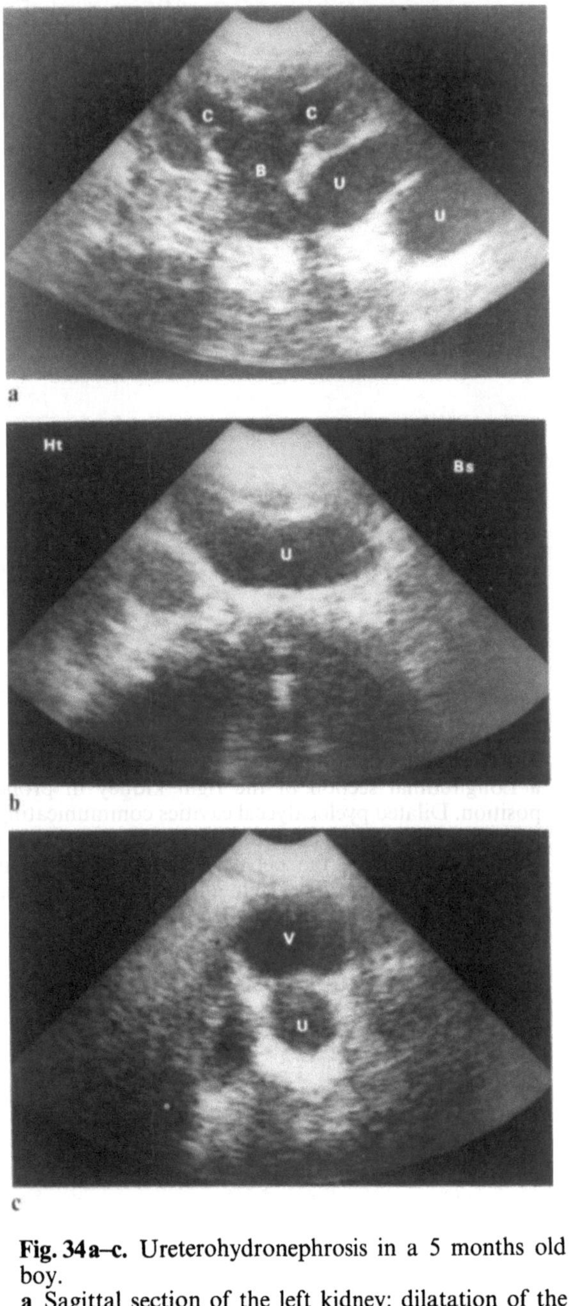

Fig. 34a–c. Ureterohydronephrosis in a 5 months old boy.
a Sagittal section of the left kidney: dilatation of the small calyces *(C)* and of the pelvis *(B)* which is in continuity with a dilated sinuous ureter *(U)*.
b Longitudinal section of the left flank in right lateral decubitus position: the left ureter is dilated in its lumbar region *(U)*.
c Transverse section of the bladder (V): image of the dilated left ureter *(U)* in a retrovesical position.

Among the malformative uropathies as causes of ureterohydronephrosis are the following entities:

1. The obstacles at the level of the ureterovesical junction – stenosis, simple ureterocele, isolated abnormal insertion of the ureter or a urinary tract duplication.
2. Bladder outlet obstructions will be discussed later.
3. The prune-belly syndrome is an association of hypoplasia or aplasia of the abdominal muscles, bilateral cryptorchidism, and anomalies

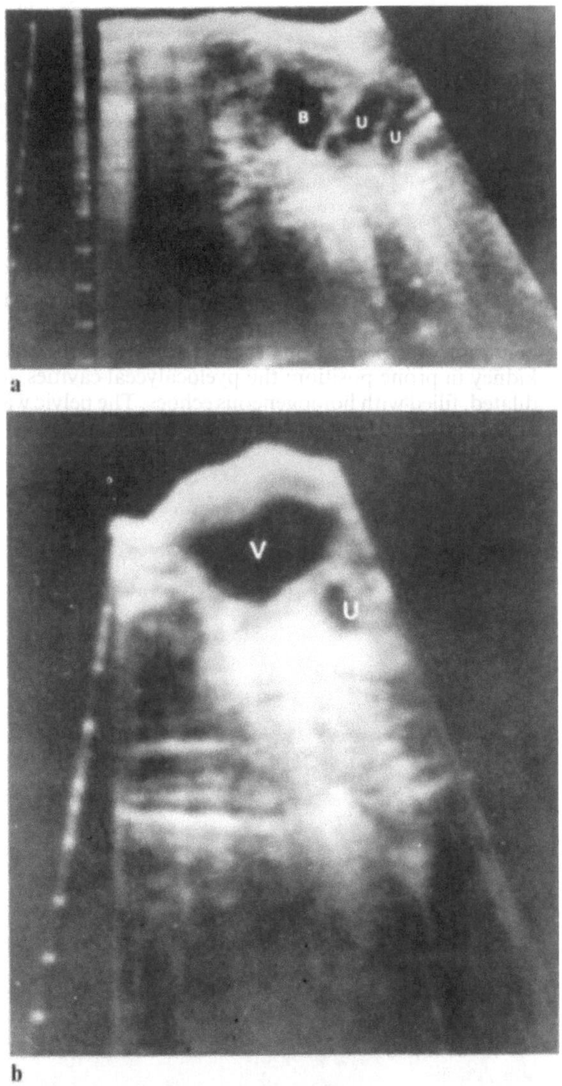

Fig. 35a and b. Ureterohydronephrosis in a 9 days old boy. **a** Longitudinal section of the left kidney in prone position. The dilated tortuous ureter *(U)* is situated under the dilated pelvis *(B)*.
b Tranverse section of the bladder *(V)* showing left round liquid image in a retrovesical position *(U)* and dilatation of the lower abdominal portion of the ureter.

of the urinary tract of variable severety. US examination permits diagnosis of the following: (a) Dysplastic kidneys without appreciable parenchyma: these forms are usually lethal; (b) Marked dilatation of the ureter in contrast with moderate dilatation or absence of dilatation of the pyelocalyceal cavities (Fig. 36); (c) Intermediate forms.

The differential diagnosis of ureterohydronephrosis should be considered in the following situations:

1. The diagnosis of a ureteral dilatation whatever the degree does not signify that an obstruction exists and in all cases a cystography is necessary to eliminate a vesicoureteral reflux.
2. A pelvic mass compressing the excretory tract should be systematically looked for while undertaking an US examination of the lower urinary tract.
3. In cases of moderate excretory tract dilatation one should consider the possibility of an increased diuresis whether pathological or induced by the use of furosemide. In the same way, a urinary tract infection may result in moderate dilatation of the entire excretory tract due to atony.
4. When the ureteral dilatation is severe, the US image of a dilated tortuous ureter is misleading and may cause confusion with a multicystic dysplasia or with a cystic lymphoma (Fig. 48).

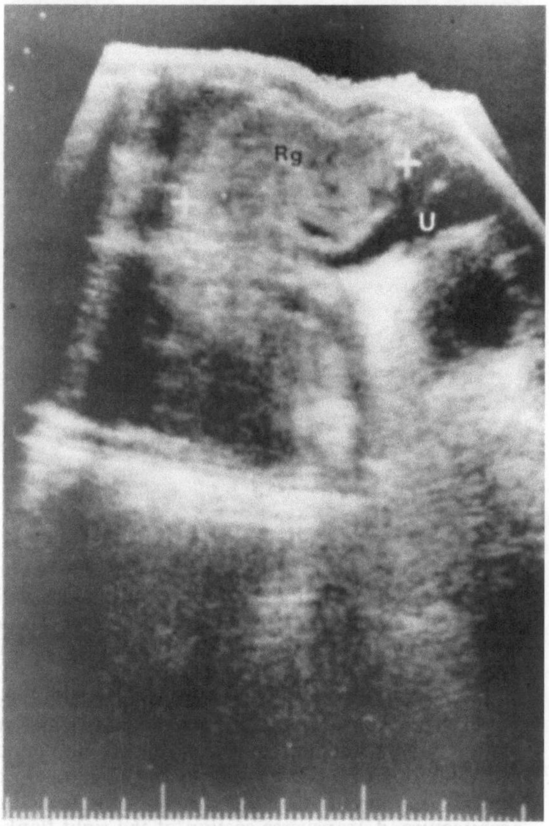

Fig. 36. "Prune-belly syndrome" in a 1 day old boy. Bivalve section of the left kidney *(Rg)*. The ureteral dilatation *(U)* contrasts with the absence of pyelocalyceal dilatation.

4.4 Bladder Outlet Obstruction

The diagnosis depends on the association of bladder anomalies and a dilatation of the overlying excretory tract.

4.4.1 The Bladder

The bladder wall is abnormal and may be several millimeters thick. It is moderately echogenic and irregular on its inner surface (Fig. 37). The bladder capacity is abnormal: either considerably increased, in which case it is not unusual for the bladder dome to reach the umbilicus (Fig. 38), or diminished with a cavity that is difficult to visualize surrounded by a very thick wall (Fig. 39). The bladder empties poorly. In the very young child, the bladder remains full for the duration of the examination whereas normally one notes numerous mictions.

4.4.2 The Consequences of Bladder Outlet Obstruction on the Upper Urinary Tract

Sections of the lower abdomen show a variable dilatation of the lower ureters, either moderate (Fig. 40) or severe, in which case one may suspect an associated vesicoureteral reflux (Fig. 41). The ureters are tortuous and are manifested by numerous juxtaposed liquid images all about equal in diameter.

Sections of the upper apparatus show a moderate or severe dilatation of the pyelocalyceal cavities and of the first part oft the ureter. The renal parenchymal thickness is reduced and the corticomedullary differentiation has disappeared. Ultrasonography does not allow definition as to wheter the renal parenchyma is dysplastic or not.

In the neonatal period, one should systematically look for an associated liquid effusion either perirenal or intraperitoneal.

4.4.3 Possible Etiologies

In boys during the first year of life, posterior urethral valves are the most common cause of

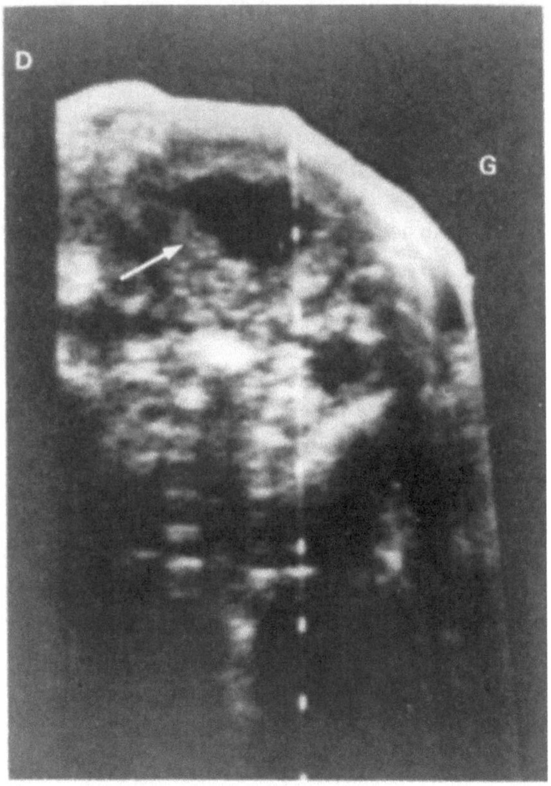

a

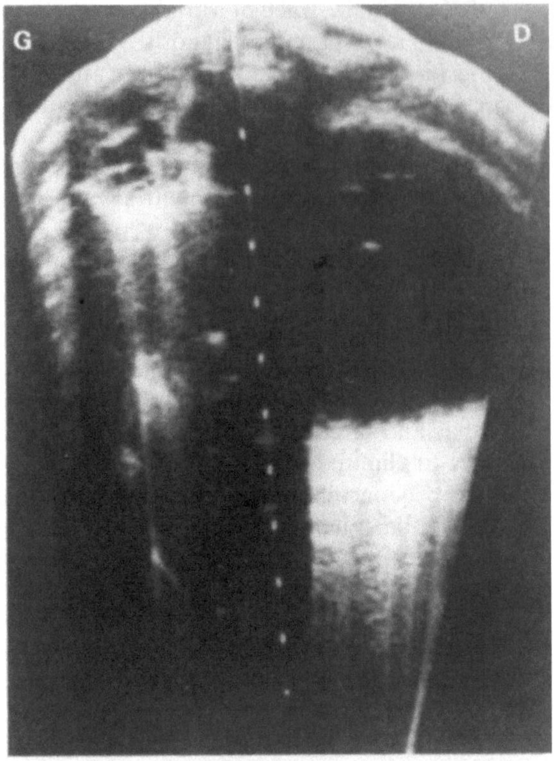

c

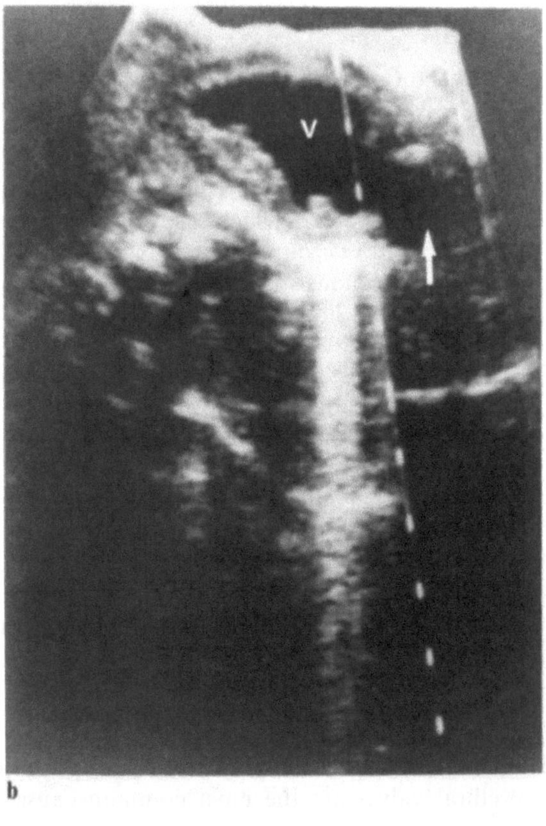

b

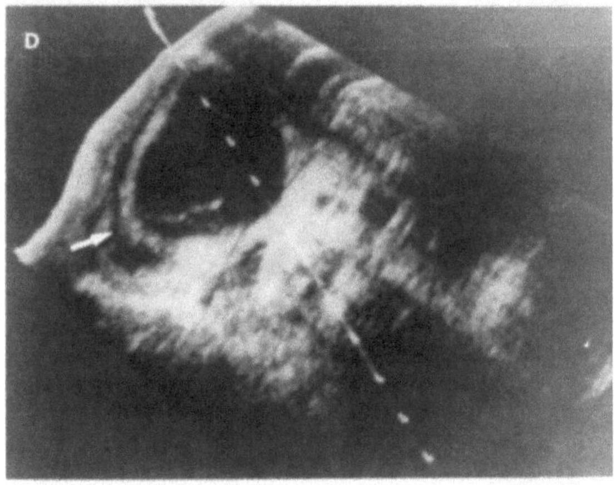

d

Fig. 37 a–d. Posterior urethral valves in a 1 day old boy. **a** Transverse section of the bladder. The bladder wall is thickened (*arrow*) and irregular on its inner surface. **b** Medial longitudinal section of the bladder *(V)* showing thickening and irregularities of the bladder wall. The liquid image towards the lower part of the bladder may be the dilated posterior urethra (*arrow*). **c** Transverse section of both lumbar fossae in prone position: moderate dilatation of the left pyelocalyceal cavities. On the right is a voluminous liquid mass without definite architecture. **d** Transverse section of the right flank in supine position. Round liquid image surrounded on its anteroexternal portion by a crescent-shaped layer of liquid (*arrow*). Ruptured hydronephrosis was diagnosed.

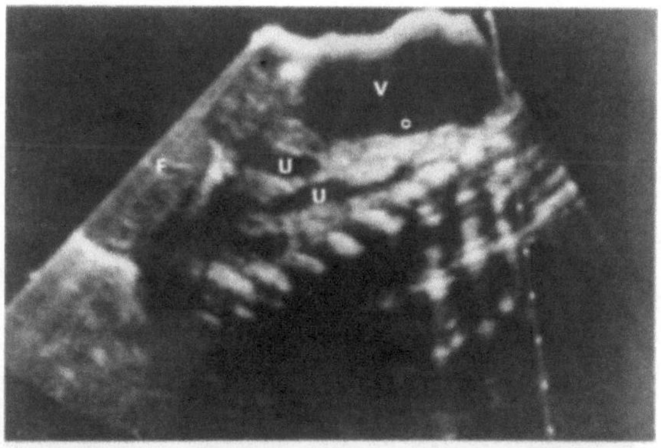

a

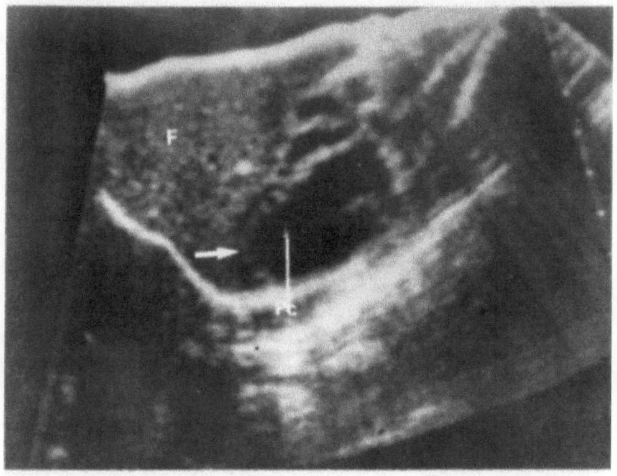

b

Fig. 38 a and b. Posterior urethral valves in a 1 day old boy. **a** Longitudinal section in supine position: the bladder *(V)* extends higher than the umbilicus and its lumen is irregular. The tubular retrovesical liquid images *(U)* correspond with a moderately dilated and sinuous ureter. *F*, Liver. **b** Longitudinal section of the right kidney in supine position: the pyelocalyceal cavities *(Pc)* are significantly dilated and the renal parenchymal thickness is reduced to a few millimeters. The perirenal layer of liquid (*arrow*) corresponds with extravasad urine. There is no ascites.

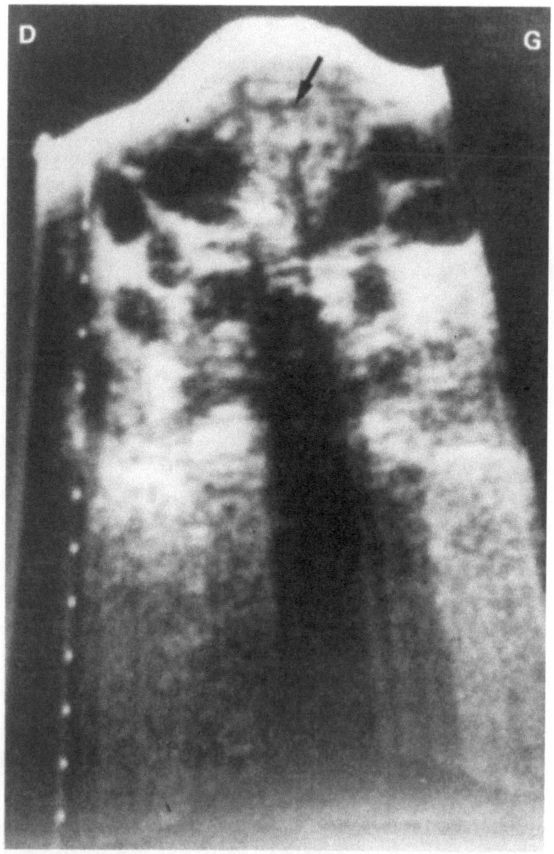

Fig. 39. Posterior urethral valves in a 3 days old boy. Transverse section of the bladder: the bladder lumen (*arrow*) is rarely visible in the middle of the thickened walls, the numerous round retro- and laterovesical liquid images correspond with the section through moderatly dilated ureters which are tortuous and folded on themselves.

bladder outlet obstruction. These infants have renal failure to a greater or lesser degree. An IV pyelogram is a risk in that one may decompensate a precarious renal function without gaining much information. In a newborn with suspicion of posterior urethral valves, US examination is the first step. The results are usually sufficiently typical to make the diagnosis. Sometimes one can even visualize the dilated posterior urethra under the bladder. The next step is a cystogram which visualizes the posterior urethral valves and searches for a vesicoureteral reflux which is frequently associated.

The other causes of bladder outlet obstruction are rare at this age, whether it be a ureterocele (either in a single ureter of a duplicated pyelon) prolapsing into the urethra during miction, diverticula of the anterior urethra, or urethral atresia.

Abnormalities other than malformative uropathies can result in difficulties with bladder emptying. The neurogenic bladder has of course an identical appearance to bladder outlet obstruction in the older child, but the clinical context is usually helpful. This problem is not encountered in the neonatal period because the bladder wall is never thickened and trabeculated due to neurological involvement as it is in urethral malformations. A bladder tumor is rare in childhood; regional tumor (neuroblastoma, rhabdomyosarcoma) can be identified on US. The diagnosis of

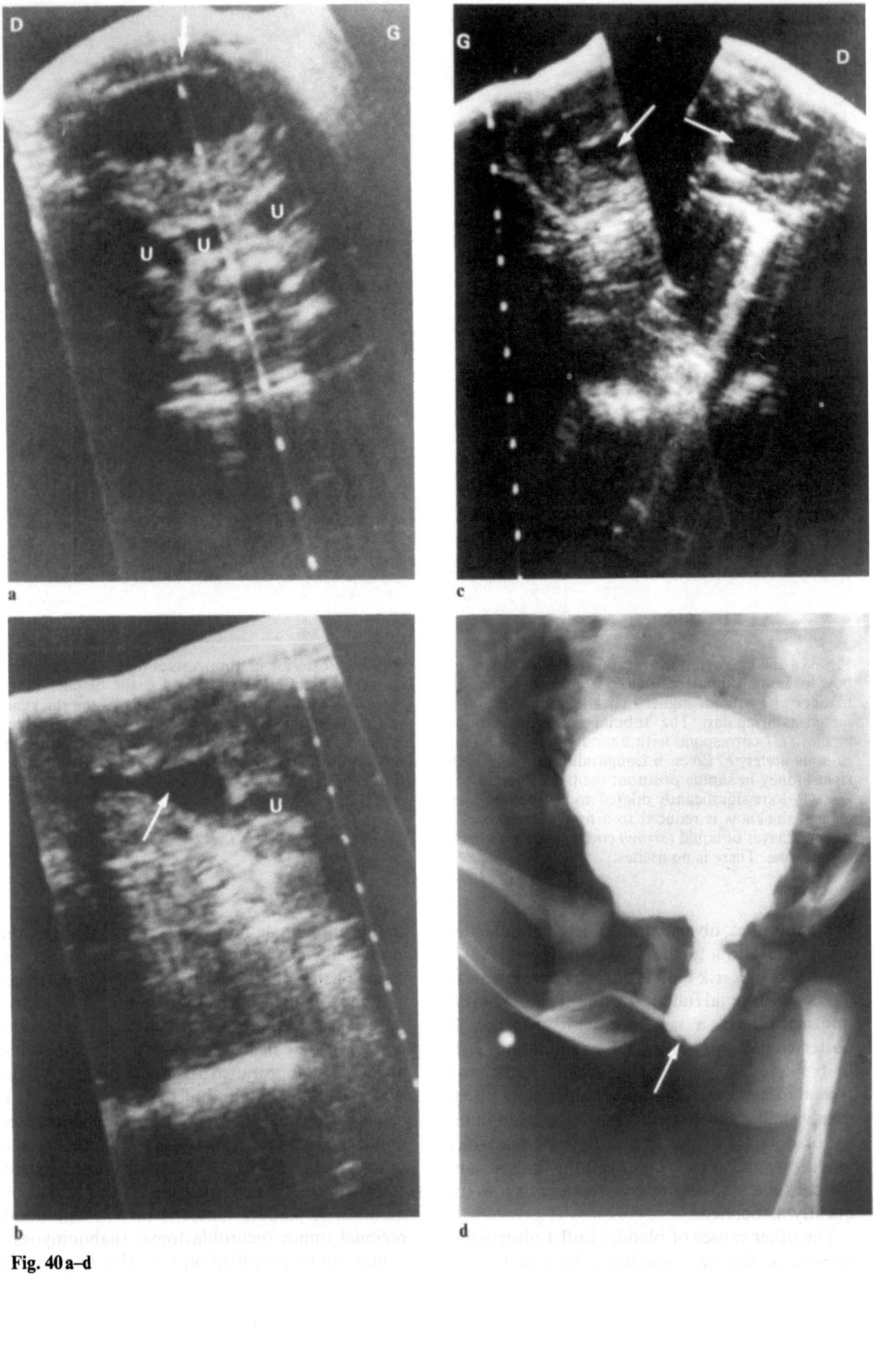

Fig. 40 a–d

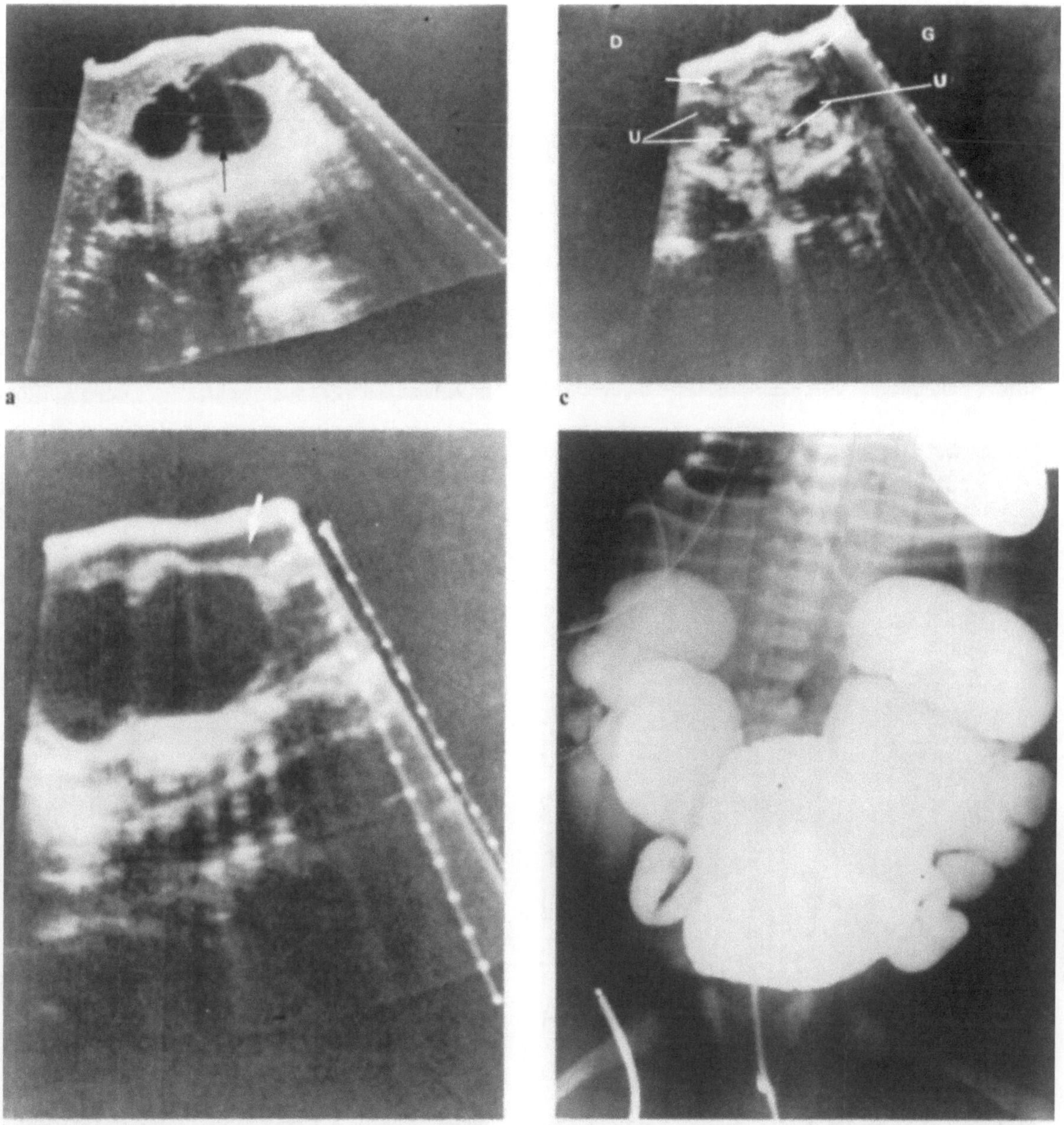

◄ **Fig. 40 a–d.** Posterior urethral valves in a 3 weeks old boy.
a Transverse section of the bladder: the thickness and irregularity of the bladder wall (*arrow*) suggest the diagnosis of bladder outlet obstruction. The multiple retrovesical liquid images correspond with the dilatation of the lower ureters *(U)*. **b** Longitudinal section of the left kidney in prone position: moderate dilatation of the pyelocalyceal cavities (*arrow*) and of the initial part of the ureter *(U)*. Renal parenchymal thickness remains satisfactory. **c** Transverse section of both lumbar fossae in prone position: moderate bilateral dilatation of the excretory tracts (*arrows*). **d** Voiding cystogram: posterior urethral valves (*arrow*) there is no associated vesicoureteral reflux.

Fig. 41 a–d. Posterior urethral valves in a 1 day old boy.
a Longitudinal section of the right flank in supine position: severe hydronephrosis (*arrow*). *F*, Liver.
b Longitudinal section of the left flank in supine position: a layer of ascites is clearly visible (*arrow*) in front of the very dilated left pyelocalyceal cavities.
c Transverse section of the bladder: the bladder lumen is diminished and the thickened bladder wall is outlined by ascites on its external surface (*arrows*). The dilated tortuous pelvic ureters form retro- and laterovesical round liquid images *(U)*.
d Retrograde cystogram: bilateral massive vesicoureteral reflux.

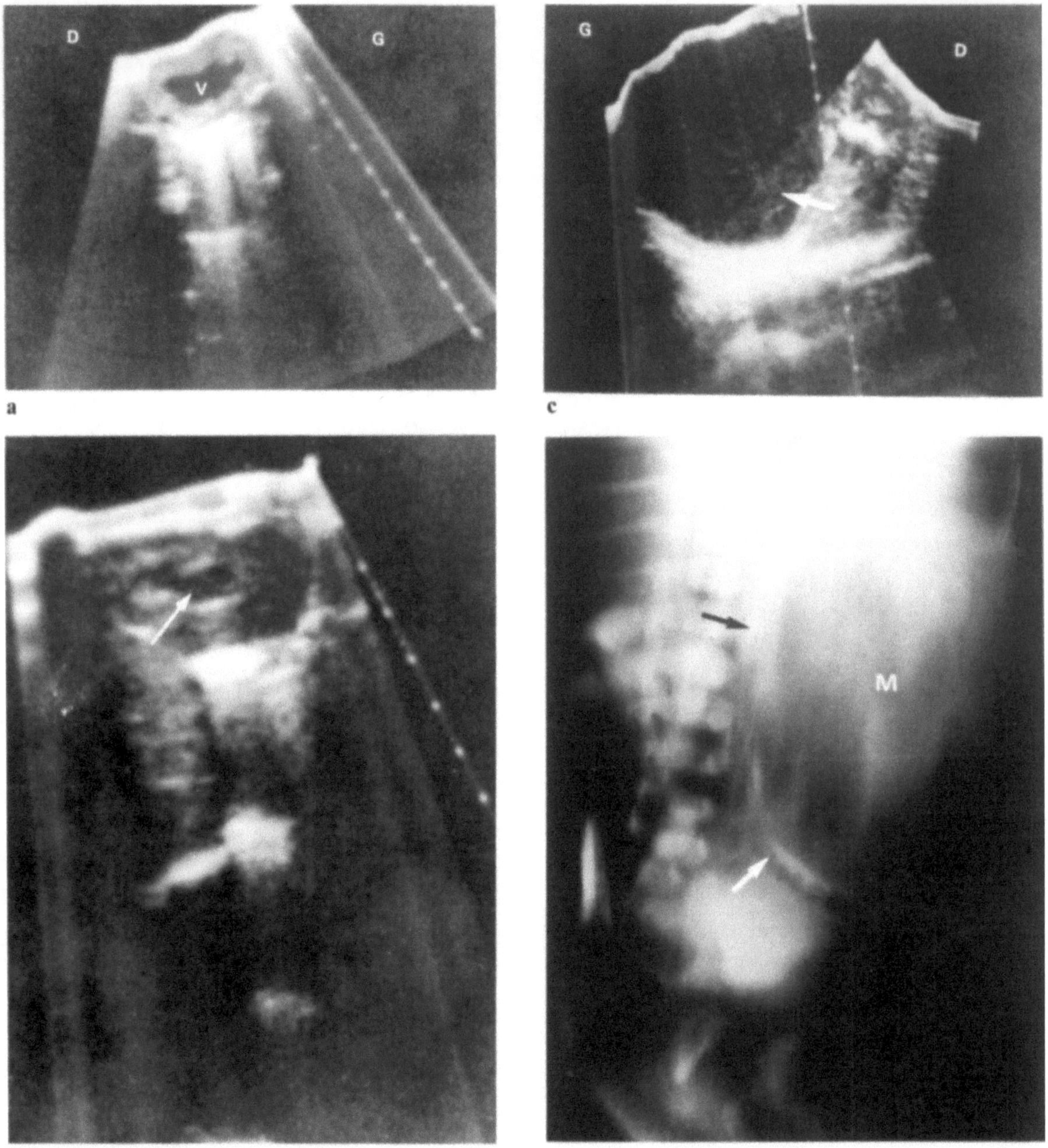

Fig. 42 a–d. Bladder outlet obstruction and diverticula of the anterior urethra in a 12 days old boy. **a** Transverse section of the bladder *(V)* in supine position: the bladder wall is thickened and irregular on its inner surface. **b** Longitudinal section of the right kidney in prone position: moderate dilatation of the pyelocalyceal cavities (*arrow*). **c** Transverse section of both lumbar fossae in prone position: voluminous mass in the left lumbar fossa: a liquid mass yet containing numerous echoes (*arrow*). **d** IV urography, tomogram: the mass *(M)* extends and displaces the left pyelocalyceal cavities (*arrows*). At surgery, urinoma secondary to a rupture of a middle-group calyx was found.

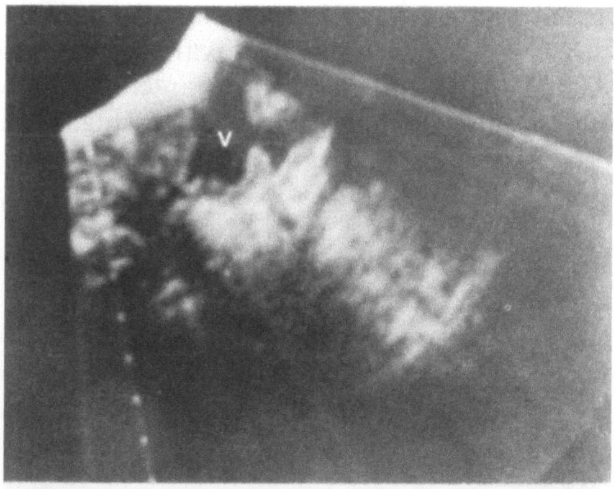

a

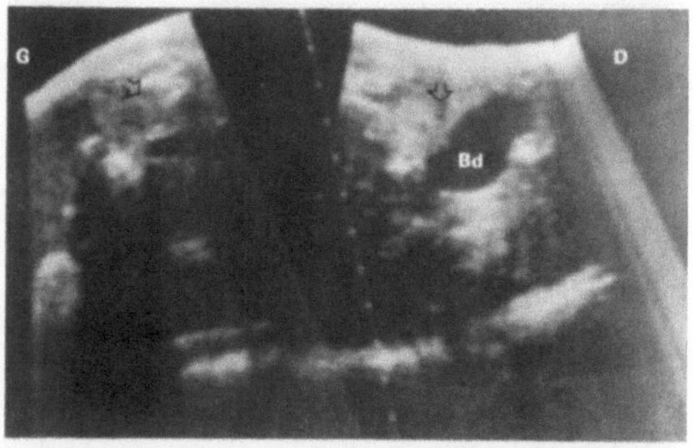

b

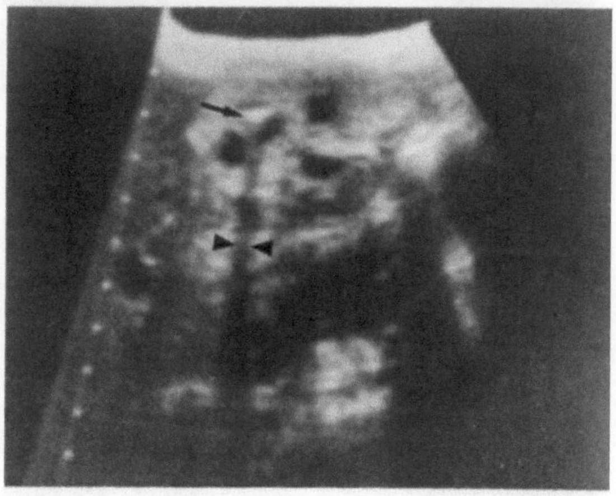

c

Fig. 43a–c. Bladder outlet obstruction, sequelae of posterior urethral valves, and renal failure lithiasis in a 8 years old boy.
a Longitudinal section of the bladder *(V)*. The bladder wall is thick and irregular.
b Transverse section of both lumbar fossae in prone position: the right pelvis is dilated *(Bd)* and the renal parenchyma is unusually echogenic bilaterally (*arrows*).
c Longitudinal section of right kidney in supine position: the dilated calyceal cavities are surrounded by a very echogenic parenchyma. The bright echo followed by an acoustic shadow (*arrowheads*) situated in a calyx of the upper group (*arrow*) corresponds with a lithiasis.

The effusion may involve the peritoneum in the form of urinary ascites, which is easily recognized on US examination. The dilatation of the pyelocalyceal cavities is evident. One must therefore look for abnormalities in the lower urinary tract.

In the older child, the complications are dominated by renal failure and lithiasis (Fig. 43).

4.5 Duplication of the Excretory Tract

Anatomically, duplication of the excretory tract consists of the presence of two pelves and two ureters. There are simple duplications, i.e., without functional side effects, and complicated duplications. The complications of excretory tract duplication are associated with the abnormal insertion of the ureters (Fig. 44). The ureter of the upper *pelvis* has a lower insertion than normal or even a totally ectopic insertion in the bladder bladder neck anomalies or urethral polyps, is made on a voiding cystogram.

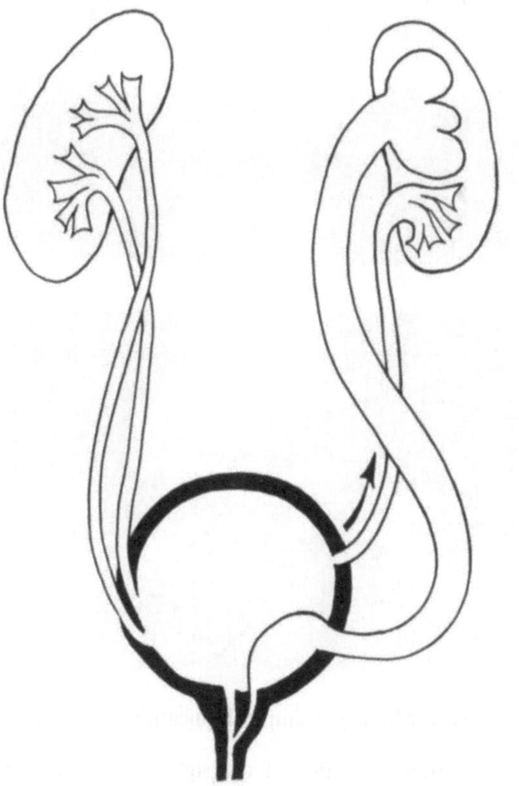

Fig. 44. Diagram of excretory tract duplication. On the right, simple duplication. On the left, ureterocele and dilatation of the excretory cavities of the upper pelvis. Reflux into the lower pelvic cavities.

The malformative uropathies responsible for bladder outlet obstruction may develop certain complications. In the neonatal period, one may encounter extravasation of urine due to rupture of the excretory tract. The effusion may be perirenal. When small in volume, it can only be diagnosed on US examination. A layer of liquid exists in a crescent shape around the kidney whose dilated cavities are easily identified (Fig. 38).

In other cases a voluminous urinary pseudocyst causes a flank mass. This is manifested by a vast cavity with a clear outline, purely echo-free, consistent with liquid, or containing echoes consistent with deposits secondary to urinary stasis (Fig. 42c).

The pyelocalyceal cavities and the ureter on the affected side are not identifiable because the excretory tract, laminated by the mass, is no longer dilated and the urinoma plays a decompressive role. On IV pyelogram the urinoma stretches the pyelocalyceal cavities of the ipsilateral kidney, displaces them antero-medially, and in this way may mimic a tumor (Fig. 42d).

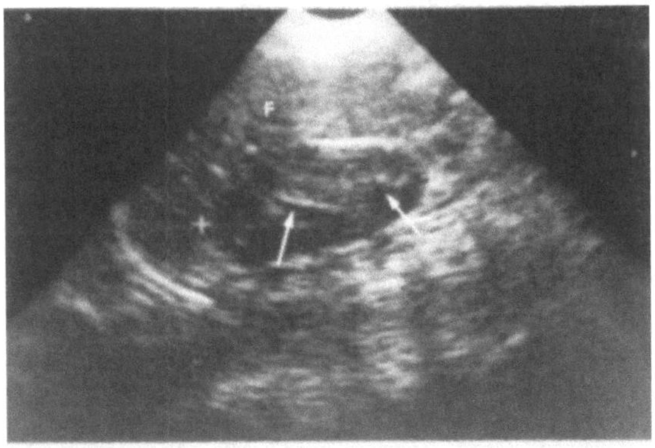

a

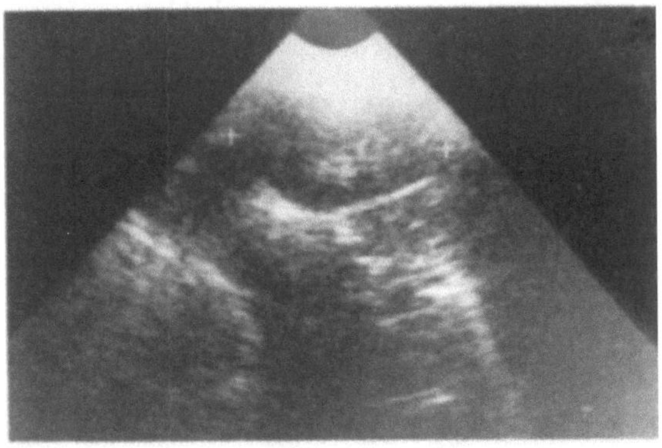
b

Fig. 45a and b. Right simple duplication in a 1 year old girl.
a Longitudinal section of the right kidney in supine position. *F*, Liver.
b Longitudinal section of the left kidney in prone position: the right kidney is longer and thinner than the left. On the right, the central echo is elongated and the thin excretory cavities seem to be separated (*arrows*).

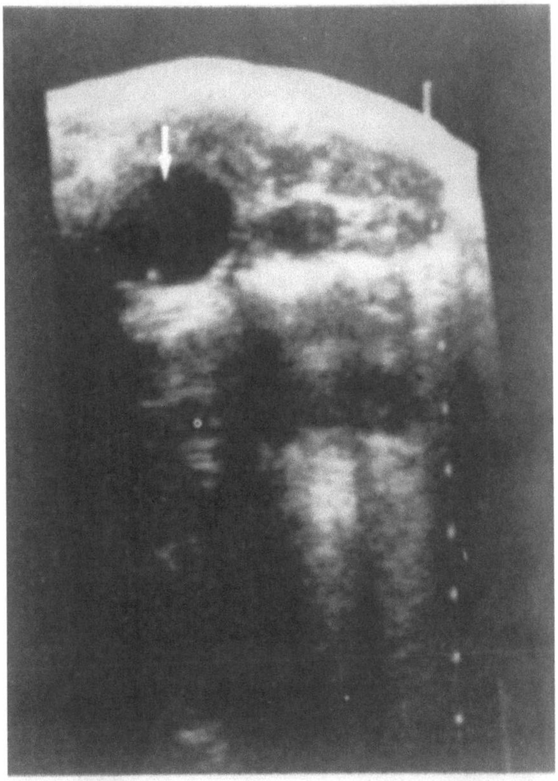
a

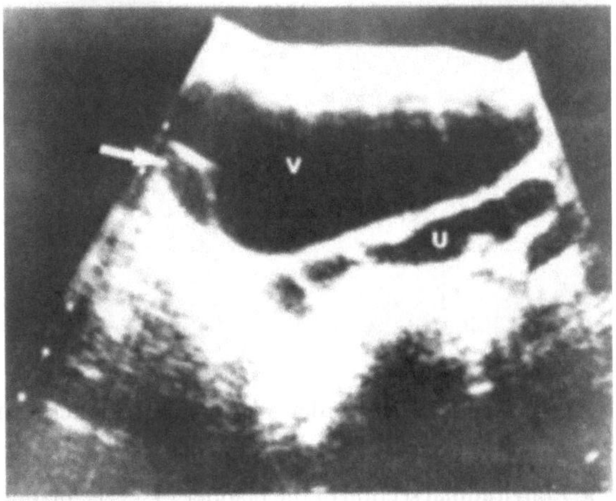

b

Fig. 46a and b. Right duplication with ureterocele in a 20 months old girl.
a Longitudinal section of the right kidney in prone position: there is a round liquid cavity at the upper pole of the right kidney (*arrow*). **b** Right paramedian longitudinal section of the bladder *(V)*: the ureter of the upper pelvis is dilated *(U)* and there is a ureterocele (*arrow*).

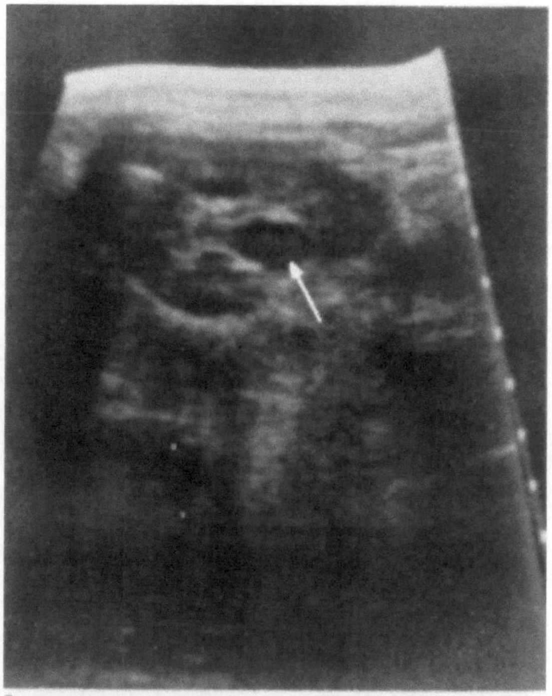

a

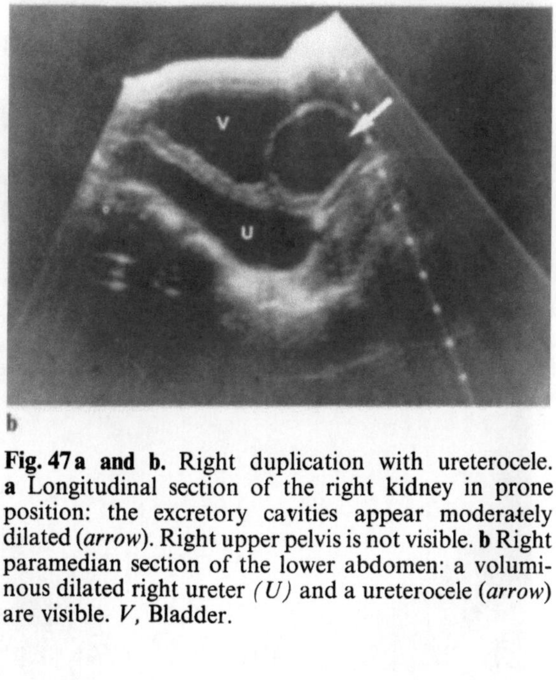

b

Fig. 47 a and b. Right duplication with ureterocele. **a** Longitudinal section of the right kidney in prone position: the excretory cavities appear moderately dilated (*arrow*). Right upper pelvis is not visible. **b** Right paramedian section of the lower abdomen: a voluminous dilated right ureter *(U)* and a ureterocele (*arrow*) are visible. *V*, Bladder.

neck, urethra, or vagina where in addition there is a ureterocele. In all these cases, an obstacle to the evacuation of urine exists and the overlying excretory tract is dilated. The ureter of the inferior *pelvis* is inserted higher than normal and is often refluxing.

The noncomplicated duplication is seen on US as a kidney with an increased longitudinal diameter and with a central pyelovascular zone divided into two (Fig. 45). Such a division is not typical only of duplication and may be seen in the case of Bertin septal hypertrophy.

In complicated duplication with ureterocele, the longitudinal section of the kidney shows an upper pyelocalyceal system which is dilated, sometimes reduced to a single liquid cavity (Fig. 46 a) extended by a dilated tortuous ureter in an anterior position. The cavities of the inferior *pelvis* are often moderately dilated. At the level of the lower abdomen, there is a ureteral dilatation and, in the bladder, a round image, variable in size with thin walls: the ureterocele (Fig. 46 b).

The upper pelvis is sometimes completely destroyed. The diagnosis is therefore made by visualization of a dilated ureter in its lumbar and pelvic portions associated with a ureterocele (Fig. 47). In the absence of a ureterocele and in the case of severe ureteral dilatation, multilocular liquid images extend from the lumbar to the retrovesical region. If there is doubt about a diagnosis of cystic lymphangioma, transcutaneous puncture with injection of contrast medium confirms the presence of a megaureter (Fig. 48).

Apart from the lesions already mentioned, excretory tract duplication may be associated with other anomalies: one of the duplicated pelves may be associated with a multicystic dysplasia or an anomaly of the ureteropelvic junction (Fig. 49).

Acknowledgements. We thank Dr. M.D. Cordier, Dr. D. Picamoles and Dr. P. Picamoles who performed some of the US examinations, the photographs of which appear in this chapter.

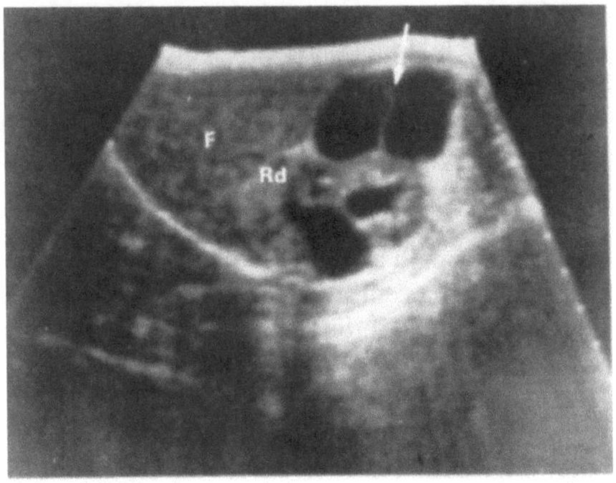

a

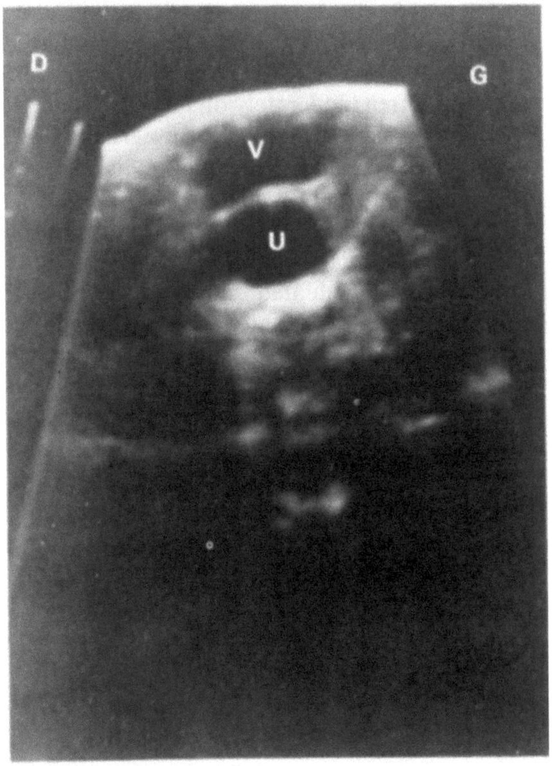

b

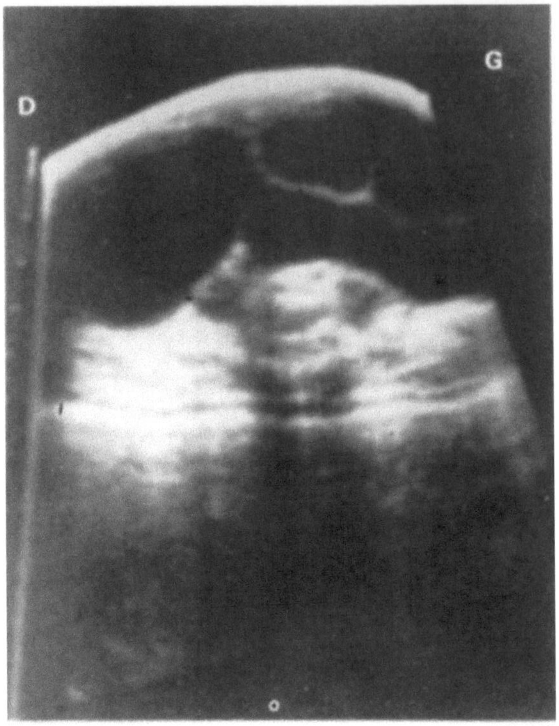

c

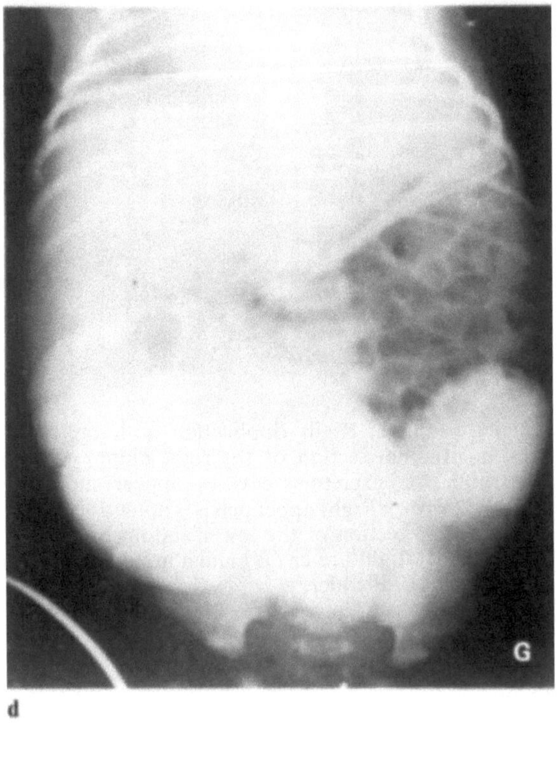

d

Fig. 48 a–d. Right duplication with vaginal insertion of the upper pelvic ureter in a 1 day old girl. **a** Longitudinal section of the right kidney in supine position: right renal *(Rd)* excretory cavities are dilated and in front of the kidney there is a loculated liquid structure with thin walls (*arrow*). *F*, Liver. **b** Transverse section of the abdomen at the level of the umbilicus showing voluminous loculated liquid mass (corresponding with the megaureter of the upper right pelvis). **c** Transverse section of the bladder *(V)*: large ureter of the right upper pelvis *(U)*. **d** Opacification by percutaneous puncture of the right superior pelvis: the enormous folded ureter occupies the majority of the abdominal cavity.

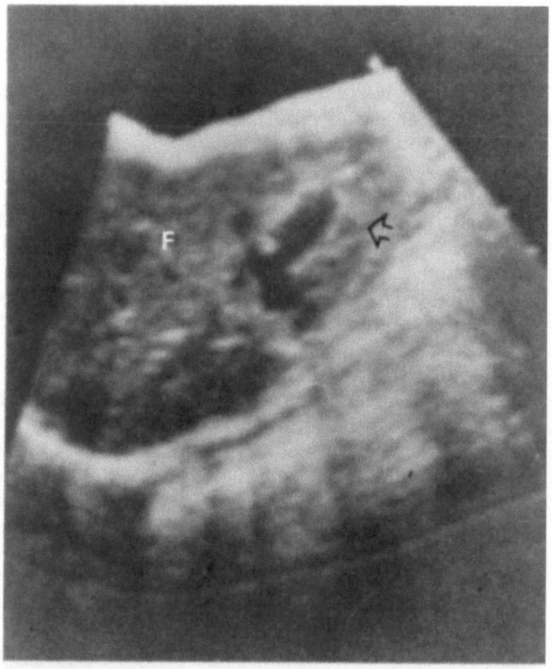

a

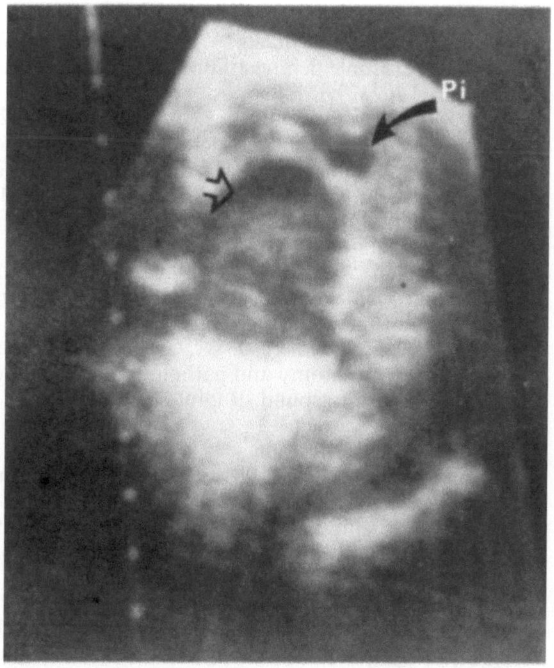

c

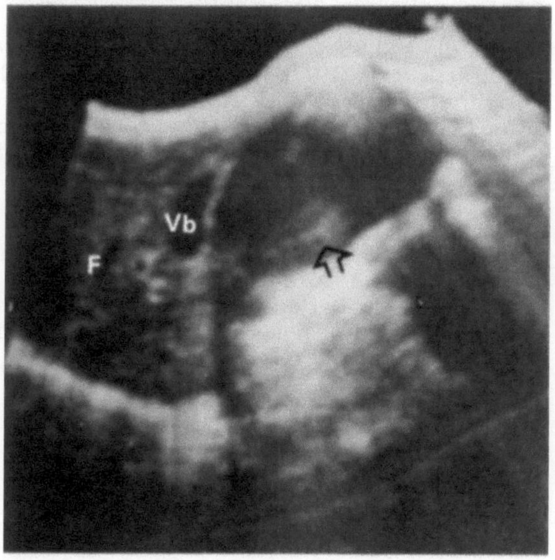

b

Fig. 49 a–c. Duplication of the right excretory tract with anomaly of the ureteropelvic junction in the upper half of the kidney in a 9 months old boy.
a Longitudinal section of the right flank in supine position showing lower pole of the kidney (*arrow*) with moderately dilated excretory cavities. *F*, Liver.
b More internal but otherwise indentical section. There is a voluminous single liquid mass with duplication of the excretory tract (*arrow*). *F*, Liver; *Vb*, Gallbladder.
c Transverse section of the right lumbar fossa in prone position. Lower pelvis is moderately dilated *(Pi)* anterointeriorly; upper pelvis is reduced to a single cavity in which a liquid interface (*arrow*) can be seen. The ureter is not visible.
At surgery, stenosis of the ureteropelvic junction was found in the upper pelvis of a duplicated excretory tract, the urinary stasis accounting for the presence of echoes in the pelvis.

References

General Review

Behan M., Wixson D., Kazam E. (1979). Sonographic evaluation of the nonfunctionning kidney. J. Clin. Ultrasound 7:449–458

Sanders R.C. (1975). Renal ultrasound. Radiol. Clin. N. Amer. 13:417–434

Sty J.-R., Starshak R.-J. (1981). Sonography of pediatric urinary tract abnormalities. Sem. ultrasound 11:71–87

Teele R.-L. (1977). Ultrasonography of the genito urinary tract in children. Radiol. Clin. N. Amer. 15:109–128

Weill F., Bihr E., Rohmer P., Zeltner F. (1981). L'ultrasonographie rénale. Vigot édit., Paris

Weitzel D., Troeger J., Straube E. (1977). Renal sonography in pediatric patients: a comparitive study between sonography and urography. Pediat. Radiol. 6:19–26

Normal Kidney

Cook J.-H. III, Rosenfield A.-T., Taylor K.-J.-W. (1977). Ultrasonic demonstration of intra renal anatomy. A.J.R. 129:831–835

Haller J.-O., Berdon W.-E., Friedman A.-P. (1982). Increased renal cortical echogenicity: a normal finding in neonates and infants. Radiology 142:173–174

Kaufman R.-A., Dunbar J.-S., Gole D.-E. (1981). Normal dilatation of the proximal ureters in children. A.J.R. 137:945–949.

Moskowitz P.-S., Carroll B.-A., McCoy J.-M. (1980). Ultrasonic renal volumetry in children: accuracy and simplicity of method. Radiology 134:61–64

Rosenfield A.-T., Taylor K.-J.-W., Crade M., de Graaf C.-S. (1978). Anatomy and pathology of the kidney by gray scale ultrasound. Radiology 128:737–744

Multicystic Dysplastic Kidney

Baudain Ph., Crouzet A. (1981). Le rein multikystique. Feuil. Radiol. 21:295–306

Greene L.-F., Feinzaig W., Dahlin D.-C. (1971). Multicystic dysplasie with special reference of the controlateral kidney. J. Urol. 105:482–487

Neuenschwander S., Cordier M.-D., Montagne J.-Ph. (1981). "Gros rein" unilatéral néonatal: approche échotomographique du diagnostic. Ann. Radiol. 24:141–146

Stuck K.-J., Koff S.-A., Silver T.-M. (1982). Ultrasonic features of multicystic dysplastic kidney: expanded diagnostic criteria. Radiology 143:217–221

Hydronephrosis

Chopra A., Teele R.-L. (1980). Hydronephrosis in children: narrowing the differential diagnosis with ultrasound. J. Clin. Ultrasound 8:473–478

Coleman B.-G., Arger P.-H., Mulhern C.-B. Jr., Pollack H.-M., Banner M.-P. (1981). Pyohydronephrosis: sonography in the diagnosis and manafement. A.J.R. 137:939–943

Haasch E. (1978). Ultrasound scanning for monitoring childhood hydronephrosis. J. Clin. Ultrasound 6:156–159

Marshall F.-F., Jeffs R.-D., Smolev J.-K. (1980). Neonatal bilateral ureteropelvic junction obstruction. J. Urol. 123:107–109

Ralls P.-W., Esensten M.-L., Boger D. (1980). Severe hydronephrosis and severe renal cystic disease: ultrasonic differentiation. A.J.R. 134:473–475

Ralls P.-W., Halls J. (1981). Hydronephrosis, renal cystic disease and renal parenchymal disease. Sem. Ultrasound 11:49–60

Ureterohydronephrosis

Garris J., Kangarloo H.„ Sarti D., Sample W.-F., Smith L. (1980). The ultrasound spectrum of Prune Belly syndrome. J. Clin. Ultrasound 8:117–120

Lebowitz R.-L., Griscom N.-T. (1977). Neonatal hydronephrosis: 146 cases. Radiol. Clin. N. Amer. 15:49–59

Bladder Outlet Obstruction

Diard F., Eklof O., Lebowitz R., Maurseth K. (1981). Urethral obstruction in boys caused by prolapse of simple ureterocele. Pediat. Radiol. 11:139–142

Morgan C.-L. Jr., Grossman H. (1978). Posterior urethral valves as a cause of neonatal uriniferous perirenal pseudocyst (urinoma). Pediat. Radiol. 7:29–32

Morris L.-C., Ahmed S. (1981). Posterior urethral valves presenting as an abdominal mass lesion due to perirenal urinoma. Ann. Radiol. 24:151–156

Scott T.-W. (1976). Urinary ascites secondary to posterior urethral valves. J. Urol. 116:87–91

Excretory Tract Duplications

Mascatello V.-J., Smith E.-H., Carrera G.-F., Berger M., Teele R.-L. (1977). Ultrasonic evaluation of the obstructed duplex kidney. A.J.R. 129:113–120

Rose J.-S.„ McCarthy J., Yeh H.-S. (1979). Ultrasound diagnosis of ectopic ureterocele. Pediat. Radiol. 8:17–20

Lithiasis

Edell S., Zegel H. (1978). Ultrasonic evalution of renal calculi. A.J.R. 130:261–263

Pollack H., Arger P.-H., Goldberg B.-B. (1978). Ultrasonic detection of nonopaque renal calculi. Radiology 127:233–237

Chapter 9

Ultrasound in Pediatric Nephrology

L. Garel and D. Pariente

1 Introduction

Our institution is the main center for kidney transplantation in France, and we therefore have had the opportunity to study routinely by ultrasound end-stage kidneys in children for several years. Most renal biopsies in our hospital are now performed after sonographic localization of the kidneys, and we have accumulated results of US examinations of numerous kidney diseases.

In almost all cases, pathological correlations were available, either from percutaneous renal biopsies or the removed right kidney at the time of renal transplantation. It became obvious that the diagnostic value of US was generally underestimated, which encouraged us to share our experience in that field.

2 Technical Considerations and Normal Anatomy (Fig. 1)

Longitudinal and transverse prone scans do not need any comment. However, the value of supine or axillary scans must be emphasized to evaluate the right kidney through the liver and the left kidney through the spleen. These parenchyma are used to assess the echogenicity of the renal cortex, which is less echoic than the adjacent liver or spleen. In our experience, this rule has only a few exceptions in some newborns (especially in premature babies).

With a short-focused high frequency transducer, corticomedullary differentiation is always visible in a normal pediatric kidney. Conversely, its absence is always indicative of an abnormal renal parenchyma.

The US examination should then establish:

1. The length, width, and thickness of the kidneys;
2. The status of the central echoes. It is always important to know the degree of hydration of the patient and the degree of bladder filling;
3. The status of the corticomedullary differentiation (preservation, disparition, specific modification);
4. The renal cortex echogenicity (as compared to liver and/or spleen);
5. The bladder volume.

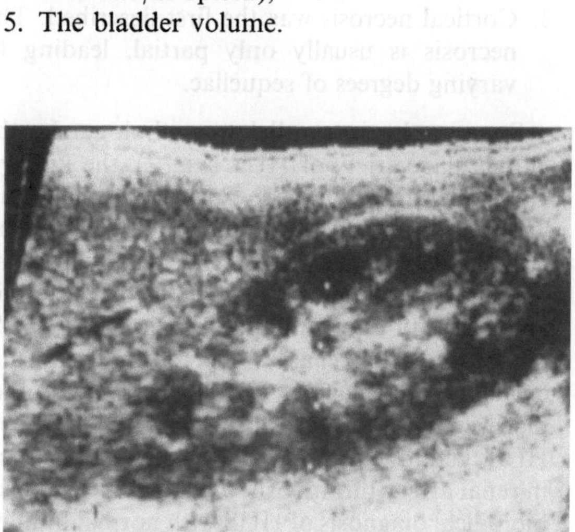

Fig. 1. Normal right kidney in a longitudinal supine scan. Renal cortex is less echoic than the liver. Anechoic medullary pyramids surround the sinusal echoes.

Very often, at the end of the examination, the contours of the kidneys will be drawn on the skin to guide percutaneous biopsy.

3 Acute Renal Failure

Acute renal failure is rare in children. Three groups of causes should be considered: glomerular and vascular diseases (60% of the cases), acute tubulonephritis (30% of the cases), and urinary obstruction (10% of the cases).

3.1 Hemolytic-Uremic Syndrome (HUS)

HUS is the main etiology of acute renal failure in infants and three pathological lesions may be seen:

1. Glomerular thrombotic microangiopathy, by far the most frequent, occurs mainly in children below the age of 2 years: its prognosis is usually good.
2. In arterial thrombotic microangiopathy, the thrombosis involves main arterial branches; it occurs essentially in older children, and the outcome is very poor.
3. Cortical necrosis was the first described. The necrosis is usually only partial, leading to varying degrees of sequellae.

Sonography is parallel to pathology. In the glomerular variety of HUS (Fig. 2), the kidneys are moderately enlarged. Corticomedullary differentiation is too apparent because of the increased echogenicity of the cortex, while the medullary pyramids are normal. Such a pattern in an oliguric or anuric infant is diagnostic of HUS. US examination enables the return to normal cortical echogenicity to be followed, which takes place within a few weeks. In the arterial type of HUS the kidneys are sonographically normal, as in renal artery thrombosis. Thus a clinical and/or biological diagnosis of HUS with normal kidneys at US examination implies a prognosis which is very bad. The diagnosis of partial cortical necrosis is often impossible in the acute phase of HUS. Later, the kidneys decrease in size with variable areas of cortical thinning.

We have studied 22 cases of HUS and found that US is very reliable in differentiating glomerular and arterial forms of HUS. Fifteen patients were below 2 years of age; among the seven older patients, six cases of terminal uremia occurred rapidly.

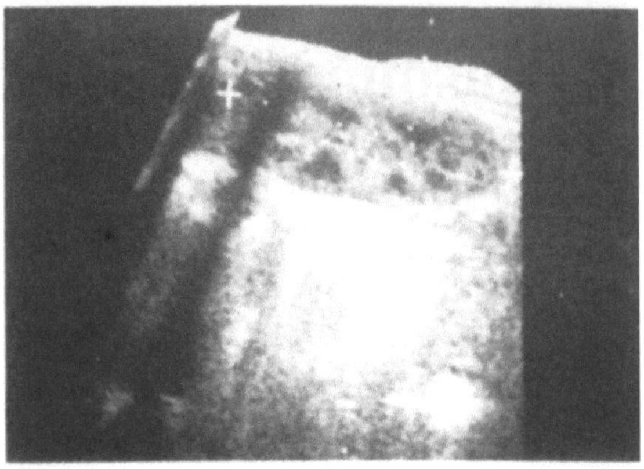

a

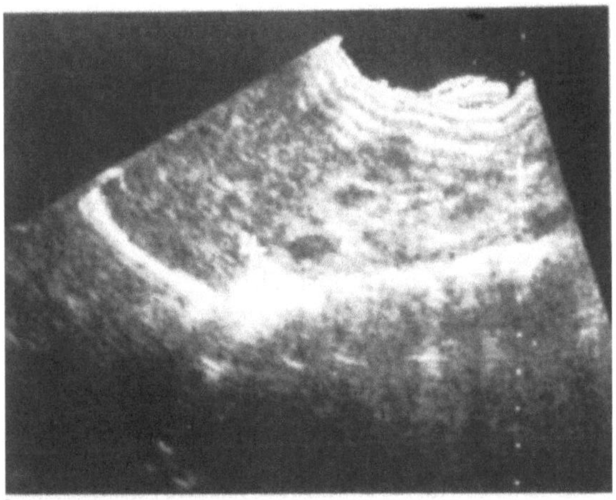

b

Fig. 2 a and b. Hemolytic uremic syndrome (glomerular type).
a Longitudinal prone scan of the left kidney; **b** Longitudinal supine scan of the right kidney.
The kidney is moderately increased in size and cortical echogenicity is more pronounced than normally.

3.2 Renal Vein Thrombosis (RVT)

In primary RVT in newborns (7 cases), the usual pattern is:

1. A definite increase in renal volume (rather than in renal length). The kidney becomes ovoid. Because of the parenchymal pressure, the sinus is no longer visible (Fig. 7).
2. A "patchwork" parenchymal echostructure, with areas of hyperechogenicity (fresh blood) and decreased echogenicity (edema). Some pyramids may remain visible in focal zones of unaffected parenchyma (Fig. 7).

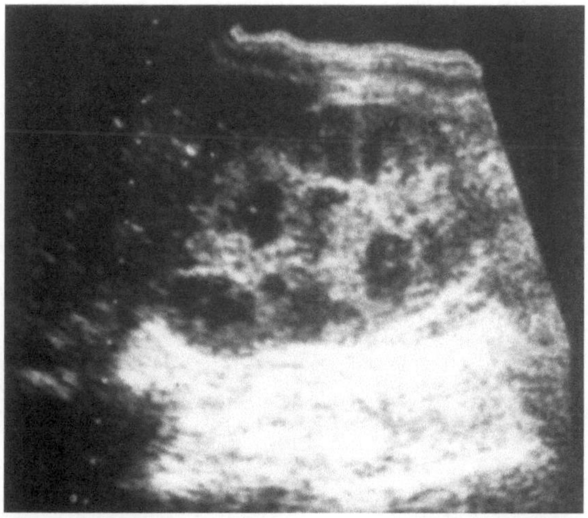

Fig. 3. Shock kidney in acute phase. Longitudinal supine scan of the right kidney. Hyperechoic cortex (the setting of the gain is such that the liver is almost anechoic). Enlarged medullary pyramids.

One should know that this "basic pattern" may vary: the renal cortex may appear globally hypoechoic if the examination takes place soon after the thrombosis has occurred (Fig. 5), and conversely, in massive hemorrhagic infarct, the entire kidney becomes extremely echoic (Fig. 6).

Initially the renal vein thrombus is not sonographically visible; IVC thrombus is extremely rare (one case in a patient with bilateral RVT) Later, these thrombi may calcified. The course varies from one case to another; follow-up examinations should note kidney size, parenchymal echostructure, and possible calcifications (Fig. 8). In several

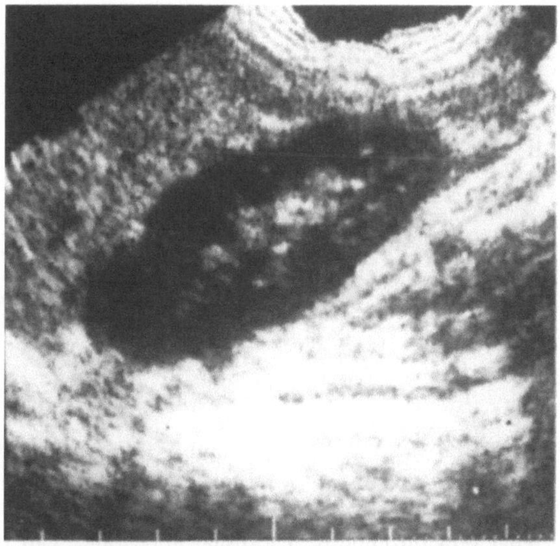

Fig. 5. Right renal vein thrombosis at an early stage. Longitudinal supine scan shows increased renal length with hypoechoic cortex and still visible pyramids. The examination was performed 3 h after the cardiac catheterization that caused the venous thrombosis.

of our cases, a reappearing corticomedullary differentiation preceded urographic secretion (Fig. 9).

In our experience, sonography did not permit differentiation of nephrotic syndrome complicated by RVT (4 cases) from nephrotic syndrome with non-RVT acute evolutive bout. Only the opacification of the IVC by showing the absence of renal vein wash-out permits this differentiation.

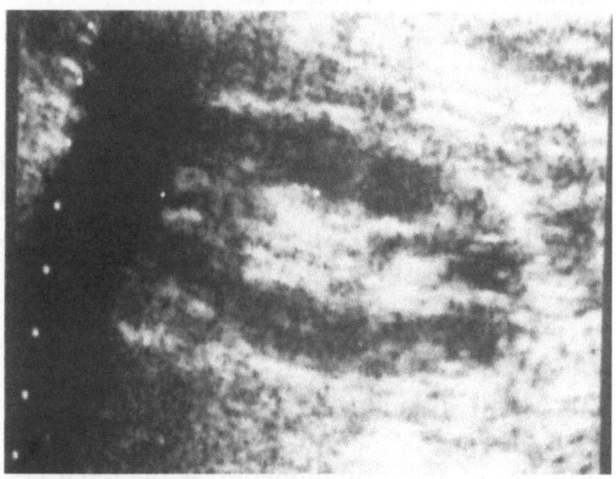

Fig. 4. End-stage massive cortical necrosis. Longitudinal prone scan of right kidney. The base of the pyramids is adjacent to the renal outline, which seems to be calcified sonographically. Radiography of the abdomen showed no calcification.

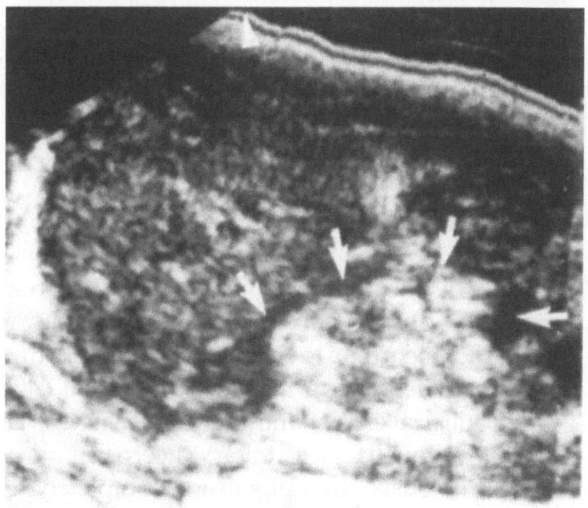

Fig. 6. Right renal vein thrombosis with massive infarction. Longitudinal supine scan shows the kidney to be globally hyperechoic (*arrows*). The patient died 2 days later.

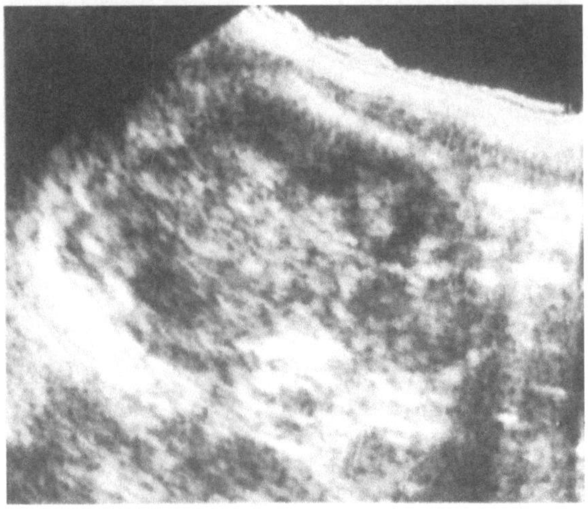

Fig. 7. Longitudinal axillary scan of a patient with right renal vein thrombosis. The usual appearance can be seen: swollen kidney with obliteration of the central echoes and "patchwork" echostructure made up of focal areas of edema and hemorrhage.

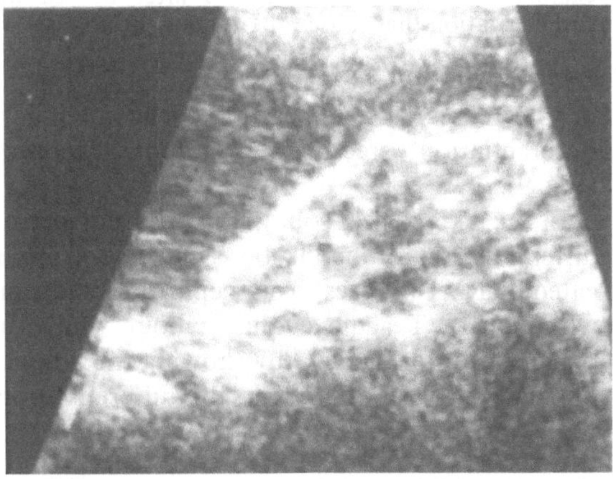

Fig. 8. Longitudinal supine scan of a patient who had right renal vein thrombosis 5 years earlier. Small kidney with calcified cortex. The cortical rim of calcium was apparent on a roentgenogram.

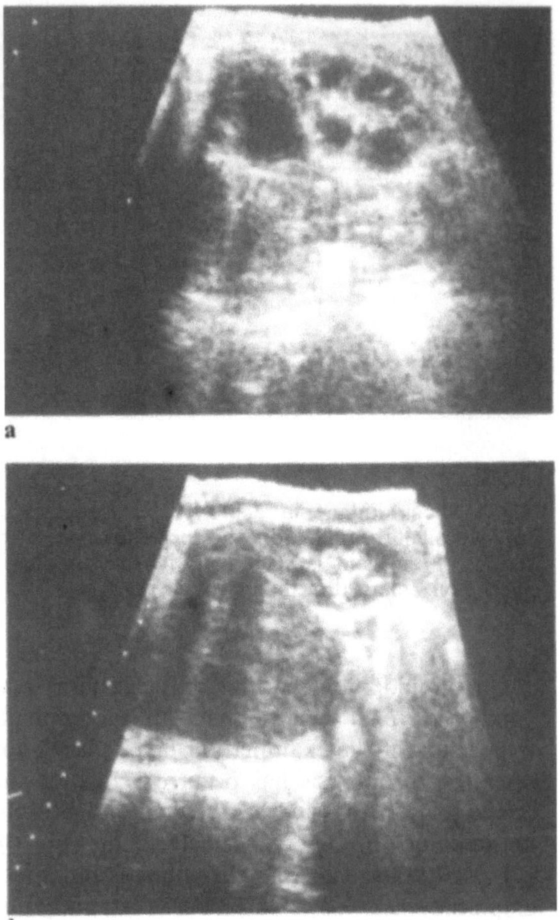

a

b

Fig. 9 a and b. Left renal vein thrombosis with associated adrenal hemorrhage (day 15).
a Longitudinal prone scan of the left kidney; **b** right kidney. Left medullary pyramids are large compared to the normal right kidney. The adrenal hemorrhage is still visible. Six days later (day 21), the right kidney was secreting normally during IVP.

3.3 Shock Kidneys (9 cases)

Under this heading, we include all the renal manifestations that occur during shock and are not RVT. According to the severity of shock, these renal manifestations will be rapidly lethal (massive cortical necrosis) and factors of varying degrees of sequellae (medullary necrosis, partial cortical necrosis), or will subside completely.

In the acute phase, the kidneys are usually enlarged, but above all their cortex has become much more echoic than normally. Medullary pyramids are prominent (Fig. 3); the measurement of cortical thickness is important to recognize medullary and/or cortical necrosis and to follow the renal sequellae on repeated examinations (Fig. 4). In their usual presentation, RVT, medullary necrosis, and transient shock kidney are thus sonographically distinct.

3.4 Acute Tubulonephritis

In cases of acute tubulonephritis the renal US is normal. In cases resulting as a complication of dehydration (five cases), the pattern is thus different from RVT. Most cases are the result of toxic intake, mostly drugs.

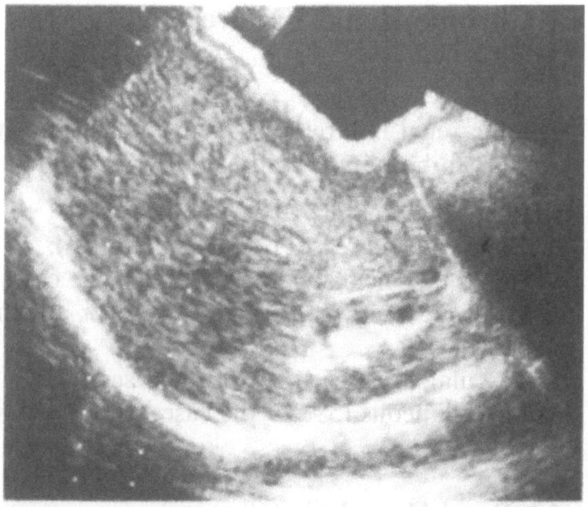

a

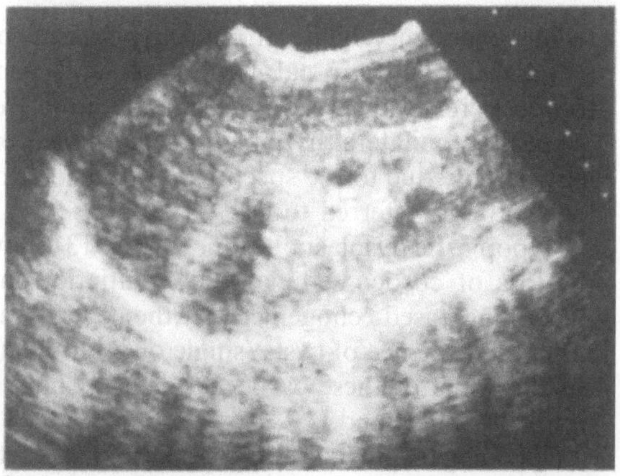

b

Fig. 10a and b. Longitudinal supine scans of the right kidney in cases of acute glomerulonephritis **(a)** and steroid-resistant nephrotic syndrome **(b)**. These frequent conditions have the same pattern of an hyperechoic cortex in enlarged kidneys.

3.5 Acute Glomerulonephritis (AGN) (44 cases) and Nephrotic Syndrome (NS) (57 cases)

AGN and NS are usually seen in children older than those with HUS. The US appearance is similar to all glomerulopathies: definite increased renal length due to increased cortical thickness, the latter being more echoic than the adjacent parenchyma, and the renal pyramids are normal (Fig. 10). The histological subtype of AGN cannot be inferred from the US appearance nor can the corticosensitivity or corticoresistance of NS. Mention should be made of congenital NS; the Finnish type resembles recessive polycystic kidneys in infants older than 3 months, as previously pointed out. Another variety of congenital NS is mesangial sclerosis, in which the medullary pyramids are normal; in contrast, in the other form the bright echonephrogram is seen throughout the entire parenchyma. Mesangial sclerosis can be associated with male pseudohermaphroditism and Wilms' tumor, the so-called Drash triad (Fig. 17).

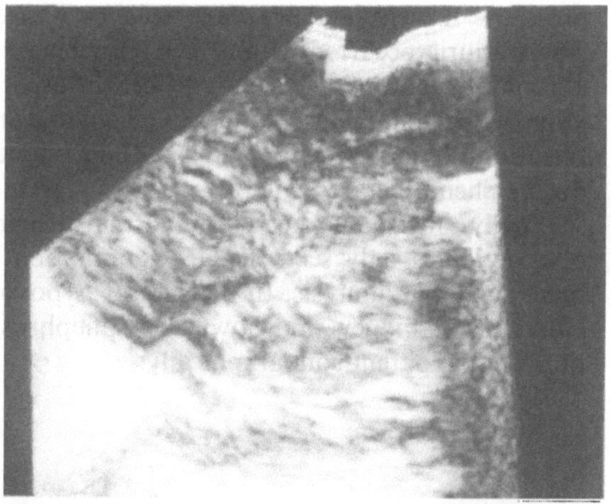

Fig. 11. Potter's syndrome with kidneys of normal size. Right kidney seen on a longitudinal supine scan. In this anuric newborn with bilateral pneumothorax, pathology showed extensive cortical dysplasia. Aortography via the umbilical artery displayed normal renal arteries. In our patients, and to the contrary of recent literature, cortical hyperechogenicity was rarely seen in normal neonatal kidneys (less than 5% of the cases).

3.6 Renal Agenesis (Potter Syndrome)

Bilateral absence of the kidneys is easy to recognize, provided the sonographer is familiar with the size and pseudo-kidney appearance of fetal adrenal glands. We have seen two cases of anuric newborns with Potter's facies where US showed kidneys of normal size. The echogenicity of the cortex was, however, abnormally high. Aortography, via an umbilical catheter, showed in both cases the presence of renal arteries. In these cases, extreme cortical dysplasia was a functional equivalent of renal agenesis (Fig. 11).

3.7 Urinary Obstruction

Obstruction is rarely a cause of acute renal failure in childhood. Lymphomas deserve a special mention because lymphomatous masses often compress the ureters, and we have seen two cases where anuria occurred within 12 h. Other mechanisms of renal insufficiency are seen in association with lymphomas: diffuse parenchymal infiltration, hyperuricemia, and xanthine stones during chemotherapy (Fig. 12).

Finally, one should keep in mind that urinary obstruction is only seen on US examination if there is enough diuresis. In the case of hypovolemia and/or kidney shut-down, hydronephrosis may be inapparent sonographically.

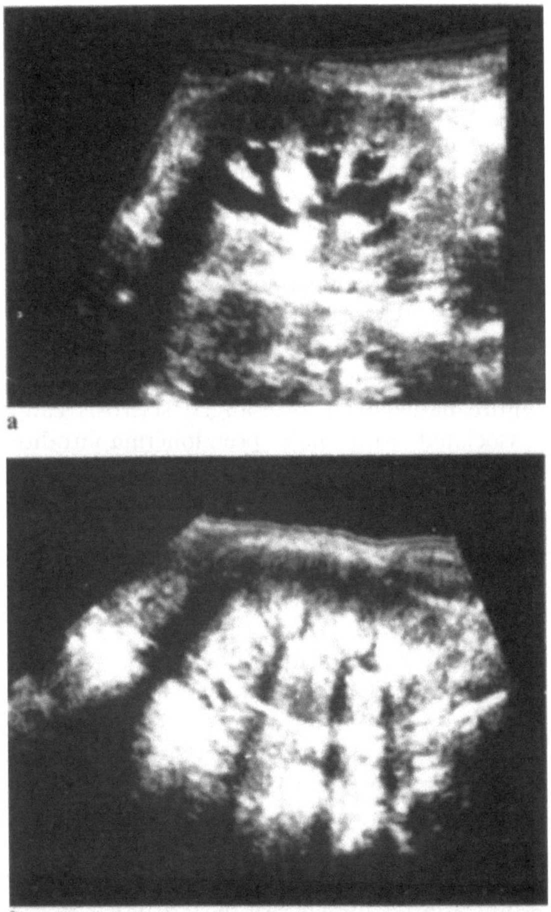

a

b

Fig. 12 a and b. Xanthine stone occurring during the chemotherapy of a Burkitt lymphoma in a 10-year-old patient presenting initially with moderate renal insufficiency. Renal failure subsided rapidly under chemotherapy and recurred 5 days later.
Longitudinal prone scans of the left kidney at the time of presentation **(a)** and after 5 days of chemotherapy **(b)**. **a** Dilatation of the calyces by the lymphomatous pelvic masses without parenchymal involvement. **b** Absence of dilatation; three (radiolucent) renal stones are present.

4 Chronic Renal Failure

Chronic renal failure is frequent in children. Its causes can be summarized as follows:

1. Renal hypoplasia (20% of the cases);
2. Glomerular diseases (25% of the cases);
3. Hereditary nephropathies (20% of the cases);
4. Urinary tract malformations (20% of the cases);
5. Vascular diseases (10% of the cases);
6. Miscellaneous (5% of the cases).

4.1 Renal Hypoplasia (68 cases)

In our experience bilateral renal hypoplasia (or the association of renal hypoplasia and controlateral renal agenesis) is three time more frequent than unilateral hypoplasia. That, however, may be only due to the specificity of the nephrologic patients referred to us.

Hypoplastic dysplastic[1] kidneys (Fig. 13) show the loss of corticomedullary differentiation, an overall increased echogenicity of the cortex, and often the presence of cysts (single or multiple) (6 cases). Some of these cystic hypoplasias have a familial background.

Oligomeganephronia (10 cases), before reaching a terminal stage, is characterized by a limited number of large pyramids (Fig. 14). This appearance is typical of the pathologic features that gave its name to the entity (the nephrons and the tubes are very few but very large).

The sonographic appearance of end-stage nondysplastic renal hypoplasia is nonspecific; the echostructure is so modified by the parenchymal fibrosis that it becomes extremely difficult to distinguish the kidney from adjacent digestive organs.

4.2 End-Stage Kidneys

Small dedifferentiated echoic kidneys are seen with all fibrotic end-stage kidneys, whatever the initial cause (Fig. 15).

[1] In our group, the only definition of renal dysplasia is histological, i.e., the necessary association of primitive tubes and cartilage inclusions. We have already mentioned the possibility of severe dysplasia without hypoplasia.

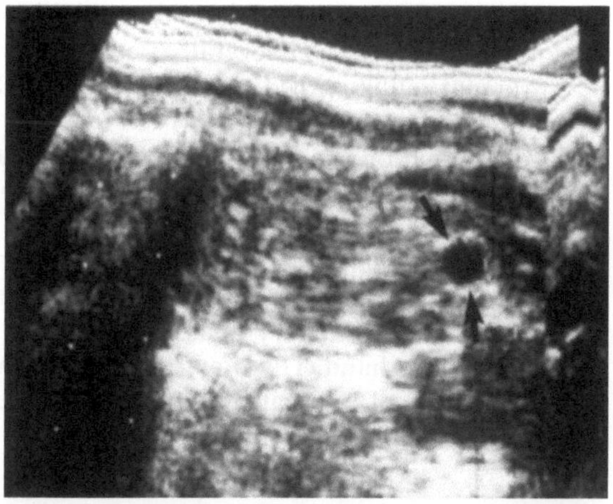

Fig. 13. Hypoplasia with dysplasia. Longitudinal prone scan of left kidney. No corticomedullary differentiation is apparent; there is a 6 mm cyst at the lower pole of this 4 cm long kidney.

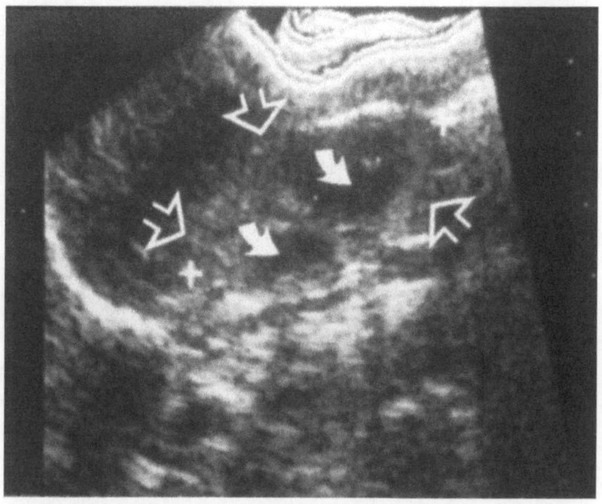

Fig. 14. Patient with oligomeganephronic hypoplasia. Longitudinal supine scan of the right kidney. There are only two medullary pyramids (*filled white arrows*) of increased volume in a 38 mm kidney (*open arrows*).

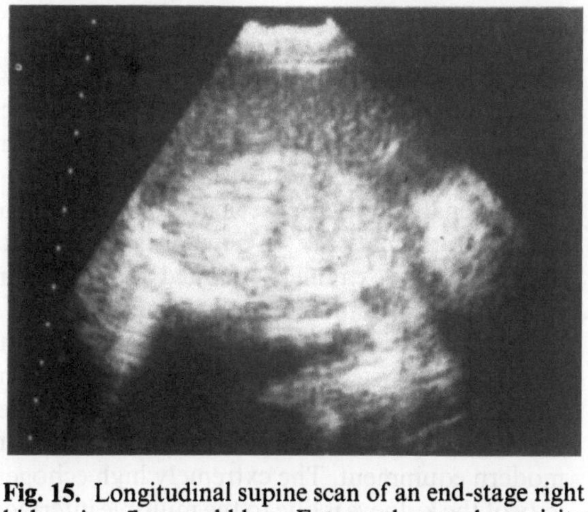

Fig. 15. Longitudinal supine scan of an end-stage right kidney in a 7-year-old boy. Extreme hyperechogenicity of a 6-cm kidney (neonatal medullary necrosis).

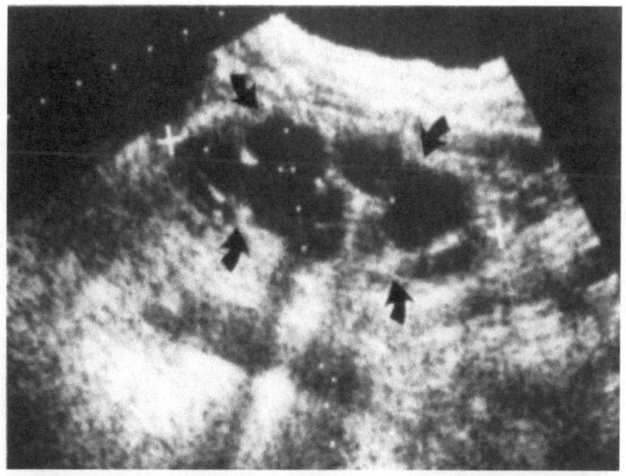

Fig. 16. End-stage left kidney on a longitudinal supine scan.
Multiple macrocysts in both kidneys were apparent before the initiation of periodic dialysis (*arrows*). The patient had two biopsies that confirmed nephrotic syndrome. He was lost to follow-up for 8 years and then returned with terminal renal failure. To the contrary of what has been shown in adults, the presence of cysts in nephritic end-stage kidneys in children is exceedingly rare (apart from juvenile nephronophtisis). This case is the only one with such a pattern in the series of 250 patients with terminal uremia who underwent transplantation in our institution, with pathological study of the nature of the removed right kidney.

In contrast to adult patients, extensive cysts are extremely rare in children with end-stage kidneys except in juvenile nephronophthisis. This was clearly shown by Habib's group (Hopital des Enfants Malades, Paris): among 250 right kidneys removed at the time of kidney transplantation in children with terminal renal failure, only one of those filled with numerous macrocysts was a biopsy proven NS (Fig. 16) and not nephronophthisis (cf. cystic hereditary diseases).

4.3 Glomerular Diseases

They may be recognized as long as the medullary pyramids remain visible. A special remark should be made regarding Schönlein-Henoch purpura with renal involvement: these patients are carefully monitored by successive renal biopsies to infer a prognosis from the glomerular involvement. They should also undergo US follow-ups, because subepithelial hemorrhage may cause subsequent severe obstruction which is not always clinically apparent.

Mesangial sclerosis leads to early terminal failure; its association with ambiguous genitalia (3 cases) and/or Wilms' tumors (2 cases) is well-known (Fig. 17).

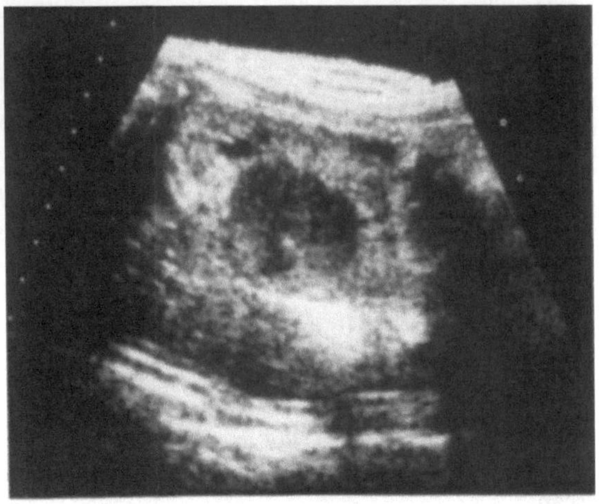

a

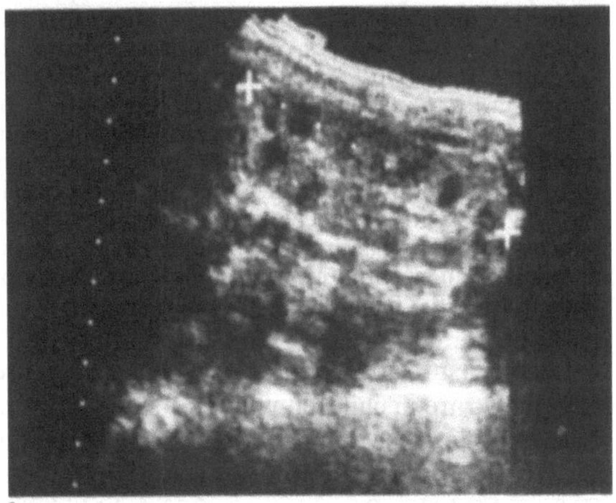

b

Fig. 17 a and b. Drash triad in an anuric 8-month-old baby with pseudohermaphroditism (same patient as in Fig. 7 of Chap. 10). Longitudinal prone scans:
a Wilms' tumor is present in the central portion of the right kidney.
b Mesangial sclerosis is apparent in the left kidney. The kidney is slightly enlarged (76 mm), corticomedullary differentiation is very apparent because of the hyperechogenicity of the cortex.

4.4 Chronic Pyelonephritis

Frequently encountered (30 cases of bilateral involvement, 7 cases of unilateral involvement, 4 cases on a single kidney, 7 cases with high blood pressure), chronic pyelonephritis always raises the question of the respective roles of vesicoureteral reflux, previous renal hypoplasia, and associated parenchymal dysplasia.

Several sonographic points should be considered:

1. There is no relation between the grading of vesicouretral (V U) reflux and renal ultrasound. We have seen several cases of severe intrarenal reflux with normal kidneys on US initially.
2. US examination is a good way to follow renal development. In one of the latter cases, the kidney became atrophic within a year.
3. Parenchymal scars are seen less well sonographically than urographically; clubbed calyces may simulate medullary cysts.
4. On the other hand, US is worthwhile for the examination of cortical regenerating nodules that often simulate tumors in IVP (Fig. 18).

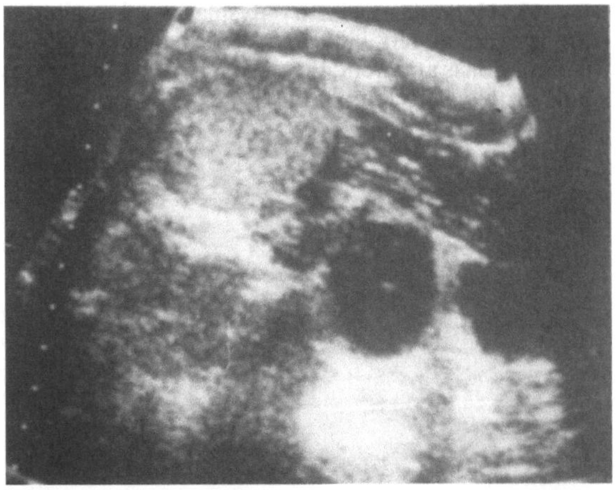

Fig. 18. Chronic pyelonephritis. Longitudinal prone scan of the left kidney through the renal pelvis shows a cortical nodule located at the upper pole. These regenerating nodules can be hypo- or hyperechoic.

4.5 Cystic Hereditary Diseases

4.5.1 Recessive Polycystic Kidneys (RPK)

RPK is also called hepatorenal polycystic disease for it is characterized pathologically by the association of renal cysts arising from the tubules and hepatic cysts arising from the biliary ducts.

Two renal patterns are seen at US depending on the age of the patients. In newborns and infants, the kidneys are extremely enlarged and the parenchymal echostructure is deeply modified: there is an extremely bright echonephrogram throughout, with loss of corticomedullary differentiation and of the central echoes complex, and a limited number of small macrocysts is usually seen with modern equipment. The extremely high echogenicity of the kidneys is due to the multiple interfaces between the cysts. In this age group, pathologi-

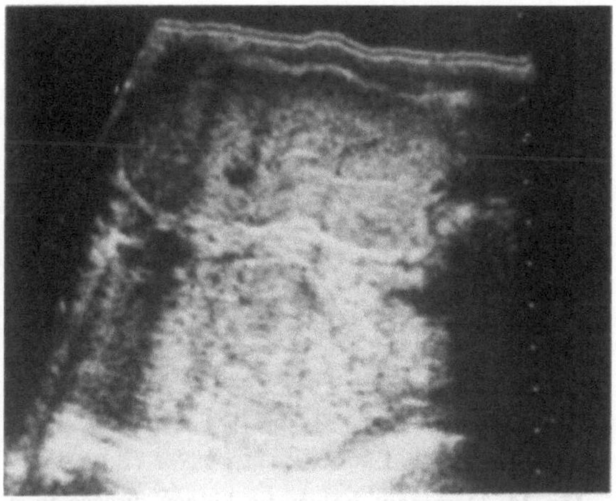

Fig. 19. Recessive polycystic disease in neonate (longitudinal axillary scan). Both kidneys are extremely enlarged, touching one another at the midline; bright echonephrogram is seen throughout the whole parenchyma. The corticomedullary differentiation and renal sinus are no longer visible. A macrocyst is apparent in the upper kidney.

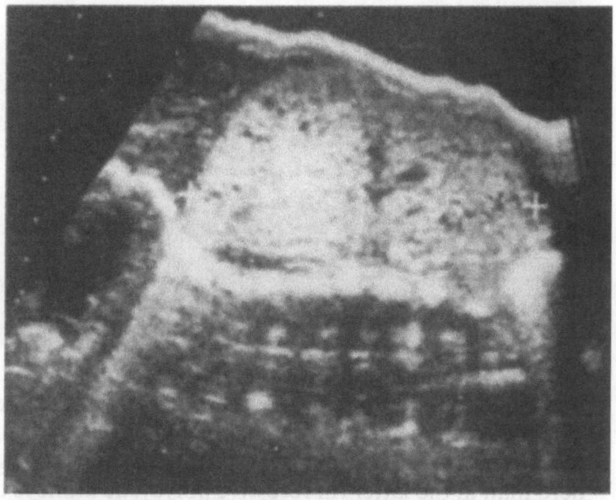

Fig. 20. Recessive polycystic kidneys in a neonate. Longitudinal supine scan of the right kidney. In this 11 cm hyperechoic kidney, several macrocysts are visible.

cally the cysts, although tubular in location, extend to the convexity of the kidney, which explains this diffuse sonographic pattern (Figs. 19 and 20).

In older children, the appearance is different: the kidneys remain enlarged, but the increased echogenicity is predominant (Fig. 21) in or confined to (Fig. 22) the medullary pyramids; renal macrocysts are smaller than 2 cm in diameter, and in our experience they do not increase in size as the child grows. Biliary cysts are often demonstrated in this age group in front of the portal radicles (Fig. 23).

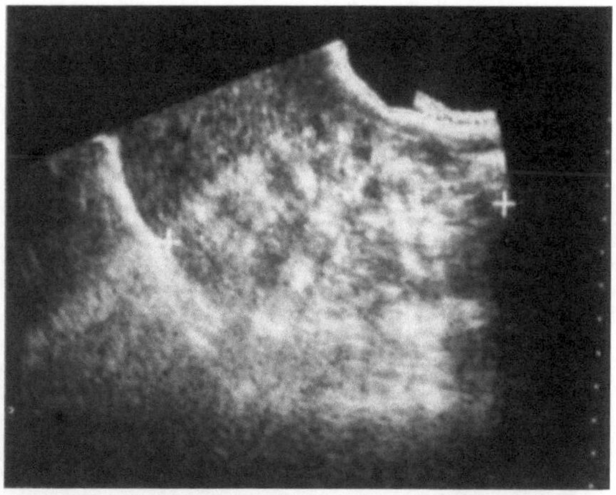

Fig. 21. Recessive polycystic kidneys in a 7-year-old patient. Longitudinal supine scan of the right kidney. The hyperechogenicity is more apparent in the medulla. The kidney remains huge.

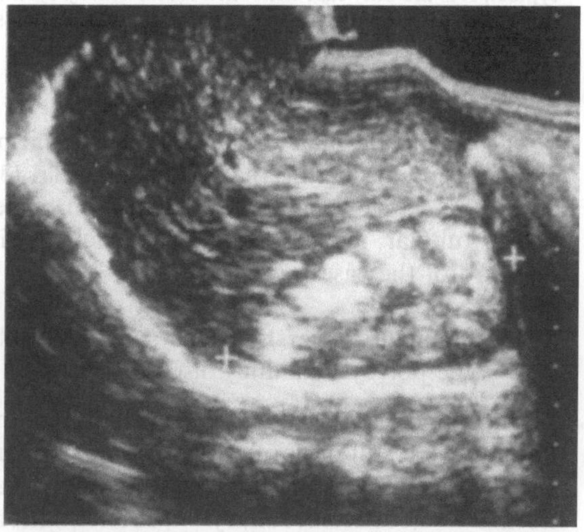

Fig. 22. Recessive polycystic kidneys in a 5-year-old girl. Right kidney seen on a longitudinal supine scan. Reserved intrarenal anatomy in an enlarged kidney. The hyperechoic pyramids reflect to tubular location of the cysts.

Hepatic involvement is generally inapparent clinically in patients with pronounced renal involvement and vice versa; severe hepatic involvement (often called congenital hepatic fibrosis) leads to portal hypertension. While studying the kidneys of patients with congenital hepatic fibrosis, we thought at first that sonography was normal because kidney size was often normal and most medullary pyramids were normally echolucent. However, by scanning the kidneys very carefully it appeared that a few pyramids were echoic. This partially abnormal echonephrogram propably reflects the partial tubular involvement.

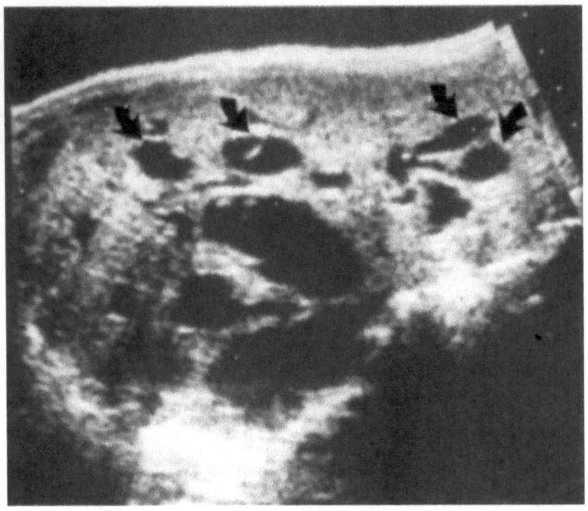

Fig. 23. Recessive polycystic disease in a 4-year-old girl. A right subcostal scan shows large biliary cysts (*arrows*). Large cysts are also visible in the posterior part of the liver. The echographic appearance of the kidneys is quite typical. It is the only case with such severe biliary cysts in our series of patients with recessive polycystic kidneys.

The diagnostic value of US in RPK should be emphasized considering that in our material (30 cases) the classic urographic presentation of delayed tubular opacification was lacking in onethird of the cases.

4.5.2 Dominant Polycystic Kidneys (DPK, adult type polycystic kidney disease)

In the four cases that we have seen in children, the kidneys were still of normal size and apart from the few macrocysts the intrarenal anatomy was normal (corticomedullary differentiation) (Fig. 24). As in adults, US may show cysts that are not visible urographically. The limited number of cases of DPK in our material is at least partially due to the reluctance of the clinicians and geneticians in our institution to examine systematically the offspring of an affected family: (because of the inevitable feelings of guilt and anxiety of the parents).

In a newborn, the urographic and sonographic patterns were similar to a form of RPK, although some macrocysts were bigger than 2 cm in diameter. In such clinical cases, US of the parent's kidneys is the diagnostic key (Fig. 25).

4.5.3 Hereditary Syndromes with Renal Cysts

There are numerous syndromes of this type, two of which are relevant here. In tuberous sclerosis renal macrocysts may be seen from birth (Fig. 26).

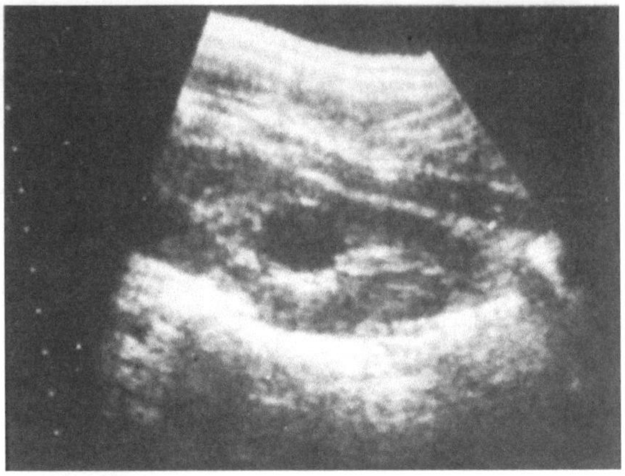

Fig. 24. Dominant polycystic kidney disease in a 6-year-old patient. Longitudinal prone scan of the left kidney. Single 2 cm cyst in an otherwise normal kidney.

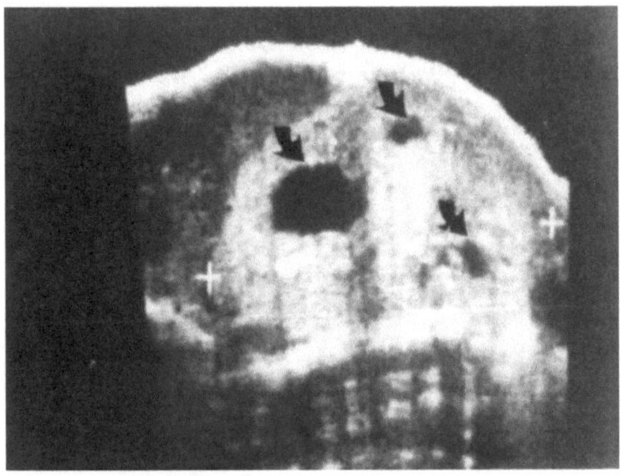

Fig. 25. Dominant polycystic kidney disease in a neonate. Longitudinal supine scan of the right kidney. The hyperechogenicity of the parenchyma is similar to a recessive form, but the macrocysts (*arrows*) appear larger here than in the latter (in recessive polycystic kidneys the cysts do not exceed 2 cm in diameter).

In Laurence-Moon-Bardet-Biedl syndrome (4 cases), the obesity of the patients results in a poor quality examination, but small medullary cysts can usually be demonstrated.

4.5.4 Juvenile Nephronophtisis (recessive medullary cystic disease of childhood)

Juvenile nephronophtisis represents 15% of the renal diseases leading to kidney transplantation in our institution. Its diagnosis may be difficult because genetic data are lacking in 50% of the cases, and renal biopsy may only display a chronic tubulointestitial nephritis as the medullary cysts are missed on a random biopsy. The main clinical feature of nephronophtisis is the asymptomatic

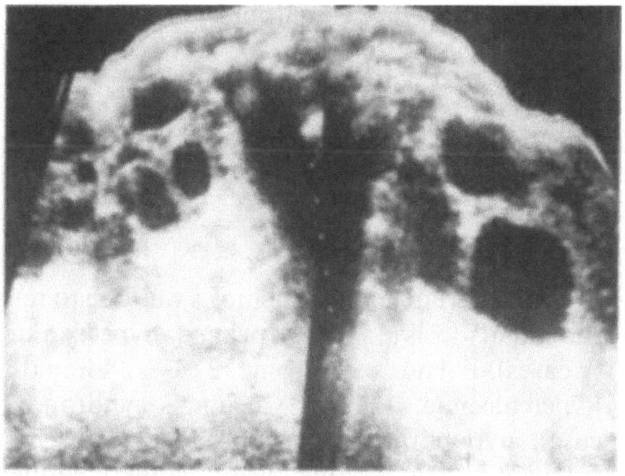

Fig. 26. Tuberous sclerosis in a 6-month-old baby girl. Transverse prone scan of both kidneys. Multiple renal cysts are demonstrated. The suggestive neurological symptoms appeared later.

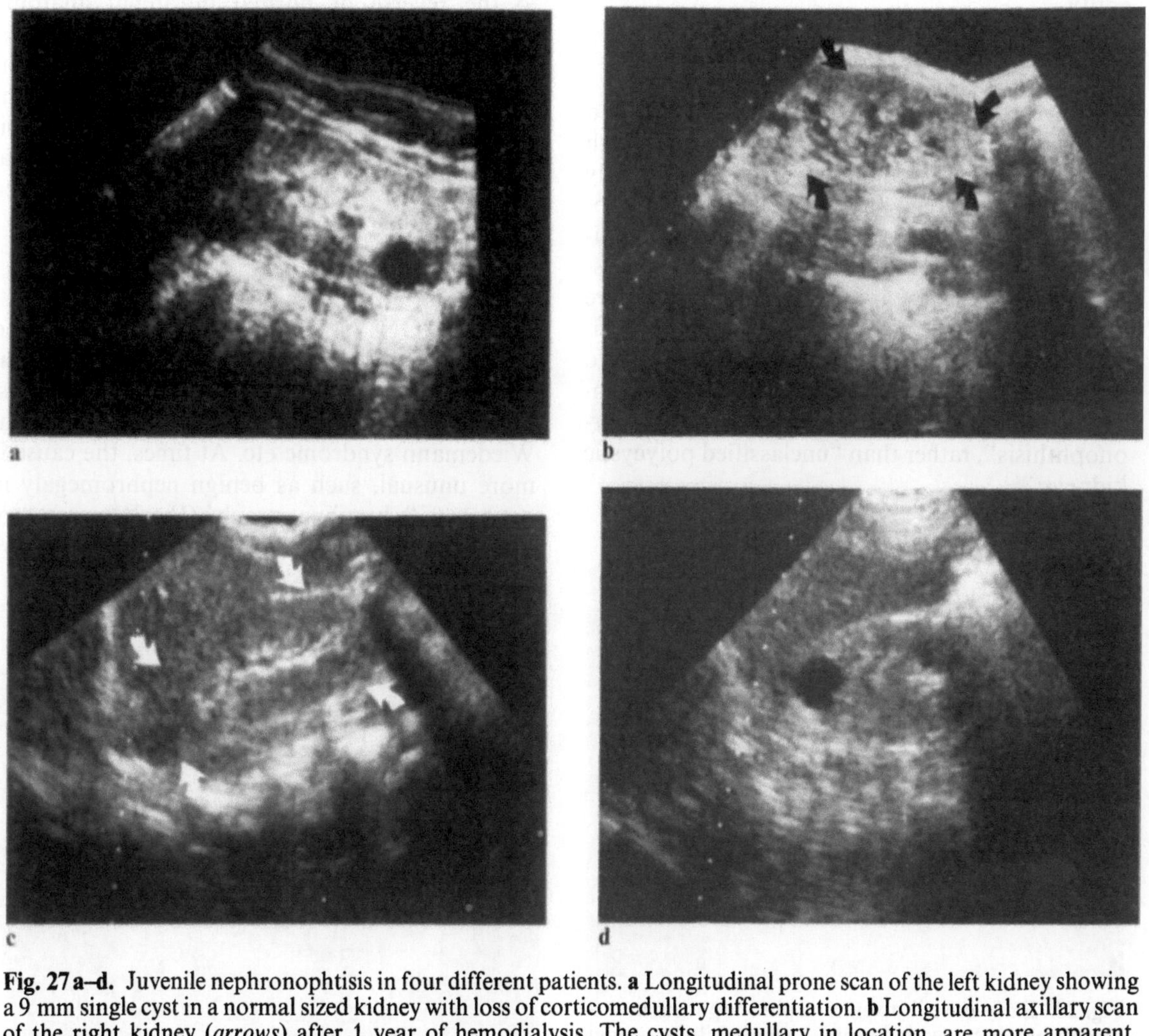

Fig. 27 a–d. Juvenile nephronophtisis in four different patients. **a** Longitudinal prone scan of the left kidney showing a 9 mm single cyst in a normal sized kidney with loss of corticomedullary differentiation. **b** Longitudinal axillary scan of the right kidney (*arrows*) after 1 year of hemodialysis. The cysts, medullary in location, are more apparent. **c** Longitudinal supine scan of the right (*arrows*) in a 4-year-old asymptomatic patient. There is complete loss of corticomedullary differentiation and increased parenchymal echogenicity. No cyst is present at this stage. **d** Sister of patient in **c.** Severe uremia. Longitudinal supine scan of the right kidney. A cyst is clearly seen in the upper pole. In patients with terminal renal failure, the presence of small medullary or corticomedullary cysts in almost normal-sized kidneys without corticomedullary differentiation is very suggestive of juvenile nephronophtisis.

period extending from birth to the age of 3–5 years. From that age the disease will then develop to chronic failure and terminal uremia. Characteristic features of the disease as shown by US (Fig. 27) in a series of 20 patients are: (a) a normal kidney length (which is extremely unusual in terminal uremia); (b) a loss of corticomedullary differentiation, the sinus remaining apparent; (c) an increased parenchymal echogenicity; (d) above all, cysts, either medullary or corticomedullary, small in size, and limited in number. Periodic dialysis will often increase the size of these cysts.

We have already mentioned the rarity of extensive cysts in end-stage kidneys in children outside juvenile nephronophtisis. US can therefore make an important contribution to the diagnosis of this entity.

4.5.5 Unclassified Hereditary Cystic Disease

We have studied by US four patients who had terminal kidney failure very early in life (at birth or in infancy) whose kidneys were not, or only moderately, enlarged and were filled with macrocysts (Fig. 28). Such a presentation is thus clinically and sonographically different from polycystic kidney diseases. Pathologically the cysts were associated with extensive tubulointerstitial fibrosis. Because of the histological similarity to nephronophthisis, Habib has suggested (Hannover, 1983) the term "early-onset juvenile nephronophthisis", rather than "unclassified polycystic kidneys."

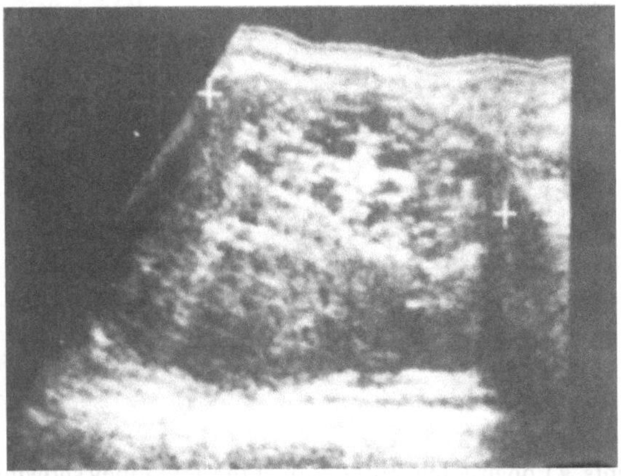

Fig. 28. "Early-onset" juvenile nephronophtisis in a 9-month-old baby with terminal renal failure. Longitudinal prone scan of the right kidney. Several macrocysts are seen in a slightly enlarged (72 mm) kidney. This pattern is thus different from recessive and dominant polycystic kidneys. A first stillborn baby had the same lesions.

4.6 Miscellaneous Conditions

4.6.1 Renal Artery Thrombosis

The kidney is sonographically normal for several weeks and then shrinks considerably.

4.6.2 Nephrocalcinosis

In our material, nephrocalcinosis was due to renal tubular acidosis (15 cases), primary hyperoxaluria (9 cases), Bartter's syndrome (2 cases), idiopathic hypercalcemia (1 case), Cushing's syndrome (1 case), hypoparathyroidism (1 case). The most frequent and suggestive pattern is the medullary form of nephrocalcinosis, where the pyramids become more echogenic than the cortex, leading to the reverse of normal intrarenal anatomy (Fig. 29). Posterior shadowing is sometimes present, depending on the amount of calcium. Nevertheless, US is far more sensitive than X-rays in the search for nephrocalcinosis. Nephrocalcinosis may also be cortical or corticomedullary in location and may be associated with calculi (especially in primary hyperoxaluria) (Fig. 30).

4.6.3 Nephromegalies

Besides AGN, NS, lymphomas, leukemias and solid tumors, there are numerous causes of enlarged kidneys: polycystic disease, amyloidosis, sickle cell disease, hyperalimentation, Beckwith-Wiedemann syndrome etc. At times, the cause is more unusual, such as benign nephromegaly in patients with hemihypertrophy (Fig. 31) or nephromegaly in Wiskott-Aldrich syndrome. We have

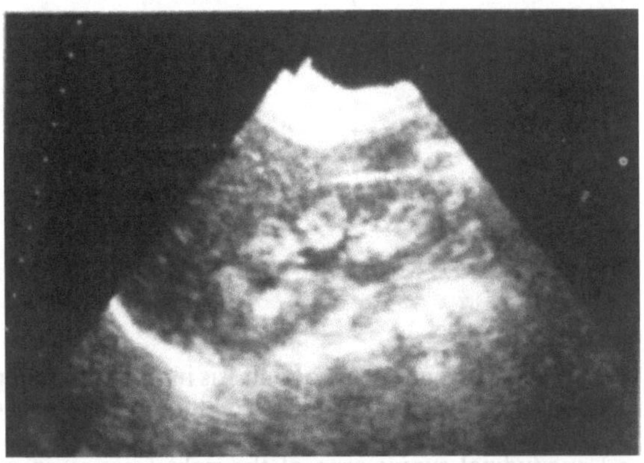

Fig. 29. Medullary nephrocalcinosis. (Renal tubular acidosis) seen in a longitudinal supine scan of the right kidney. Reversed intrarenal anatomy in a normal-sized kidney. There is no posterior shadowing in this case.

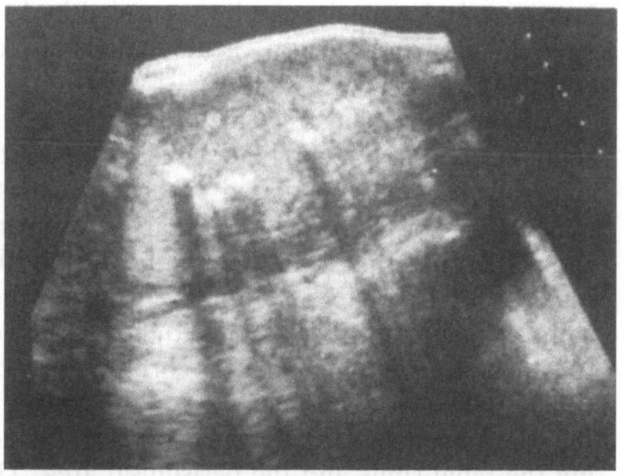

Fig. 30. Recurrent hyperoxaluria in a transplanted kidney. Global nephrocalcinosis (cortical and medullary) associated with stones. Primary hyperoxaluria is the second cause of nephrocalcinosis in children after renal tubular acidosis.

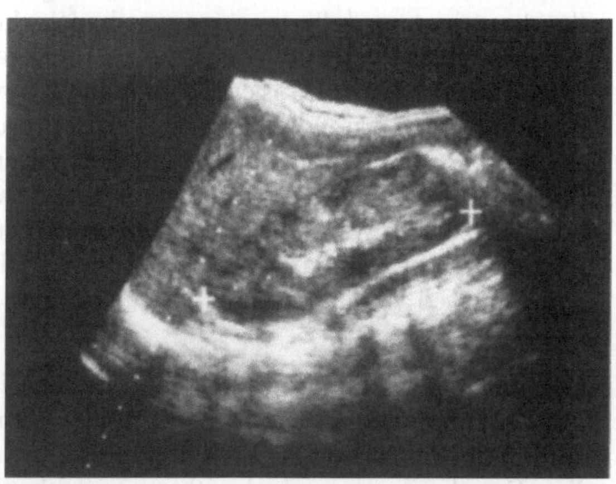

Fig. 31. Benign nephromegaly in a newborn with hemihypertrophy. Longitudinal supine scan of the right kidney. Normal corticomedullary differentiation in a 8.6 cm kidney. Normal pathology at surgical biopsy. No change during sonographic follow-ups.

even seen a case of marked nephromegaly in a child undergoing periodic dialysis for several years (Fig. 32).

4.6.4 Cystinosis (8 cases)

Cystinosis on the other hand shows considerable atrophy of the kidneys under hemodialysis.

4.6.5 Corticomedullary and Perimedullary Dotted Line

Interlobar and arcuate vessels run between and around the medullary pyramids. They are usually visible as a small single or double echoic dots

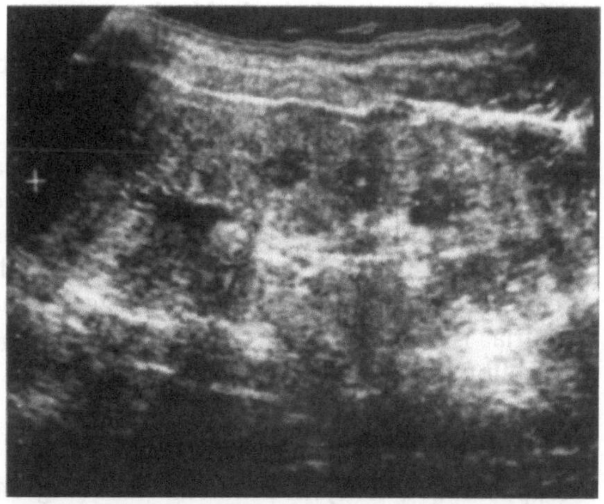

Fig. 32. Extreme nephromegaly (16 cm) with preserved corticomedullary differentiation in a child undergoing dialysis for 4 year. Longitudinal prone scan of the left kidney. Renal biopsy was not performed because of coagulation disorders. Probable storage disease.

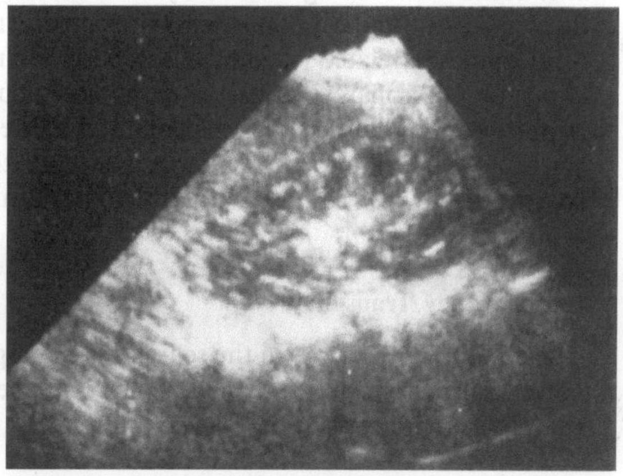

Fig. 33. Pseudoxanthoma elasticum in a 10-year-old hypertensive patient. Longitudinal supine scan of the right kidney showing increased marking of the arcuate vessels at the base of the pyramids. Normal arteriogram; superficial temporal artery biopsy showed calcifications in the medial elastic membrane.

between the pyramids (interlobar arteries) and at their base (arcuate arteries).

We have seen seven patients with high blood pressure and high level of renin where renal angiography was normal, and where US showed excessive intrarenal vascular landmarks. Superficial temporal artery biopsy and renal biopsy proved this pattern to be caused by fibrosis and calcifications in the wall of small arteries. Small vessel calcifying arteritis appears to be a cause of renovascular hypertension in children only displayed by US (Fig. 33).

4.6.6 Transient Anuria in the Newborn

Transient anuria in the newborn is well known by neonatologists. US shows a very specific pattern: the kidneys are of normal size and the cortex is also normal, but the medullary pyramids appear very echogenic. This increased medullary echogenicity subsides within a few days, from the base to the apex of the pyramids, parallel to the reappearing diuresis. This change suggests that anuria is related to a transient tubular obstruction.

4.6.7 Acute Bacterial Focal Nephritis (3 cases)

It appears as a noncystic intrarenal mass (Fig. 34), US being performed in cases of long-duration fever and/or flank pain. Like renal abcesses (4 cases), acute bacterial focal nephritis is treated medically, US following the return to normal of the kidney. Urinary infection is not always present, some cases being secondary to hematogenous spread. Similarly, anuria may occur during septicemia (unrelated to shock) the latter being clinically not apparent at first (4 cases): the acute nephritis is then diffuse and the enlarged kidneys show a marked increased echogenicity of the cortex that will subside gradually under antibiotics.

4.6.8 Kidney Transplant

The contribution of US in the search for urologic complications is well known. Let us recall here that hydronephrosis (due to ureteroureteral or ureterovesical stenosis) can be concealed by kidney shut-down (due to acute rejection for example).

The literature has stressed the value of US in acute rejection (Fig. 35): increased kidney size, enlarged pyramids, increased cortical thickness, hypoechoic or hyperechoic focal areas. One should certainly insist on the modification of the renal sinus. In acute rejection, the central echocomplex is no longer visible due to the pressure of the edematous parenchyma; in chronic rejection (the so-called vascular rejection) on the contrary, the central echoes are more pronounced, including the renal sinus and the perisinusal area. The "excessive" central echoes reflect the thickening of the wall of main renal artery branches seen in chronic rejection.

In several patients with acute rejection, the cortex was subdivided into two zones (Fig. 36): the deep, juxtamedullary cortex was hyperechogenic, whereas the rest of the cortex was normal. This appearance was transient. Although we have no pathological proof (most biopsies do not reach the deep cortex) it seems likely that this pattern illustrates the different perfusion of these two cortical zones. We have also seen this perimedullary "ring" in native kidneys with partially compromised vascularization.

Diagnostic plans taking into account kidney size and renal echostructure are a very useful working tool in our institution, as shown in the following list. For the items marked with an asterisk, the

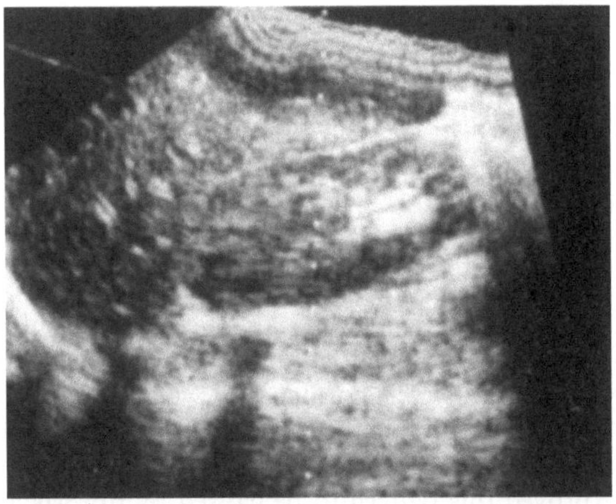

Fig. 34. Acute focal bacterial nephritis in a 10-year-old girl. Longitudinal supine scan of the right kidney shows enlargement of the upper pole with localized mass effect on the sinus. There was complete recovery under IV administration of antibiotics.

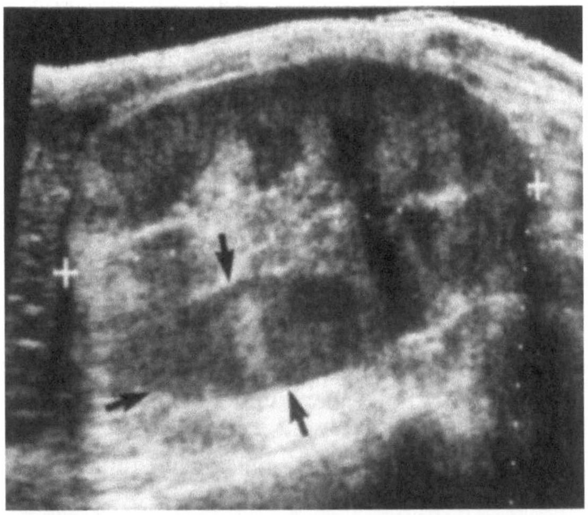

Fig. 35. Acute rejection of a renal transplant. Swollen, ovoid transplant and hypoechoic focal area (*arrows*). The modifications of the central sinus echoes are the most reliable features of rejection.

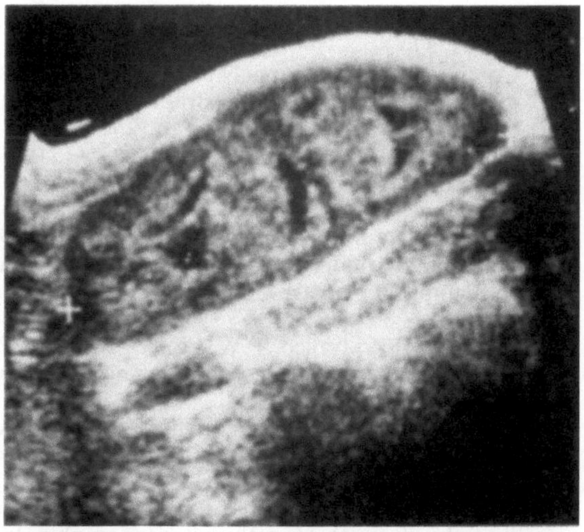

Fig. 36. Renal transplant with "perimedullary crown" pattern. After several episodes of acute rejection, two different zones of cortical echoes were noted: one peripheral and one central. This pattern may reflect the different vascularization of the superficial and deep cortices.

renal cortical echogenicity is superior to hepatic and/or splenic echogenicity.

Enlarged kidneys

Loss of corticomedullary differentiation (CMD)
- RVT*
- RPK (newborns; infants)*
- Congenital NS of Finnish type (infant, older than 3 months)*
- Storage and infiltrative disease*

Reversed CMD
- RPK (children)

Preservation of CMD
- RVT (early stage)
- AGN*
- NS (except congenital Finnish type NS)*
- Shock kidneys*
- Glomerular HUS*

Small kidneys

Loss of CMD
- End stage kidneys*
- Dysplastic hypoplastic kidneys*

Preservation of CMD
- Oligomeganephronia (early stage)*
- Simple hypoplasia

Normal or only slightly modified renal length

Loss of CMD
- Juvenile nephronophthisis (+medullary cysts)*

Reversed CMD
- Medullary nephrocalcinosis
- Transient anuria in the newborn

Preservation of CMD
- ATN
- Renal artery thrombosis and arterial HUS
- Small vessel calcifying arteritis (corticomedullary dotted line)

There is no doubt that in pediatric nephrology pathology has the final word; however, a definite advantage of US over renal biopsy is the visualization of the entire kidney whereas the latter shows only a small part of the "puzzle" and therefore can miss specific lesions.

References

General references

1. Royer P., Broyer M., Habib R., Mathieu H. (1973). Néphrologie Pédiatrique. Flammarion Ed. Paris
2. Edelman C.M. (1979). Pediatric kidney disease. Little Brown and Company, Boston
3. Cook J.H., Rosenfield A.T., Taylor K.J.W. (1977). Ultrasonic demonstration of intrarenal anatomy. A.J.R. 129:831
4. Haller J.O., Berdon W.E., Friedman A.P. (1982). Increased renal echogenicity: a normal finding in neonates and infants. Radiology 142:173–174
5. Moskowitz P.S., Carroll B.A., McCoy J.M. (1980). Ultrasonic renal volumetry in children: accuracy and simplicity of method. Radiology 134:61
6. Garel L., Lallemand D., Kalifa G. (1981). Radiologie de l'insuffisance rénale de l'enfant. E.P.U., Journées de Radiologie, Paris
7. Rosenfield A.T., Taylor K.J.W., Crade M., de Graaf C.S. (1978). Anatomy and pathology of the kidney by gray-scale ultrasound. Radiology 128:737
8. Rosenfield A.T., Siegel N.J. (1981). Renal parenchymal disease: histopathologic-sonographic correlation. A.J.R. 137:793

Acute renal failure

1. Garel L., Habib R., Babin C., Lallemand D., Sauvegrain J., Broyer M. (1983). Hemolytic-uremic syndrome. Diagnostic and prognostic value of ultrasound. Ann. Radiol. 26:169–174
2. Rosenberg E.R., Trought W.S., Kirks D.R. (1980). Ultrasonic diagnosis of renal vein thrombosis in neonates. A.J.R. 134:35
3. Braun B., Weileman L.S., Weigand W. (1981). Ultrasonographic demonstration of renal vein thrombosis. Radiology 138:157
4. Silverman P.M., Carroll B.A., Moskowitz P.S. (1980). Adrenal sonography in renal agenesis and dysplasia. A.J.R. 134:600
5. Hoffman J.C., Schnur M.J., Koenigsberg M. (1982). Demonstration of renal papillary necrosis by sonography. Radiology 145:785

6. Hricak H., Romanski R.N., Eyler W.R. (1982). Renal sinus during allegraft rejection: sonographic and histopathologic findings. Radiology 142:693
7. Avni F., Spehl - Robberecht M., Lebrun D., Gomes H., Garel L. (1983). Transient acute tubular disease in the newborn: characteristic ultrasound pattern. Ann. Radiol. 26:175–182

Miscellaneous conditions

1. Le Quesne G.W. (1978). Assessment of glomerulonephritis in children by ultrasound. In ultrasound in Medicine. Ed. White D., Lyons E.A., New York, Plenum Press
2. Kay C.J., Rosenfield A.T., Taylor K.J.W. (1979). Ultrasonic characteristics of chronic atrophy pyelonephritis. A.J.R. 132:47
3. Pariente D. (1981). Contribution de l'échographie à l'étude des maladies kystiques héréditaires des reins de l'enfant. Thèse, Paris, Necker Enfants Malades
4. Artaud J., Broussin B., Cadier L., Diard F. (1980). Aspects échographiques des polykystoses hépatorénales récessives chez ll'enfant. J. Radiol. 61:243–249
5. Thomas J.L., Summer T.E., Crowe J.E. (1978). Neonatal detection and evaluation of infantile polycystic disease by gray-scale echography. J.C.U. 6:295
6. Boal D.K., Littlewood-Teele R. (1980). Sonography of infantile polycystic kidney disease. A.J.R. 135:575–580
7. Rosenfield A.T., Siegel N.J., Kappelman N.B. (1977). Gray-scale ultrasonography in medullary cystic disease of the kidney and congenital hepatic fibrosis with tubular ectasia: new observations. A.J.R. 129:297–303
8. Rosenfield A.T., Lipson M.H., Wolf B., Taylor K.J.W., Rosenfield N.S., Hendler E. (1980). Ultrasonography and nephrotomography in the diagnosis of dominantly inherited polycystic kidney disease. Radiology 135:423–427
9. Stapleton F.B., Johnson D., Kaplan G.W. (1980). The cystic renal lesion in tuberous sclerosis. J. Ped. 97:574–579
10. Cacciarelli A.A., Young N., Levine A.J. (1978). Gray-scale ultrasonic demonstration of nephrocalcinosis. Radiology 128:459
11. Shuman W.P., Mack L.A., Rogers J.V. (1981). Diffuse nephrocalcinosis: hyperechoic sonographic appearance. A.J.R. 136:830
12. Wilson D.A., Wenzl J.E., Altschuler G.P. (1979). Ultrasound demonstration of diffuse cortical nephrocalcinosis in a case of primary hyperoxaluria. A.J.R. 132:659
13. Glazer G.M., Callen P.W., Filly R.A. (1982). Medullary nephrocalcinosis: sonographic evaluation. A.J.R. 138:55–57
14. Sauvegrain J., Garel L., Pariente D. (1983). Sonography of nephrocalcinosis in Cushing syndrome (letter). A.J.R. 140:833–834
15. Subramanyan B.R. (1981). Renal amyloidosis in juvenile rheumatoid arthritis: sonographic features. A.J.R. 136:411
16. Rosenfield A.T., Glickman M.G., Taylor K.J.W., Grade M., Hodson J. (1979). Acute focal bacterial nephritis (acute lobar nephromia). Radiology 132:553
17. Lee J.K.T., McClennan B.L., Meson G.L. (1980). Acute focal bacterial nephritis. Emphasis on gray-scale sonography and computed tomography. A.J.R. 135–87
18. Frick M.P., Feinberg S.B., Sibley R., Idstrom M.E. (1981). Ultrasound in acute renal transplant rejection. Radiology 138:657
19. Graif M., Silon M., Strauss S., Manor A., Itz Y. (1982). Congenital nephrosis: ultrasonographic features. Pediatr. Radiol. 12:154–155
20. Garel L., Sauvegrain J., Filiatrault D. (1983). Dominant polycystic kidney disease in a neonate. Ann. Radiol. 86:183–186
21. Garel L., Habib R., Pariente D., Broyer M., Sauvegrain J. Juvenile nephronophtisis: a pathognomonic sonography appearance in children with severe uremia. Radiology (in press)

Chapter 10

Retroperitoneal Tumors

L. Garel, P. Devred, and J. Leclere

1 Material

The diagnosis of a retroperitoneal tumor is mainly based on the data obtained simultaneously by the IVP (AP and lateral) sonography and the biological tests (especially cathecolamines assays). CT is extremely valuable in assessing the extent of the process and in following the course of the disease under appropriate treatment.

Table 1. Cases studied.

Renal tumors			
Malignant		*Benign*	
Wilms' tumor	139	Mesoblastic nephroma	5
Hypernephroma	7	Neurofibroma	1
Sarcoma	3	Multilocular cyst	3
Lymphoma	12	Hydatid cyst	3
Leukemia	4	Angiomyolipoma	6
		Simple cyst	7
		Lymphangioma	1
		Cavernous angioma	2
		(Multicystic dysplasia 40)	
		(Polycystic kidney disease 35)	
		(Abscess 8)	
Extrarenal tumors			
Malignant		*Benign*	
Neuroblastoma	165	Pheochromocytoma	6
Sarcoma	5	Lymphangioma	6
Adrenal endocrine tumors	5	Adrenal hemorrhage	10
Adenopathies	25	Lipoma	2
Adrenal lymphoma	1	Schwannoma	1
		(Psoas hemorrhage 4)	
		(Psoas abscess 1)	
		(Urinoma 6)	

Our sonographic material of retroperitoneal tumors has been gathered over the last 4 years and includes patients examined in three institutions: Hôpital des Enfants-Malades (Paris), Institut Gustave Roussy (Paris), and Hôpital la Timone (Marseille) (see Table 1).

2 Technical Aspects

The US examination of a retroperitoneal tumor should include, if possible, longitudinal and transverse scans in supine, prone, and lateral decubitus positions. One should note, in particular:

1. The tumor size;
2. The tumor contours (well demarcated or not);
3. The tumor echostructure (echogenicity, cystic areas, calcifications);
4. The tumor interface from adjacent parenchymas;
5. The state of the liver, pancreas, and kidney;
6. The relations between the tumor and the vascular landmarks (IVC, aorta and branches, portal trunk and feeding veins, renal veins);
7. The presence of enlarged lymph nodes.

The examination should be performed in a systematic fashion; follow-up examinations, in fact, will be compared to the initial baseline study.

Our purpose, in this chapter, is only to mention some practical diagnostic features of US. We do not intend to compare US with other imaging modalities, nor to discuss extensively the literature.

3 Malignant Tumors

3.1 Wilms' Tumor

Most Wilms' tumors appear as a large mass, more than 10 cm in diameter in our 139 cases. The tumor is round or oval, well defined, often encapsulated, of solid, medium echogenicity usually with intratumoral cystic areas (Fig. 1 a).

The tumor is continuous with the normal renal parenchyma (Fig. 1 b and c). There are no enlarged nodes and no calcifications. Generally speaking, Wilms' tumors displace adjacent parenchymas and vessels without infiltrating them (Fig. 2). We have seen only two cases of tumoral extension into the IVC (Fig. 39) and in both cases the right atrium was free of tumor.

According to the European protocol for Wilms' tumors (International Society for Pediatric Oncology), most cases undergo 5 weeks of chemotherapy before surgery. Under chemotherapy the volume of the tumor decreases rapidly and notably (Fig. 3), often with evidence of intratumoral necrosis. Sometimes the size of the mass does not change, but the internal echostructure is greatly modified, illustrating the efficiency of chemotherapy (Fig. 4). Several specific points deserve a comment.

3.1.1 Bilateral Wilms' Tumors (12 cases)

In twothirds of our cases, Wilms' tumors were initially bilateral (Fig. 5), in the remaining four cases the other kidney was affected secondarily (in one case 8 years after the first tumor). Bilateral Wilms' tumors raise the question of an underlying

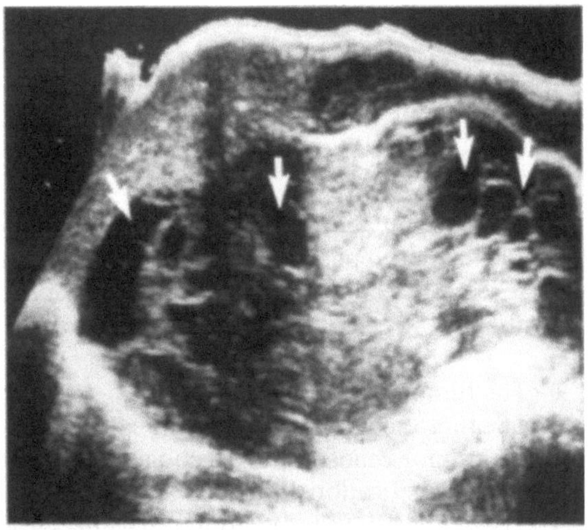
a

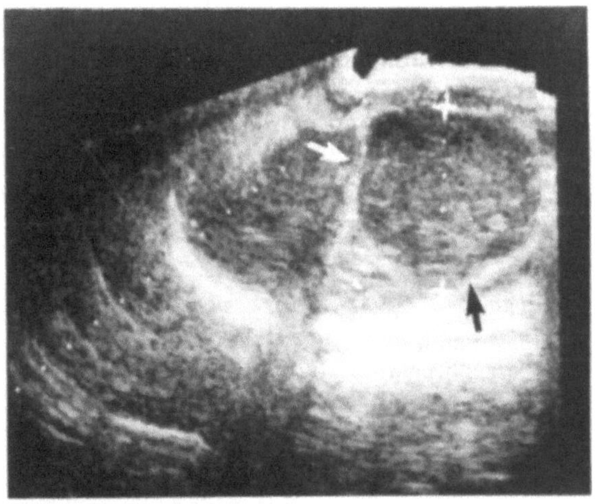
c

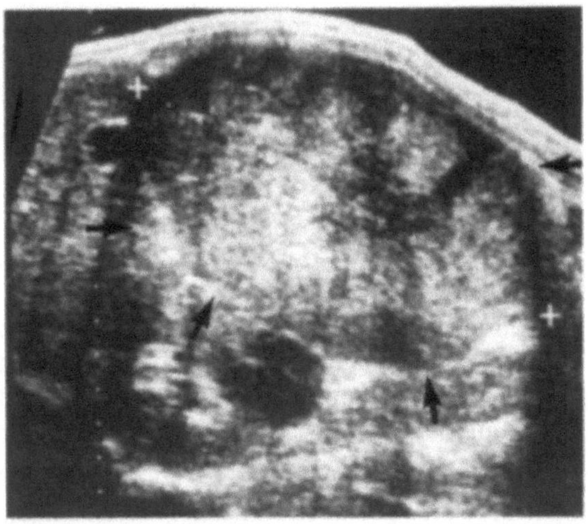
b

Fig. 1 a–c. Sonographic features of Wilms' tumor in three different patients.
a Longitudinal supine scan of the right upper quadrant in an 8-month-old girl. Large solid mass with several cystic components (*arrows*).
b Longitudinal supine scan of the right kidney in a 9-year-old patient showing 13 cm well circumscribed solid tumor (*arrows*) developed anteriorly from the lower aspect of the kidney.
c Longitudinal axillary scan of the left kidney in a 16-month-old girl. 5 cm solid tumor in continuity upwards and posteriorly with the normal renal parenchyma (*arrows*). The peripheral capsule, the intratumoral cystic areas, and the continuity with the normal kidney are hallmarks of Wilm's tumor.

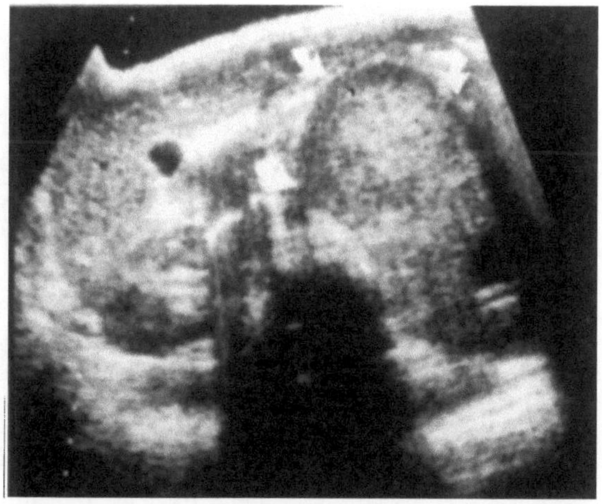

Fig. 2. Transverse supine scan showing a solid tumor arising from the anterior side of the left kidney in a 6-year-old child. The mass displaces the left lobe of the liver, the stomach, and the aorta. Wilms' tumor does not behave as an infiltrative neoplasm: for example, there is no local extension to the liver in Wilms' tumors.

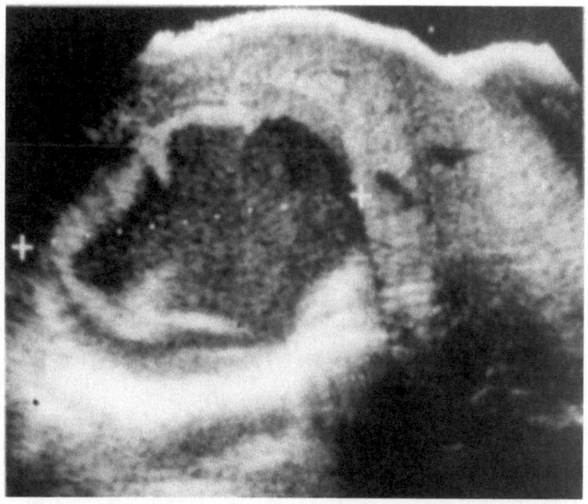

Fig. 4. Right Wilms' tumor after preoperative chemotherapy (transverse supine scan). No clinical reduction in size of the mass. The tumor is almost entirely necrotic. The efficiency of chemotherapy is only assessed by the modifications of the tumoral echostructure.

nephroblastomatosis which can only be assessed by multiple surgical biopsies.

3.1.2 **Nephroblastomatosis** (6 cases)

Sonographic features of nephroblastomatosis appear variable in our cases. In the diffuse variety, the kidneys are markedly enlarged, with irregular contours and cortical nodules that can be hypo-, iso-, or hyperechogenic. Corticomedullary differentiation is no longer visible and intratumoral cysts are possible (Fig. 6). It is usually impossible to differentiate by US simple nephroblastomatosis from nephroblastomatosis complicated by foci of a Wilms' tumor. Normal renal US does not rule out microscopic nephroblastomatosis and secondary development of Wilms' tumor.

Other associations are classic: hemihypertrophy, Beckwith-Wiedeman syndrome, aniridia, glomerular diseases (especially mesangial sclerosis). In the sonographic followup of these patients at risk we have not seen tumors that were not obvious clinically.

Drash triad is the association of mesangial sclerosis, male pseudohermaphroditism, and

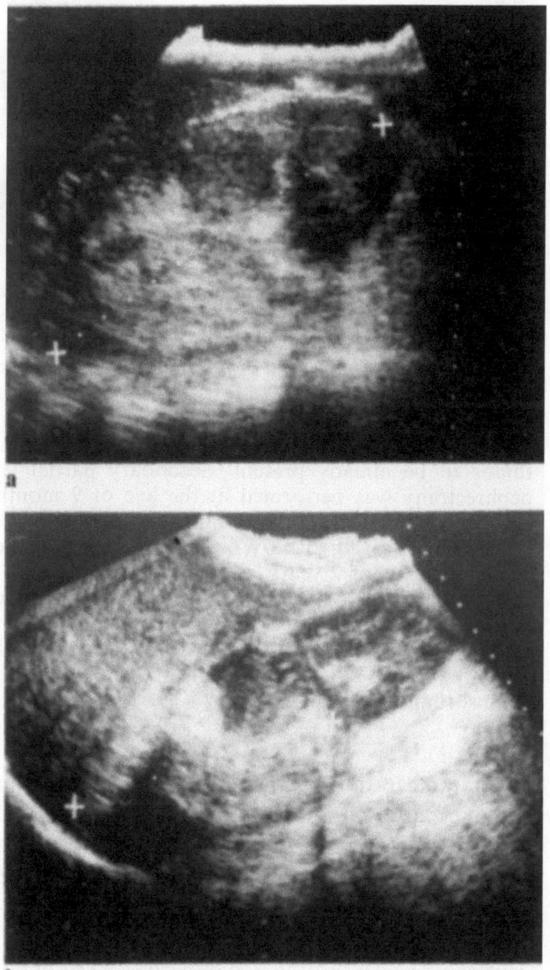

a

b

Fig. 3 a and b. Upper pole Wilms' tumor in a 3-year-old patient seen on longitudinal supine scans of the right kidney.
a Initially; **b** After chemotherapy. The tumor is smaller, the interface with the normal renal parenchyma is sharply delineated. (One notes again the separation from the adjacent liver.)

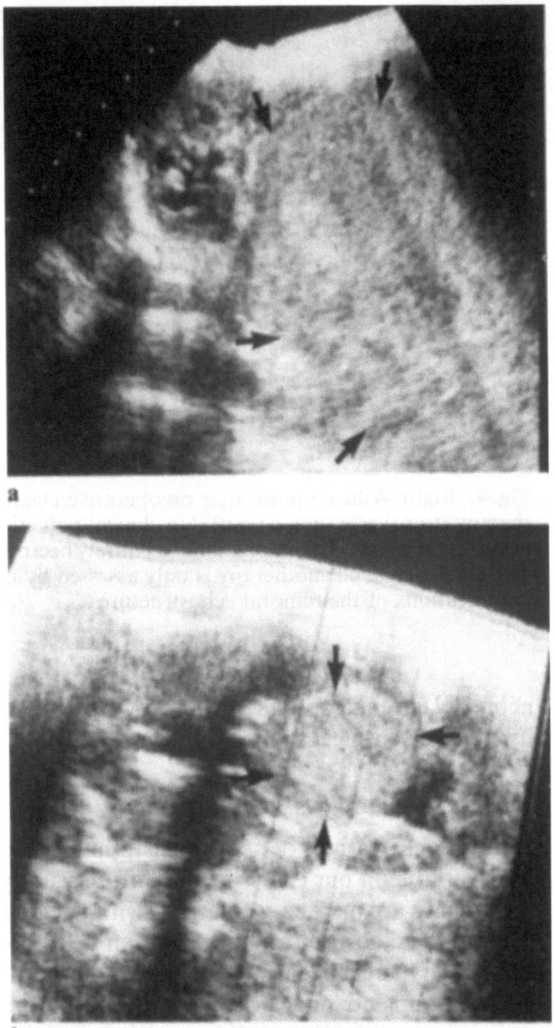

a

b

Fig. 5 a and b. Bilateral Wilms' tumor in a 13-month-old girl seen on longitudinal axillary scans.
a Right kidney. Huge inferior tumor, distinct from the normal kidney (*arrows*).
b Left kidney with a 2 cm nodule impinging upon the sinus (*arrows*). After chemotherapy, a right nephrectomy was performed followed by a partial left nephrectomy.

Wilms' tumor. In the two "complete" cases that we have seen, sonography was performed for different clinical indications: one patient presented with anuria (Fig. 7) and the second case was kept under observation for ambiguous genitalia with proteinuria.

Upper pole Wilms' tumors are often difficult to study, especially on the left side. The two calcified Wilms' tumors in our series arose from the upper pole of the kidney. One of these, on the left, was

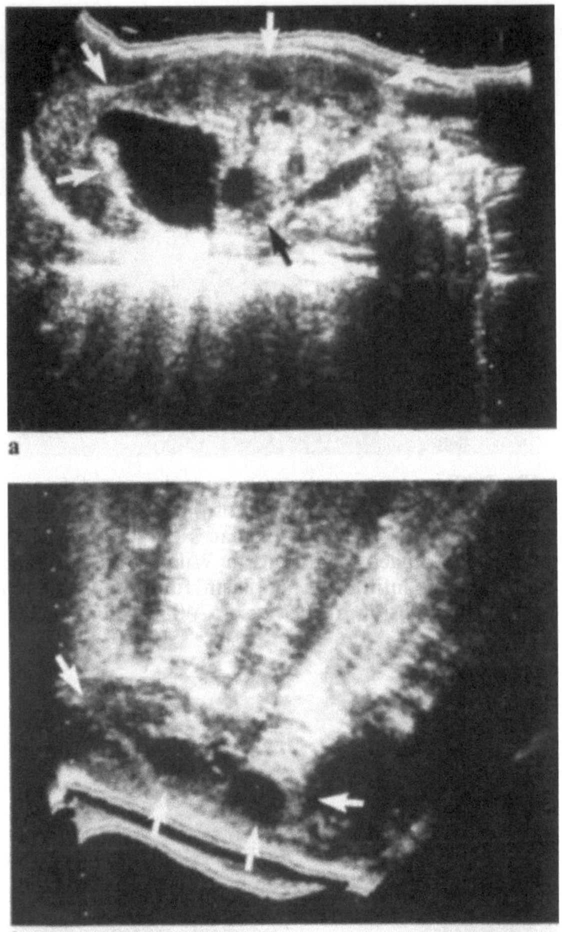

a

b

Fig. 6 a and b. Nephroblastomatosis in a 15-day-old infant. **a** Longitudinal supine scan of the right kidney infant.
a Longitudinal supine scan of the right kidney (*arrows*).
b Longitudinal prone scan of the left kidney (*arrows*). Unequal kidney size. Both kidneys show evidence of cysts. Right nephrectomy showed Wilms' tumor to be already present. Secondary partial left nephrectomy was performed at the age of 9 months because of an upper pole nodule picked up by US (which also proved to be Wilms' tumor). No further evidence of tumor 2 years later.
Nephroblastomatosis can be solid or cystic. US is of great help in ruling out recessive polycystic kidneys, the most common cause of bilateral neonatal nephromegaly. Only surgical biopsies will confirm the presence of a Wilms' tumor.

considered initially as a nonsecreting neuroblastoma because of the spatial relationship of the tumor to the pancreas (Fig. 8). In one case, the tumor appeared extrarenal and may have developed on a supernumary kidney (Fig. 9).

Some Wilms' tumors are *poorly demonstrated IVP,* while US easily displays the mass: these include silent kidneys (7 cases) and those with anterior or posterior origin of the tumor. The smallest tumor in our series falls into such a group (Fig. 10). Conversely the large centrorenal Wilms' tumors appear as an entirely tumoral kidney without evidence of normal parenchyma (Fig. 11).

Metastases that are well demonstrated and followed by US are in hepatic (7 cases) and peritoneal (5 cases) sites (Fig. 13). Hepatic metastases often occur early in the course of the disease, but sometimes later (5 years after nephrectomy in one case). Surgery is indicated in the case of a single lesion. When multiple, US can follow their involution (Fig. 12). Peritoneal metastases are secondary to the rupture of the tumor capsule either initially or at surgery: they occur therefore early.

Local recurrences after nephrectomy (4 cases) can easily be overlooked by US because of the displacement of the colon into the renal fossa. CT is then of great value.

3.2 Neuroblastoma

Suprarenal neuroblastomas are also large tumors, but usually not as large as Wilms' tumors. Above all, the tumor has ill-defined contours, no capsule,

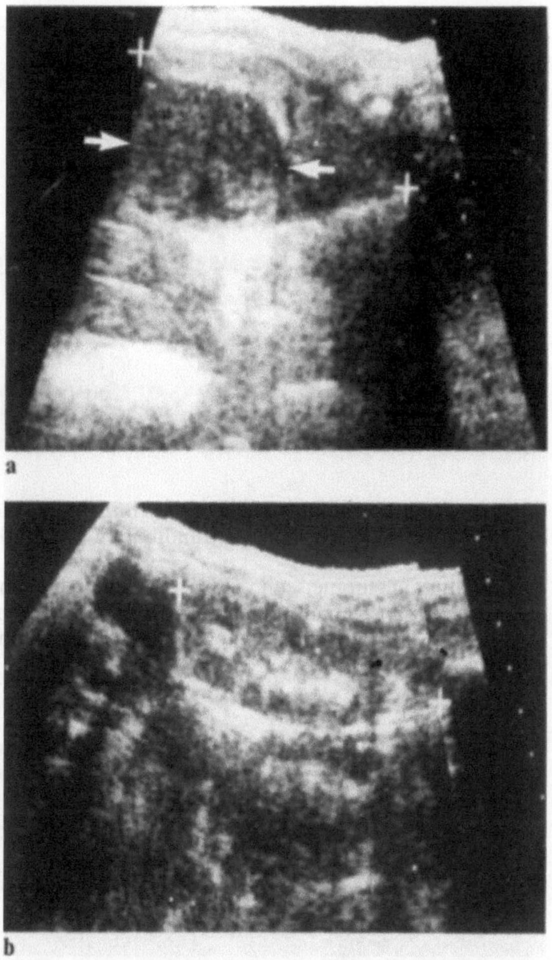

Fig. 7 a and b. Anuria in an 8-month-old patient with posterior hypospadias (longitudinal prone scans).
a Right kidney: 4 cm anterior Wilm's tumor (*arrow*).
b Left kidney: moderately enlarged (79 mm) kidney with normal pyramids and increased cortical echogenicity (same patient as in Fig. 16 of Chap. 9). The association between glomerular diseases and Wilms' tumors is are (30 reported cases) but classic.

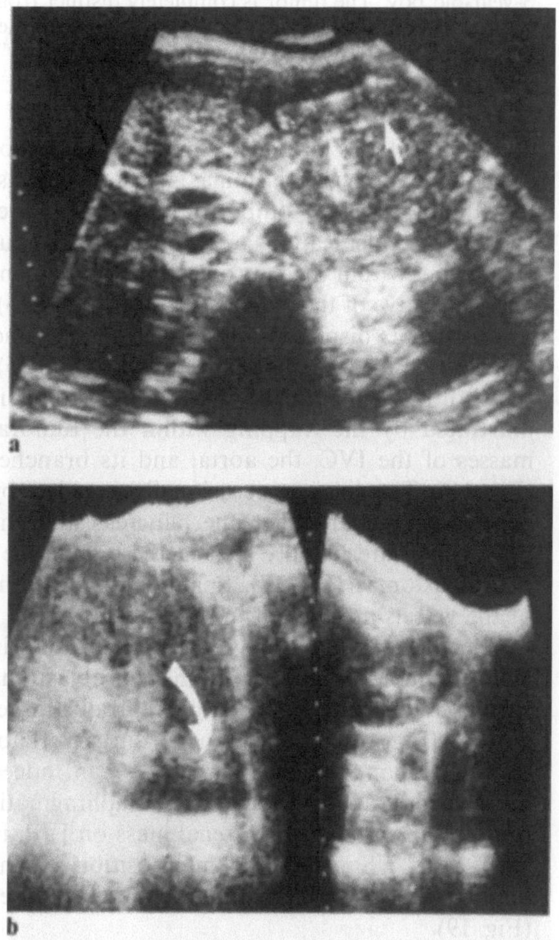

Fig. 8 a and b. Calcified left upper polar Wilms' tumor in a 4-year-old girl. Negative catecholamines.
a Transverse supine scan in the celiac region. The tumor displaces the pancreas forward (*arrows*), a feature suggestive of a neuroblastoma.
b Transverse prone scan. The left kidney is displaced medially (*arrow*), although suprarenal neuroblastomas usually displace the kidney laterally. The exact diagnosis was made at surgery.

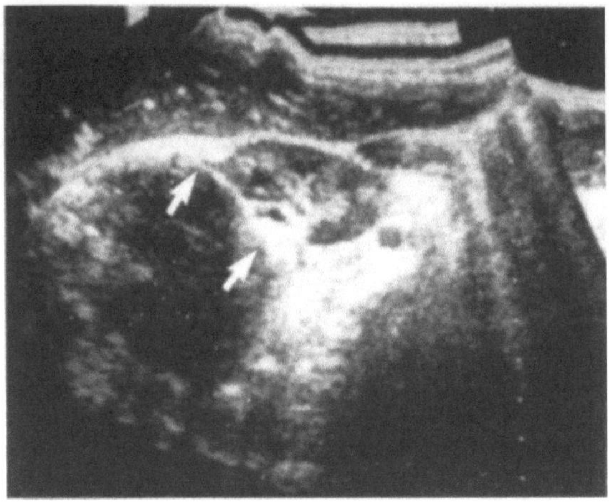

Fig. 9. Longitudinal supine scan of the right kidney in a 3-year-old boy. The tumor is completely distinct from the kidney. Surgical report of a Wilms' tumor "either extrarenal" or "developed on a supernumary kidney".

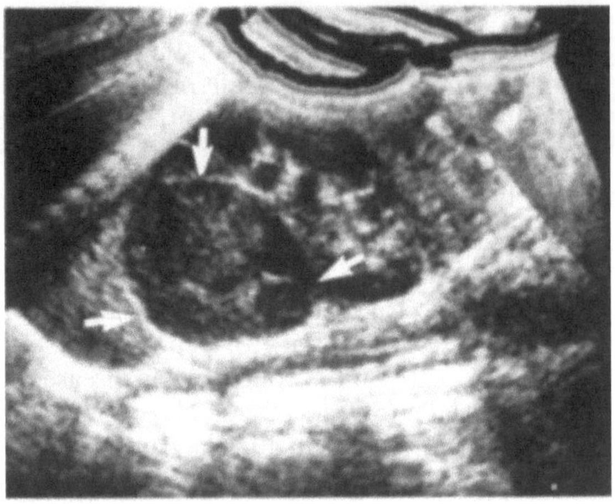

a

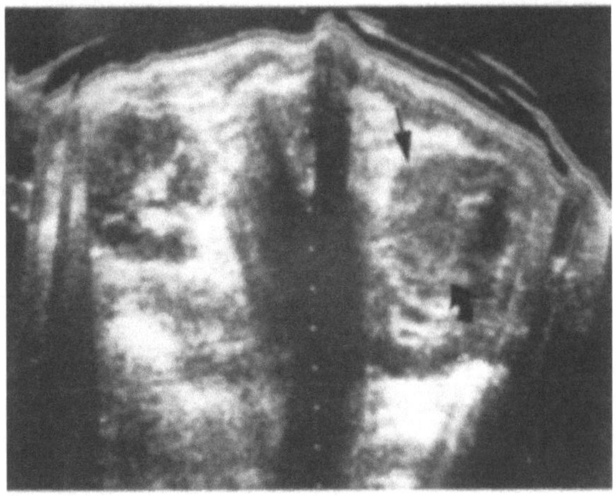

b

Fig. 10 a and b. Palpable right kidney in a 3-year-old girl. On the IVP the upper infundibulum was only slightly narrowed.
a Longitudinal supine scan of the left kidney; **b** Prone transverse scan. Small tumor (*arrows*), perfectly encapsulated, arising from the posterior aspect of the kidney.

and often extends beyond the midline. The echostructure of a neuroblastoma is heterogeneous; intratumoral cystic components are very rare. Evidence of calcifications or echoic areas without shadowing within the neuroblastoma is frequent and suggestive of the diagnosis (Figs. 14 and 15). The kidney is displaced inferiorly, laterally, and anteriorly. Enlarged nodes are common (Fig. 15); the infiltrative nature of the neuroblastoma is illustrated by the trapping within the tumoral masses of the IVC, the aorta, and its branches (Fig. 16). The liver is occasionally invaded by contiguity; in particular, the pancreas and the celia region are literally split in these "midline" neuroblastomas (Fig. 17). Spatial modifications of the vessels are present in 80% of the cases.

Chemotherapy is usually less efficient than in Wilms' tumors. In some cases, the neuroblastoma shrinks and becomes more echoic centrally (target pattern) (Fig. 18): it is then time for surgery. If not operated upon, the residual tumors can indeed grow again rapidly. Some supradiaphragmatic tumors can simulate an adrenal mass on IVP; in such cases US shows the interposition of the diaphragm between the tumor and the kidney (Fig. 19).

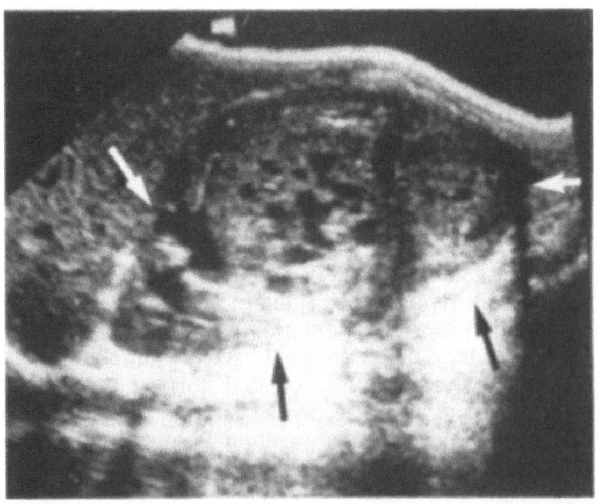

Fig. 11. Right centrorenal Wilms' tumor (outlined by *black and white arrows*) in 2-year-old patient (longitudinal supine scan). Its size of 12 cm is common for a Wilms' tumor. Several internal cysts are present. A peripheral hypoechoic halo can also be seen.

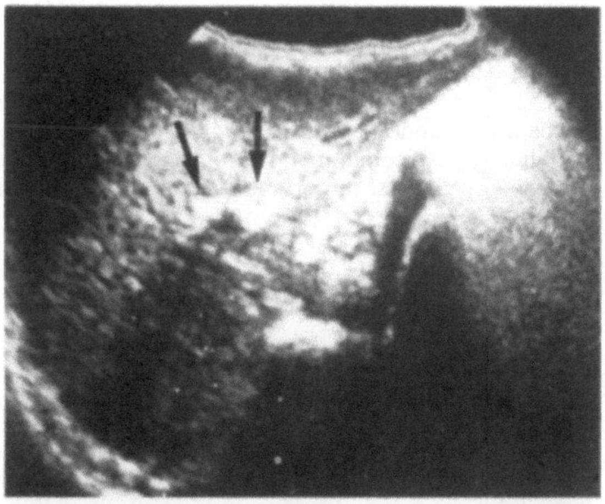

Fig. 12. Hepatic metastases from Wilms' tumor after chemotherapy (transverse supine scan). At biopsy the bright spots (*arrows*) only consisted of fibrous tissue and calcium deposits. The sonographic follow-up of such metastases appears very valuable in the assessment of their nonevolutivity.

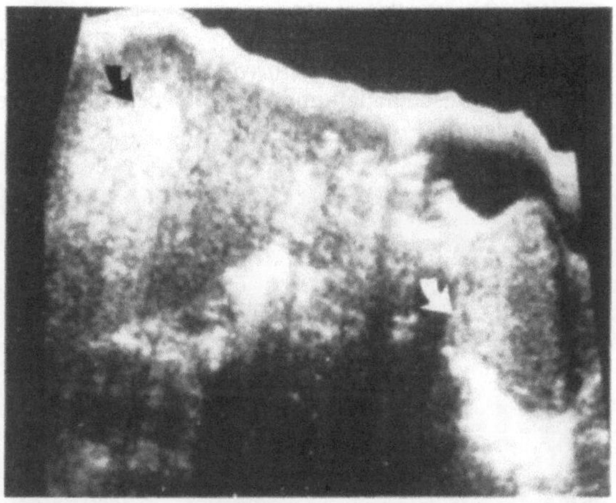

Fig. 13. Left nephrectomy for Wilms' tumor in a 4-year-old girl. Tumoral rupture at surgery. Hepatomegaly 1 month later (longitudinal scan to the right of the midline). Hepatic (*black arrow*) and Douglas' peritoneal recess (*white arrow*) metastases. Complete disappearance of the metastases under chemotherapy, which was confirmed during a surgical examination.

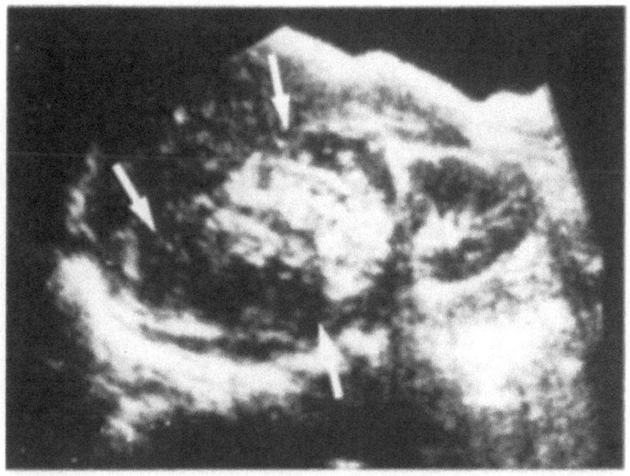

a

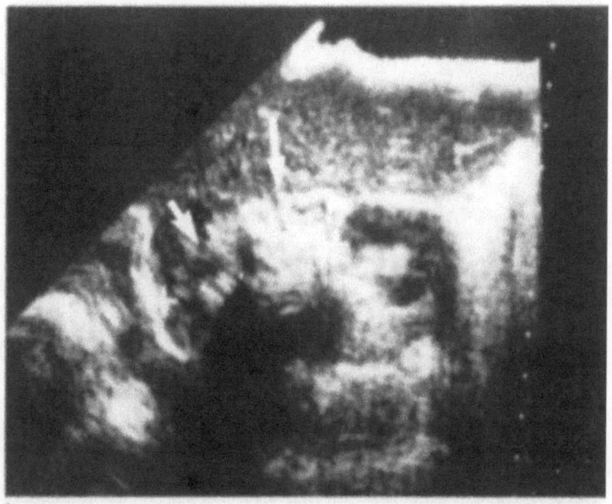

b

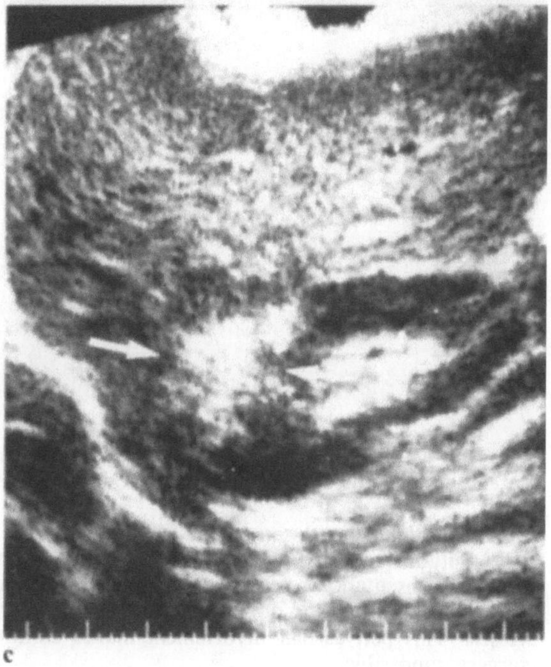

c

Fig. 14. Calcified right suprarenal neuroblastoma (*arrows*) seen on longitudinal supine scans in a 1-year-old boy. ▶
a Initially; **b** After 2 months of chemotherapy; **c** After 4 months of chemotherapy. The efficiency of chemotherapy, although often less active than in Wilms' tumor, is here quite impressive. A right nephrectomy was still necessary because of the tumoral infiltration of the upper pole of the kidney.

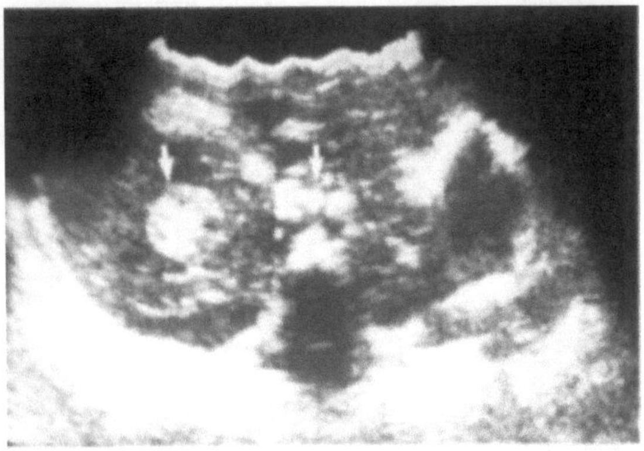

◀ **Fig. 15.** Right suprarenal neuroblastoma in a 15-month-old girl (transverse supine scan). The right paraspinal mass contains a very echoic nodule (*arrow* at left). There is also evidence of calcified inter-aorticocaval nodes (*arrow* at right). These enlarged lymph nodes are common in neuroblastomas and represent one of its most important diagnostic sonographic features.

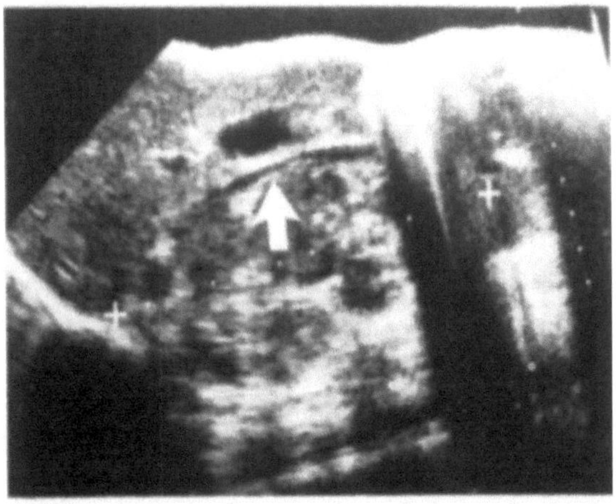

a

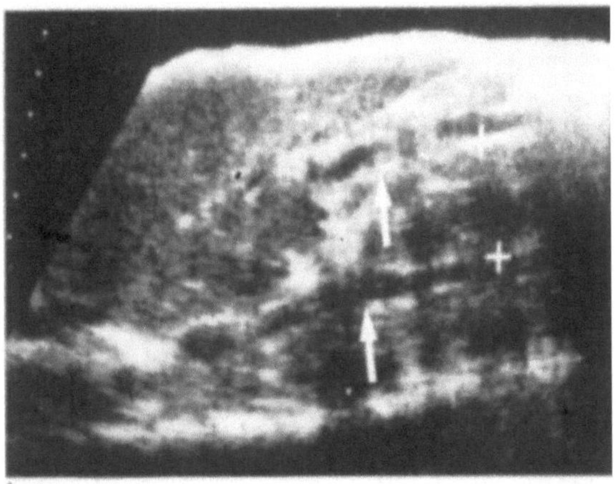

b

Fig. 16. "Midline" neuroblastoma in a 4-year-old girl, spreading around retroperitoneal and abdominal vessels.
a Longitudinal supine scan on the IVC (*arrow*);
b Longitudinal supine scan on the aorta (*top arrow*) and superior mesenteric vessels (*bottom arrow*). Anterior displacement of the IVC, aorta, and superior mesenteric vessels. This perivascular involvement makes curative surgery impossible.

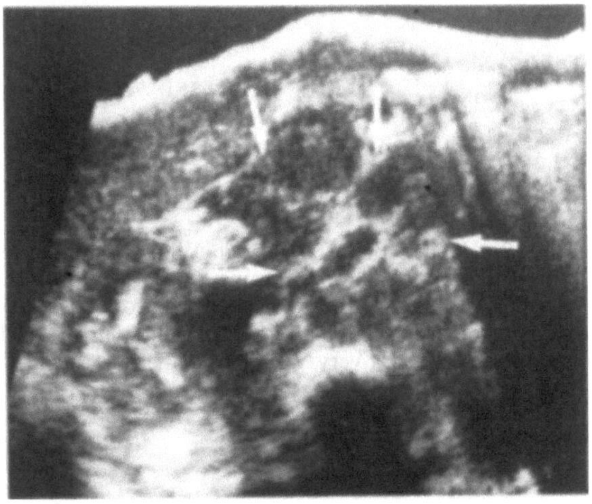

Fig. 17. "Midline" neuroblastoma in a 5-year-old patient seen on a transverse supine scan. "Blown-up" appearance of the pancreas (*arrows*). It is impossible to outline the vascular landmarks of the celiac and pancreatic regions.

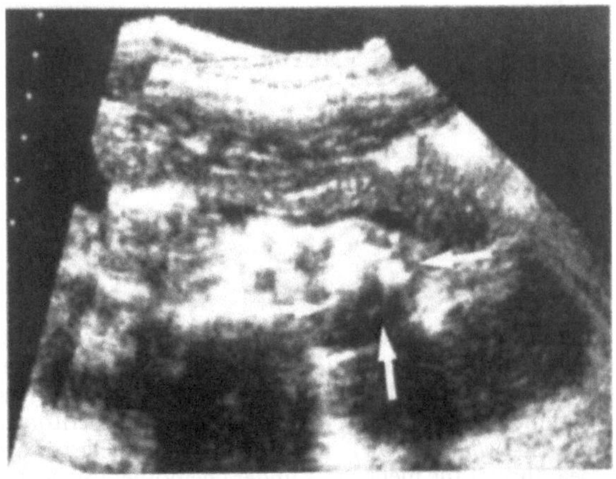

Fig. 18. Left suprarenal neuroblastoma after chemotherapy in a 5-year-old patient. Target-like pattern of the residual calcified tumor (*arrows*). The splenic vein lies anterior to the mass, the aorta and mesenteric vessels medially.

Subrenal neuroblastomas develop in the psoas: only the lower pole of the kidney is thus displaced laterally, anteriorly, and upwards. Sonography, in such locations, is more successful through an anterior or an axillary approach rather than in prone position (Fig. 20).

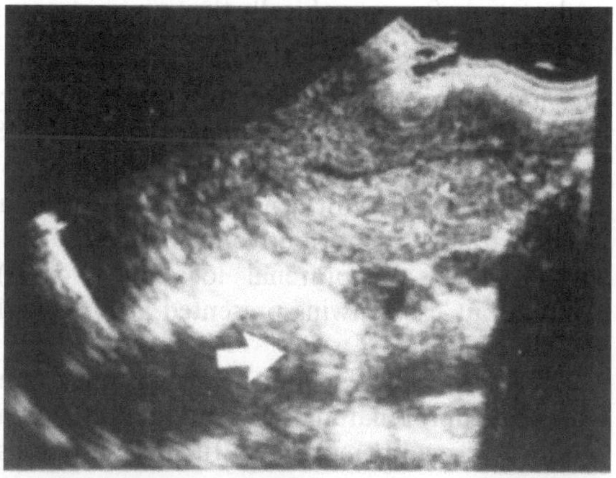

a

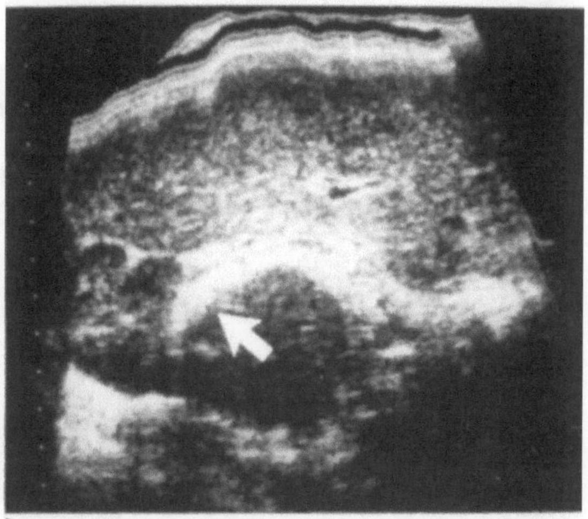

b

Fig. 19 a and b. Right supraphrenic neuroblastoma in a 4-year-old boy. The diaphragm, invaded by the tumor, is seen between the kidney and the mass (*arrows*).
a Longitudinal supine scan of the right kidney;
b Right subcostal supine scan.
Conventional radiology is unable to differentiate such a supradiaphragmatic tumor from a suprarenal tumor, US is therefore extremely valuable in imaging the diaphragm.

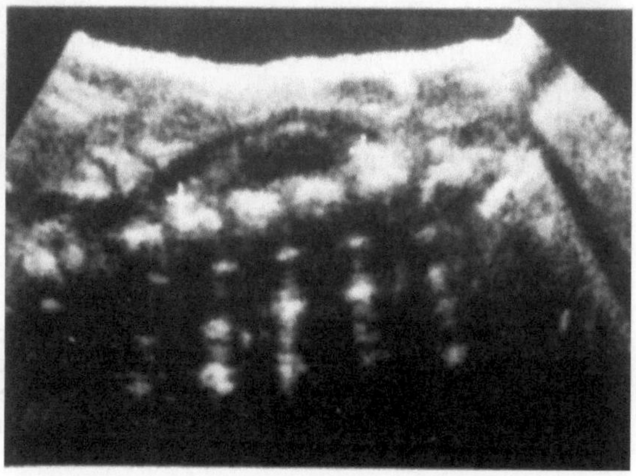

◄ **Fig. 20.** Left subrenal neuroblastoma in a 2-month-old infant (longitudinal supine scan on the left of the midline). The aorta is displaced anteriorly from the spine by a tumoral component between the two calipers.

Neuroblastomas can present with normal IVP. This concept is classic for the left side (Fig. 21) where the adrenal is often prerenal. Supine scans display the mass extending from the anterior side of the left kidney to the posterior border of the tail of the pancreas which can be pushed anteriorly.

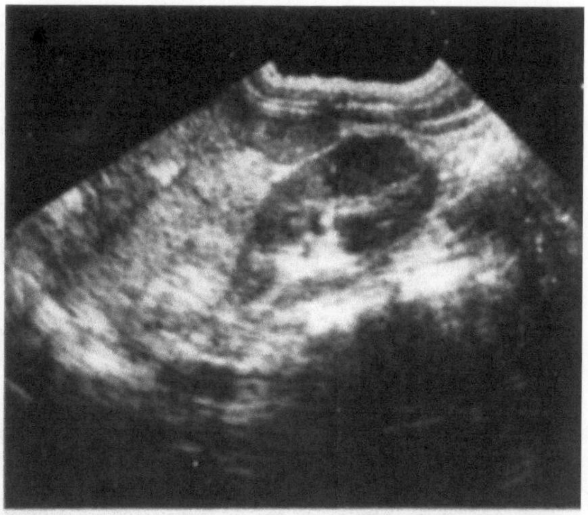

a

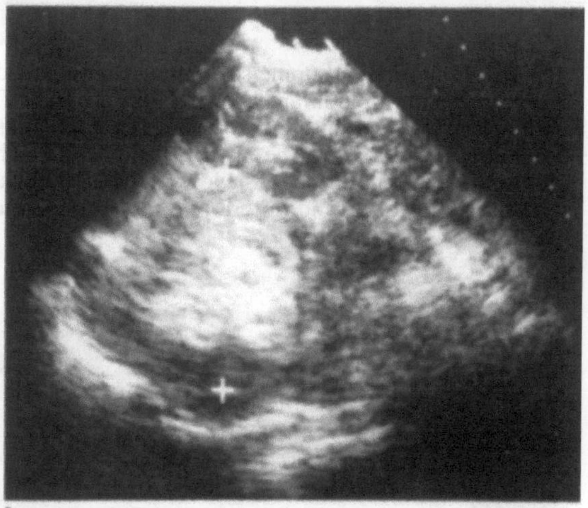

b

Fig. 21 a and b. Left prerenal neuroblastoma in a 10-year-old boy presenting with bone metastases. Normal IVP.
a Left longitudinal axillary scan;
b Longitudinal prone scan on the left kidney.
There is a 7-cm hyperechoic mass in front of the anterior side of the kiddney extending laterally to the spleen. The anterior surface of the left kidney is not deformed by the neuroblastoma.

Although infrequent, the prerenal location of neuroblastoma is also possible on the right side (Fig. 22).

Neuroblastomas that develop in the renal sinus (4 cases) can be urographically misleading and simulate a pelvi-ureteral obstruction or a renal malrotation. Sonographically the tumor impinges upon the renal pelvis (Fig. 23).

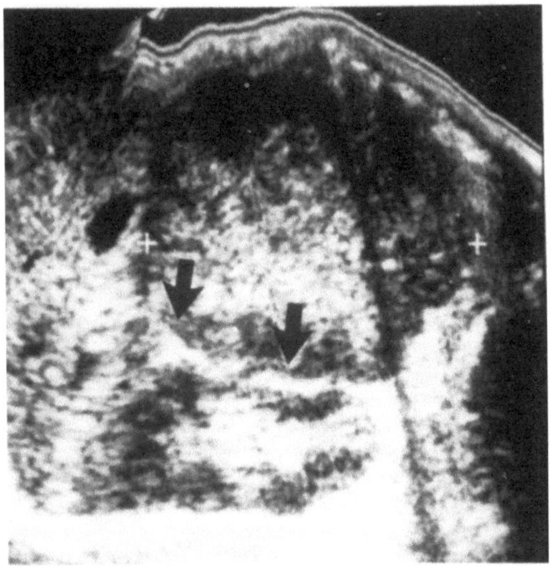

Fig. 22. Longitudinal supine scan along the right kidney in a 2-month-old infant showing a Equivocal IVP right prerenal neuroblastoma. There is a 6 cm mass extending posteriorly to the anterior side of the right kidney (*arrows*), upwards to the lower edge of the liver and the gallbladder, and anteriorly to the abdominal wall.

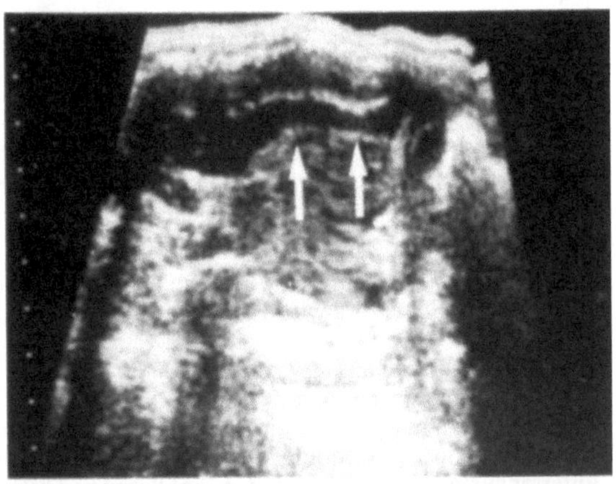

Fig. 23. Palpable "enlarged" kidney in a 7-month-old baby. Malrotation of the left kidney on the IVP. Longitudinal prone scan of the left kidney shows sinusal tumor impinging upon the renal pelvis (*arrows*). On the aortography performed by IV route, this 5-cm neuroblastoma was located between the renal pelvis posteriorly and the aorta anteriorly. A left nephrectomy was necessary.

Neonatal neuroblastomas are rare: approximatelly half of the cases present as Pepper syndrome. US shows an enlarged liver, either infiltrated or nodular (Fig. 24) with a normal-sized aorta. In some patients the primitive neuroblastoma is visualized in a suprarenal location (2 cases). Among our cases, twins presented at birth with Pepper syndrome.

Other cases of neonatal neuroblastomas present as a suprarenal mass raising the differential with an adrenal hemorrhage. In such situations,

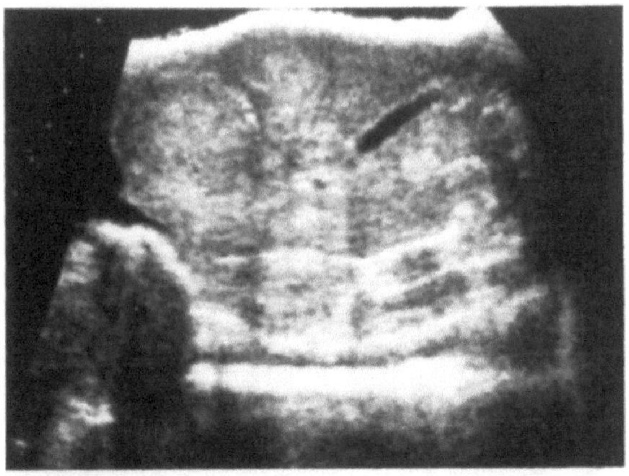

a

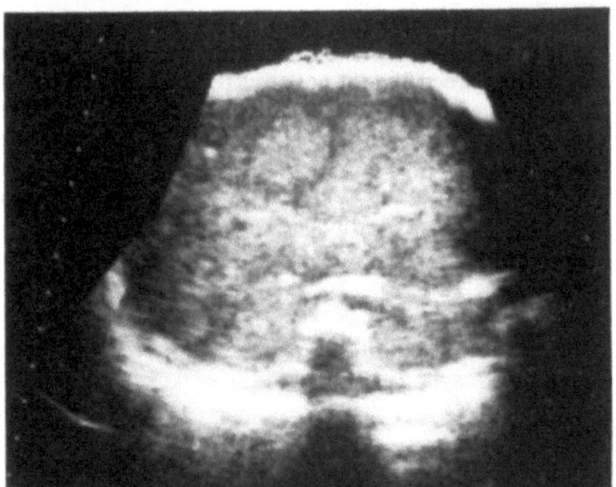

b

Fig. 24 a and b. Neonatal Pepper syndrome.
a Longitudinal supine scan along the gallbladder;
b Transverse supine scan of the liver.
Presence of echoic hepatic nodules. No primary tumor found. On complementary scans, the aorta was of normal caliber (different therefore from the enlarged aorta and enlarged celiac trunk encountered in hypervascular hepatic angiomas).

one should repeat the US examination 1 week later as the neuroblastoma remains solid on the second examination (Fig. 40). We have seen a case of bilateral neonatal nonsecreting neuroblastoma with no change in the internal echogenicity at the follow-up examination. We only found one exception to this rule in neonatal suprarenal masses.

3.3 Other Malignant Renal Tumors

Hypernephromas (7 cases) do not seem to have specific sonographic features that differentiate them from Wilms' tumors. It is known that hematuria is more frequent as a symptom in hypernephromas. At times, this diagnosis may be considered in the case of inefficiency of preoperative chemotherapy (when the diagnosis of Wilms' tumor has been wrongly made).

Renal involvement of lymphoma (12 cases) *and acute leukemia* (4 cases). Usually the involvement is that of hypoechoic solid masses, variable in number and size from one patient to another. These hypoechoic tumors are very characteristic of lymphoma (Fig. 25). Renal involvement can be part of a widespread form or can be the single initial location of the process. These anechoic parenchymal defects should not be confused with cysts.

Sometimes the kidneys appear diffusely infiltrated, symmetrically or not, with increased echogenicity of the parenchyma. Dilatation of the renal collecting system by pelvic or lumbar masses is frequent; obstructive anuria may occur within 24 h.

The possibility of lithiasis complicating chemotherapy has been mentioned in the chapter on medical conditions of the kidney (Fig. 12 in Chap. 9).

Renal sarcomas are rare (3 cases). They infiltrate the whole parenchyma without necessarily modifying the renal contours (Fig. 26).

3.4 Other Malignant Extrarenal Tumors

Retroperitoneal sarcomas (5 cases) rapidly invade the kidney and can then have a pattern similar to that of Wilms' tumor.

Adrenal tumors (5 cases) are often hormone-producing neoplasms and therefore seen in a suggestive clinical setting: Cushing syndrome, precocious puberty (Fig. 27). They can be small.

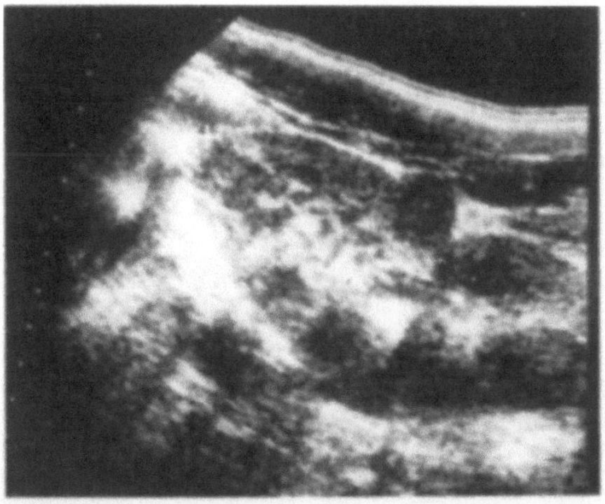

a

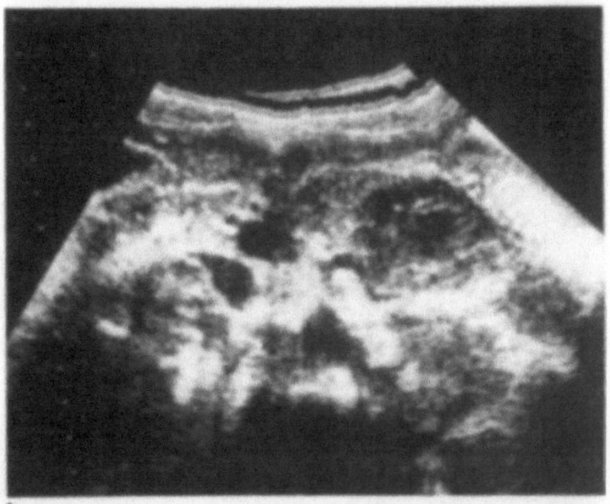

b

Fig. 25 a and b. Burkitt's lymphoma in a 15-year-old patient.
a Longitudinal prone scan of the left kidney. Several hypoechoic nodules are seen, bulging along the renal contours.
b Transverse supine scan of the pancreas showing enlarged lymph nodes behind the IVC and a lymphomatous mass in the tail of the pancreas (immediately in front of the splenic artery seen here arising from the celiac trunk).

Sarcomas of the posterior parietal muscles were seen in two cases. In one case the psoas was involved and in the other the quadratus lumborum.

Enlarged lymph nodes are seen mainly in lymphomas (Fig. 28) and testicular tumors. Adenopathies are recognized by their vascular connection rather than by their echostructure (classically made of low to medium homogeneous echoes). We have seen a case of recurrent Burkitt's lymphoma of the gastrointestinal tract with involvement of both adrenals (Fig. 29).

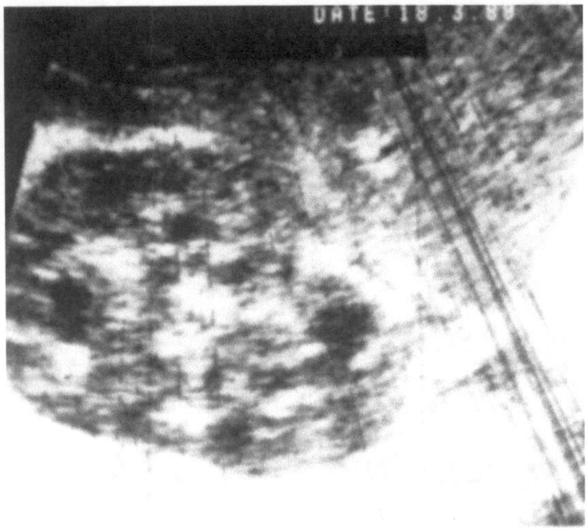

◀ **Fig. 26.** Right renal sarcoma in a 6-month-old infant with multiple pulmonary metastases (right subcostal scan). The whole kidney is infiltrated without modification of its contours.

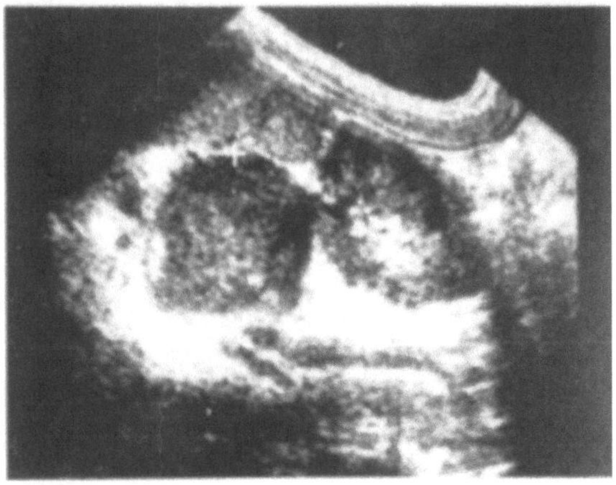

Fig. 27. Heterosexual precocious puberty in a 7-year-old girl (left longitudinal axillary scan). A 5 cm mass (calipers) extending from the anterior surface of the left kidney to the spleen: virilizing adrenocortical tumor.

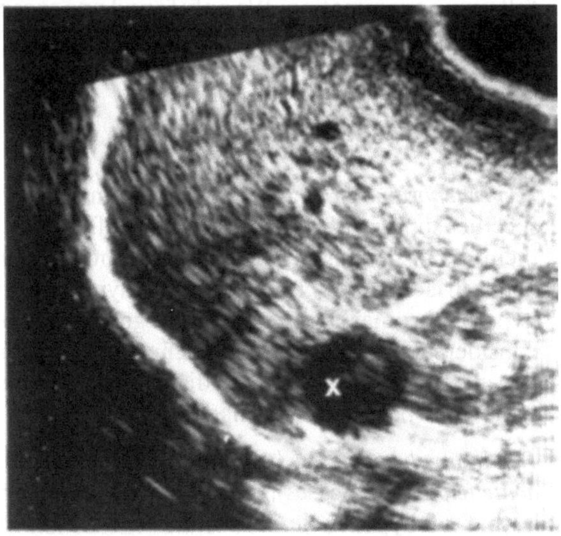

a

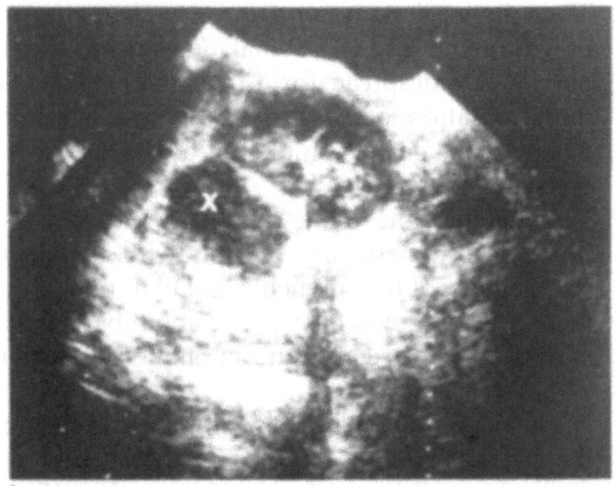

b

Fig. 29 a and b. An autistic 13-year-old boy operated upon for Burkitt lymphoma of the gastrointestinal tract (right hemicolectomy). Routine sonogram 6 weeks after surgery.
a Longitudinal supine scan on the right kidney;
b Left longitudinal axillary scan.
Lymphomatous hypoechoic masses in both adrenals (*x*), which completely disappeared under chemotherapy.

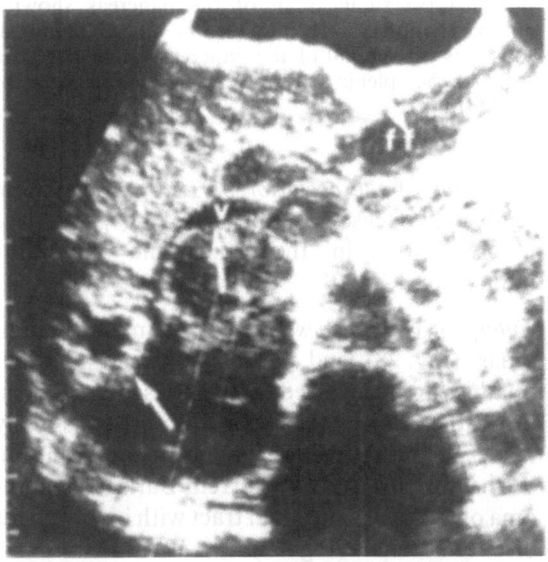

◀ **Fig. 28.** Hodgkin's disease in a 14-year-old girl (transverse supine scan). Large adenopathies displacing the aorta and IVC (*v*), pushing the right kidney away from the spine (*arrows*). Nodes are also present in the hepatic pedicle. Involvement of the liver is seen in the left lobe (*ff*).

4 Benign Tumors

4.1 Tumors of the Kidney

The high frequency (30%) of controlateral abnormalities (renal hypoplasia, megaureter, etc.) explains why multicystic dysplasia has been included in the chapter on urology rather than in this chapter.

Mesoblastic nephroma (renal hamartoma, Bolande's tumor) is readily recognized in the newborn (4 cases) because of the rarity of malignant renal tumors in this age group. In three cases, the tumor was well defined (Fig. 30), in the fourth the tumor presented as a multinodular involvement of the entire kidney. In one older child, the sonographic pattern was similar to a Wilms' tumor with areas of cystic changes.

Multilocular cysts comprise numerous cysts with thick septae (2 cases) or a few large cysts (1 case). In a 2-year-old boy, the cyst developed on the lower pole of a duplex kidney. An associated Wilms' tumor can be found in multilocular cysts (Fig. 31).

Angiomyolipomas (6 cases) belong to the spectrum of tuberous sclerosis. The presence of fat within the tumors explains their hyperechogenicity. Angiomyolipomas appear more often as discrete masses, at times as a diffuse fatty infiltration. In the previous chapter the possibility of multiple cysts in tuberous sclerosis patients was mentioned (Fig. 26, Chap. 9).

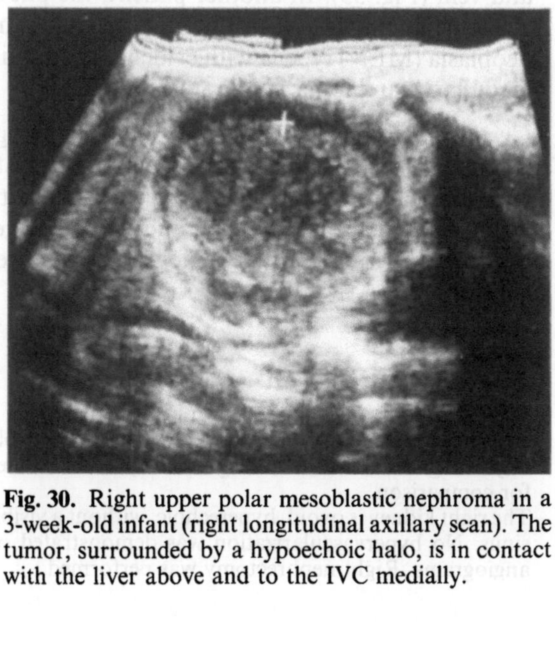

Fig. 30. Right upper polar mesoblastic nephroma in a 3-week-old infant (right longitudinal axillary scan). The tumor, surrounded by a hypoechoic halo, is in contact with the liver above and to the IVC medially.

Hydatid renal cysts are quite rare. In two patients, liver and lung cysts coexist with the renal involvement. In one patient (Fig. 32), however, the kidney was the only involved parenchyma.

Simple cysts (7 cases) are usually picked up on routine IVP or sonogram performed for nonrelated symptoms.

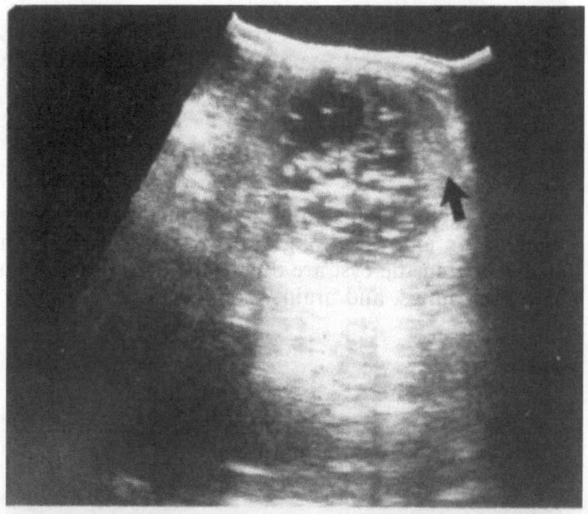

a

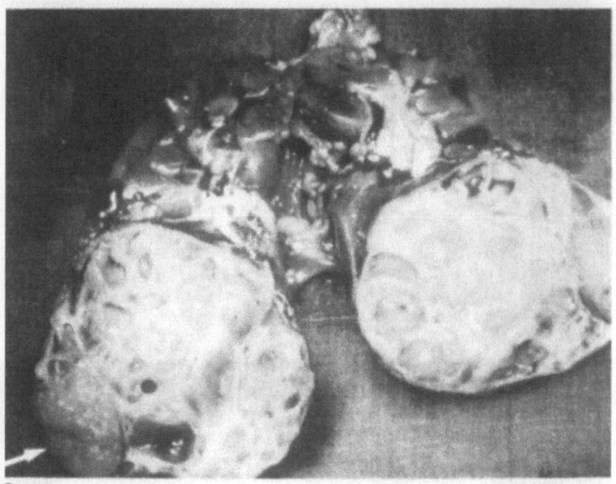

b

Fig. 31 a and b. Left multilocular renal cyst in a 17-month-old patient.
a Longitudinal prone scan. Thick internal septae are seen in a pluricystic mass (*arrow*). **b** Gross pathology of the removed left kidney. A small Wilms' tumor was present at the lower aspect of the multilocular cyst (*arrow*). This was correlated only retrospectively with the sonogram (**a**). Sonographically one cannot differentiate between simple multilocular cyst and multilocular cyst with foci or nodules of Wilms' tumor in the septare (the so-called multicystic Wilms' tumor).

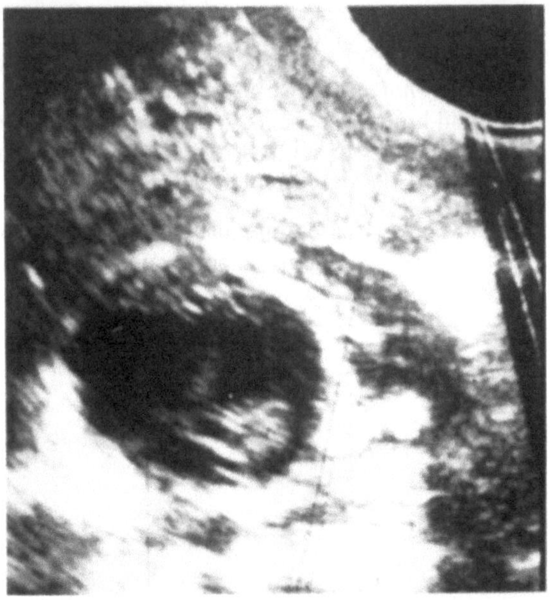

Fig. 32. Right renal hydatid cyst in a patient investigated for enuresis (longitudinal supine scan). The echoes within the cyst are due to the membrane folds. The liver, lungs, and brain were normal.

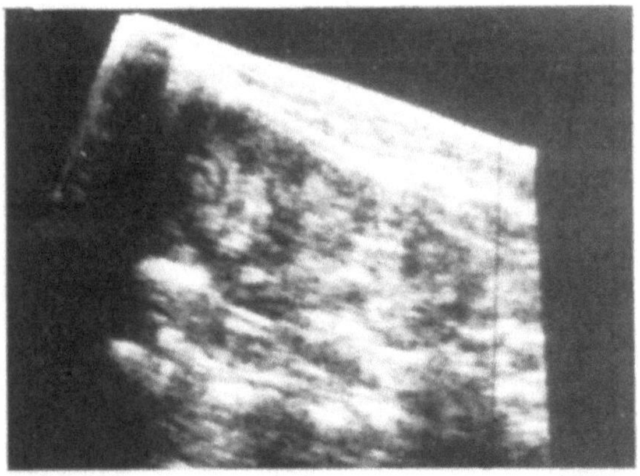

a

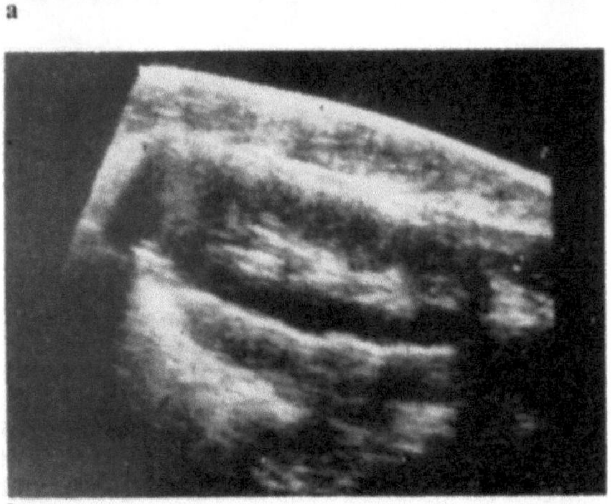

b

Some remarks should be made regarding three unusual benign tumors:

1. Two cases of *cavernous angiomas* of the kidney were obvious on sonograms (Fig. 33), while IVP and angiography were noncontributory.
2. *An intrarenal neurofibroma,* without evidence of neurofibromatosis, was only recognized at pathology in a 6-year-old boy operated upon with the initial diagnosis of Wilms' tumor.
3. In a 10-year-old girl, a multicystic mass in the right kidney coexisting with a few cysts in the opposite kidney proved to be an *intrarenal lymphangioma.*

4.2 Extrarenal Tumors

Adrenal secreting tumors have already been mentioned. The difficulty in assessing the malignant or benign nature of such tumors is well known.

Pheochromocytomas (6 cases) were always found in hypertensive patients. In four cases, IVP was normal. In two patients, three secreting tumors were present (Fig. 34). This emphasizes the need for a complete evaluation in a patient with an obvious tumor; in particular, the left prerenal region and the retrocaval area must be carefully scanned.

The echogenicity was homogeneous in five cases. In only one patient, the large size of the mass accounts for some necrotic areas. In one case of a single lesion, the retrocaval pheochromocytoma was located between the right renal artery and vein (Fig. 35). In another patient, the pheochromocytoma was part of a multiple endocrine neoplasia (MEN) type II with evidence of thyroid medullary carcinoma.

Cystic lymphangiomas (6 cases) are easily recognized in their usual pattern of multiple cysts with internal septae. However, they are prone to acute inflammatory changes and hemorrhage, resulting in less suggestive sonographic features (Fig. 36).

Fig. 33 a and b. Longitudinal prone scans showing a cavernous angioma of the right kidney in a 4-year-old boy with gross hematuria. **a** Right kidney; **b** Left kidney for comparison.
The right kidney is ovoid, hyperechoic, without a visible sinus. No hypervascularization was demonstrated on angiograms. Right nephrectomy was performed.

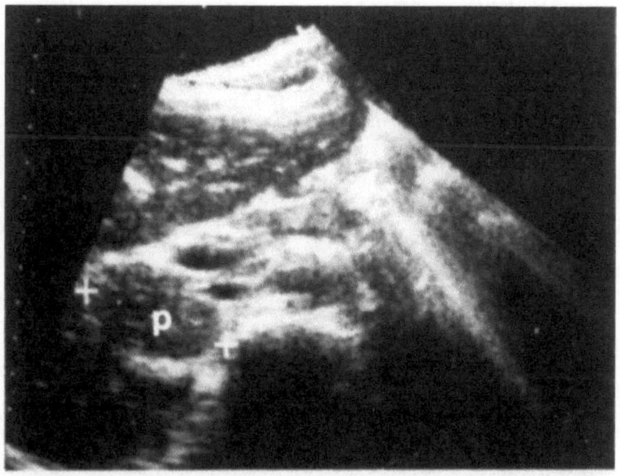

a

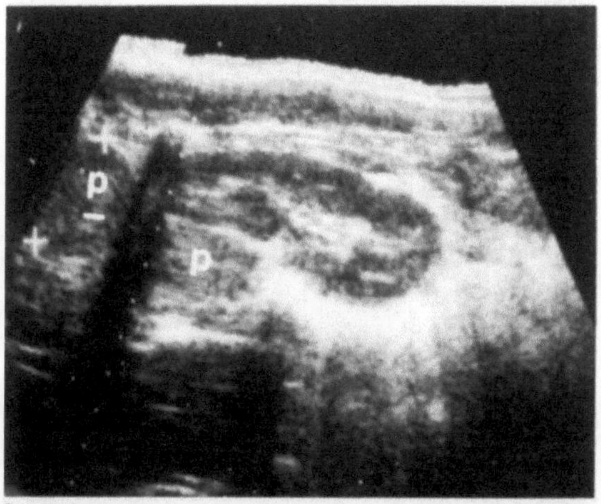

b

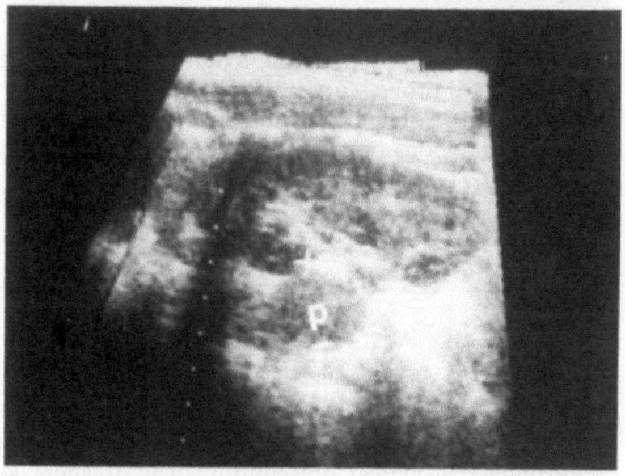

c

Fig. 34 a–c. Arterial hypertension in a 10-year-old boy.
a Transverse supine scan;
b Longitudinal prone scan on the right kidney;
c Longitudinal prone scan on the left kidney.
Three pheochromocytomas (*p*) are present: above the right kidney, behind the IVC, and in front of the right and left kidneys. The three tumors were removed at the same surgical intervention.

Retroperitoneal lipomas (2 cases) are basically recognized on plain film of the abdomen.

Adrenal hemorrhage (10 cases) can be echoic initially and become cystic on a second examination 1 week later (Fig. 40). On follow-up studies, the cyst decreases in size with peripheral calcifications. We have seen only one case of a large echoic right adrenal hemorrhage that did not become cystic, nor decrease significantly in size over a 3-month period. Surgery was performed to rule out a congenital neuroblastoma; pathology disclosed a "typical" noncalcified adrenal hemorrhage.

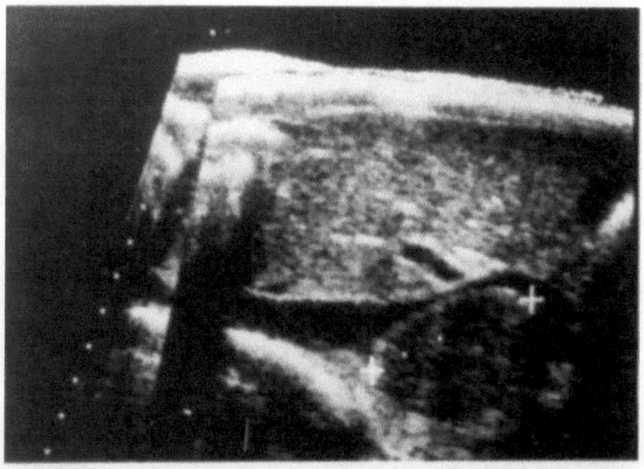

a

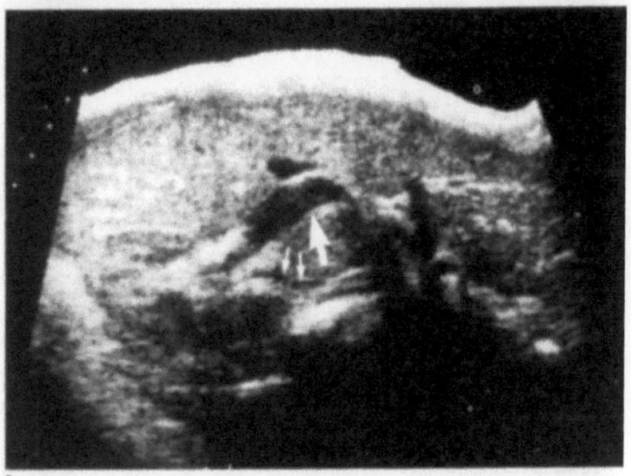

b

Fig. 35 a and b. Paroxystic hypertension in a 10-year-old girl. Normal IVP.
a Longitudinal supine scan along the IVC;
b Right subcostal scan.
A retrocaval (*large arrow*) pheochromocytoma is demonstrated; the right renal artery is posterior to the tumor (*small arrows*). Two urographically silent regions are often involved in pheochromocytomas: the suprarenal retrocaval region and the left prerenal juxtasinusal region. Sonography is of particular help in the study of these locations.

Benign neurogenic tumors in our series are illustrated by a single case of schwannoma. Ganglioneuromas are less common in the abdomen than in the thorax and represent the maturation of neuroblastic cells.

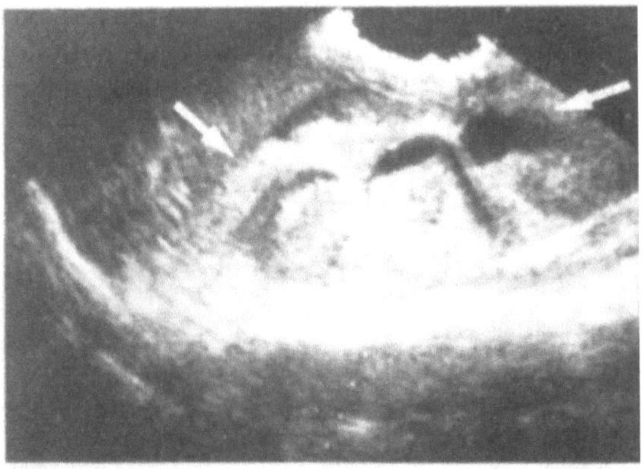

a

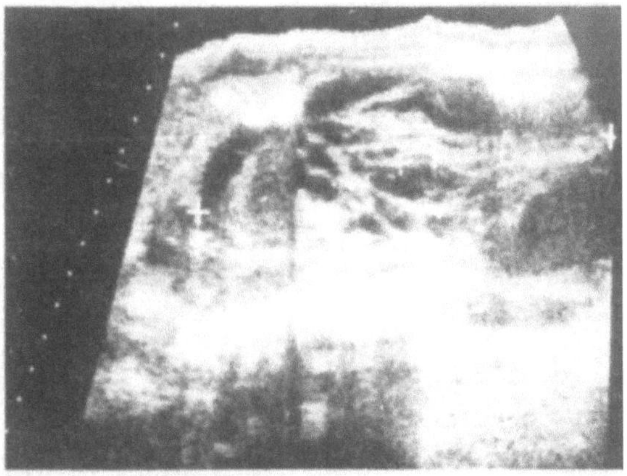

b

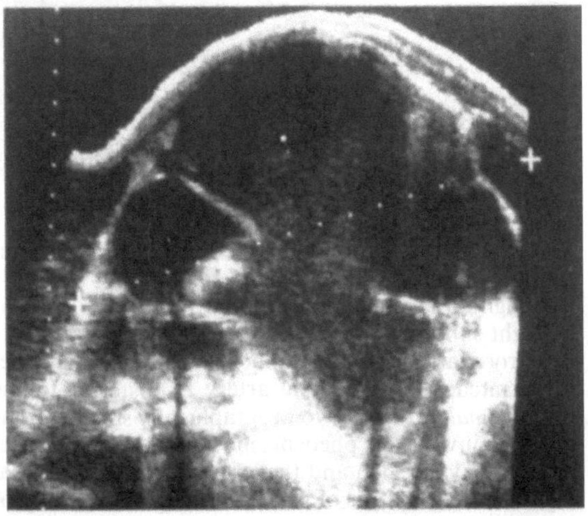

c

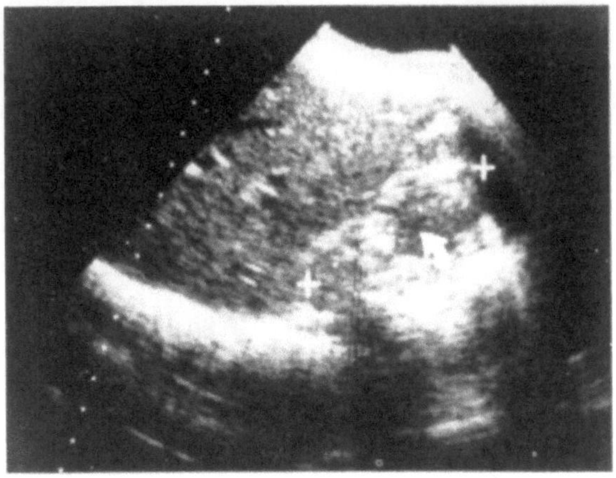

Fig. 37. Right pseudotumoral cortical nodule in a 14-year-old patient with chronic pyelonephritis. Longitudinal supine scan. The nodule appears hypoechoic (*arrow*) as compared to the remaining parenchyma, which is not always the case.

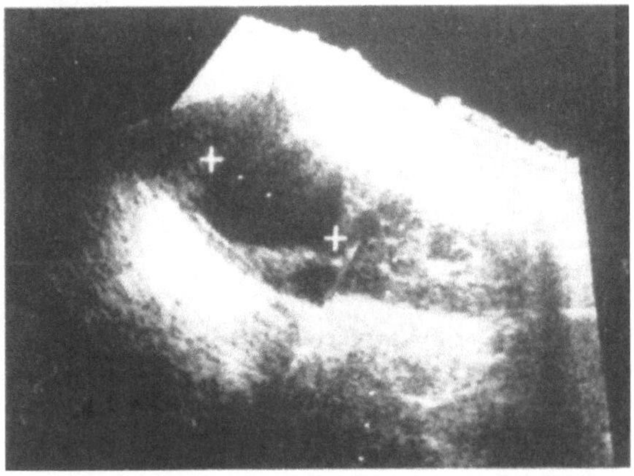

Fig. 38. Long duration fever in an 11-year-old girl. No urinary symptoms or infection. Routine sonogram with a longitudinal prone scan of the left kidney. Abscess of the upper pole of the left kidney. Complete recovery after percutaneous puncture and therapy of antibiotic.

Fig. 36a–c. Right retroperitoneal lymphangioma in a 3-year-old boy (longitudinal scans of the right flank).
a Initially the clinical presentation was of acute appendicitis; the lymphangioma (*arrows*) appears mostly echogenic because of internal debris.
b After 4 days of steroids.
c After 1 month of steroids, preoperatively. The multicystic pattern with internal septae is now very suggestive of lymphangioma.
One should note the atypical sonographic appearance of lymphangiomas when they present during an acute inflammatory or hemorrhagic episode.

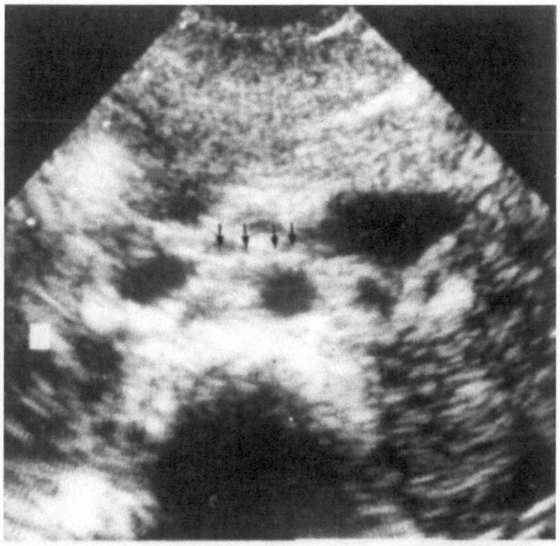
a

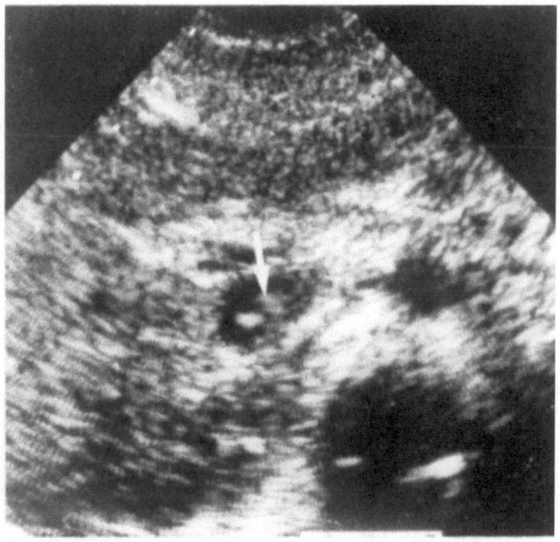
b

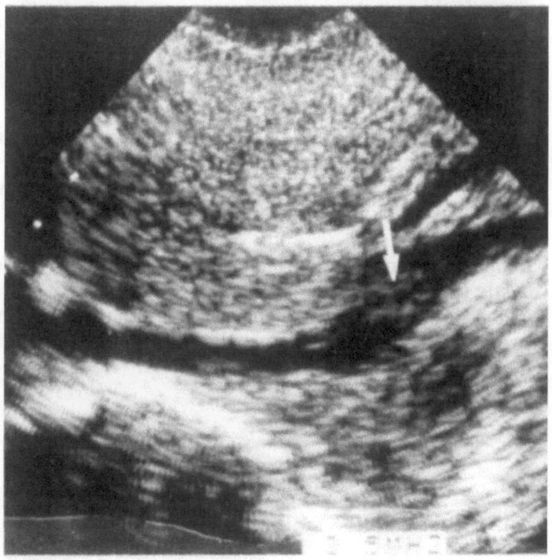
c

Fig. 39a–c. Left Wilms' tumor in a 4-year-old child.
a Transverse supine scan: Thrombus into the left renal vein (*arrows*) with distal dilatation.
b and c Transverse and longitudinal supine scans along the IVC showing extension of the thrombus into the lumen of the IVC (*arrows*).

5 Differential Diagnosis

Some entities can, at times, be confused with true tumors.

Cortical nodules in abnormal kidneys (chronic pyelonephritis, renal dysplasia) represent localized compensatory hypertrophy (5 cases). These nodules are often mistaken for Wilms' tumors (Fig. 37).

Recessive polycystic kidney disease (RPKD) is the most common cause of bilateral nephromegaly in newborns and infants. Renal echogenicity is markedly and globally increased and permits by itself the differentiation between RPKD and nephroblastomatosis.

Dominant (adult-type) polycystic kidneys are only occasionally seen in children. The exact nature of the cysts is assessed by the routine renal sonograms of the parents.

Renal abscesses (5 cases) and *focal bacterial nephritis* (3 cases) can similate a necrotic tumor (Fig. 38). The causal infectious agent can be identified by a guided puncture, for urinary tract

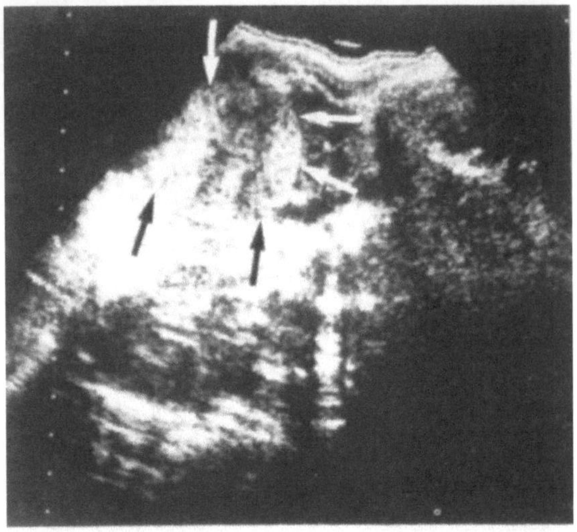

a

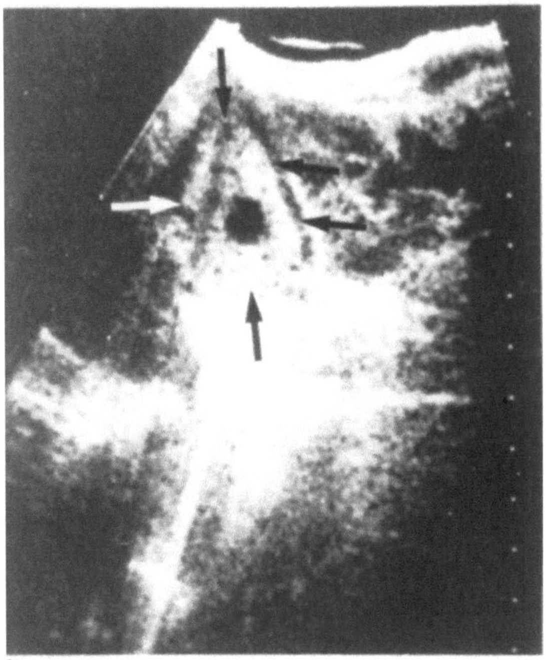

b

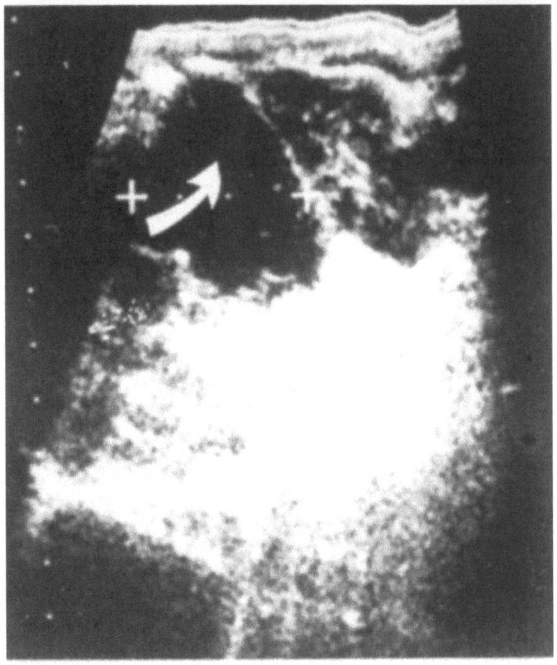

c

Fig. 40 a–c. A second, delayed sonogram is valuable in neonatal suprarenal masses.
a Neonatal nonsecreting neuroblastoma (*arrows*). There was no change in the echogenicity of the tumor 8 days later.
b and c Adrenal hemorrhage, initially echoic **(b)**, later cystic **(C)**.
The 8-day delay between the two examinations has no prognostic significance in the case of congenital neuroblastoma.

infection was absent in most of our cases. Sonography assesses the renal recovery during antibiotic therapy.

Psoas hematomas in known hemophilia patients (4 cases) are easily recognized.

Similarly, *urinomas* following trauma or secondary to posterior urethral valves are readily linked to their cause.

Obviously the sonographic features of retroperitoneal tumors must always be correlated with clinical and biological data. In our experience US is quite competitive with CT in determining the stage of retroperitoneal tumors. US is extremely valuable in following the efficiency of chemotherapy in nonoperated patients.

References

General references

1. Schweisguth O. (1979). Tumeurs solides de l'enfant. Flammarion. Médecine Sciences. Paris
2. Cadier L., Broussin B., Calabet A., Baudain Ph., Diard F. (1982). Apport de l'échographie dans l'étude des tumeurs rétropéritonéales de l'enfant. J. Radiol. 63:15–23

3. Garel L., Lallemand D., Lacombe P., Chereau O., Sauvegrain J. (1982). The renal sinus: an important anatomical landmark in children. Ann. Radiol. 25:1:65–71
4. Gore R.M., Callen P.W., Filly R.A. (1982). Displaced retroperitoneal fat: sonographic guide to right upper quadrant mass localization. Radiology 142:701–705
5. Padovani J., Raybaud C., Faure F., Devred Ph., Bernard J.L., Simonin G. (1981). Interest of CT in retroperitoneal masses in childhood. Ann. Radiol. 24:1:18–24

Wilms' tumors and other renal tumors

6. Jaffe M.H., White S.J., Silver T.M., Heidelberger K.P. (1981). Wilms tumor: ultrasonic features, pathologic correlation, and diagnostic pitfalls. Radiology 140:147
7. Kaufman R.A., Holt J.F., Heidelberger K.P. (1978). Calcification in primary and metastatic Wilms tumor. A.J.R. 130:783–785
8. Rosenfield N.S., Shimkin P., Berdon W.E. (1980). Wilms tumor arising from spontaneously regressing nephroblastomatosis. A.J.R. 135:381
9. Goldman S.M., Garfunkel D.J., Oh K. S., Dorst J.P. (1981). Drash syndrome: male pseudohermaphroditism, nephritis, and Wilms tumor. Radiology 141:87
10. Filiatrault D., Garel L., Tournade M.F., Zucker J.M. (1982). Echographic Aspects of Hepatic metastases of nephroblastomas. Ped. Radiol. 12:72–77
11. Slovis T.L., Philippart A.L., Cushing B., Das L., Perlmutter A.D., Reed J.O., Wilner H.I., Kroovand R.L., Farooki Z.Q. (1981). Evaluation of the inferior vena cava by sonography and venography in children with renal and hepatic tumors. Radiology 140:767
12. Madewell J.E., Goldman S.M., Davis C.J., Hartman D.S., Feigin D.S., Lichtenstein J.E. (1983). Multilocular cystic nephroma: a radiographic pathologic correlation of 58 patients. Radiology 146:309–322
13. Hartman D.S., Lesar M.S.L., Madewell J.E. (1981). Mesoblastic nephroma: radiologic-pathologic correlation of 20 cases. A.J.R. 136:69
14. McAlister W.H., Siegel M.J., Askin F., Shackelford G.D. (1979). Congenital mesoblastic nephroma. Radiology 132:356
15. Andre C., Garel L., Sauvegrain J. (1983). Ultrasound of renal lymphoma in children: a report of 9 cases. Ann. Radiol. 25:6:385–394
16. Shirkhoda A., Staab E.V., Mittelstaedt C.A. (1980). Renal lymphoma imaged by ultrasound and gallium 67. Radiology 137:175
17. Hartman D.D., Goldman S.M., Friedman A.C., Davis C.J., Madewell J.E., Sherman J.L. (1981). Angiomyolipoma: ultrasonic-pathologic correlation. Radiology 139:451
18. Scheible W., Ellengogen P.H., Leopold G.R., Siao N.T. (1978). Lipomatous tumors of the kidney and adrenal: apparent echographic specifity. Radiology 129:153
19. Carlson D.H., Carlson D., Simon H. (1978). Benign multilocular cystic nephroma. A.J.R. 131:621–625
20. Gordon R.L., Pollack H.M., Popky G.L., Duchett J.W. (1979). Simple serous cysts of the kidney in children. Radiology 131:357
21. Banner M.P., Pollack H.M., Chatten J. (1981). Multilocular renal cysts: radiologic-pathologic correlation. A.J.R. 136:239

Extrarenal tumors

22. Berger D.E., Kuhn J.P., Numschauer R.W. (1978). Computed tomography and ultrasound in the diagnosis and management of neuroblastoma. Radiology 128:633–667
23. Haller J.O., Berdon W.E., Baker D.H., Kassner E.G. (1977). Left adrenal neuroblastoma with normal appearing urogram. A.J.R. 129:1051–1055
24. Hamdouch M., Hartmann O., Garel L., Sauvegrain J. (1982). Radiological diagnosis and particularities of neonatal neuroblastomas (Pepper's syndrome excluded).: 25 cases. Ann. Radiol. 25:1:5–11
25. Yeh H.S., Mitty H.A., Rose J., Wolf B.S., Gabrillove J.L. (1978). Ultrasonography of adrenal masses. I. Usual features. Radiology 127:467–474. II. Unusual manifestations. Radiology 127: 475–483
26. Bernardino M.E., Goldstein M.H., Green B. (1978). Gray-scale ultrasonography of adrenal neoplasms. A.J.R. 130:741–744
27. Leonidas J.C., Brill P.W., Bhan I., Smith T.H. (1978). Cystic retroperitoneal lymphangioma in infants and children. Radiology 127:203–208
28. Mineau D.E., Nixon G.W. (1978). Retroperitoneal lipoma in a child. Radiology 126:456
29. Kangerloo H., Sukow R.J., Sample W.f., Lipson M., Smith L.E. (1977). Ultrasonographic evaluation of juxta-diaphragmatic masses in children. Radiology 125:785
30. Currarino G., Pinckney L.E. (1981). Renal displacement caused by a supradiaphragmatic paraspinal Ewing-like sarcoma and simulating and adrenal mass. Radiology 139:603
31. Metreweli C., Garel L., Montagne J.Ph. (1981). Echographic aspects of neonatal adrenal hemorrhage. Ann. Radiol. 24:1:13–17

Chapter 11

Pelvic Echography

C. André and B. Le Bihan

Everyone agrees that echography is an interesting tool in the study of pelvic pathology in children. Its indications are numerous in girls, less in boys. It is a painless and inoffensive method to explore almost all pelvic organs at the same time and it avoids pelvic irradiation.

In this chapter we do not aim to give an exhaustive review of pathology but to bring practical solutions to current clinical situations.

1 Technique

Pelvic echography is a simple, painless method similar to the one used in adults and in general neither sedation nor retention is needed. The only difficulty lies in getting the indispensable full bladder which pushes the gas filled intestines back out of the pelvis allowing good ultrasonic transmission and creating an acoustical "window" – "the bigger the window the better the view". The bladder is also an important anatomical landmark. Bladder-filling is difficult to achieve in children younger than 2 years; the solution is to give the child a bottle and to be patient. A diuretic can be given.

The study is performed in the dorsal position and starts by transverse views to locate the uterus, then longitudinal views along its axis. Ovaries are studied first longitudinally then transversally.

A manual or preferably automatic sectoral balayage apparatus is used. A 5 MHz transducer is usually enough to study a child's pelvis. However, a 3.5 MHz transducer is preferable in adolescents. It is better to use a real-time apparatus to differentiate the intestinal mobolity when looking at the bowel content, as gas and stool in the rectosigmoid can simulate a tumor. During the study, a water enema can easily avoid this mistake.

2 Normal Echographic Anatomy

It is very important to know normal anatomy but also the variations with age, particularly in the pelvic area which is deeply modified around puberty.

The bladder is the first organ to recognize. When full, its shape is obvious: triangular in the longitudinal view and trapeze-like transversally. It is echo-free with posterior enhancement and thin walls as seen in liquid structures.

The vagina is rapidly recognized in the longitudinal views. It is seen as a tubular medial shape directly behind and below the bladder reaching behind the pubis. Its walls do not give much echo and surround a dense linear central echo which is the virtual cavity.

The uterus follows the vagina, directly behind the bladder on which it leaves a pring (Fig. 1). The uterus is usually medial, sometimes deviated laterally. Its axis is better seen on transverse views (Fig. 2). In children it usually leans forward, rarely backward. Its echostructure is solid, homogeneous with a low echo and its contours are regular. Its cavity is virtual and seen as an axial line where the walls meet. Size and shape vary with age (Fig. 3).

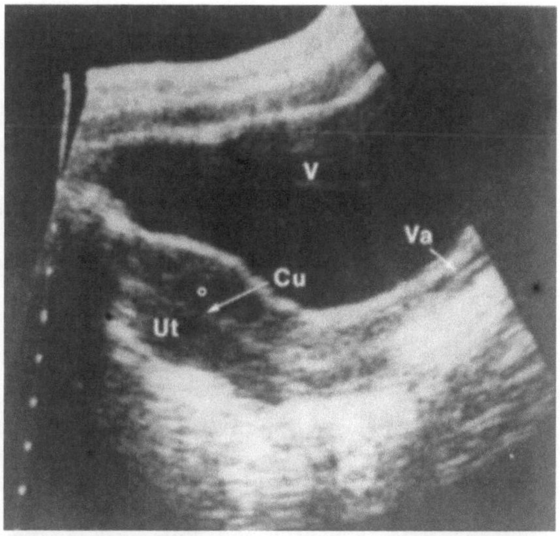

Fig. 1. Medial longitudinal view of vagina and postpubertal uterus. The well developed body of the uterus makes an imprint of the posterior side of the bladder. Dense axial echo is uterine and vaginal cavities.
V, Bladder; *Va*, Vagina; *Ut*, Uterus; *Cu*, Uterine cavity.

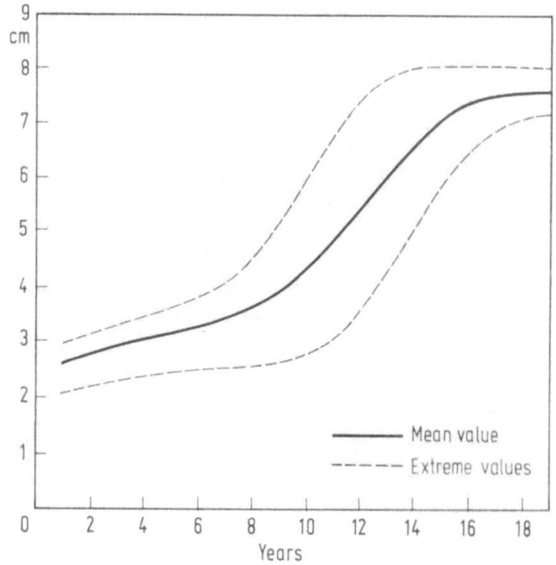

Fig. 3. Uterine growth according to age. Before 3 months of age the uterine growth is related to the maternal hormones. Before puberty, the growth is slow (min. 3.1 cm). At puberty, this growth is accelerated and there is a high spectrum of values.

Prepubertal uterus is tear drop-shaped (Figs. 4 and 5). Neck and isthmus are more developed than the body as they make up twothirds of uterine volume. The neck is twice as thick as the body. It is 2.5–3.5 cm long (mean 3.1 cm) and the body is 0.5–1 cm thick (mean 0.8 cm). Uterus size remains the same until puberty. Then, with the production of estrogens, the uterus, mostly the body, increases in length and thickness and becomes pear-shaped. The postpubertal uterus is 5–8 cm long (mean 6.7 cm) with a body thickness of 2–4 cm (mean 3 cm).

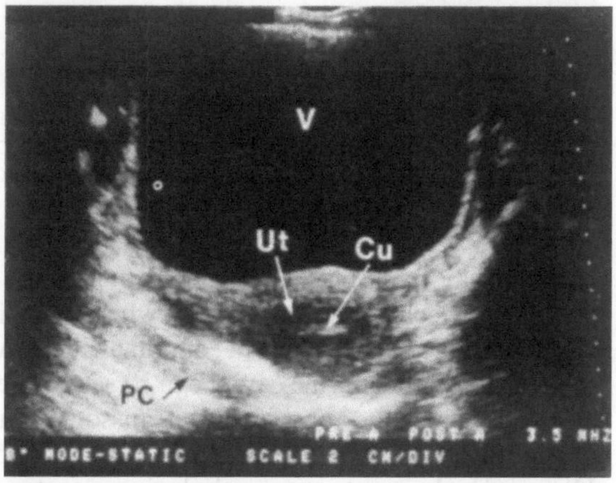

Fig. 2. Transverse view of uterus. The axis of the uterus is better seen on this view through the uterus.
V, Bladder; *Ut*, Uterus; *Cu*, Uterine cavity; *Pc*, Pubococcygeal muscle.

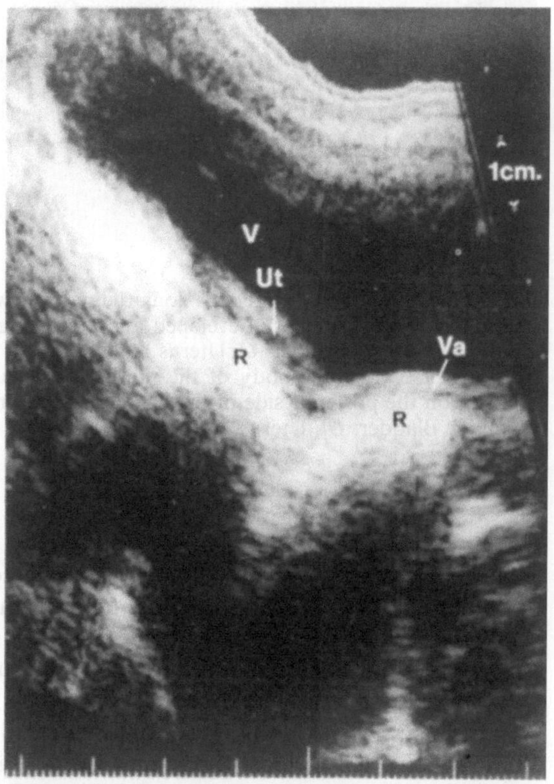

Fig. 4. Nonpubertal uterus: a medial transverse view. Uterus is 3 cm long. Uterus body is not as thick as neck.
V, Bladder; *Ut*, Uterus; *Va*, Vagina; *R*, Rectum.

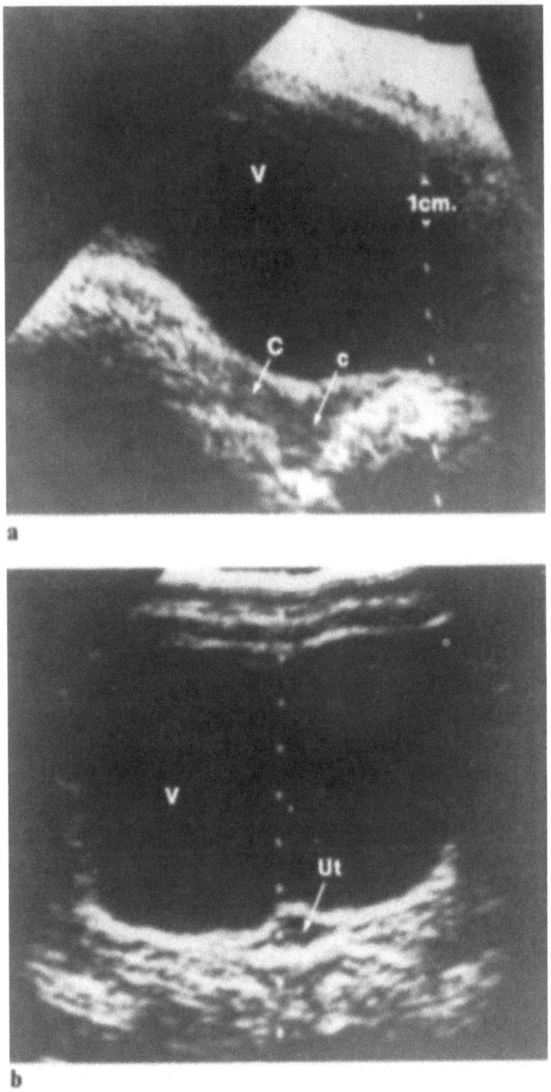

Fig. 5. a Nonpubertal uterus: longitudinal view. Isthmus and neck are very developed and are thicker than the body. *V*, Bladder; *C*, Uterus body.
b Transverse view: the body of the uterus makes an imprint on the posterior side of the bladder. It is 1 cm thick. *V*, Bladder; *Ut*, Uterus.

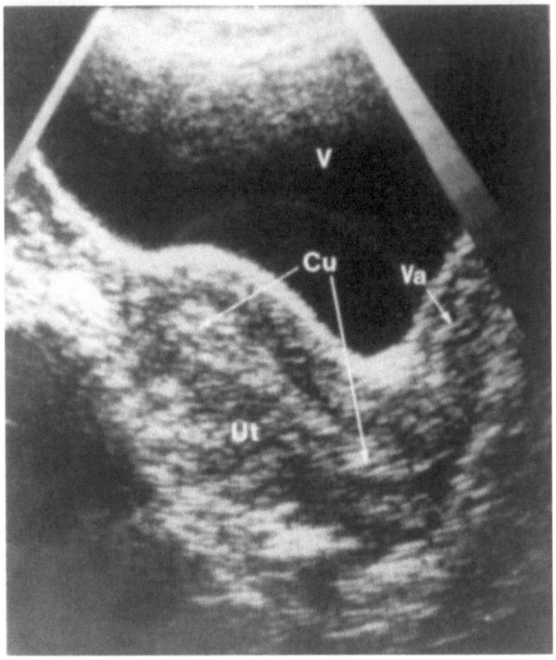

Fig. 6. Variations during menstrual cycle. Longitudinal view of uterus. Medial linear echo can become very thick especially before menstruation. This is plain endometrial hyperplasia. It can look like decidual reaction in extrauterine pregnancy.
V, Bladder; *Va*, Vagina; *Ut*, Uterus; *Cu*, Uterine cavity.

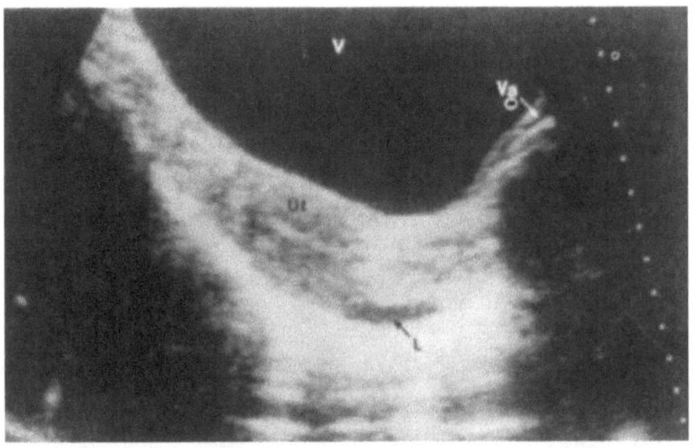

Fig. 7. Variations during menstrual cycle: longitudinal view of the pelvis. Presence of liquid in the pouch of Douglas at the time of ovulation, which is short-lived. *V*, Bladder; *Va*, Vagina; *Ut*, Uterus; *L*, Liquid.

In the neonatal period the uterus is stimulated by maternal hormones and becomes tubular: the body is as thick as the neck, sometimes thicker. In 4–6 weeks hormones diminish and the uterus rapidly reduces to prepubertal size.

The postpubertal uterus varies physiologically during menstrual periods. In the first half of the cycle the central echo can be invisible. After ovulation, the echo becomes obvious, sometimes 2–3 cm thick just before menstruation because of endometrial hyperplasia (Fig. 6). Sometimes a circular low echo zone can be seen where there is vascular engorgement in the endometrium. At menstruation the uterine cavity can be seen either as a thick echo zone or as a central transsonic zone depending on the presence of clots or fresh blood. Uterus size does not vary much during menstrual periods. Sometimes at the time of ovulation and even in prepubertal girls some liquid can be seen in the pouch of Douglas (Fig. 7), which is rapidly

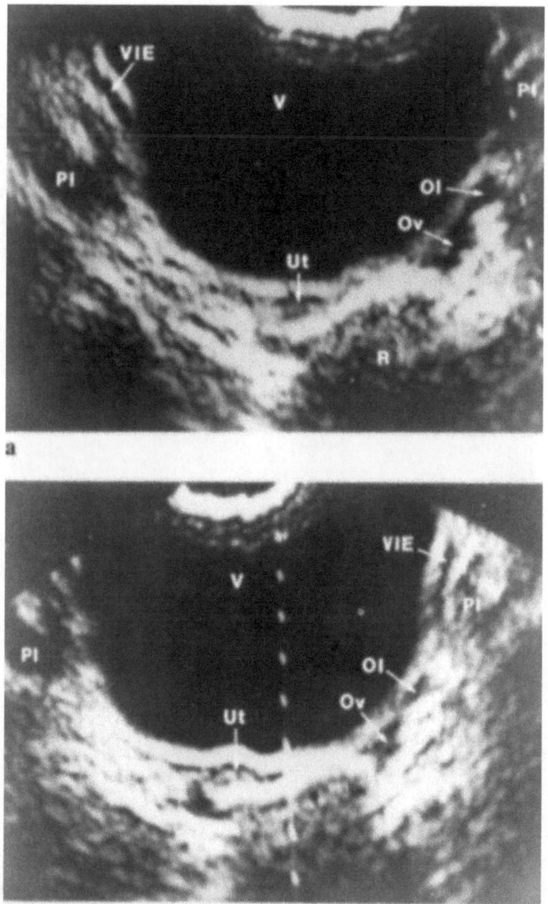

Fig. 8 a and b. Transverse view in a 7-year-old girl showing lateral walls of the pelvis which are often hard to visualizes. Large psoas iliac muscles are easily seen; external iliac vessels are on their internal side. Internal obturator muscle underneath is visible on the left side only. Ovary is below and inward in front of internal iliac vessels. Pubococcygeal muscle of the deep perineum is harder to see.
V, Bladder; *Ut*, Uterus; *Ov*, Ovary; *PI*, Psoas iliac muscle; *OI*, Internal obturator muscle; *R*, Rectum; *VIE*, External iliac vessel.

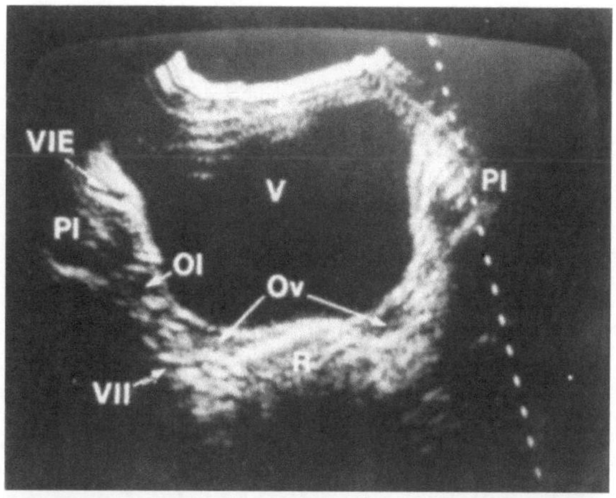

Fig. 9. Lateral walls of the pelvis on a transverse view. The ovaries are easily seen inside and below the internal obturator muscle.
V, Bladder; *Ov*, Ovaries; *R*, Rectum; *OI*, Internal obturator muscle; *VII*, Internal iliac vessel; *VIE*, External iliac vessel; *PI*, Iliopsoas muscle.

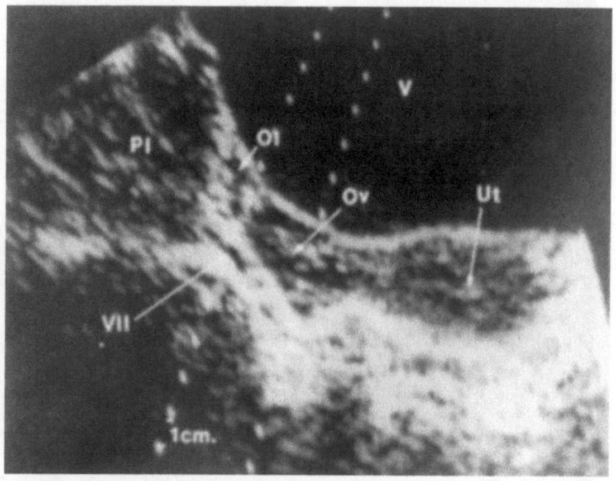

Fig. 10. Transverse view of postpubertal ovary posterior to the bladder, outward from uterus, inward from internal obturator muscle, in front of internal iliac
V, Bladder; *Ut*, Uterus; *Ov*, Ovary; *PI*, Iliopsoas muscle; *OI*, Internal obturator muscle; *VII*, Internal iliac vessels.

resorbed. Also in young girls who are not yet continent some urine can be seen in the posterior vaginal pouch. This liquid zone must not be mistaken for liquid in the pouch of Douglas: it never lies higher than the uterus neck even in the Trendelenburg position.

The fallopian tubes are not visible normally. Ovaries are the hardest pelvic organs to see especially before the age 5 years. To identify ovaries one must first know and see the lateral pelvic walls. This is often difficult due to their small size and bad bladder filling before 2 years of age or because of intestinal gas – the echographists' worst enemy.

Pelvic walls are echographycally made of three symmetrical muscular groups seen on transverse views (Figs. 8 and 9); from front to back and from outside to inside, there is the psoas iliac muscle (thick, solid, low echo), then the smaller internal obturator muscle, and the pubococcygeus muscle.

Iliac vessels lie inside the muscular wall: the external iliac vessels lie medial to the ilio psoas muscle, the internal iliac vessels lie iliac medial to the internal obturator muscle.

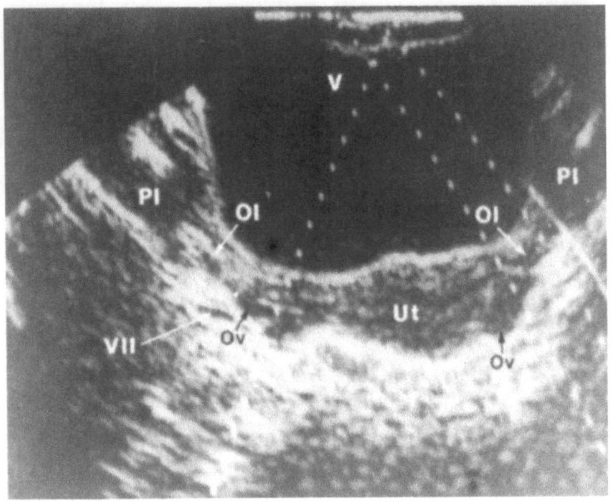

Fig. 11. Ovaries on a transverse view. Left ovary is next to the uterus wall.
V, Bladder; *Ut*, Uterus; *Ov*, Ovary; *PI*, Iliopsoas muscle; *OI*, Internal obturator muscle; *VII*, Internal iliac vessels.

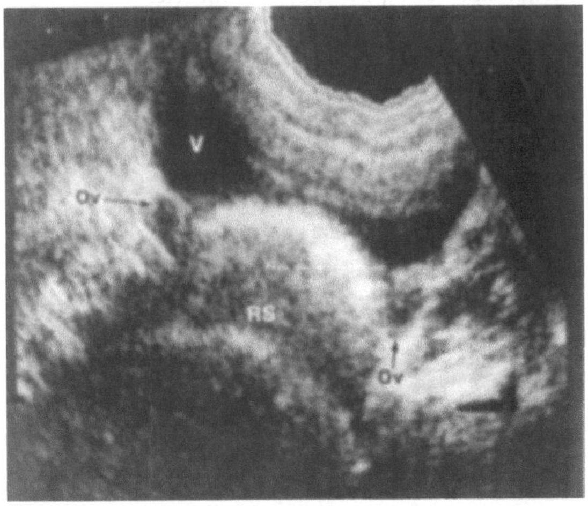

Fig. 12. Transverse view of prepubertal ovaries in a 2-year-old girl. Rarely seen before 5 years of age. They are small oval masses less than 1 cm^3. *V*, Bladder; *Ov*, Ovary; *RS*, Rectosigmoid with gas.

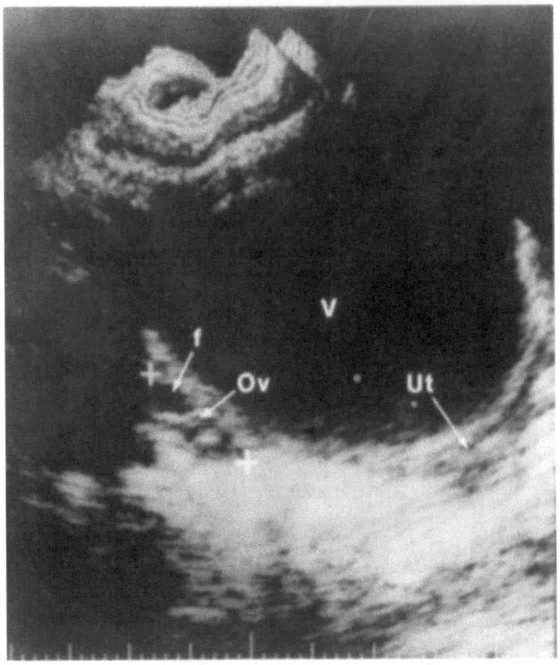

Fig. 13. Postpubertal ovaries in a transverse view. The ovaries measure 2.2 cm. A follicle can be seen less than 1 cm. *V*, Bladder; *Ut*, Uterus; *Ov*, Ovary; *f*, Follicle.

The ovaries are next to the uterus in the ovarian fossa, which echographycally on transverse views is limited forward by the bladder, medially by the uterus, externally by the internal obturator muscle and backward by internal iliac vessels (Figs. 10 and 11). Actually, the position varies with bladder filling and stool and gas in the rectosigmoid intestine. It varies mostly with the uterus position: when it is deviated laterally, the ovary on that side can be behind or even on top of the uterus. Maximum bladder filling may then be necessary to be able to see it. In the neonatal period, ovary migration can be incomplete and they can be found at the lower end of the kidney.

Ovaries are small, oval masses with solid echostructure. Longitudinal and transverse views necessary to determine the size of the ovaries three-dimensionally. Ovary volume can be calculated as an ellipse.
$V = \frac{1}{2} (X \times Y \times Z)$,
where V = volume; X = length; Y = width; Z = thickness.

When the ovary is small, it is sometimes difficult to measure the three dimensions: it can be considered as a sphere where the diameter is measured. Thus pubertal ovary volume is 0.3–0.9 cm^3 (mean 0.5 cm^3) (Fig. 12). If it exceeds 1 cm^3, puberty has begun, as prepubertal volume increase is small.

At puberty, ovaries increase rapidly and postpubertal volume is 1.8–5.3 cm^3 (mean 4 cm^3). The volume should always be below 6 cm^3. The echostructure changes from homogeneous to heterogeneous. In the first half of the menstrual cycle follicles can be seen as small liquid shapes, with a maximum diameter of 2 cm (Figs. 13, 14, and 15). The appearance of the corpus luteum varies greatly.

The main indications of pelvic echography in children can be seen in Table 1 and are discussed below.

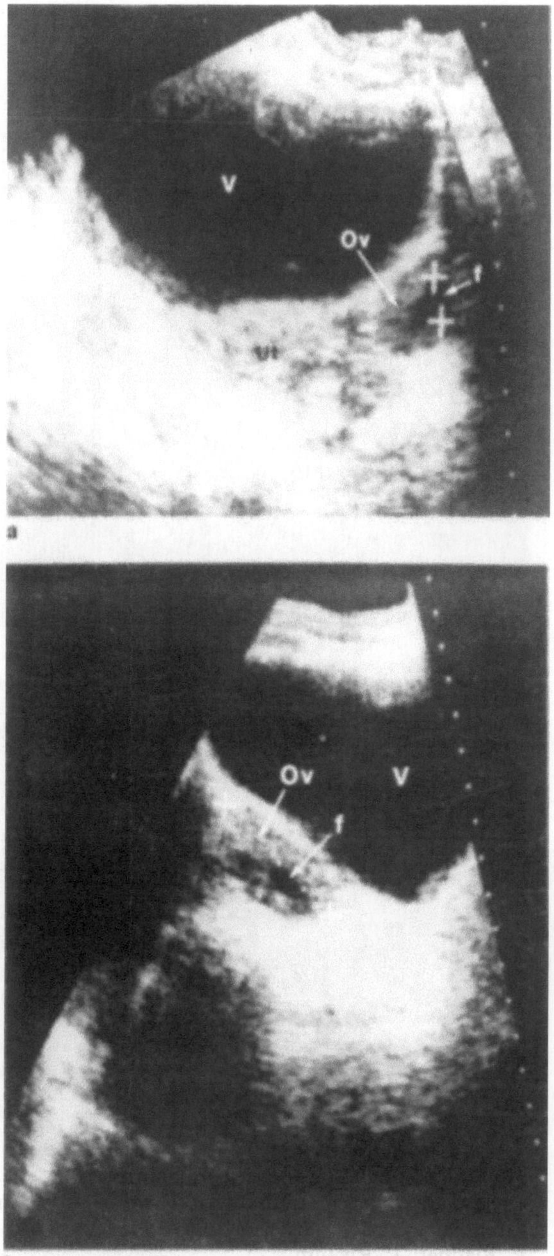

Fig. 14. a Postpubertal ovaries in a 14-year-old girl. Transverse view Ovary is 2.2 cm wide. There is a follicle less than 1 cm.
b Longitudinal view. Both views enable the three dimensions to be measured so that ovary volume can be calculated: V = ½ (length × width × thickness).
V, Bladder; *Ov*, Ovary; *f*, Follicle; *Ut*, Uterus.

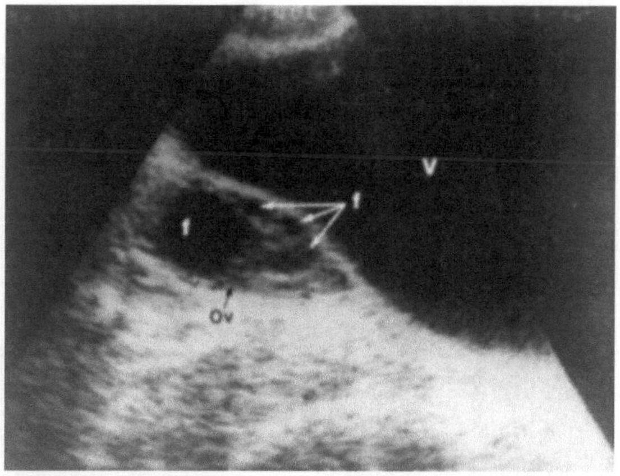

Fig. 15. Longitudinal view of postpubertal ovary. Ovary is 4 cm long. There is a large mature follicle (2 cm in diameter) visible just before ovulation.
V, Bladder; *Ov*, Ovary; *f*, Follicle.

Table 1. Clinical indications for pelvic echography in children.

Sexual ambiguity
Precocious puberty
Delayed puberty
Menstrual pathology: Primary and secondary amenorrhea
Pelvic masses
Polymalformations
Abdominopelvic pain
Abnormal vaginal discharge

3 Sexual Ambiguities

It is important to assign a sex as rapidly as possible to a newborn with sexual ambiguity. Clinically, external genital organs can be defined according to Prader's stages and other malformations are looked for. As part of the radiological study, genitography and echography are easily and rapidly obtained. Pelvic echography aims to confirm the presence or absence of a uterus or vagina. These organs are often better seen on transverse views (Fig. 16) after an often long and strenuous study because of size and insufficient bladder filling during the first days of life. In the case of male pseudohermaphroditism, rectal gas next to the back of the bladder confirms the absence of a uterus (Fig. 17). In this type of malformation there is always a more or less sizable utricle rarely seen on echography.

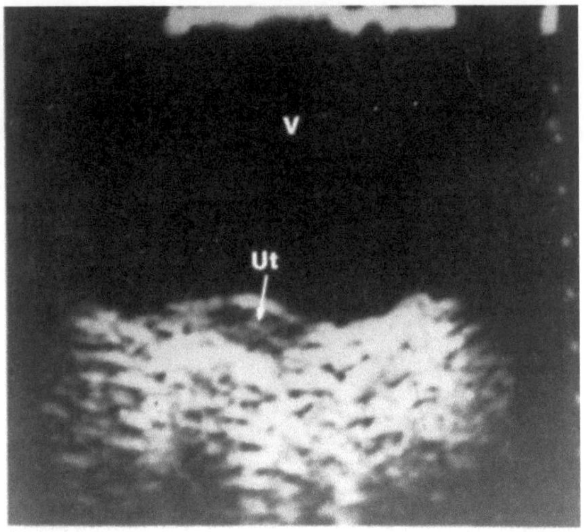

a

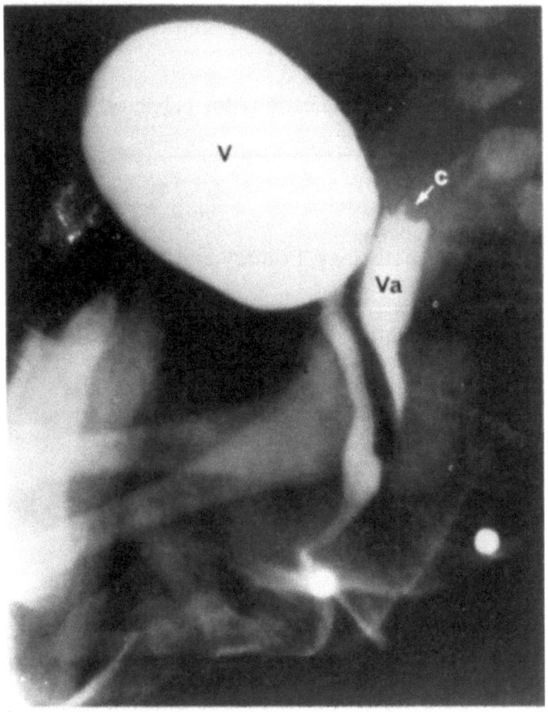

b

Fig. 16a and b. Female pseudohermaphroditism.
a Transverse view: in a newborn it is difficult to see pelvic walls. Uterus is better seen on transverse view making an imprint of posterior side of bladder.
b Genitography. Prader stage IV. Opacification through only perineal hole shows vaginal cavity at the bottom of which uterus neck makes typical imprint. *V*, Bladder; *Va*, Vagina; *C*, Uterus neck; *Va*, Vagina

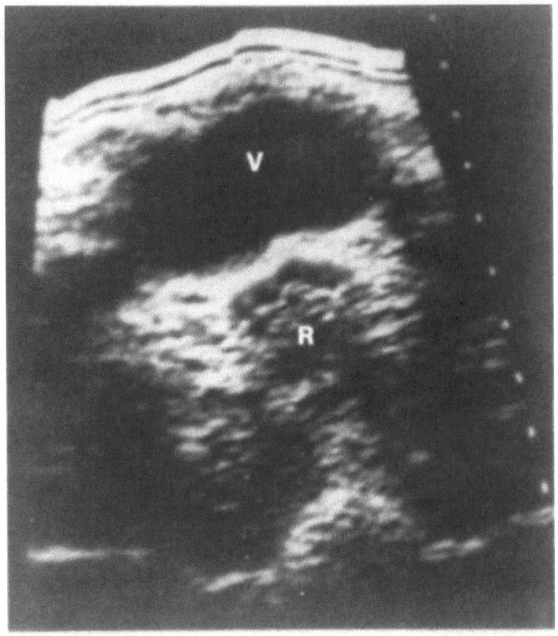

a

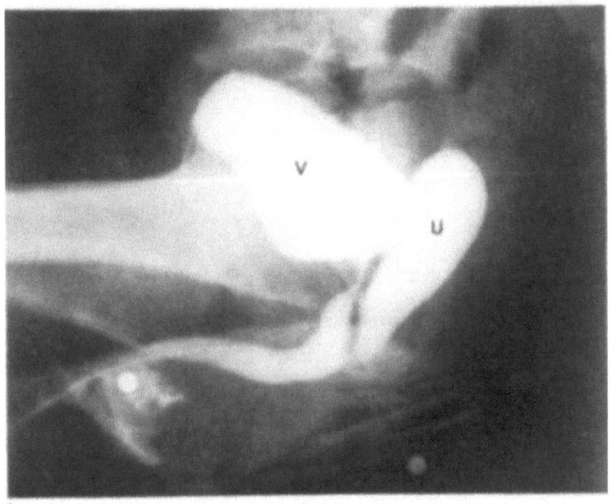

b

Fig. 17 a and b. Male pseudohermaphroditism.
a Transverse view of the pelvis. There is no uterus: rectal gas is next to posterior side of bladder. *V*, Bladder; *R*, Rectum.
b Genitography. Vulviform hypospadias; urethra opacification shows large utricle with no uterus neck imprint. *V*, Bladder; *U*, Utricle

A total of 80% of all sexual ambiguities are female pseudohermaphroditism mostly due to congenital surrenal hyperplasia. Another possible etiology is fetal virilization by maternal hormones (drugs taken during pregnancy or virilizing tumor of the mother). Male pseudohermaphroditism is rarer and due either to a testosterone synthesis defect caused by enzyme deficiency or more often to incomplete androgen receptivity dysfunction. If the defect is complete, it can be due to a feminizing testicle which is never revealed by neonatal sexual ambiguity. True hermaphroditism is exceptional.

4 Precocious Puberty

Precocious puberty is defined as secondary sexual traits appearing before 8 years of age in girls and 10 years of age in boys. It is three times more frequent in girls than in boys, but in girls it is rarely due to a lesion (6% of cases). True precocious puberty is always isosexual, due to primary hypothalamohypophyseal dysfunction. False precocious puberty is either iso sexual or heterosexual due to primary gonadal or adrenal dysfunction. Table 2 shows the etiologies in girls.

Pelvic echography is now part of any check-up for precocious puberty: it was performed in 62 girls from 1 to 8 years of age, presenting with simple mammary bulging to more or less complete harmonious development of secondary sexual traits. The degree of estrogen impregnation is judged on morphology and size of uterus.

The uterus is normal in size and shape in the case of premature thelarche (20 cases) or premature adrenarche (9 cases), but in most true cases of precocious puberty, there is a significant increase in the size of the uterus for the age of the patient.

Compared to other types of studies such as rectal examination, hormonal dosage, and cytological studies, there is now some doubt about

Table 2. Etiologies of sexual precocity in girls.

True precocious puberty
- Idiopathic: 90% of cases
- Tumors: hamartoma, astrocytoma, pinealoma
- Hydrocephaly of any cause
- Inflammatory causes: meningitis, encephalitis, arachnoiditis
- Head trauma
- General diseases: Recklinghausen disease; tuberous sclerosis of Bourneville; McCune-Albright syndrome
- Endocrine causes: hypothyroidism; primary adrenal insuffiency
- Paraneoplastic: HCG secreting teratoma

Isosexual precocious pseudopuberty
- Exogenous hyperestrogens: drugs, food, cosmetics
- Endogenous hyper estrogens: feminizing tumor of the adrenal gland, exceptional
- Ovarian feminizing tumor; rare: granulosa tumor, thecoma, teratoma, choriocarcinoma, chorio epithelioma, benign ovarian cyst

Heterosexual early pseudopuberty
- Adrenal causes: congenital adrenal hyperplasia; virilizing adrenal tumor (corticosurrenaloma)
- Gonadic causes: virilizing ovarian tumor: arrhenoblastoma

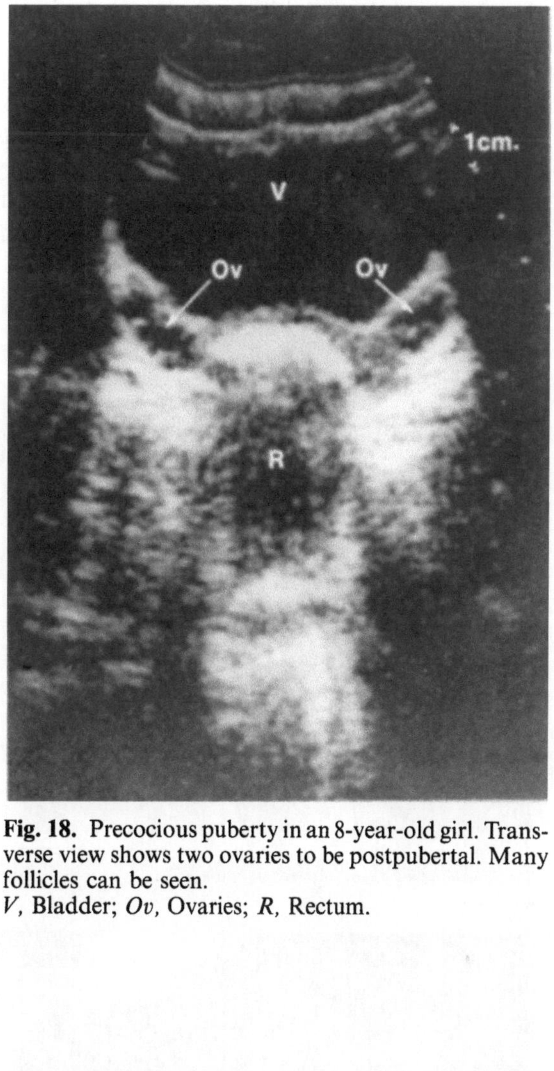

Fig. 18. Precocious puberty in an 8-year-old girl. Transverse view shows two ovaries to be postpubertal. Many follicles can be seen.
V, Bladder; *Ov*, Ovaries; *R*, Rectum.

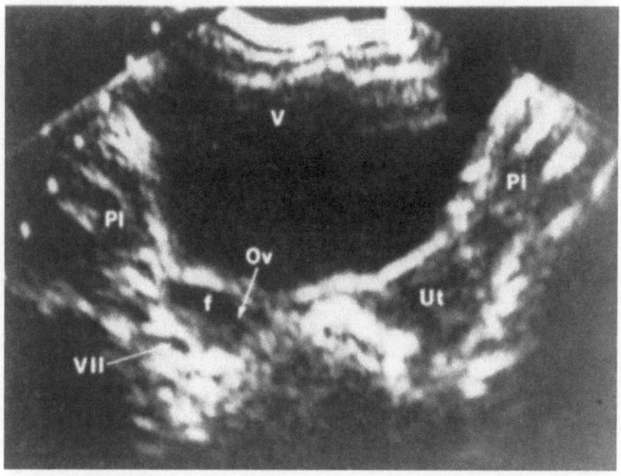

Fig. 19. Precocious puberty in a 5-year-old girl. Transverse view. Uterus body is to the left side, well developed, and 2 cm thick. Right ovary is postpubertal size and a follicle is seen.
V, Bladder; *Ut*, Uterus; *Ov*, Ovary; *f*, Follicle; *PI*, Iliopsoas muscle; *VII*, Internal iliac vessel.

the place and dependability of echography in the appreciation of hormone impregnation.

Easily repeated successive echographical studies can be used to follow hormonal therapy or uterus involution in the case of treated precocious puberty. Echography can also be used to study and measure ovaries: volume over 1 cm^3 is a sign of starting puberty (Figs. 18 and 19). During precocious puberty with a recognized cause, functional ovary cysts that are transitory can sometimes be seen. Exceptionally, a primary secreting ovarian tumor is found to be the cause of precocious puberty. The most frequent is the granulosa tumor with a variable echostructure – either solid, liquid, or mixed (Fig. 20).

There is no indication from echography in boys with precocious puberty. On the other hand, adrenal gland echography is an important part of isosexual precocious puberty survey in boys and heterosexual in girls when looking for congenital adrenal gland hyperplasia or virilizing corticoadrenal tumor.

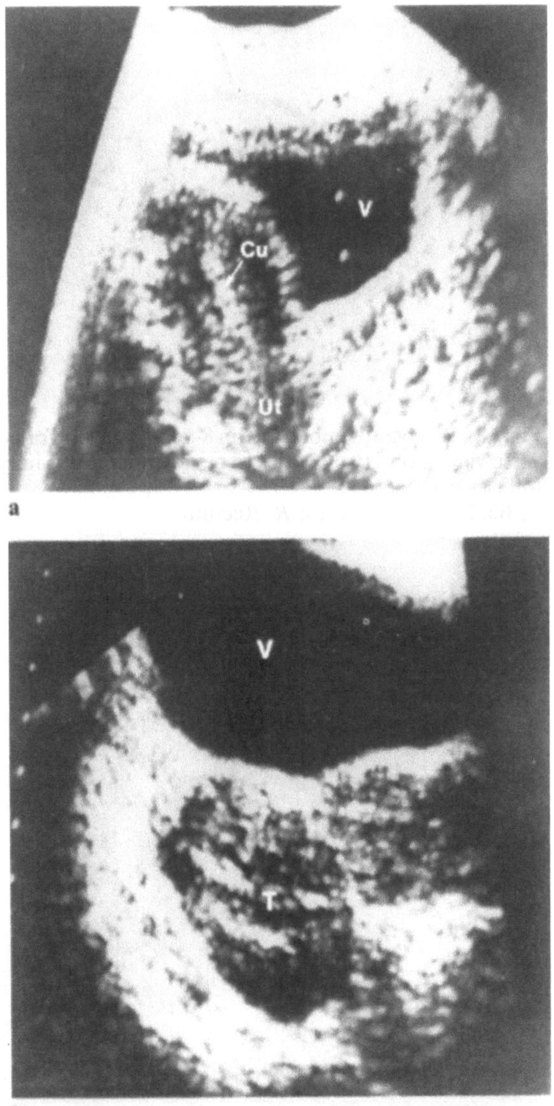

Fig. 20 a and b. Precocious puberty in a 7-year-old girl.
a Longitudinal view. Large postpubertal uterus.
V, Bladder; *Ut*, Uterus; *Cu*, Uterus cavity.
b Paramedial longitudinal view showing solid, heterogeneous mass 5 cm in diameter: it is a secreting tumor of the ovary. *V*, Bladder; *T*, Tumor.

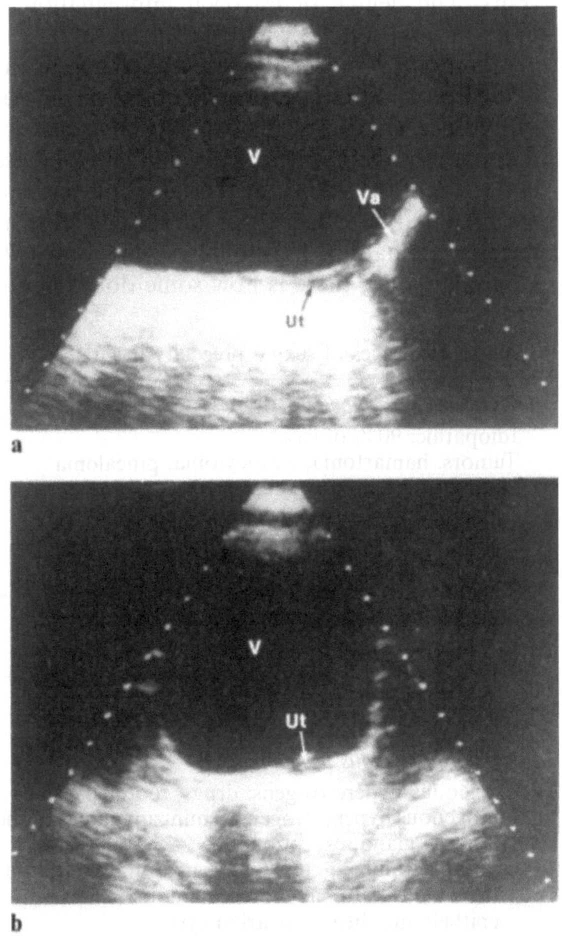

Fig. 21 a and b. Turner gonadic dysgenesis in a 15-year-old girl.
a Longitudinal view of the pelvis. Uterus is small, 3.4 cm long, prepubertal.
b Transverse view. Ovaries are not seen.
V, Bladder; *Ut*, Uterus; *Va*, Vagina.

5 Delayed Puberty

Delayed puberty is defined as secondary sexual traits appearing at 15 years of age in girls and 17 years in boys. Pelvic echography then has precise and limited indications. It again shows the degree of hormonal impregnation as judged by the shape and size of the uterus. If there is a marked absence of development of internal genital organs with often nonidentifiable ovaries less than 1 cm^3 in size, two etiologies are possible – either gonadic dysgenesis such as Turner's syndrome (Fig. 21) or hypogonadotrophic hypogonadism whatever the cause. The role of echography as a means of following up uterus maturation under hormone therapy must again be emphasized.

On the other hand, confirmation of the partial development of the internal genital organs contrasting with prepubertal external genitalia reassuringly shows only benign delayed puberty.

6 Menstrual Problems

Gynecological pathology in children is more limited than in adult women ; however, pelvic echography should often be used.

6.1 Primary Amenorrhea

The etiologies are given in Table 3. Echography is used to check the internal genital organs in young girls presenting with primary amenorrhea.

First, one looks for hematocolpos, i.e., menstrual blood retention by an obstacle: it is most often a nonperforated hymen, in which case the hymen is blue and bulges; it is rarely a vaginal diaphragm. Vaginal atresia is seen earlier in life in the neonatal period together with other malformations. Clinically, pelvic pain is present and characteristically repeats itself. Untreated, the accumulation of blood will lead to hematometria and hematosalpinx. Using echography hematocolpos is diagnosed by the presence of a medial liquid mass behind the bladder extending behind the pubis in place the vagina, which is no longer recognizable (Fig. 22). This mass can be totally transonic or produce tiny echoes from the sedimentation of liquid levels. At the top of this mass lies the uterus. It is normal if there is an hematocolpos, or dilated and full of blood if it is an hematometrocolpos.

Table 3. Etiology of primary amenorrhea: 3 cases.

1. Presence of harmonious feminine sexual traits
US can rule out any abnormality of the internal genitalia
Hematocolpos due to
Fusion of the labia
Hymen imperforation
Vaginal diaphragm
Vaginal atresia
Absence of uterus
Rokitanski-Küster-Hauser syndrome
Feminizing testicle
General causes
Psychological (anorexia nervosa)
Endocrine
2. Nonpuberty
Primary hypergonadotrophic hypogonadism
Gonadic dysgenesia: Turner syndrome
Castration through radiotherapy or surgery
Secondary hypogonadotrophic hypogonadism
Lesional causes: tumors, meningitis
Olfactogenital dysplasia of the de Morsier's syndrome (z), Laurence-Moon-Biedl syndrome
Functional; severe general diseases, endocrine diseases (hypothyroid, Cushing, anorexia nervosa)
3. Presence of secondary sexual traits with signs of virilization
Ovarian and adrenal causes

If the uterus is not seen during the ultrasonic examination, a feminizing testicle with uterine agenesis must be considered, i.e., agenesis of the top two thirds of the vagina and the absence of ovaries. Sometimes, however, echography reveals two pelvis masses where the ovaries should be. This can be confusing because these masses are actually cryptorchid testes. In Rokitanski-Küster-Hauser syndrome, the absence of a uterus is found along with vaginal agenesis and malformation of the urinary tract.

6.2 Secondary Amenorrhea

One should first eliminate a pregnancy whether normal or ectopic. Some authors in North America look for pregnancy in any young girl with pelvic pain, pelvic mass, or amenorrhea. The uterus increases, becomes rounder, and contains a small round mass that later becomes oval: this is the gestational pouch surrounded by trophoblast (Fig. 23). Inside this pouch the embryo is visible after 6 weeks of amenorrhea as a small linear

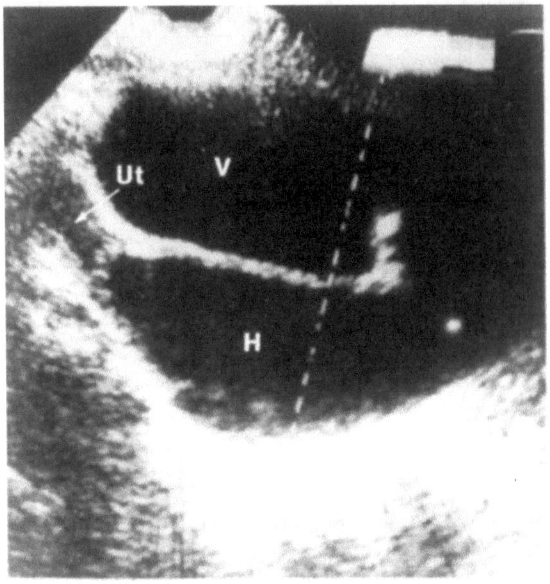

a

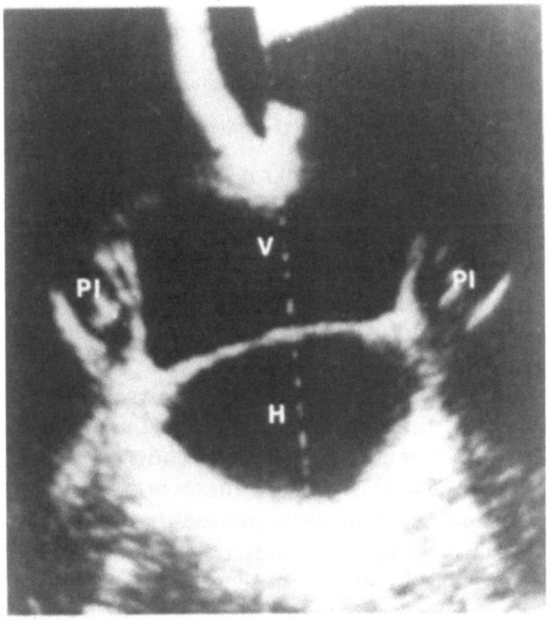

b

Fig. 22 a and b. Hematocolpos. **a** Longitudinal view: retrovesical liquid mass extending behind the pubis. On top is nondilated uterus.
b Transverse view: medial liquid mass.
V, Bladder; *H*, Hematocolpos; *PI*, Iliopsoas muscle; *Ut*, Uterus.

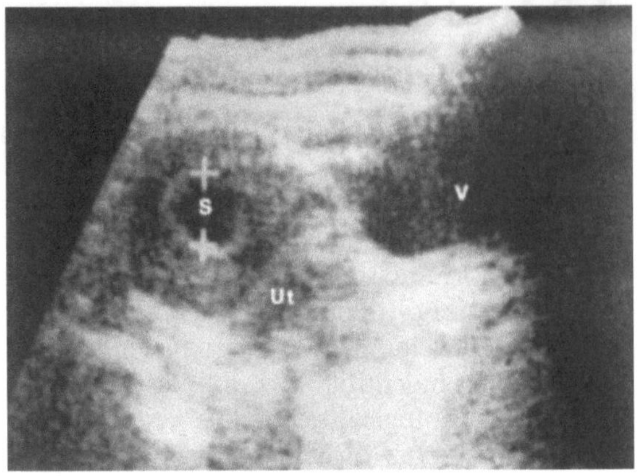

Fig. 23. Early intrauterine pregnancy in a 15-year-old girl. Paramedial longitudinal view. Uterus body is round. Ovular pouch (*S*) is seen as a liquid intracavity form with dense echo as the trophoplast.
V, Bladder; *Ut*, Uterus.

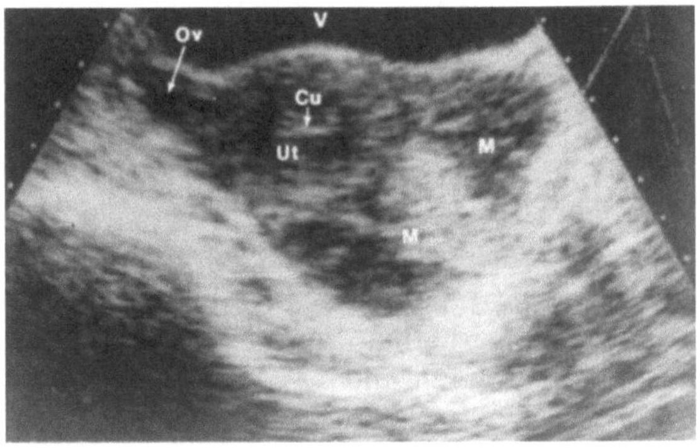

Fig. 24. Extrauterine cavity: transverse view. Right ovary is seen. There is an heterogeneous mass of the left side which is the extrauterine pregnancy in the left fallopian tube.
V, Bladder; *Ut*, Uterus; *Cu*, Uterine cavity; *Ov*, Ovary; *M*, Mass.

dense echo. In the first trimester, gestational age can be calculated by measuring the oval pouch and the embryo. Later, the embryo is easily recognized and biparietal diameter can be measured. Often at the start of pregnancy many luteal ovarian cysts can be seen, which cause pelvic pain.

Diagnosis is more difficult in the case of an ectopic pregnancy. Before the age of 15, diagnosis is difficult and it is important to have it in mind as "one only finds what one looks for". The uterus is slightly increased, nongravid, with a thickening of the lumen which is reaction of the decidual. A latero-uterine mass is present with a complex echostructure mixed with imprecise boundaries (Fig. 24). Egg and embryo are exceptionally seen. If the pregnancy is terminated, one finds liquid in the pouch of Douglas which facilitates diagnosis and should lead to celioscopy (Fig. 25). A dose of positive human chorionic gonadotropin 10 days after conception helps in the diagnosis of an ectopic pregnancy.

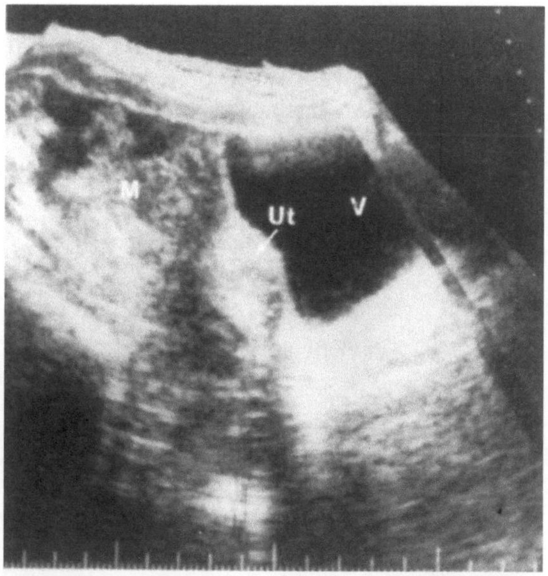

Fig. 25. Split extrauterine pregnancy in a 15-year-old girl. Longitudinal view of the pelvis: uterus is seen and its cavity is virtual. There is an heterogeneous mass plunging into the pouch of Douglas with the split extrauterine pregnancy with hemoperitoneum.
V, Bladder; *Ut*, Uterus; *M*, Mass.

6.3 Stein-Leventhal Syndrome

Most often oligomenorrhea with hirsutism and obesity are present. In addition to biological results, echography is typical by showing two large ovaries whose volume is two or three times normal. Echostructure is heterogeneous with many fine echo lines created by microcysts (Fig. 26). If pelvic echography is normal, the adrenal glands must be examined to look for an extragonadic cause for the hyperandrogenia.

6.4 Endometriosis

Endometriosis can be seen in children with abdominal and pelvic pain, dysmenorrhea, or even a pelvic mass. It can be found anywhere: on the peritoneum, uterosacral ligaments, and ovaries. Uterine endometriosis or adenomyosis is indetectable on echography. Outside the uterus, one can see cysts, without echo but with thick irregular walls; sometimes septa or dense echoes due to clots can be identified. This is not typical and can also be found in pelvic abscesses and some ovarian tumors.

7 Pelvic Masses

To diagnose pelvic masses one must be as quick, as dependable, and as low as possible in cost and irradiation, which is why in most cases IVP with total body opacification and echography are enough. These can be performed in any order, although in postpubertal girls it is preferable to start by echography in case of pregnancy.

Echography is fundamental to the diagnosis of pelvic masses: transverse views show their position medially. Healthy organs outside the mass have to be found in order to find its origin. Echography shows its outlines, echostructure

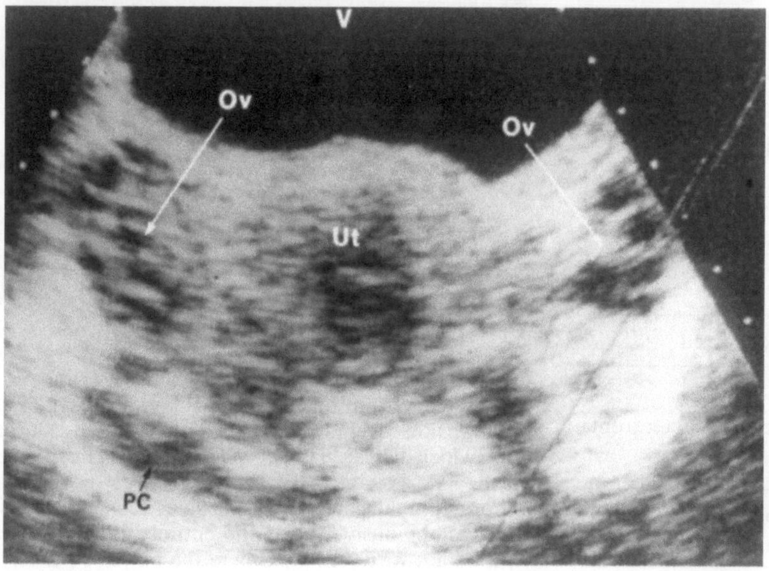

Fig. 26. Stein-Leventhal syndrome. Transverse view showing two large ovaries 4 cm wide. They are heterogeneous with numerous cysts, variable in size. The bigger cysts are visible, the others are seen as fine echo lines.
V, Bladder; *Ut*, Uterus; *Ov*, Ovary; *Pc*, Pubococcygeal muscle.

(solid, liquid, or mixed) and the shape of its wall. Such results considered in relation to the child's age and sex lead to diagnosis. Now one must emphasize the determinant role of puncture during echography in cases where it may be used. During the examination one looks for ascites, hepatic metastases, and renal participation. It is very difficult to look for retroperitoneal adenopathies.

Often diagnosis is complex and other studies should be carried out: barium enema, vaginography, bone tomographies, CAT scan, and arteriography. Nowad ays CAT scan is better in finding pelvic mass extension rather than making the actual initial diagnosis. It is more efficient in showing relation to big vessels, extension to viscera or bone than conventional studies. CAT scan is better in diagnosing pelvic wall lesions while echography is essential in the follow-up of masses undergoing chemotherapy: different views give tridimensional measurements before and after treatment. Observation of tumor volume reduction and necrosis helps in the choice of the best time to operate. After surgery, echography is part of follow-up because it is more easily performed and repeated in comparison with CAT scan.

7.1 Pelvic Neonatal Masses (Table 4)

A pelvic mass in a newborn is always abdominal and pelvic. If it is a liquid mass, one must eliminate urinary tract pathology such as an enlarged bladder due to urethral valves in boys or prune-belly syndrome (abdominal wall muscle aplasia). One must be able to recognize a bladder diverticulum, a congenital megaureter, or a large multicystic kidneys reaching into the pelvis, which is why echography of the kidney is so important. When the digestive tract is dilated and full of liquid there can be some confusion.

Table 4. Pelvic masses in newborns.

	Liquid	Solid or mixed
Frequent	Eliminate a large bladder Ovarian cysts Hydrocolpos	Sacrococcygeal teratoma
Rare	Rectal duplication Anterior meningocele	Neuroblastoma Pelvic kidney

A liquid mass in a newborn girl is an ovarian cyst unless proven otherwise (Fig. 27). Antenatal echography shows a more or less sizable pure liquid mass. At birth it is clinically mobile. Postnatal echography shows the mass and helps in the search for urinary tract compression. It is

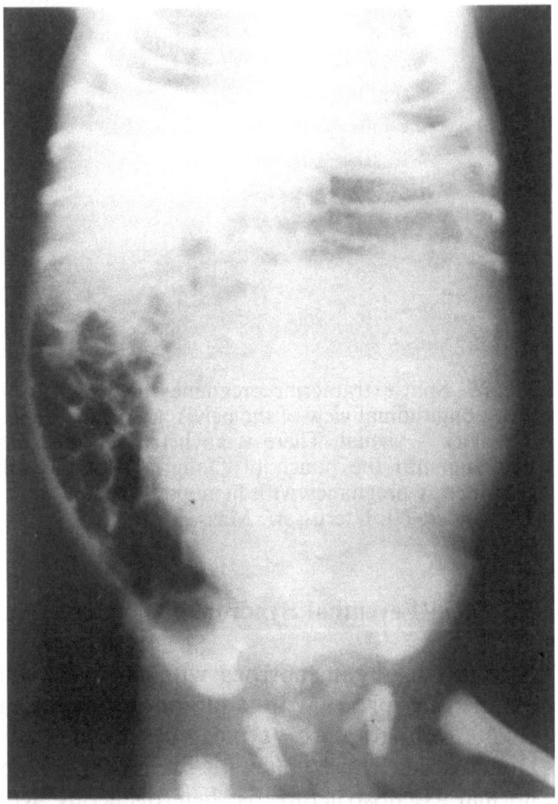

a

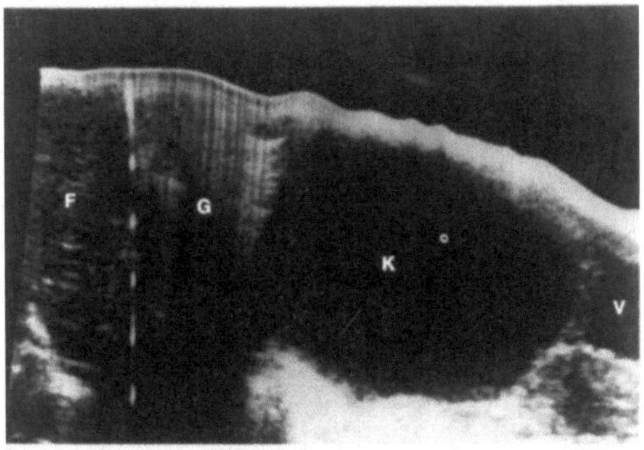

b

Fig. 27a and b. Ovarian cysts.
a Roentgenogram on the second day of life. A cystic mass was discovered during the antenatal US examination which displaced the bowel loops and is clearly seen on the left.
b Longitudinal view on the right side showing the mass, which is obviously mobile and entirely liquid.
V, Bladder; *K*, Cysts; *G*, Gas in the bowel; *F*, Liver.

important to know the different aspects of ovarian cysts on echography. It can be partitioned and can look like cystic lymphangioma inside or outside the peritoneum down to the pelvis (Fig. 28). Sometimes there is intracystic sludge with dense slow-moving echoes which are cholesterol crystals or blood due to spontaneous or traumatic intracystic hemorrhage (Fig. 29).

Hydrocolpos is a medial, nonmobile abdominal and pelvic mass in a newborn girl with other congenital malformations: anal imperforation, malformative uropathy, cardiopathy, or spinal malformation. Hydrocolpos or hydrometrocolpos is secondary to a vaginal obstacle such as a diaphragm or atresia. Cervical glands overstimulated by maternal estrogens in the first weeks of life lead to secretion accumulation. Echography is similar to hematocolpos as described above. It is different from an ovarian cyst in that it is medial, behind the bladder going downward. The vagina is not in the correct position. The uterus is visible at the top of the mass, and its cavity is normal or dilated (Fig. 30).

Other neonatal liquid masses are unusual: anterior sacral meningocele is a caudal meningeal hernia across a sacral defect. This presacral, retrorectal mass is seen as a cyst on echography. Sacral spine deformity is typical. Rectal duplication is similar on echography; its wall can be calcified.

Among solid or mixed neonatal masses, sacrococcygeal teratomas are most frequent. Diagnosis is easy when the extrapelvic part is large and palpable at the buttock. The intrapelvic part can be compressive. Simple abdominal X-ray examination shows typical presacral and rectrorectal calcifications with sacrococcygeal malformations. The echostructure is mixed, cystic with more or less echogenous zones that are connective, fatty, or calcic structures. Rarely it is only cystic and then impossible to differentiate from rectal duplication or anterior meningocele (Fig. 31). The

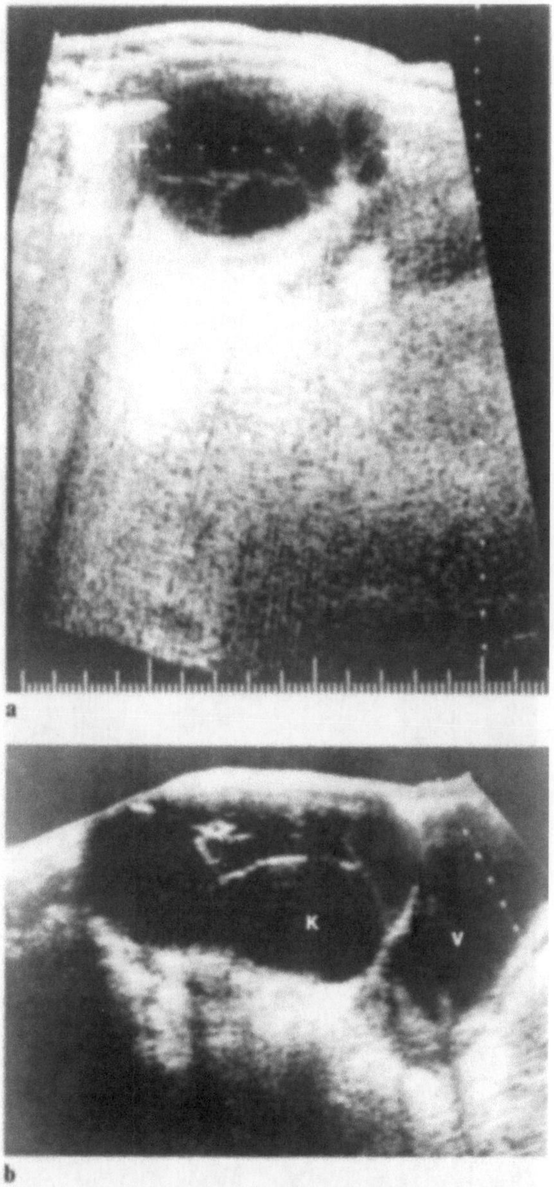

Fig. 28 a and b. Partitioned ovarian cyst. **a** Paramedial longitudinal view. Thick partitions.
b Medial longitudinal view. Large benign multilobed cystadenoma of the left ovary. *V*, Bladder; *K*, Cyst.

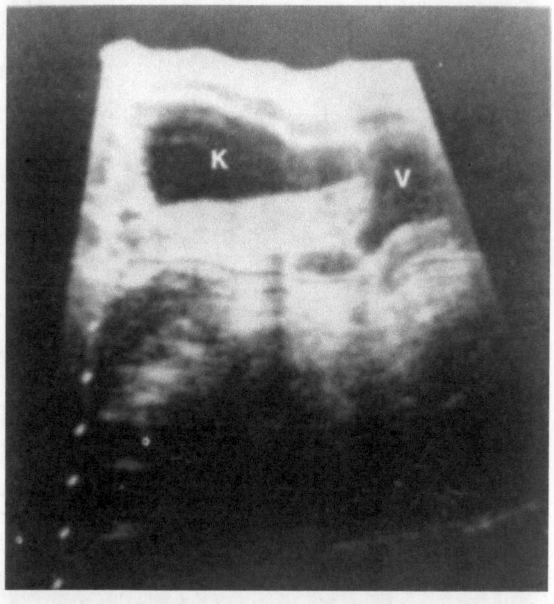

Fig. 29. Longitudinal view showing ovarian cyst with liquid over liquid echo. It is a necrosed cyst, free in the peritoneum of a newborn. *V*, Bladder; *K*, Cyst.

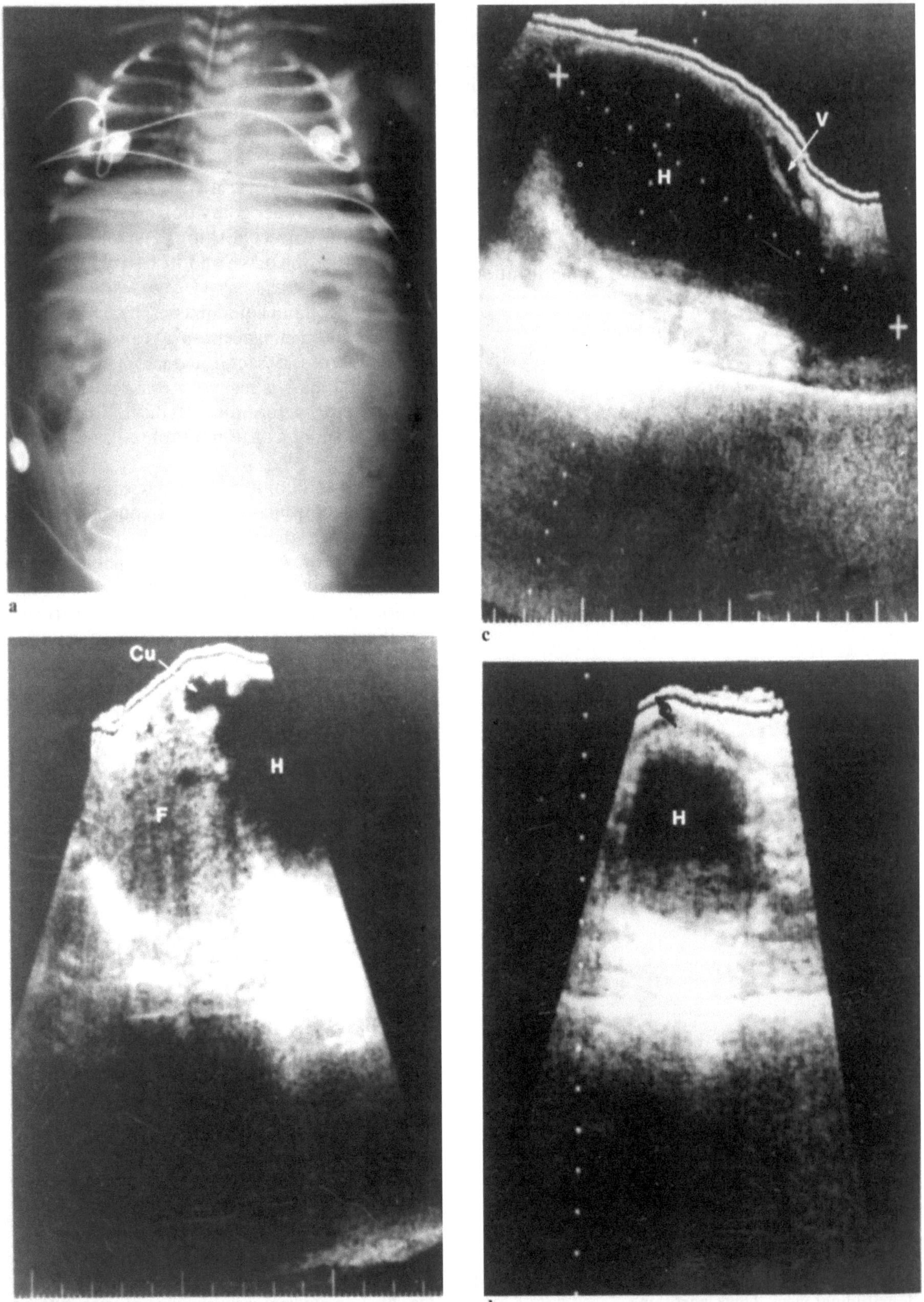

Fig. 30 a–d

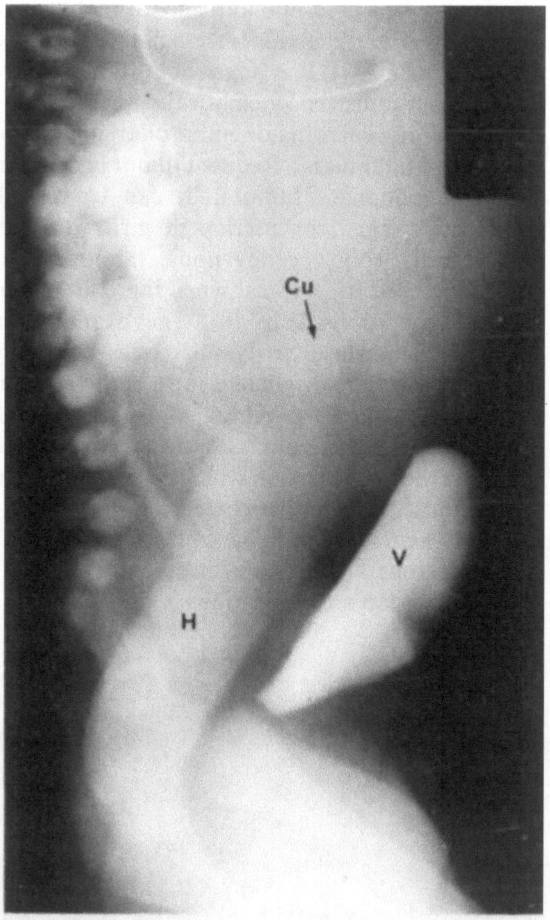

e

Fig. 30 a–e. Hydrocolpos.
a Abdominal roentgenogram in a newborn girl with a large abdominopelvic mass causing respiratory distress. Aspiration of 350 cc liquid with mucus. Mass is medial and pushes back intestine.
b Longitudinal view: small bladder against a large liquid mass behind the pubis. *V*, Bladder; *H*, Hematocolpos. **c** Longitudinal view on top of the mass: uterus cavity (*Cu*) is dilated and communicates with hydrocolpos (*H*). *F*, Liver. **d** Transverse view: fine downward echoes inside liquid mass. **e** IVP side view: X ray examination produced similar results to echography. *V*, Bladder; *H*, Hydrocolpos; *Cu*, Uterine cavity.

predominantly solid echostructure should bring to mind malignant teratoma (less than 40% of cases) but one should avoid histological diagnosis on echography (Fig. 32). In this type of tumor, CAT scan is better in showing fatty tissue, small calcifications, and its relation to bone. A mixed echostructure differentiates sacrococcygeal teratoma from pelvic neuroblastoma which is solid, echogenous, and homogeneous outside calcifications. An increase in urinary catecholamines confirms the diagnosis.

7.2 Pelvic Masses Outside the Neonatal Period (Table 5)

The etiologies are the same as in the neonatal period, while ovarian cysts are frequent especially at puberty whether they are organic or functional.

Hematocolpos has been described in the section on primary amenorrhea. Hydrosalpinx can be seen after puberty: it follows a badly treated genital infection (staphylococcus, streptococcus) leading to occlusion of the fallopian tubes and dilatation of their distal portion. Echography shows a typical laterouterine, often bilateral, liquid oval mass (Fig. 33). Here again fine echoes can be present inside this liquid mass as in pyosalpinx. The most frequent pelvic abscess found in children is appendicular or postoperative. It rarely follows Crohn's disease. Its echostructure is liquid or mixed. Its wall is thick, irregular, badly defined, heterogeneous inside. Liquid in the pouch of Douglas is often found. It can be more difficult to diagnose an abscess when there is pelvic inflammation with a decrease in uterus echogenicity and loss of wall and pelvic organ contours.

There are many different solid or mixed masses. Ovarian teratomas are frequent, especially in girls after puberty. They are asymptomatic for a long time and finally present as a large pelvic or abdominopelvic palpable mass. They are rarely found when there is acute torsion. In 10% of cases, diagnosis can be made if the abdominal X-ray examination shows calcifications on bone (Fig. 34). These calcifications are present in 50%–80% of ovarian teratomas. They are echographically typical and no different from sacrococcygeal teratomas (Figs. 35 and 36). Echostructure

Table 5. Pelvic masses outside the neonatal period [Eliminate intrauterine pregnancy (IUP) and extrauterine pregnancy (EUP)].

Liquid	Solid or mixed
Ovarian cyst (+ + +)	Ovarian teratoma
Hematocolpos	Rhabdomyosarcoma
Abscess	Neuroblastoma, ganglioneuroma
Hydrosalpinx	Abscess
Rectal duplication	Tumor or inflammatory adenopathy
Anterior meningocele	Bone tumors (Ewing, chondrosarcoma)
	Chordoma
	Lipoma
	Pelvic kidney

is mixed; when predominantly solid, malignancy with ascites and hepatic metastases should be suspected (Fig. 37). It is bilateral in 10% or more of cases and must be sytematically sought.

Rhabdomyosarcoma or embryonal sarcoma of the urogenital sinus is a frequent tumor in children (10% of malignant tumors). It can be vesical, prostatic, vaginal, or uterine in girls. It is an intervesical, solid, echogenous homogeneous mass (Fig. 39). It is typical when there are endovesical vegetations (Fig. 38). The examination looks for metastases to lymph nodes especially when the sarcoma originated in the prostate, but hepatic metastases should also be considered. Sometimes these sarcomas develop from perineal tissue or the pelvic wall in which case CAT scan is better for the study of its extension.

Pelvic neuroblastomas account for 4% of all neuroblastomas. They are retrorectal often with small punctuated calcifications.

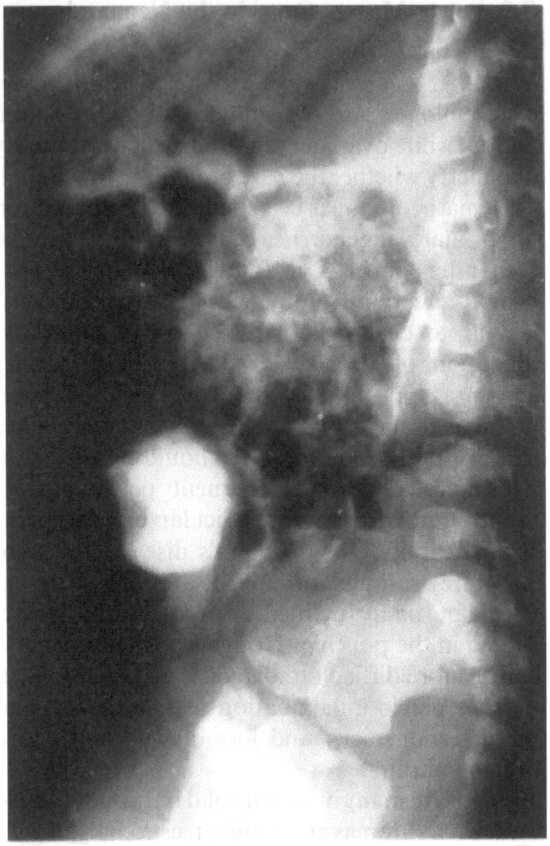

▲a ▼c

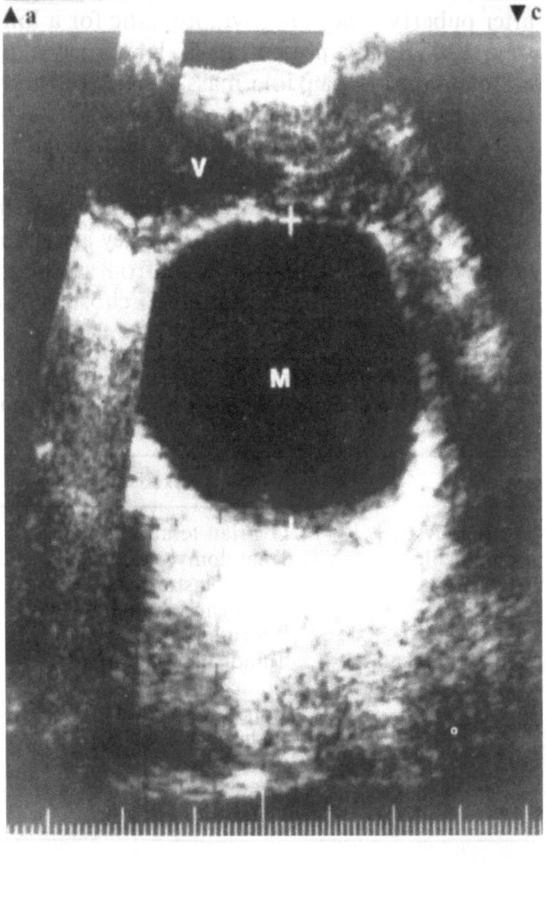

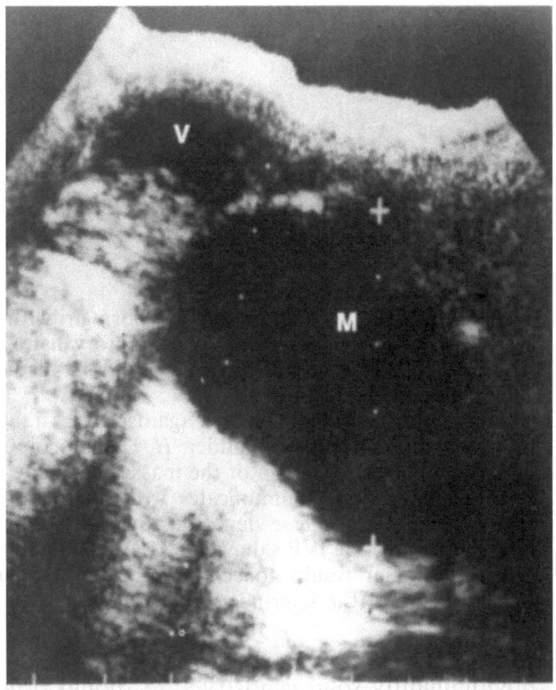

b

Fig. 31 a–c. Sacrococcygeal teratoma in a 2-month-old baby.
a IVP, side view: pelvic noncalcified mass pushing ureters forward and bladder upward. Rectum is not seen.
b Longitudinal view: totally cystic, large mass below the bladder.
c Transverse view: same appearance. Teratomas are often totally cystic similar at that age to rectal duplication or anterior meningocele. Their frequency guides diagnosis. *V*, Bladder; *M*, Mass.

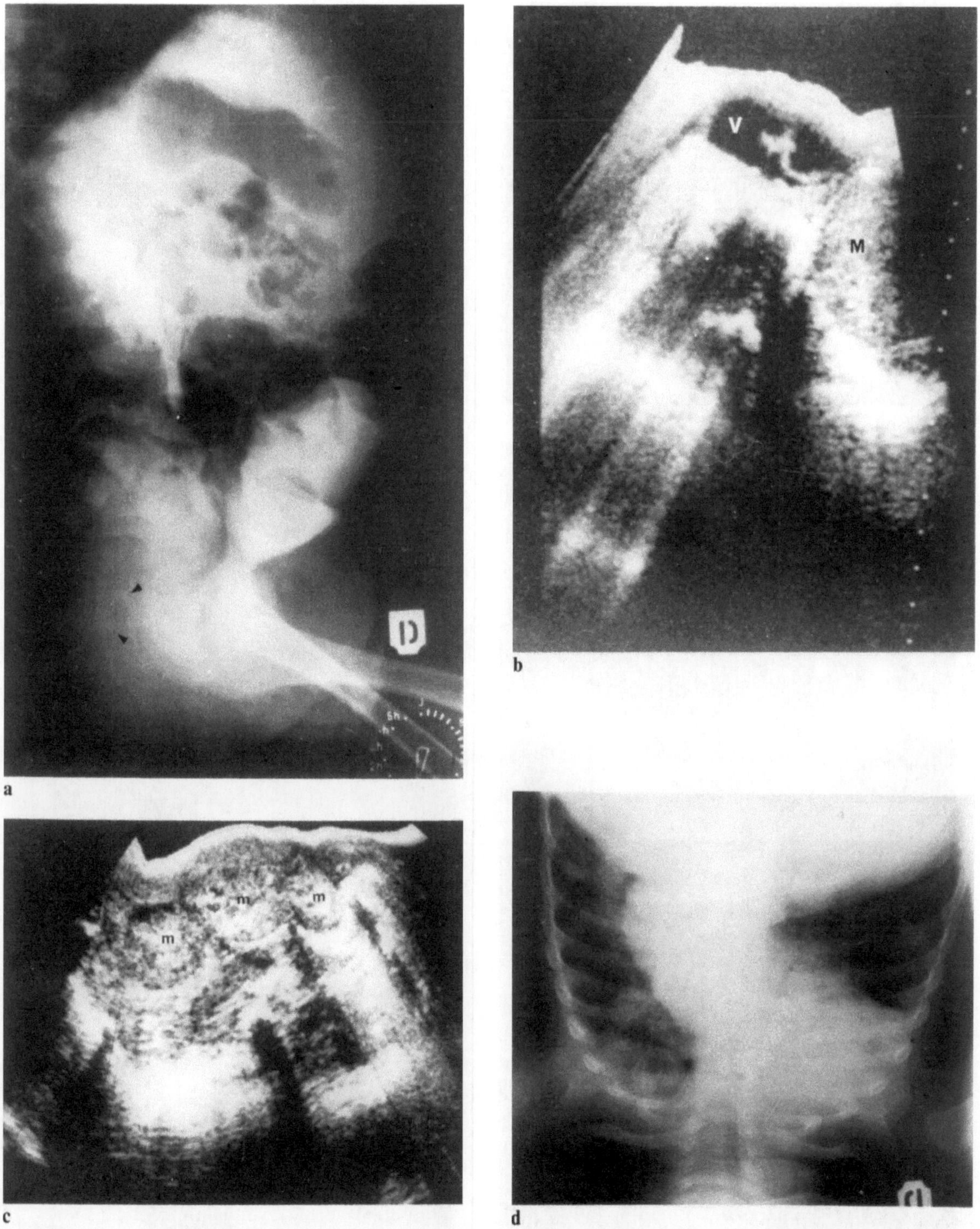

a b c d

Fig. 32 a–d. Sacrococcygeal teratoma in a 6-month-old baby. **a** IVP side view: exo- and endopelvic mass extending to buttock, with calcifications (*arrows*). Ureterohydronephrosis is present above. **b** Longitudinal view: solid, echogenous mass (*M*) under bladder (*V*). Vesical sound is in place. **c** Recurrent view below liver: many hepatic metastases (*m*) with same echostructure as pelvic teratoma. **d** Thorax with many pulmonary metastases. It is a degenerated sacrococcygeal teratoma.

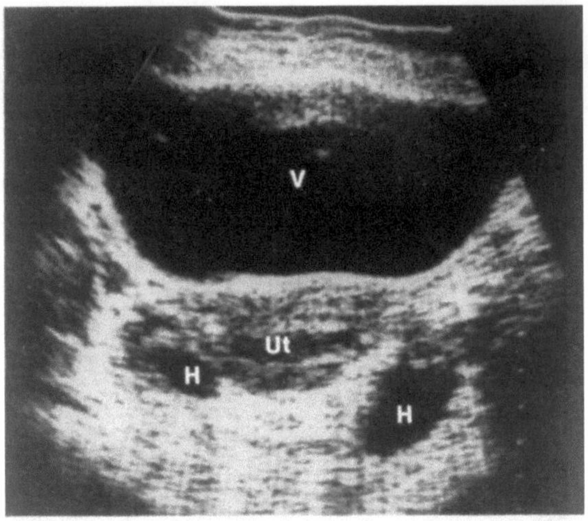

a

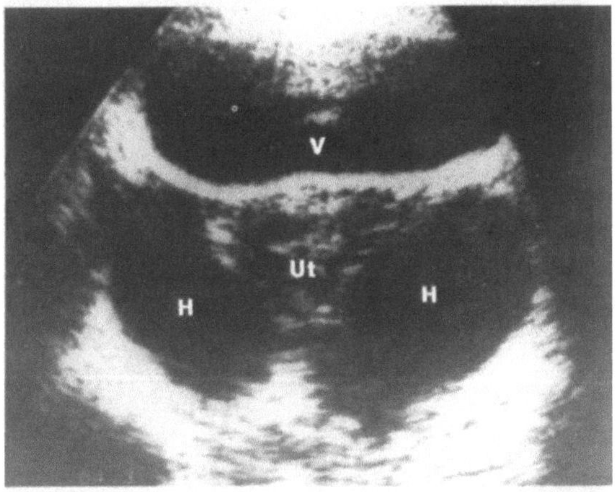

b

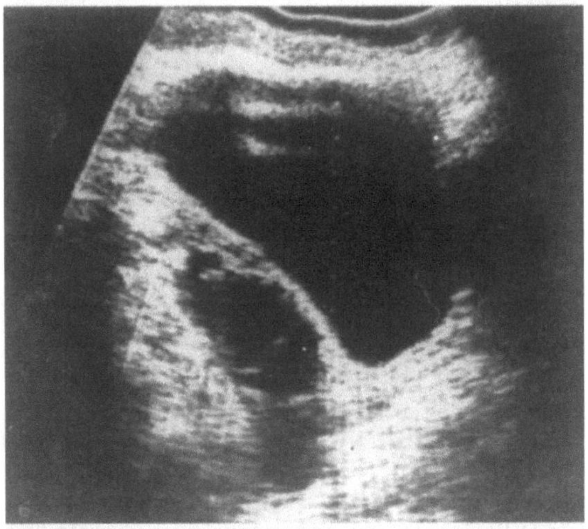

c

Fig. 33 a–c. Hydrosalpinx.
a Transverse view: two oval liquid masses; small bilateral hydrosalpinx. **b** Transverse view: typical very large bilateral hydrosalpinx. *V*, Bladder; *Ut*, Uterus; *H*, Hydrosalpinx.
c Longitudinal view: echo lines in the liquid mass correspond to dilated and sinuous fallopian tube.

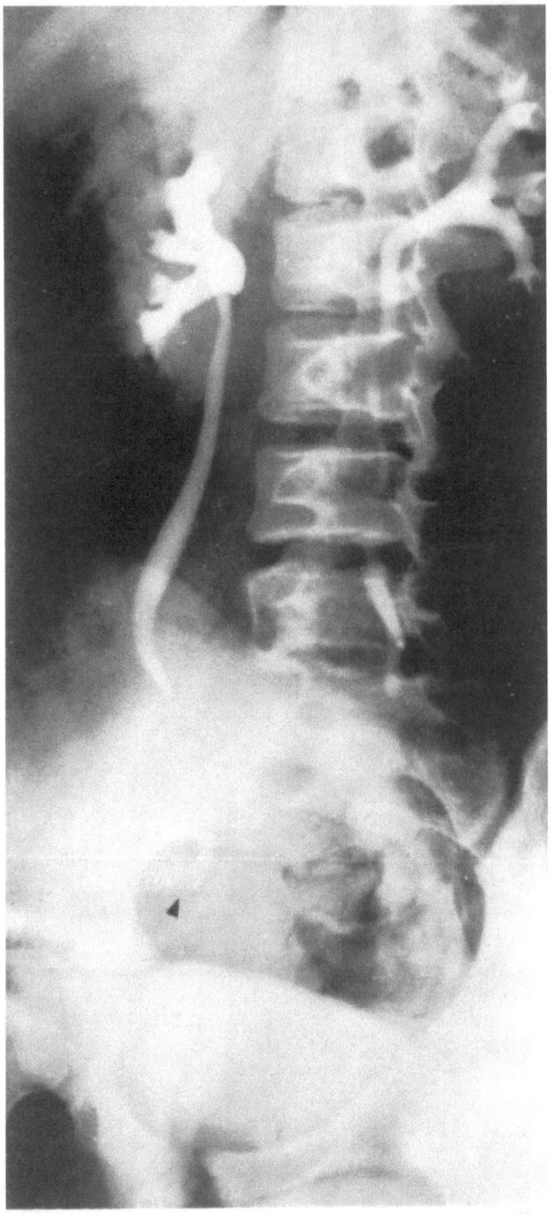

▲a ▼b

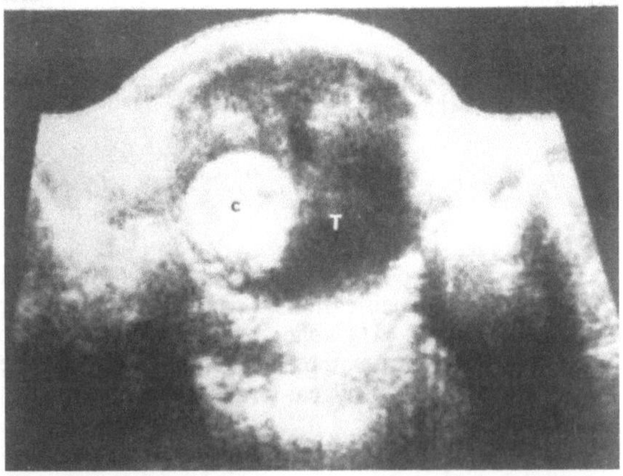

Fig. 34 a and b

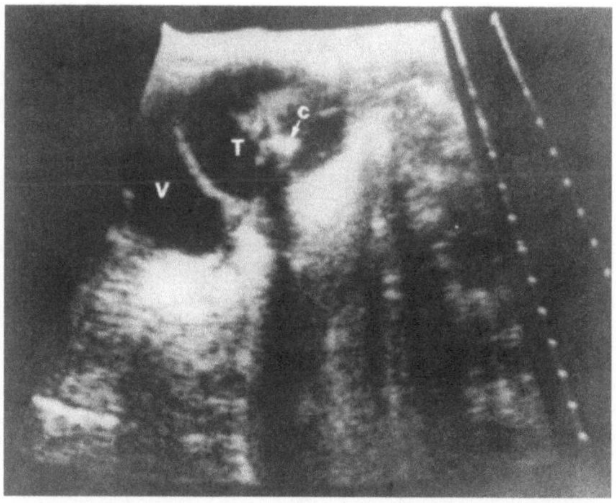

Fig. 35. Ovarian teratoma (*T*). Left oblique view. Mixed cystic echostructure with echo zones that are connective, fatty, and calcic tissue.
V, Bladder; *c*, Calcification.

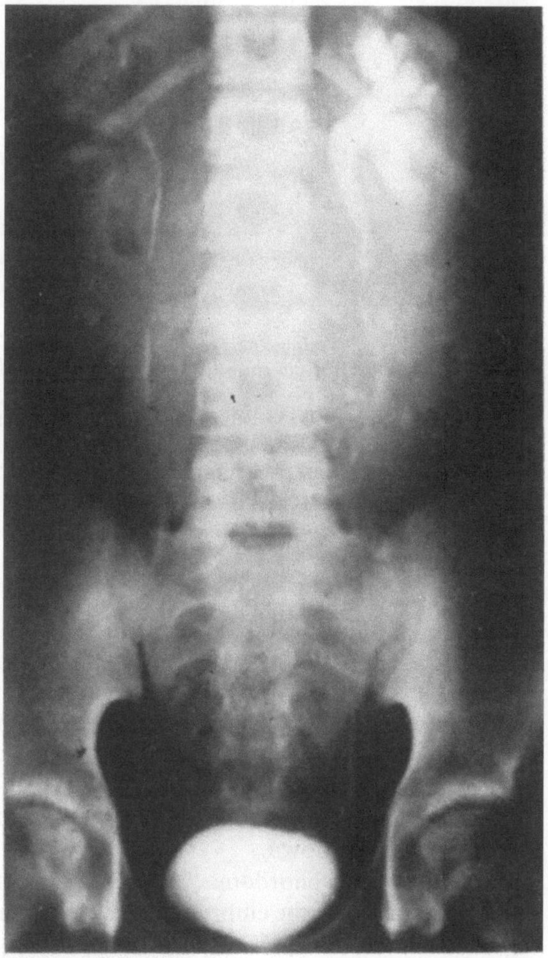

a

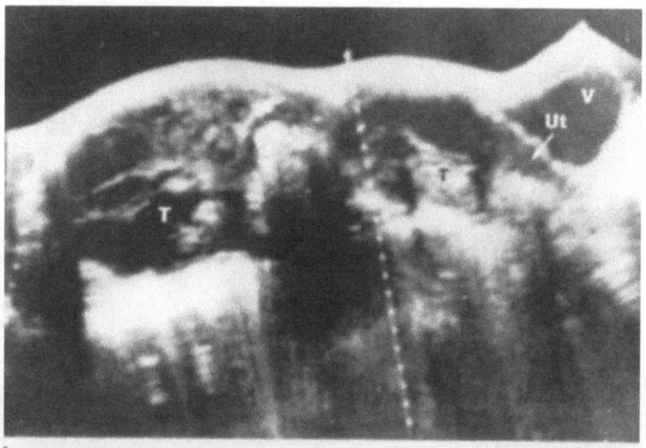

b

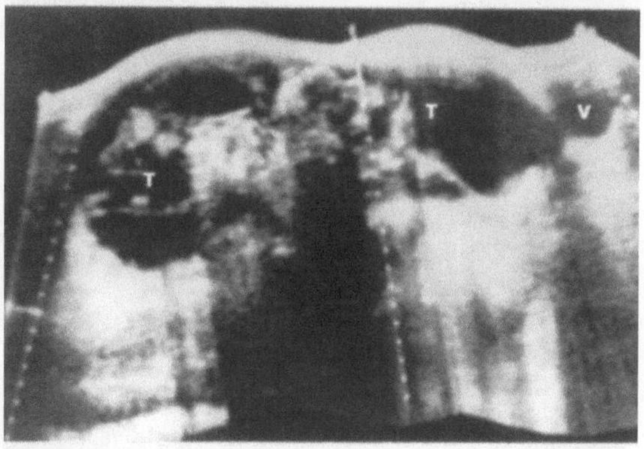

c

Fig. 36 a–c. Ovarian teratoma in a 12-year-old girl.
a IVP, front view: large calcified slightly compressive mass.
b and c Medial and paramedial longitudinal views: mixed typical echostructure with mature 4 kg ovarian teratoma (*T*). *V*, Bladder; *Ut*, Uterus

◄ **Fig. 34 a and b.** Dermoid cyst in an 11-year-old girl. **a** IVP: typical calcification (*arrow*) inside a liquid mass. It is a bony tumor. **b** Transverse view: mixed cystic mass with high echogenic area and a shady cone that corresponds to calcification. *T*, Tumor; *c*, Calcification.

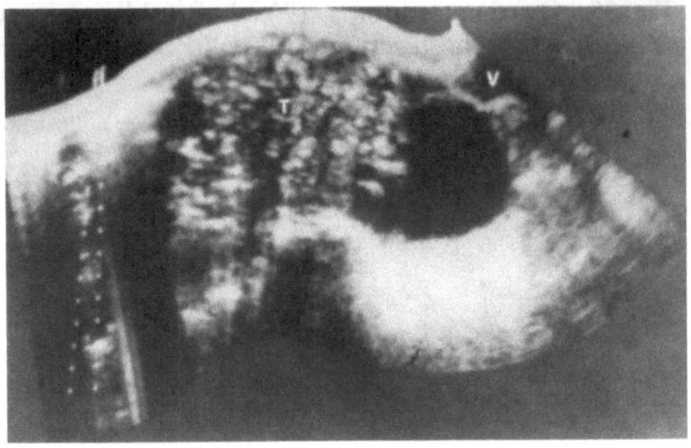

Fig. 37. Degenerated ovarian teratoma (*T*) on a paramedial longitudinal view. Predominantly solid echostructure with calcifications. *V*, Bladder.

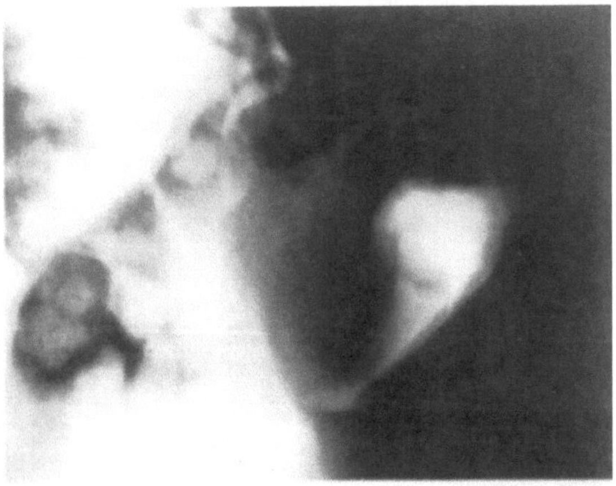

a

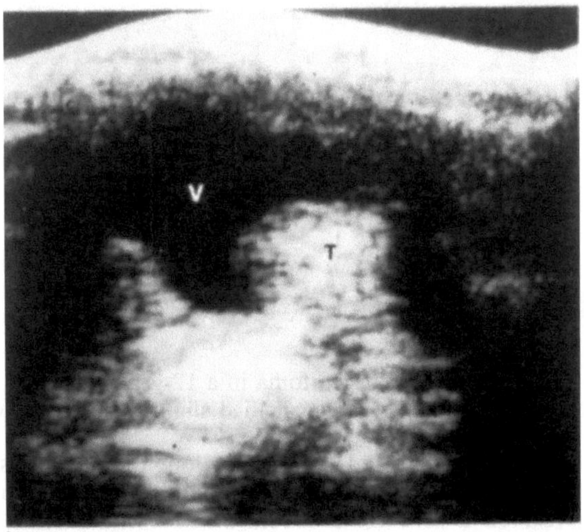

b

Fig. 38 a and b. Vesicoprostatic rhabdomyosarcoma in a 1-year-old boy.
a IVP, side view: noncalcified intervesicorectal mass.
b transverse view of bladder (*V*): typical intervesical bulging tumors (*T*).

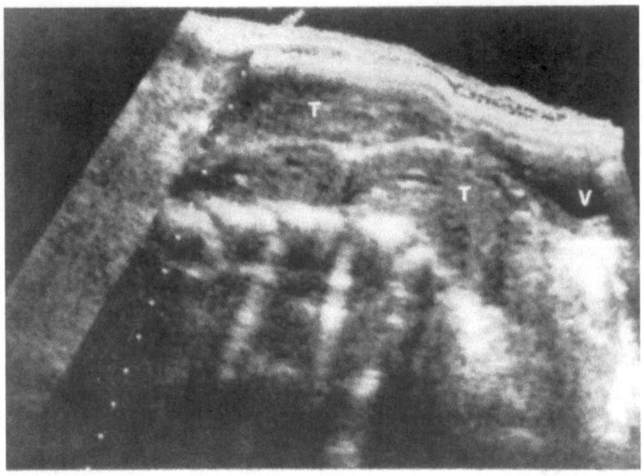

a

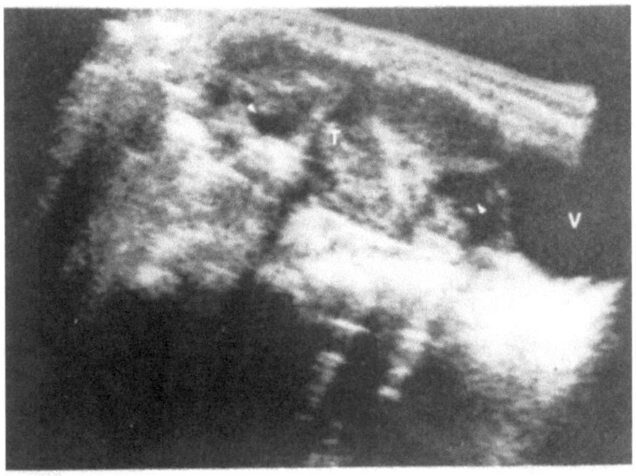

b

Fig. 39 a and b. Uterine rhabdomyosarcoma in a 1-year-old girl.
a Longitudinal view: large echogenous, homogeneous mass. *V*, Bladder; *T*, Tumor.
b Longitudinal view after chemotherapy: slight reduction and necrosed zones. Child underwent surgery.

Lymphomas are ileocecal, visible in the pelvis or as iliac adenopathies. They are typically homogeneous, low echo, or nonecho solid masses with polycystic contours if they are ganglia. A complete extension study should look for hepatic, splenic, or renal participation. It is difficult to find retroperitoneal adenopathies and here echography can let us down.

Sacrococcygeal chordoma is a rare medial tumor, arising from the embryonic remains of the notochord. It is seen typically as a medial osteolysis in the first sacral scans with an intra- or extraspinal anterior, rarely posterior, mass; 20% of chordomas are calcified. Echography shows a mixed, partially cystic mass.

The possibility of a pelvic kidney must always be considered (Fig. 40).

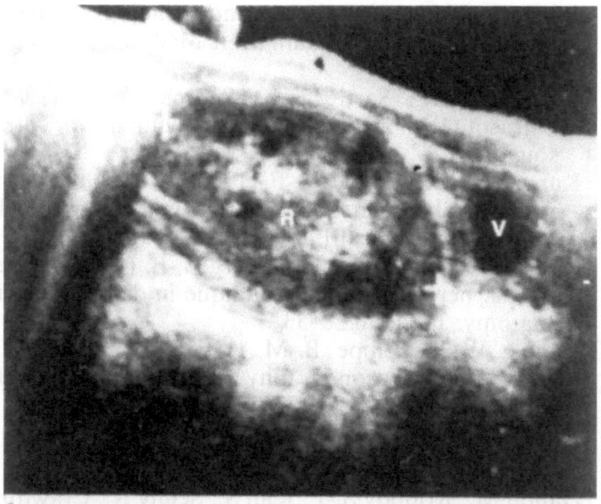

a

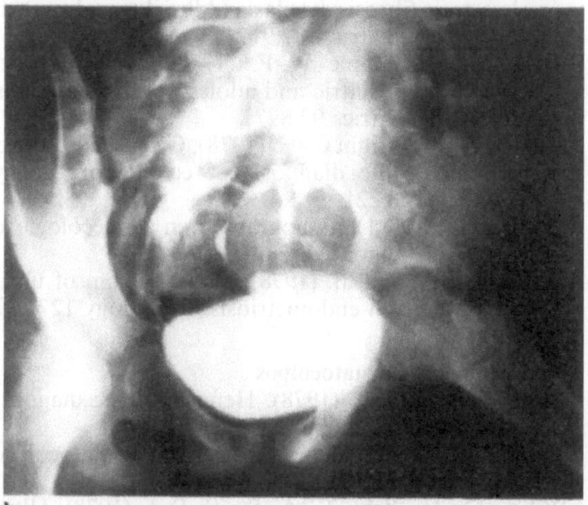

b

Fig. 40 a and b. Pelvic kidney found on systematic clinical examination.
a Longitudinal view: typical kidney *(R)* under the bladder (*V*).
b IVP horseshoe pelvic kidney.

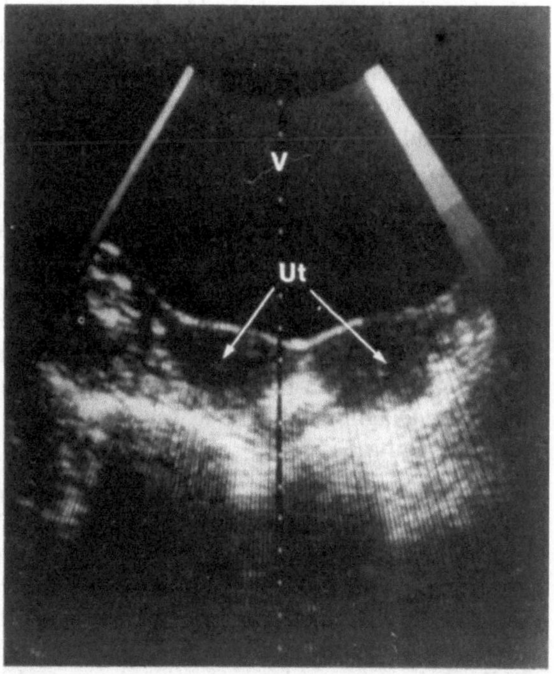

a

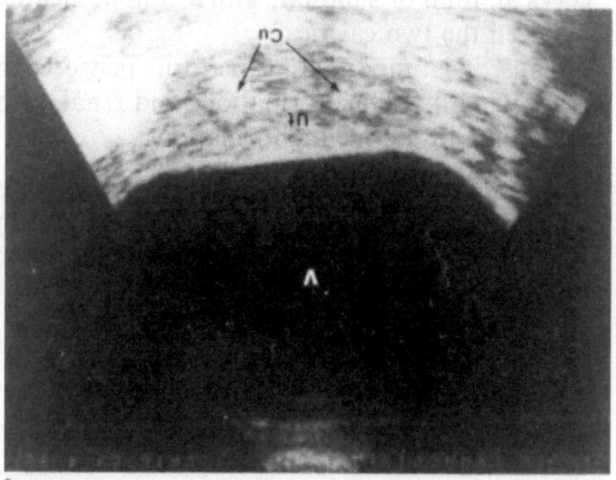

b

Fig. 41 a and b. Uterus malformation.
a Two-horned uterus: back wall hernia of the bladder (*V*) between two hemiuteruses (*Ut*).
b Partitioned uterus: one uterus (*Ut*) with two separate cavities (*Cu*) but no outside ridge and no posterior bladder hernia. *V*, Bladder

8 Congenital Malformations

Congenital urinary tract anomalies are rarely discovered in children as they are nonsymptomatic. They should be considered when certain urinary polymalformations are present such as renal, anorectal, or spinal agenesis. They are due to a defect in müllerian duct development. We will discuss only the most frequent malformations.

Uterine aplasia. Bilateral complete aplasia has only been confirmed in major polymalformations that are incompatible with life. Bilateral incomplete aplasia is represented by Rokitansky-Küster-Hauser Syndrome with the absence of vagina and normal fallopian tubes and ovaries. Echography shows the absence of the vagina and uterus, and ovaries can sometimes be seen. Malformative uropathy (20% of case) should be looked for. Unilateral aplasia or unicorn uterus is often associated with renal aplasia on the same side as the uterus horn aplasia. The uterus seem long and thin and to one side.

Uterine duplication and double horn uterus. In 10%–20% of cases this malformation is associated with renal agenesis and müllerian duct defect. On echography, two hemi-uteruses with two virtual lumens can be seen on transverse views. Typically posterior bladder wall hernia is present medially (Fig. 41 a). Furthermore, the axis of the two hemi-uteruses diverge. Transverse views behind the pubis differentiate a two-horn bicervical, bivaginal uterus from a unicervical uterus by the number of lumens visible. The two cavities can communicate or unilateral cervical and vaginal aplasia can be present causing hematometria. Diagnosis is difficult because there is a normal vagina beside it.

Partitioned uterus. This is due to a fault in medial wall resorption and does not bring about modification of the outside morphology of the uterus. Echography shows the uterus to have two lumens separated by an anteroposterior dense wall with no posterior bladder wall hernia (Fig. 41 b). This wall can be more or less extensive, corporeal or cervical, total or subtotal, with a communication between the two cavities.

Thus, it is important to perform pelvic echography in all polymalformations and renal echography in all uterine malformations.

Abnormal vaginal discharge. There are three causes in girls that can be seen on echography: intravaginal foreign body, vaginal rhabdomyosarcoma, and precocious puberty.

References

Normal US anatomy

Emans J.-H., Goldstein P.-D. (1977). Pediatric and adolescent gynecology. Little Brown and Company. Boston

Gates G.-F. (1978). Atlas of abdominal ultrasonography in children. Churchill livingstone. New York

Hall D.-A., Hann L.-E., Ferrucci J.-T. and al. (1979). Sonographic morphology of the normal menstrual cycle. Radiology. 133:185

Haller J.-O., Shkolnik A. (1981). Ultrasound in pediatrics. Clinic in diagnostic Ultrasound n° 8. Churchill Livingstone. New York

Haller J.-O., Kassner E.-G., Staiano S. and al. (1978). Ultrasonic diagnosis of gynecologic disorders in children. Pediatrics 62:339

Haller J.-O., Schneider M., Kassner E.-G. and al. (1977). Ultrasonography in pediatric gynecology and obstetrics. A.J.R. 128:423

Job J.-C., Pierson M. (1978). Endocrinologie pédiatrique et croissance. Flammarion Medecine. Sciences. Paris

Kangarloo M., Sarti D.-A., Sample W.-F. (1980). Ultrasound in pediatric pelvis. Seminars in Ultrasound 1:51

Kangarloo M., Sample W.-F. (1980). Ultrasound of the pediatric abdomen. A correlative imaging approach. Year Book Medical Publishers. Chicago

Rubin C., Kurtz A.-B., Goldberg B.-B. (1978). Water enema: new ultrasound technique in defining pelvic anatomy. J.C.U. 6:28–33

Sample W.-F., Lippe B.-M., Gyepes M.-T. (1977). Gray-scale ultrasonography of the normal female pelvis. Radiology 125:477

Endocrine and puberty disorders

Danon M., Robboy S.-J., Kim S., Scully R., Crawford J.-D. (1975). Cushing syndrome, sexual precocity and poly ostotic fibrosis dysplasia (Albright syndrome) in infancy. J. Pediatrics. 87:917

Lippe B.-M., Sample W.-F. (1978). Pelvic ultrasonography in pediatric and adolescent endocrine disorders. J. Pediatrics 92:897

Maklad N.-F., Wright C.-H. (1978). Gray-scale ultrasonography in the diagnosis of ectopic pregnancy. Radiology 126:221

Mauleon F. (1981). Echographie en Gynécologie et Obstétrique. Vigot, éditeur, Paris

Sandler M.-A. and al. (1978). The spectrum of ultrasonic findings in endometriosis. Radiology 127:229

Hydrocolpos – Hematocolpos

Little H.-K. and al. (1978). Hematocolpos: diagnosis made by ultrasound. J.C.U. 6:341–342

Sailer J.-F. (1979). Hematometra and hematocolpos: ultrasound findings. A.J.R. 132:1010

Wilson D.-A., Stacy T.-M., Smith E.-I. (1978). Ultrasound diagnosis of hydrocolpos and hydrometrocolpos. Radiology 128:451–454

Pelvic masses

Breen J.-L., Maxon W.-S. (1977). Ovarian tumors in children and adolescents. Clin. Obstet. Gynecol. 20:607–623

Carter B.-L. and al. (1976). Unusual pelvic masses: a comparison of CT scanning and U.S. Radiology 121:383–390

Fleischer A.-C., James A.-E., Millis J.-B., and al. (1978). Differential diagnosis of pelvic masses by gray scale sonography. A.J.R. 131:469–476

Goldberg B.-B., Pollack H.-M., Capitano M.-A., Kirkpatrick J.-A. (1975). Ultrasonography: an aid in the diagnosis of masses in pediatric patients. Pediatrics 56:421

Kirks R.-D., Merten D.-F., Grossmaann H., Bowie J.-D. (1981). Diagnostic imaging of pediatric abdominal masses: an overview. Radiol. Clinic. J. North America 19:3:427–546

Lawson T.-L., Albarelli J.-N. (1977). Diagnosis of gynecologic pelvic masses by gray scale ultrasonography; analysis of specificity and accuracy. A.J.R. 128:1003

Mittelstaedt C.-A. (1977). Gray-scalle patterns of pelvic disease in the male. Radiology 123:727–732

Reeves R.-D., Drake T.-S., O'Brien W.-F. (1980). Ultrasonographic versus clinical evaluation of a pelvic mass. Radiology (ab) 136:827

Sandler M.-A., Silver T.-M., Karo J.-J. (1979). Gray-scale ultrasonic features of ovarian teratomas. Radiology 131:705–709

Schey W.-L., Shkolnik A., White M. (1977). Clinical and radiographic considerations of sacro-coccygeal teratomas: an analysis of 26 new cases and a review of literature. Radiology 125:189–195

Siegel M.-J., McAlister W.-H., Shackelford G.-D. (1978). Radiographic findings in ovarian teratomas in children. A.J.R. 131:613–616

Walsh J.-W. and al. (1979). Gray-scale ultrasound in 204 proved gynecologic masses: accuracy and specific diagnostic criteria. Radiology 130:391–397

Werner J.-L., Taybi H. (1970). Presacral masses in childhood. A.J.R. 109:403–408

White E.-A., Filly R.-A. (1980). Cholesterol crystals as the source of both diffuse and layered echoes in a cystic ovarian tumor. J.C.U. 8:241

Inflammatory diseases of the pelvis

Doust B.-D., Quiroz F., Stewart J.-M. (1977). Ultrasonic distinction of abscesses form other intra-abdominal fluid collections. Radiology 125:213–218

Spiegel R.-M., Ben-Ora A. (1980). Ultrasound of inflammatory disease in the pelvis. S.U. 1:41

Uhrich P.-L., Sanders R.-C. (1976). Ultrasonic characteristics of pelvis inflammatory masses. J.C.U. 4:199

Congenital malformations

Fried A.-M., Oliff M., Wilson E.-A. and al. (1978). Ulterine anomalies associated with renal agenesis: role of gray-scale ultrasonography. A.J.R. 131:973

Shenker L., Brickman F.-E. (1979). Bicornuate uterus with incomplete vaginal septum and unilateral renal agenesis. Radiology 133:455

Vinstein A.-L., Franken E.-A. (1972). Unilateral hematocolpos associated with agenesis of the kidney. Radiology 102:625

Yoder I.-C., Pfister R.-C. (1976). Unilateral hematocolpos and unilateral renal agenesis: report of two cases and review of the literature. A.J.R. 127:303–308

Chapter 12

Ultrasound of the Scrotum

L. Garel

US can be very useful in children, especially in the case of a swollen, painful scrotum. It should be emphasized, however, that any clinical or sonographic indications of an acute surgical condition should lead to an exploratory operation without delay.

1 Technique

We use a 7 MHz short focused probe. The testis is immobilized either on a towel or manually. The scanning must be gentle and explore completely the testis and epididymis, in longitudinal and transverse scans. The setting should be made carefully to provide an homogeneous echostructure of the gland. The appearance of normal scrotum contents is identical to that in adults. The controlateral scrotum should always be studied comparatively.

2 Material

The number and diagnosis of the cases studied are given in the following list:

Testis torsion 6
Morgani's appendix testis torsion 10
Hydrocele 10
Cyst of the cord 2
Orchitis 4
Orchiepididymitis 2
Inguinal hernia 2
Tumors: Lymphoma 1
Pseudolymphoma 1
Recurrence of acute lymphoblastic leukemia 4
Paratesticular rhabdomyosarcome 1
Hormone secreting tumor (precocious puberty) 1
Inflammatory pseudotumor (calcified testicular parasite) 1
Ectopic testis 35.

3 Comments

The diagnosis of hydrocele is easily made (Fig. 1). Lymphoma (Fig. 2) and pseudolymphoma ap-

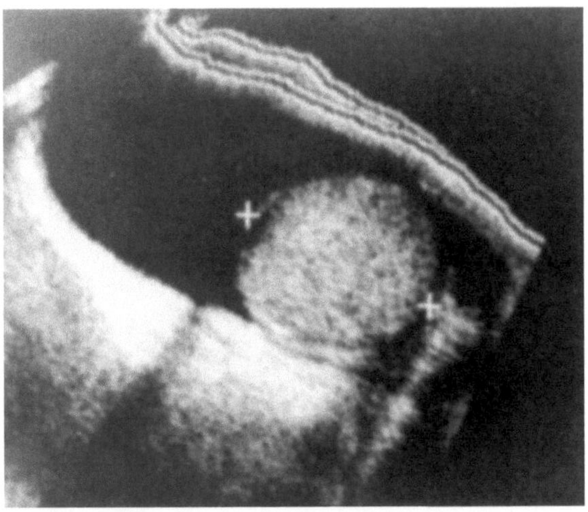

Fig. 1. A large hydrocele in a 14-year-old boy. Longitudinal scan of the right scrotum.

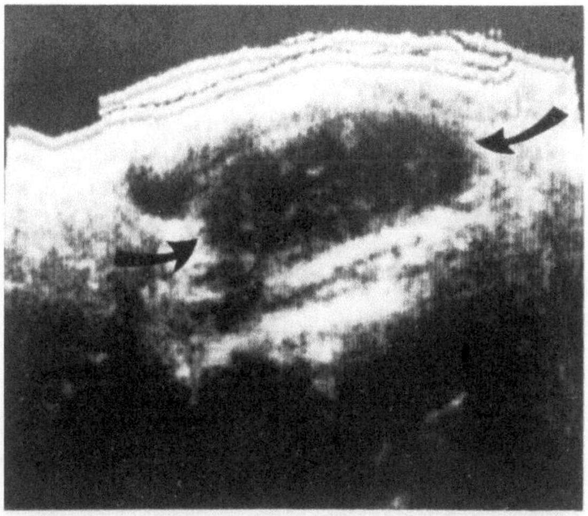

a

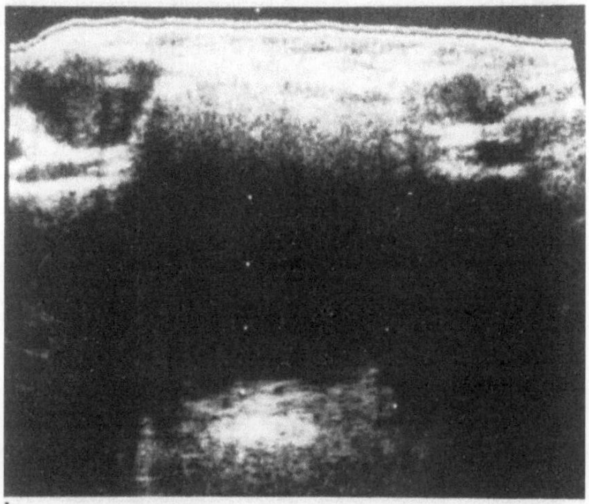

b

Fig. 2. A 9-year-old boy with a large palpable right iliac fossa mass and a small right inguinal mass.
a Longitudinal scan of the right inguinal canal.
b Transverse scan of both inguinal regions. The right testis is enlarged, its echogenicity is merkedly decreased (*arrows*). Burkitt's lymphoma of the ileocecal region and right testis. One notes the inguinal location of both glands in this patient.

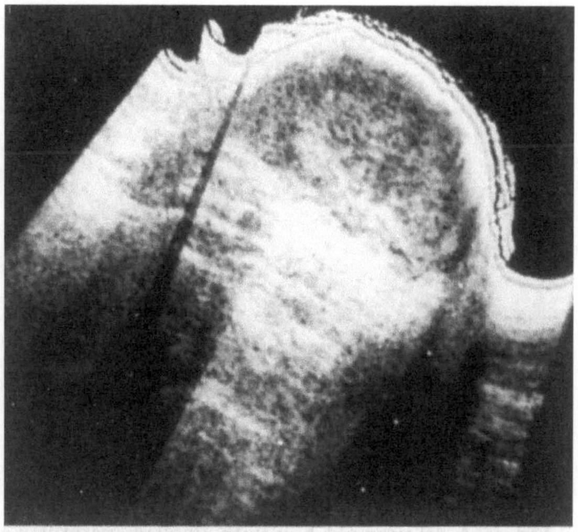

a

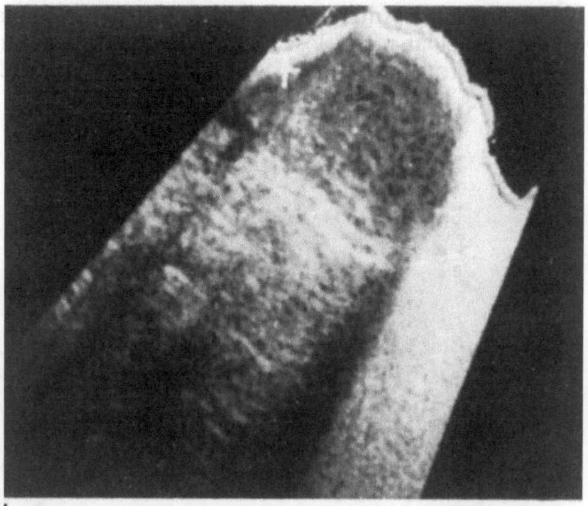

b

Fig. 3 a and b. A 10-year-old boy after, completerelase of acute lymphocytic leukemic for 3.5 years. Recent enlargement of the right testis.
a Longitudinal scan of the right testis.
b Comparative longitudinal scan of the left testis. Biopsy of right testis shows evidence of leukemic recurrence.

pear, as in other parenchymas, as hypoechogenic lesions. Testicular leukemic recurrences, on the other hand, can present only as an enlarged testis of normal echogenicity (Fig. 3).

Morgani's appendix torsion is illustrated sonographically by a normal testis topped by a small distinct mass, adjacent to the epididymis head (Fig. 4). This latter diagnosis implies, in most cases, nonsurgical treatment, emphasizing therefore the importance of its recognition.

In torsion of the testis, the gland becomes markedly swollen, hypoechoic (edematous) initially, then hyperechoic (infarcted) after a few hours (Fig. 5). The major differential diagnosis of torsion testis is represented by the inflammatory changes of orchitis, epididymitis, and orchiepididymitis. It is then important to show the involvement of both the testis and the epididymis. Obviously one can encounter equivocal cases (Fig. 6); let us repeat that any diagnostic doubt must lead to emergency surgery. The sonographic search for ectopic testes has been, in our experience, a failure in most cases with the exception only of the inguinal canal (Fig. 2).

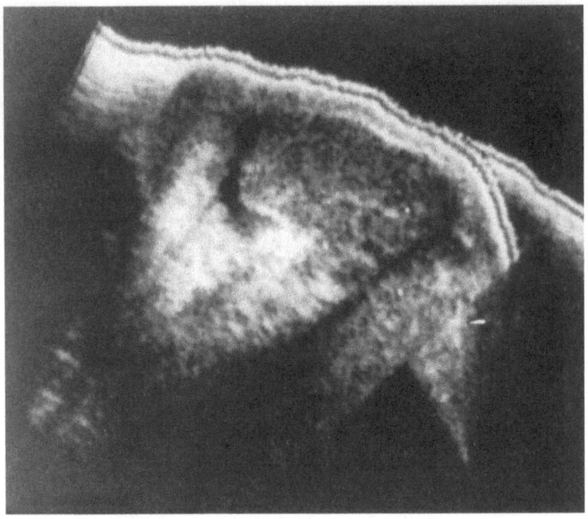

Fig. 4. A 10-year-old boy with swollen, painful right scrotum without evidence of fever (longitudinal scan). The testis is normal in size and echostructure. Small supratesticular mass close to the epididymis head and distinct from the testis itself. Morgani's appendix torsion. Conservative treatment.

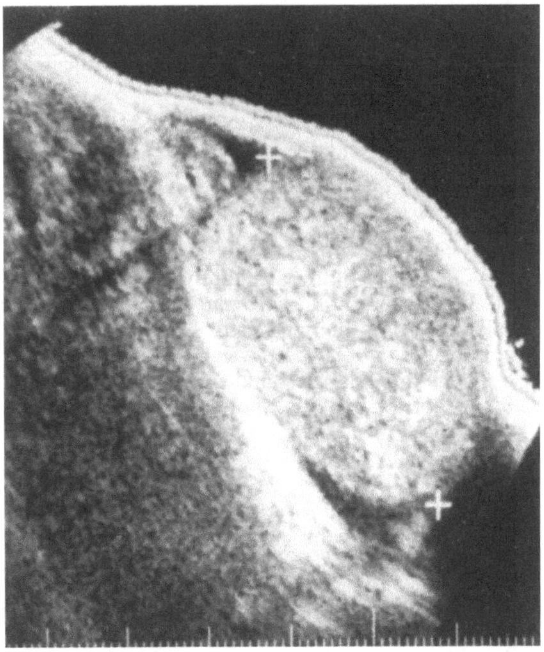

Fig. 5. Longitudinal scan in a 14-year-old boy with swollen, painful left scrotum with inflammatory changes of the skin. The left testis is considerably swollen; its echogenicity is homogeneously increased. There is a small hydrocele. At surgery, torsion testis with a blood-filled infarcted gland was present. Depending on the duration of the torsion, the sonographic pattern can vary: globally hypoechoic gland, "patchwork" echostructure, or hyperechoic parenchyma.

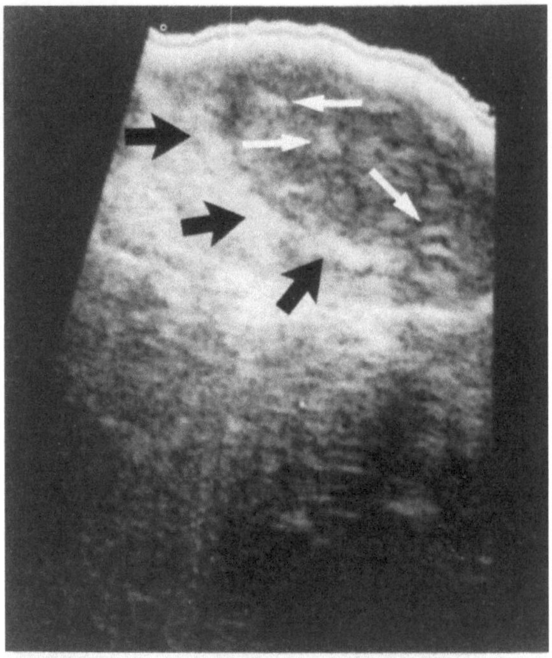

a

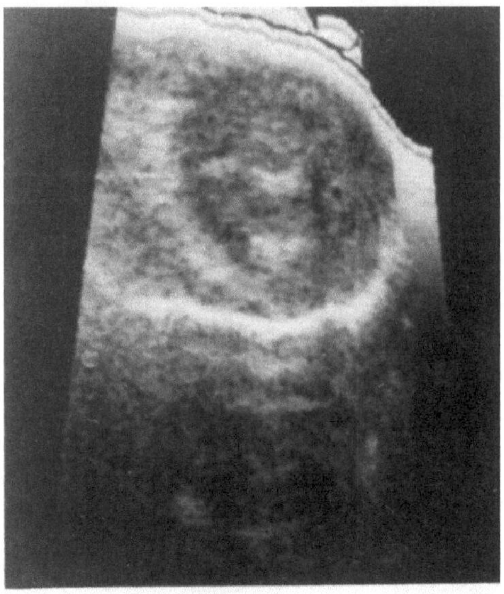

b

Fig. 6 a and b. A 5-month-old infant presenting with an enlarged left scrotum.
Longitudinal **(a)** and transverse **(b)** scans of the left scrotum. Enlarged epididymis (*black arrows*) coexisting with intratesticular hyperechoic spots (*white arrows*). At surgery an acute epididymitis with some testicular hematomas was found.

References

1. Sample W.F., Gottesmann J.E., Skinner D.G., Ehrlich R.M. (1978). Gray scale ultrasound of the scrotum. Radiology 127:255
2. Leopold G.R., Woo V.L., Scheible F.W., Nachtsheim D., Gosink B. (1979). High resolution ultrasonography of scrotal pathology. Radiology 131:719
3. Phillips G.N., Schneider M., Goodman J.D., Macchia R. (1980). Ultrasonic evaluation of the scrotum. Urol. Radiol. 1:157
4. Glazer H.S., Lee J.K.T., Leland Melson G., McClennan B.L. (1982). Sonographic detection of occult testicular neoplasms. A.J.R. 138:673–675
5. Carroll B.A., Gross D.M. (1983). High frequency scrotal pathology. A.J.R. 140:511–516

Chapter 13

Ultrasound of the Spine

L. Garel and D. Pariente

Although we have gathered little experience in this area, our first attempts at sonography of the spinal canal have been so rewarding that we wish to comment briefly on this new field of US.

1 Technical Aspects

The literature has stressed the interest of high-resolution real-time US in the investigation of the spine in infants and postoperative patients. Although less satisfactory, this can also be achieved through a contact B scanner with a 7 MHz short-focused transducer.

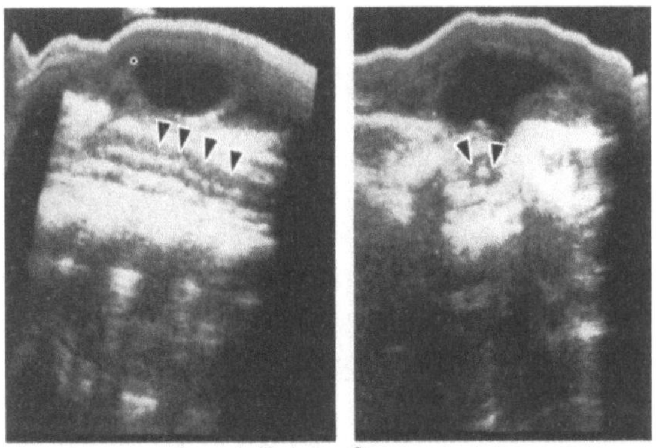

a b

Fig 1 a and b. Lumbosacral spina bifida with meningocele in a newborn.
a Longitudinal scan. The medulla (*arrows*) is seen posterior to the meningocele with its central echoic line: low fixed medulla.
b Transverse scan. The anatomical relationship between the meningocele and the medulla is well demonstrated.

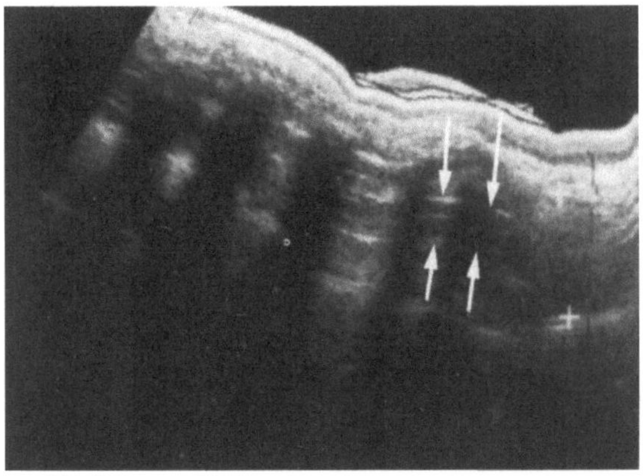

Fig. 2. Enlarged spinal canal in a newborn with a soft tissue mass in the lumbar region. Longitudinal scan. The medulla (*arrows*) is inserted on an intraspinal lipoma (calipers). The bony artifacts are due to the complete neural arches of the lumbar vertebrae.

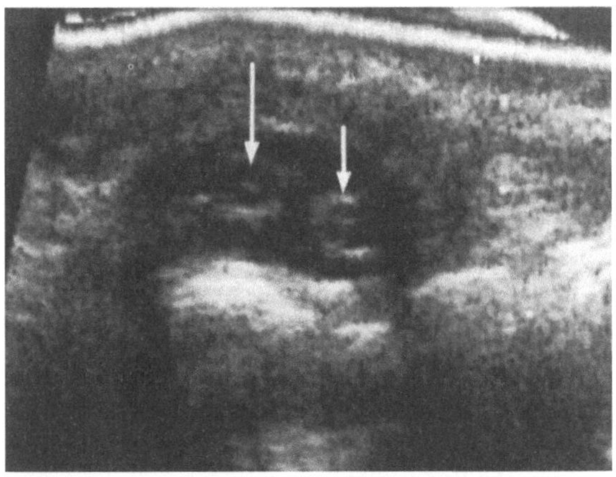

Fig. 3. Complex spinal dysraphism of the lumbar spine in a 3-month-old baby boy. Screening US examination was performed. On transverse scan two medullae are present (*arrows*). Myelography showed the presence of a nonossified spur within the canal (diastematomyelia).

2 Results

Normal anatomy has been clearly described in the recent literature. Our initial experience deals with spinal dysraphism (Figs. 1, 2, and 3). We have no experience yet with postoperative patients. It is our opinion that US of the spine can be very useful as a screening precedure in infants with neural arch defects.

References

1. Leopold G.R. (1980). Ultrasonography of superficially located structures. Radiol. Clinics N.A. 18:1:161–173
2. Miller J.H., Reid B.S., Kemberling C.R. (1982). Utilization of ultrasound in the evaluation of spinal dysraphism in children. Radiology 143:737–740
3. Braun I.F., Raghavendra B.N., Kricheff I.I. (1983). Spinal cord imaging using renal time high-resolution ultrasound. Radiology 147:459–465
4. Scheible W., James H.E., Leopold G.R., Hilton S.W. (1983). Occult spinal dysraphysm in infants: screening with high resolution real time ultrasound. Radiology 146:743–746

Subject Index

MIX
Papier aus verantwortungsvollen Quellen
Paper from responsible sources
FSC® C105338

If you have any concerns about our products,
you can contact us on
ProductSafety@springernature.com

In case Publisher is established outside the EU,
the EU authorized representative is:
Springer Nature Customer Service Center GmbH
Europaplatz 3, 69115 Heidelberg, Germany

Printed by Libri Plureos GmbH
in Hamburg, Germany